Essentials of

Anatomy and Physiology

Fourth Edition

Valerie C. Scanlon, PhD
College of Mount Saint Vincent
Riverdale, New York

Tina Sanders
Medical Illustrator
Castle Creek, New York
Formerly
Head Graphic Artist
Tompkins Cortland Community College
Dryden, New York

F. A. DAVIS COMPANY • Philadelphia

F. A. Davis Company
1915 Arch Street
Philadelphia, PA 19103

Printed in the United States of America

Last digit indicates print number: 10 9 8 7 6 5 4 3

Nursing Editor: Lisa Biello
Developmental Editor: Diane Blodgett
Production Manager: Sam Rondinelli
Cover Designer: Louis J. Forgione

As new scientific information becomes available through basic and clinical research, recommended treatments and drug therapies undergo changes. The author and publisher have done everything possible to make this book accurate, up to date, and in accord with accepted standards at the time of publication. The author, editors, and publisher are not responsible for errors or omissions or for consequences from application of the book, and make no warranty, expressed or implied, in regard to the contents of the book. Any practice described in this book should be applied by the reader in accordance with professional standards of care used in regard to the unique circumstances that may apply in each situation. The reader is advised always to check product information (package inserts) for changes and new information regarding dose and contraindications before administering any drug. Caution is especially urged when using new or infrequently ordered drugs.

Library of Congress Cataloging-in-Publication Data

Scanlon, Valerie C.
     Essentials of anatomy and physiology / Valerie C. Scanlon, Tina
Sanders.—4th ed.
          p. cm.
     ISBN 0-8036-1007-6
     1. Human physiology. 2. Human anatomy. I. Sanders, Tina.
II. Title.
QP34.5.S288 2002
612—dc21   2002073776
                                                      CIP

Preface

Traditions are signposts, markers in our lives, and it has become a most gratifying tradition for us to thank all of our colleagues in teaching who have helped make *Essentials of Anatomy and Physiology* a success. Thank you for making this fourth edition a reality, with your suggestions and use of our book for your students. If you are using our textbook for the first time, we thank you, and hope you will be pleased.

The text has been updated wherever appropriate to include recent research and to add new material. This will be apparent in the boxed inserts on pathophysiology and elsewhere in the text as well. So much of current research is at the molecular level, far beyond the scope of any introductory textbook, but we have kept to our purpose and hope to provide students with a comprehensive foundation for their future courses and their work in health care. The chemistry chapter remains important for that, as an introduction to the fundamentals of molecular biology. In Chapter 1 you will find more detailed explanations of both negative and positive feedback mechanisms in the section on homeostasis, and Chapter 3 provides a brief discussion of receptor sites. All have been kept basic, a foundation to build upon. Stem cells are discussed in Chapter 3 and in Chapter 21 as well as in Chapter 11, and prion disease is the subject of a new box in Chapter 2. Revised illustrations include the neuromuscular junction in Chapter 7, the synapse in Chapter 8, layers of the alimentary tube in Chapter 16, the nephron in Chapter 18, and water intake and output in Chapter 19.

New illustrations of anatomy include the epidermis in Chapter 5, muscles of the pelvic floor in Chapter 7, and spinal meninges and a frontal section of the brain in Chapter 8. For physiology we have added more illustrations of hormone functions in Chapter 10, the life cycle of red blood cells in Chapter 11, and distribution of blood flow in Chapter 13. Additional photographs include smoker's lung, renal blood vessels, and middle and inner ear structures. We hope you and your students will find them helpful.

Also new to this edition are end-of-chapter sections titled For Further Thought, with thought questions of several kinds, all related to basic physiology and anatomy. Detailed answers and suggestions for their use in collaborative learning may be found in the Instructor's Guide.

As always, your comments and suggestions will be most welcome, and they may be sent to us in care of the publisher: F. A. Davis Company, 1915 Arch Street, Philadelphia, PA 19103.

Valerie C. Scanlon
Dobbs Ferry, New York

Tina Sanders
Castle Creek, New York

To the Instructor

As the science and arts of medicine and health care become increasingly complex, so too does the education of those who pursue careers in nursing and other health-related fields. Human anatomy and physiology is often a first course in many education programs, and is the basis for so many of the more specialized courses. Teachers of introductory anatomy and physiology thus take on a special challenge: We must distill and express the complexities of human structure and function in a simple way, without losing the essence and meaning of the material. That is the goal of this textbook: to make this material readily accessible to students with diverse backgrounds and varying levels of educational preparation.

No prior knowledge of biology or chemistry is assumed, and even the most fundamental terms are defined thoroughly. Essential aspects of anatomy are presented clearly and reinforced with excellent illustrations. Essential aspects of physiology are discussed simply, yet with accuracy and precision. Again, the illustrations complement the text material and foster comprehension on the part of the student. These illustrations were prepared especially for students for whom this is a first course in anatomy and physiology. As you will see, these are images in which detail is readily apparent. All important parts have been labeled, but the student is not overwhelmed with unnecessary labels. Illustrations of physiology lead the student step-by-step. Wherever appropriate, the legends refer students to the text for further description or explanation.

The text has three unifying themes: the relationship between physiology and anatomy, the interrelations among the organ systems, and the relationship of each organ system to homeostasis. Although each type of cell, tissue, organ, or organ system is discussed simply and thoroughly in itself, applicable connections are made to other aspects of the body or to the functioning of the body as a whole. Our goal is to provide your students with the essentials of anatomy and physiology, and in doing so, to help give them a solid foundation for their future work, and an appreciation for the incredible living organism that is the human body.

The sequence of chapters is a very traditional one. Cross-references are used to remind students of what they have learned from previous chapters. Nevertheless, the textbook is very flexible, and, following the introductory four chapters, the organ systems may be covered in almost any order, depending on the needs of your course.

Each chapter is organized from the simple to the more complex, with the anatomy followed by the physiology. The Instructor's Guide presents modifications of the topic sequences that may be used, again depending on the needs of your course. Certain more advanced topics may be omitted from each chapter without losing the meaning or flow of the rest of the material, and these are indicated, for each chapter, in the Instructor's Guide.

Clinical applications are set apart from the text in boxed inserts. These are often aspects of pathophysiology that are related to the normal anatomy or physiology in the text discussion. Each box presents one particular topic and is referenced at the appropriate point in the text. This material is intended to be an integral part of the chapter but is set apart for ease of reference and to enable you to include or omit as many of these topics as you wish. The use of these boxes also enables students to read the text material without interruption and then to focus on specific aspects of pathophysiology. A comprehensive list of the boxes appears inside the book's front and back covers, and another list at the beginning of each chapter cites the boxes within that chapter.

Tables are utilized as summaries of structure and function, to present a sequence of events, or additional material that you may choose to include. Each table is referenced in the text and is intended to facilitate your teaching and to help your students learn.

New terms appear in bold type within the text, and all such terms are fully defined in an extensive glossary, with phonetic pronunciations. Bold type may also be used for emphasis whenever one of these terms is used again in a later chapter.

Each chapter begins with a chapter outline and student objectives to prepare the student for the chapter itself. New terminology and related clinical terms are also listed, with phonetic pronunciations. Each of these terms is fully defined in the glossary, with cross-references back to the chapter in which the term is introduced.

At the end of each chapter are a study outline and review questions. The study outline includes all of the essentials of the chapter in a concise outline form. The review questions may be assigned as homework, or used by the students as a review or self-test. Following each question is a page reference in parentheses. This reference cites the page(s) in the chapter on which the content needed to answer the question correctly can be found. The answers themselves are included in the Instructor's Guide. The questions in the sections titled For Further Thought may be used in a variety of ways, and the answers are in the Instructor's Guide.

An important supplementary learning tool for your students is available in the form of a *Student Workbook* that accompanies this text. For each chapter in the textbook, the workbook offers fill-in and matching-column questions, figure-labeling and figure-coloring exercises, and crossword puzzles based on the chapter's vocabulary list. Also included are two comprehensive, multiple-choice chapter tests to provide a thorough review for students. All answers are provided at the end of the workbook.

Ancillary materials for the teacher using this text are all on a CD-ROM: a complete Instructor's Guide, a computerized test bank, and an Image Ancillary presentation of the text illustrations. The Instructor's Guide contains expanded chapter outlines, notes on each chapter's organization and content (useful for modifying the book to your specific teaching needs), topics for class discussion, answers to the chapter review questions from the textbook, and very detailed answers to the questions in the For Further Thought sections. The computerized test bank contains more than 2600 multiple-choice questions. These questions have been organized in relation to the chapter review questions, and further explanation may be found in the Instructor's Guide. The Image Ancillary presentation contains many of the illustrations from the textbook, with suggested points for use in classroom lectures, and questions for every slide.

Suggestions and comments from colleagues are always valuable, and yours would be greatly appreciated. When we took on the task of writing and illustrating this textbook, we wanted to make it the most useful book possible for you and your students. Any suggestions that you can provide to help us achieve that goal are most welcome, and they may be sent to us in care of F. A. Davis Company, 1915 Arch Street, Philadelphia, PA 19103.

Valerie C. Scanlon
Dobbs Ferry, New York

Tina Sanders
Castle Creek, New York

To the Student

This is your textbook for your first course in human anatomy and physiology, a subject that is both fascinating and rewarding. That you are taking such a course says something about you. You may simply be curious as to how the human body functions or you may have a personal goal of making a contribution in one of the health-care professions. Whatever your reason, this textbook will help you to be successful in your anatomy and physiology course.

The material is presented simply and concisely, yet with accuracy and precision. The writing style is informal yet clear and specific; it is intended to promote your comprehension and understanding.

ORGANIZATION OF THE TEXTBOOK

To use this textbook effectively, you should know the purpose of its various parts. Each chapter is organized in the following way:

Chapter Outline—This presents the main topics in the chapter, which corresponds to the major headings in the text.

Student Objectives—These summarize what you should know after reading and studying the chapter. These are not questions to be answered, but are rather, with the chapter outline, a preview of the chapter contents.

New Terminology and Related Clinical Terminology—These are some of the new terms you will come across in the chapter. Read through these terms before you read the chapter, but do not attempt to memorize them just yet. When you have finished the chapter, return to the list and see how many terms you can define. Note those you may not be sure of and look them up. All of these terms are fully defined in the glossary.

Study Outline—This is found at the end of the chapter. It is a concise summary of the essentials in the chapter. You may find this outline very useful as a quick review before an exam.

Review Questions—These are also at the end of the chapter. Your instructor may assign some or all of them as homework. If not, the questions may be used as a self-test to evaluate your comprehension of the chapter's content. The page number(s) in parentheses following each question refers you to the page(s) in the chapter on which the content needed to answer the question correctly can be found.

For Further Thought—The heading tells you what these are for: thinking. Your instructor may use these for class discussion, and, if so, please do not ever be afraid to be wrong. Being wrong in the classroom is one of the ways each and every one of us learns. Contribute, raise your hand and speak up with your best thoughts, and listen to those of others. Together you will find the answers.

OTHER FEATURES WITHIN EACH CHAPTER

Illustrations—These are an essential part of this textbook. Use them. Study them carefully, and they will be of great help to you as you learn. They are intended to help you develop your own mental picture of the body and its parts and processes. You may not have thought of mental pictures as being important, but they are, and each new one you create is a major step in learning. Each illustration is referenced in the text, so you will know when to consult it. With a little concentration, you will have it in your mind for whenever you need it.

Boxes—Discussions of clinical applications are in separate boxes in the text so that you may find and refer to them easily. Your instructor may include all or some of these as required reading. If you are planning a career in the health professions, these boxes are an introduction to pathophysiology, and you will find them interesting and helpful.

Bold Type—This is used whenever a new term is introduced, or when an old term is especially important. The terms in bold type are fully defined in the glossary, which includes phonetic pronunciations.

Tables—This format is used to present material in a very concise form. Some tables are summaries of text material and are very useful for a quick review. Other tables present additional material that complements the text material.

Glossary—Not within the chapters but at the end, the dictionary of the book. All of the terms in bold type, as well as others, are defined here. Make use of it, rather than wonder what a word means. The sooner you have a definition firmly in your mind, the sooner it is truly part of your knowledge.

To make the best use of your study time, a *Student Workbook* is available that will help you to focus your attention on the essentials in each chapter. Also included are comprehensive chapter tests to help you determine which topics you have learned thoroughly and which you may have to review. If your instructor has not made the workbook a required text, you may wish to ask that it be ordered and made available in your bookstore. You will find it very helpful.

SOME FINAL WORDS OF ENCOURAGEMENT

Your success in this course depends to a great extent on you. Try to set aside study time for yourself every day; a little time each day is usually much more productive than trying to cram at the last minute.

Ask questions of yourself as you are studying. What kinds of questions? The simplest ones. If you are studying a part of the body such as an organ, ask yourself: What is its name? Where is it? What is it made of? What does it do? That is: name, location, structure, and function. These are the essentials. If you are studying a process, ask yourself: What is happening here? What is its purpose? That is: What is going on? And what good is it? Again, these are the essentials.

We hope this textbook will contribute to your success. If you have any suggestions or comments, we would very much like to hear them. After all, this book was written for you, to help you achieve your goals in this course and in your education. Please send your suggestions and comments to us in care of F. A. Davis Company, 1915 Arch Street, Philadelphia, PA 19103.

Valerie C. Scanlon
Dobbs Ferry, New York

Tina Sanders
Castle Creek, New York

Acknowledgments

Writing and illustrating are part of a book, yet never the whole, and we thank the editors and production staff of the F. A. Davis Company, especially:

- Lisa Biello, Nursing Editor
- Diane Blodgett, Developmental Editor
- Sam Rondinelli, Production Editor
- Michael Bailey, Director of Production
- Patti Cleary, Editor in Chief, Nursing
- Bette Haitsch, Managing Editor
- Lori Asbury, Project Manager
- Lorretta Palagi, Copy Editor
- Marie Clifton, for designing the layout of the book.
- Louis J. Forgione, for designing the cover of the book.
- Valerie extends special thanks to Dan Kaufman for the new photographs, and to her sister, Joan Scanlon, for the computer help desk that is always on call and encourages laughter.
- Tina and Valerie acknowledge, with gratitude and affection, all of the contributions made by Alan Sorkowitz; they will remain a lasting part of the book.
- Both of us extend our deepest appreciation to Neil Kelly, Director of Sales, and to all of the F.A. Davis sales representatives, whose travels and efforts have contributed so greatly to the success of this textbook. We are very grateful.

VCS

TS

To my students, past and present
VCS

To Brooks, for his encouragement
TS

Contents

CHAPTER 1

Organization and General Plan of the Body

CHAPTER 1

Student Objectives

- Define anatomy, physiology, and pathophysiology. Use an example to explain how they are related.
- Name the levels of organization of the body from simplest to most complex, and explain each.
- Define homeostasis, and use an example to explain.
- Explain how a negative feedback mechanism works, and how a positive feedback mechanism differs.
- Describe the anatomic position.
- State the anatomic terms for the parts of the body.
- Use proper terminology to describe the location of body parts with respect to one another.
- Name the body cavities, their membranes, and some organs within each cavity.
- Describe the possible sections through the body or an organ.
- Explain how and why the abdomen is divided into smaller areas. Be able to name organs in these areas.

Organization and General Plan of the Body

New Terminology

Anatomy (uh-**NAT**-uh-mee)
Body cavity (**BAH**-dee **KAV**-i-tee)
Cell (**SELL**)
Homeostasis (HOH-me-oh-**STAY**-sis)
Inorganic chemicals (**IN**-or-GAN-ik **KEM**-i-kuls)
Meninges (me-**NIN**-jeez)
Negative feedback (**NEG**-ah-tiv **FEED**-bak)
Organ (**OR**-gan)
Organ system (**OR**-gan **SIS**-tem)
Organic chemicals (or-**GAN**-ik **KEM**-i-kuls)
Pathophysiology (PATH-oh-FIZZ-ee-**AH**-luh-jee)
Pericardial membranes (PER-ee-**KAR**-dee-uhl **MEM**-brains)
Peritoneum/Mesentery (PER-i-toh-**NEE**-um/**MEZ**-en-TER-ee)
Physiology (FIZZ-ee-**AH**-luh-jee)
Plane (**PLAYN**)
Pleural membranes (**PLOOR**-uhl **MEM**-brayns)
Section (**SEK**-shun)
Tissue (**TISH**-yoo)

Related Clinical Terminology

Computed tomography (CT) scan (kom-**PEW**-ted toh-**MAH**-grah-fee SKAN)
Diagnosis (DYE-ag-**NO**-sis)
Disease (di-**ZEEZ**)
Magnetic resonance imaging (MRI) (mag-**NET**-ik **REZ**-ah-nanse **IM**-ah-jing)
Positron emission tomography (PET) (**PAHZ**-i-tron e-**MISH**-un toh-**MAH**-grah-fee)

*Terms that appear in **bold type** in the chapter text are defined in the glossary, which begins on page 521.*

The human body is a precisely structured container of chemical reactions. Have you ever thought of yourself in this way? Probably not, and yet, in the strictly physical sense, that is what each of us is. The body consists of trillions of atoms in specific arrangements and thousands of chemical reactions proceeding in a very orderly manner. That literally describes us, and yet it is clearly not the whole story. The keys to understanding human consciousness and self-awareness are still beyond our grasp. We do not yet know what enables us to study ourselves—no other animals do, as far as we know—but we have accumulated a great deal of knowledge about ourselves. Some of this knowledge makes up the course you are about to take, a course in basic human anatomy and physiology.

Anatomy is the study of body structure, which includes size, shape, composition, and perhaps even coloration. **Physiology** is the study of how the body functions. The physiology of red blood cells, for example, includes what these cells do, how they do it, and how this is related to the functioning of the rest of the body. Physiology is directly related to anatomy. For example, red blood cells contain the mineral iron in molecules of the protein called hemoglobin; this is an aspect of their anatomy. The presence of iron enables red blood cells to carry oxygen, which is their function. All cells in the body must receive oxygen in order to function properly, so the physiology of red blood cells is essential to the physiology of the body as a whole.

Pathophysiology is the study of disorders of functioning, and a knowledge of normal physiology makes such disorders easier to understand. For example, you are probably familiar with the anemia called iron-deficiency anemia. With insufficient iron in the diet, there will not be enough iron in the hemoglobin of red blood cells, and hence less oxygen will be transported throughout the body, resulting in the symptoms of the iron-deficiency disorder. This example shows the relationship between anatomy, physiology, and pathophysiology.

The purpose of this text is to enable you to gain an understanding of anatomy and physiology with the emphasis on normal structure and function. Many examples of pathophysiology have been included, however, to illustrate the relationship of **disease** to normal physiology and to describe some of the procedures used in the **diagnosis** of disease. Many of the examples are clinical applications that will help you begin to apply what you have learned and demon-strate that your knowledge of anatomy and physiology will become the basis for your further study in the health professions.

LEVELS OF ORGANIZATION

The human body is organized in structural and functional levels of increasing complexity. Each higher level incorporates the structures and functions of the previous level, as you will see. We will begin with the simplest level, which is the chemical level, and proceed to cells, tissues, organs, and organ systems. All of the levels of organization are depicted in Fig. 1–1.

CHEMICALS

The chemicals that make up the body may be divided into two major categories: inorganic and organic. **Inorganic chemicals** are usually simple molecules made of one or two elements other than carbon (with a few exceptions). Examples of inorganic chemicals are water (H_2O); oxygen (O_2); one of the exceptions, carbon dioxide (CO_2); and minerals such as iron (Fe), calcium (Ca), and sodium (Na). **Organic chemicals** are often very complex and always contain the elements carbon and hydrogen. In this category of organic chemicals are carbohydrates, fats, proteins, and nucleic acids. The chemical organization of the body is the subject of Chapter 2.

CELLS

The smallest living units of structure and function are **cells**. There are many different types of human cells; each is made of chemicals and carries out specific chemical reactions. Cell structure and function are discussed in Chapter 3.

TISSUES

A **tissue** is a group of cells with similar structure and function. There are four groups of tissues:

Epithelial tissues—cover or line body surfaces; some are capable of producing secretions with specific functions. The outer layer of the skin and sweat glands are examples of epithelial tissues. Internal epithelial tissues include the walls of capillaries (squamous epithelium) and the kidney tubules (cuboidal epithelium), as shown in Fig. 1–1.

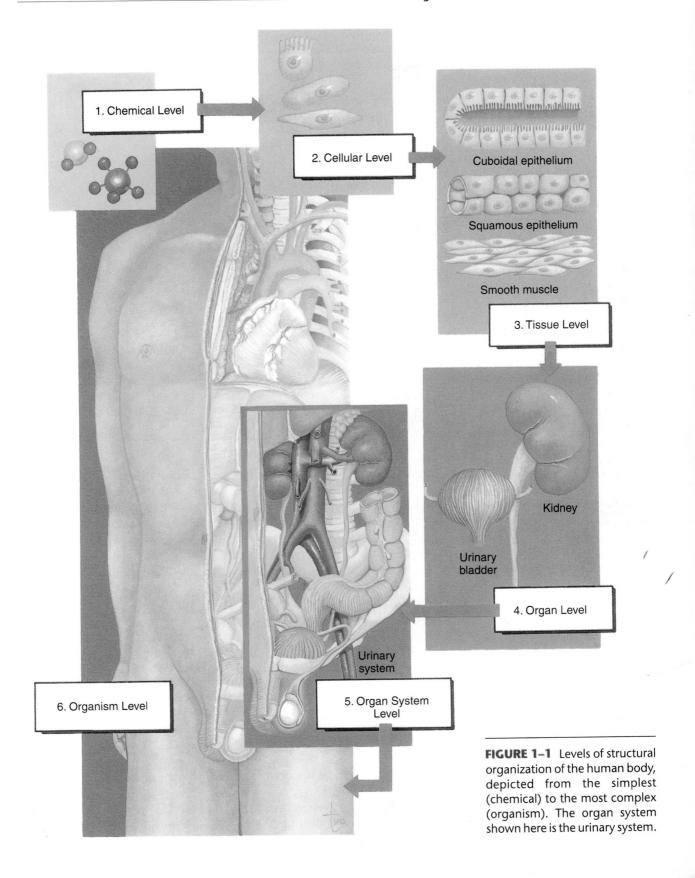

1. Chemical Level

2. Cellular Level

Cuboidal epithelium

Squamous epithelium

Smooth muscle

3. Tissue Level

Kidney

Urinary
bladder

4. Organ Level

Urinary
system

6. Organism Level

5. Organ System
Level

FIGURE 1–1 Levels of structural organization of the human body, depicted from the simplest (chemical) to the most complex (organism). The organ system shown here is the urinary system.

Box 1-1   REPLACING TISSUES AND ORGANS

Blood transfusions are probably the most familiar and frequent form of "replacement parts" for people. Blood is a tissue, and when properly typed and cross-matched (blood types will be discussed in Chapter 11) may safely be given to someone with the same or a compatible blood type.

Organs, however, are much more complex structures. When a patient receives an organ transplant, there is always the possibility of rejection (destruction) of the organ by the recipient's immune system (Chapter 14). With the discovery and use of more effective immune-suppressing medications, however, the success rate for many types of organ transplants has increased. Organs that may be transplanted include corneas, kidneys, the heart, the liver, and the lungs.

The skin is also an organ, but skin transplanted from another person will not survive very long. Several kinds of artificial skin are now available to temporarily cover large areas of damaged skin. Patients with severe burns, for example, will eventually need skin grafts from their own unburned skin to form permanent new skin over the burn sites. It is now possible to "grow" a patient's skin in laboratory culture, so that a small patch of skin may eventually be used to cover a large surface. Other cells grown in culture include cartilage, bone, pancreas, and liver. Much research is being done on liver implants (not transplants), clusters of functional liver cells grown in a lab. Such implants would reduce or eliminate the need for human donors. Tissue engineering is also being used to create arteries and urinary bladders.

Many artificial replacement parts have also been developed. These are made of plastic or metal and are not rejected as foreign by the recipient's immune system. Damaged heart valves, for example, may be replaced by artificial ones, and sections of arteries may be replaced by tubular grafts made of synthetic materials. Artificial joints are available for every joint in the body, as is artificial bone for reconstructive surgery. Cochlear implants are tiny instruments that convert sound waves to electrical impulses the brain can learn to interpret, and have provided some sense of hearing for people with certain types of deafness. Work is also progressing on the use of a featherweight computer chip as an artificial retina, on devices that help damaged hearts pump blood more efficiently, and on small, self-contained artificial hearts.

Connective tissues—connect and support parts of the body; some transport or store materials. Blood, bone, cartilage, and adipose tissue are examples of this group.

Muscle tissues—specialized for contraction, which brings about movement. Our skeletal muscles and the heart are examples of muscle tissue. In Fig. 1–1, you see smooth muscle tissue, which is found in organs such as the urinary bladder and stomach.

Nerve tissue—specialized to generate and transmit electrochemical impulses that regulate body functions. The brain and optic nerves are examples of nerve tissue.

The types of tissues in these four groups, as well as their specific functions, are the subject of Chapter 4.

ORGANS

An **organ** is a group of tissues precisely arranged so as to accomplish specific functions. Examples of organs are the kidneys, liver, lungs, and stomach. The kidneys contain several kinds of epithelial, or surface tissues, for their work of absorption. The stomach is lined with epithelial tissue that secretes gastric juice for digestion. Smooth muscle tissue in the wall of the stomach contracts to mix food with gastric juice and propel it to the small intestine. Nerve tissue carries impulses that increase or decrease the contractions of the stomach (see Box 1–1: Replacing Tissues and Organs).

ORGAN SYSTEMS

An **organ system** is a group of organs that all contribute to a particular function. Examples are the urinary system, digestive system, and respiratory system. In Fig. 1–1 you see the urinary system, which consists of the kidneys, ureters, urinary bladder, and urethra. These organs all contribute to the formation and elimination of urine.

As a starting point, Table 1–1 lists the organ systems of the human body with their general functions, and some representative organs (Fig. 1–2); these organ systems make up an individual person. The balance of this text discusses each system in more detail.

Table 1–1	THE ORGAN SYSTEMS	
System	**Functions**	**Organs***
Integumentary	• Is a barrier to pathogens and chemicals • Prevents excessive water loss	skin, hair, subcutaneous tissue
Skeletal	• Supports the body • Protects internal organs • Provides a framework to be moved by muscles	bones, ligaments
Muscular	• Moves the skeleton • Produces heat	muscles, tendons
Nervous	• Interprets sensory information • Regulates body functions such as movement by means of electrochemical impulses	brain, nerves, eyes, ears
Endocrine	• Regulates body functions by means of hormones	thyroid gland, pituitary gland
Circulatory	• Transports oxygen and nutrients to tissues and removes waste products	heart, blood, arteries
Lymphatic	• Returns tissue fluid to the blood • Destroys pathogens that enter the body	spleen, lymph nodes
Respiratory	• Exchanges oxygen and carbon dioxide between the air and blood	lungs, trachea, larynx
Digestive	• Changes food to simple chemicals that can be absorbed and used by the body	stomach, colon, liver
Urinary	• Removes waste products from the blood • Regulates volume and pH of blood	kidneys, urinary bladder, urethra
Reproductive	• Produces eggs or sperm • *In women,* provides a site for the developing embryo-fetus	*Female:* ovaries, uterus *Male:* testes, prostate gland

* These are simply representative organs, not an all-inclusive list.

HOMEOSTASIS

A person who is in good health is in a state of **homeostasis**. Homeostasis reflects the ability of the body to maintain relative stability and to function normally despite constant changes. Changes may be external or internal, and the body must respond appropriately.

Eating breakfast, for example, brings about an internal change. Suddenly there is food in the stomach, and something must be done with it. What happens? The food is digested or broken down into simple chemicals that the body can use. The protein in a hard-boiled egg is digested into amino acids, its basic chemical building blocks; these amino acids can then be used by the body to produce its own specialized proteins.

An example of an external change is a rise in environmental temperature. On a hot day, the body temperature would also tend to rise. However, body temperature must be kept within its normal range of about 97° to 99°F (36° to 38°C), in order to support normal functioning. What happens? One of the body's responses to the external temperature rise is to increase sweating so that excess body heat can be lost by the evaporation of sweat on the surface of the skin. This response, however, may bring about an undesirable internal change, dehydration. What happens? As body water decreases, we feel the sensation of thirst and drink fluids to replace the water lost in sweating. Notice that when certain body responses occur, they reverse the event that triggered them. In the example above, a rising body temperature stimulates increased sweating, which lowers body temperature, which in turn decreases sweating. Unnecessary sweating that would be wasteful of water is prevented. This is an example of a **negative feedback** mechanism, in which the body's response reverses the stimulus (in

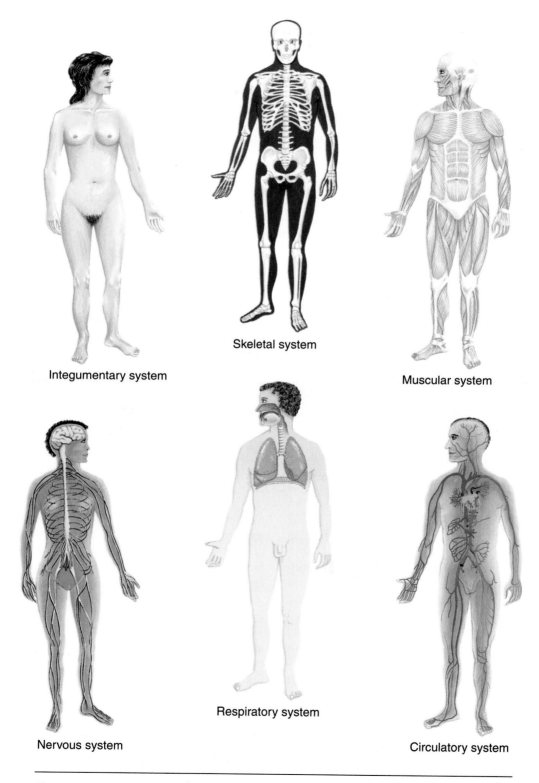

Integumentary system

Skeletal system

Muscular system

Nervous system

Respiratory system

Circulatory system

Figure 1–2 Organ systems. Compare the depiction of each system to its description in Table 1–1. Try to name at least one organ shown in each system.

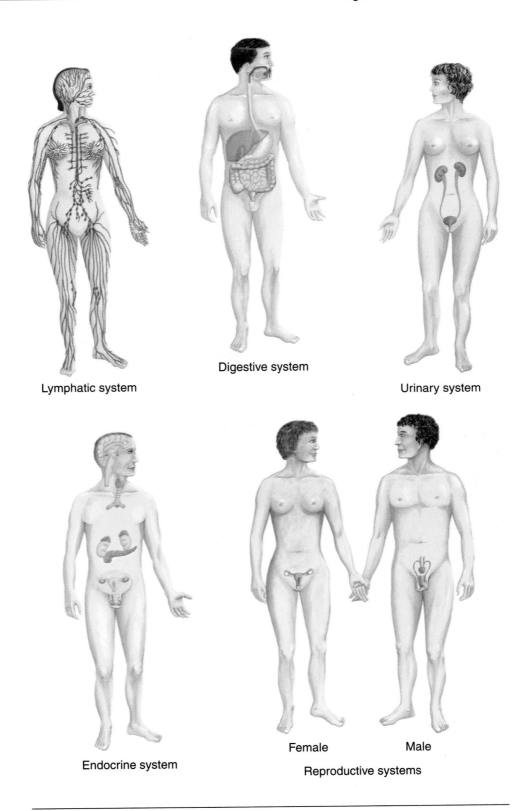

Lymphatic system

Digestive system

Urinary system

Endocrine system

Female   Male

Reproductive systems

Figure 1–2 (Continued)

effect, turning it off for a while) and keeps some aspect of the body within its normal range.

You may be wondering if there is such a thing as a positive feedback mechanism. There is, but they are rare in the body and quite different from a negative feedback mechanism. In a positive feedback mechanism, the response to the stimulus does not stop or reverse the stimulus, but instead keeps the sequence of events going. The best example is childbirth, in which the sequence of events, simply stated, is as follows: stretching of the uterine cervix stimulates secretion of the hormone oxytocin by the anterior pituitary gland. Oxytocin stimulates contraction of the uterine muscle, which causes more stretching, which stimulates more oxytocin and, hence, more contractions. The mechanism stops with the delivery of the baby and the placenta. This is the "brake," the interrupting event.

A positive feedback mechanism requires an external "brake," something to interrupt it. Blood clotting is such a mechanism, and without external controls clotting may become a vicious cycle of clotting and more clotting, doing far more harm than good (discussed in Chapter 11). It is for this reason, because positive feedback mechanisms have the potential to continue excessively and cause harm, that they are rare in the body.

Negative feedback mechanisms, however, contain their own brakes, and the body has many of them. The secretion of most hormones (Chapter 10) is regulated by negative feedback mechanisms. The regulation of heart rate (Chapter 12) and blood pressure (Chapter 13) involves several negative feedback mechanisms. The result of all of these mechanisms working together is that all aspects of body functioning are kept within normal limits, a steady state or equilibrium. This is homeostasis.

In the chapters to come, you will find many more examples. As you continue your study of the human body, keep in mind that the proper functioning of each organ and organ system contributes to homeostasis.

TERMINOLOGY AND GENERAL PLAN OF THE BODY

As part of your course in anatomy and physiology, you will learn many new words or terms. At times you may feel that you are learning a second language, and indeed you are. Each term has a precise meaning, which is understood by everyone else who has learned the language. Mastering the terminology of your profession is essential to enable you to communicate effectively with your co-workers and your future patients. Although the number of new terms may seem a bit overwhelming at first, you will find that their use soon becomes second nature to you.

The terminology presented in this chapter will be used throughout the text in the discussion of the organ systems. This will help to reinforce the meanings of these terms and will transform these new words into knowledge.

BODY PARTS AND AREAS

Each of the terms listed in Table 1–2 and shown in Fig. 1–3 refers to a specific part or area of the body.

Table 1–2	DESCRIPTIVE TERMS FOR BODY PARTS AND AREAS
Term	**Definition (Refers to)**
Axillary	armpit
Brachial	upper arm
Buccal (oral)	mouth
Cardiac	heart
Cervical	neck
Cranial	head
Cutaneous	skin
Deltoid	shoulder
Femoral	thigh
Frontal	forehead
Gastric	stomach
Gluteal	buttocks
Hepatic	liver
Iliac	hip
Inguinal	groin
Lumbar	small of back
Mammary	breast
Nasal	nose
Occipital	back of head
Orbital	eye
Parietal	crown of head
Patellar	kneecap
Pectoral	chest
Perineal	pelvic floor
Plantar	sole of foot
Popliteal	back of knee
Pulmonary	lungs
Renal	kidney
Sacral	base of spine
Temporal	side of head
Umbilical	navel
Volar (palmar)	palm

Body Parts and Areas

Anatomical position

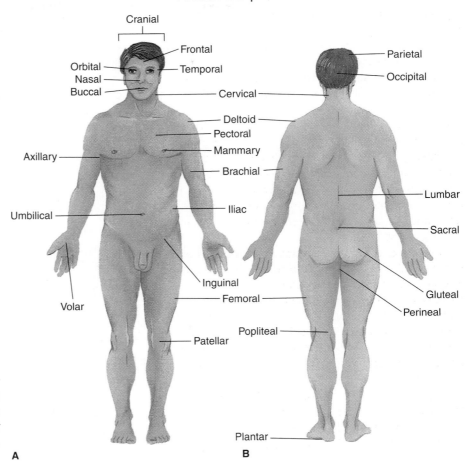

Figure 1–3 Body parts and areas. The body is shown in anatomic position. **(A)** Anterior view. **(B)** Posterior view. (Compare with Table 1–2.)   **A**   **B**

For example, the term *femoral* always refers to the thigh. The femoral artery is a blood vessel that passes through the thigh, and the quadriceps femoris is a large muscle group of the thigh.

Another example is *pulmonary*, which always refers to the lungs, as in pulmonary artery, pulmonary edema, and pulmonary embolism. Although you may not know the exact meaning of each of these terms now, you do know that each has something to do with the lungs.

TERMS OF LOCATION AND POSITION

When describing relative locations, the body is always assumed to be in **anatomic position**: standing upright facing forward, arms at the sides with palms forward, and the feet slightly apart. The terms of location are listed in Table 1–3, with a definition and example for each. As you read each term, find the body parts used as examples in Figs. 1–3 and 1–4. Notice also that these are pairs of terms and that each pair is a set of opposites. This will help you recall the terms and their meanings.

BODY CAVITIES AND THEIR MEMBRANES

The body has two major cavities: the **dorsal cavity** (posterior) and the **ventral cavity** (anterior). Each of these cavities has further subdivisions, which are shown in Fig. 1–4.

Table 1–3	TERMS OF LOCATION AND POSITION	

Term	Definition	Example
Superior	above, or higher	The heart is superior to the liver.
Inferior	below, or lower	The liver is inferior to the lungs.
Anterior	toward the front	The chest is on the anterior side of the body.
Posterior	toward the back	The lumbar area is posterior to the umbilical area.
Ventral	toward the front	The mammary area is on the ventral side of the body.
Dorsal	toward the back	The buttocks are on the dorsal side of the body.
Medial	toward the midline	The heart is medial to the lungs.
Lateral	away from the midline	The shoulders are lateral to the neck.
Internal	within, or interior to	The brain is internal to the skull.
External	outside, or exterior to	The ribs are external to the lungs.
Superficial	toward the surface	The skin is the most superficial organ.
Deep	within, or interior to	The deep veins of the legs are surrounded by muscles.
Central	the main part	The brain is part of the central nervous system.
Peripheral	extending from the main part	Nerves in the arm are part of the peripheral nervous system.
Proximal	closer to the origin	The knee is proximal to the foot.
Distal	farther from the origin	The palm is distal to the elbow.
Parietal	pertaining to the wall of a cavity	The parietal pleura lines the chest cavity.
Visceral	pertaining to the organs within a cavity	The visceral pleura covers the lungs.

Dorsal Cavity

The dorsal cavity contains the central nervous system, and consists of the cranial cavity and the vertebral or spinal cavity. The **cranial cavity** is formed by the skull and contains the brain. The **spinal cavity** is formed by the backbone (spine) and contains the spinal cord. The membranes that line these cavities and cover the brain and spinal cord are called the **meninges**.

Ventral Cavity

The ventral cavity consists of two compartments, the thoracic cavity and the abdominal cavity, which are separated by the diaphragm. The diaphragm is a large, dome-shaped respiratory muscle. It has openings for the esophagus and for large blood vessels, but otherwise is a wall between the thoracic and abdominal cavities. The pelvic cavity may be considered a subdivision of the abdominal cavity (there is no wall between them) or as a separate cavity.

Organs in the **thoracic cavity** include the heart and lungs. The membranes of the thoracic cavity are serous membranes called the **pleural membranes**. The parietal pleura lines the chest wall, and the visceral pleura covers the lungs. The heart has its own set of serous membranes called the **pericardial membranes**. The parietal pericardium lines the fibrous pericardial sac, and the visceral pericardium covers the heart muscle.

Organs in the **abdominal cavity** include the liver, stomach, and intestines. The membranes of the abdominal cavity are also serous membranes called the peritoneum and mesentery. The **peritoneum** is the membrane that lines the entire abdominal wall, and the **mesentery** is the continuation of this

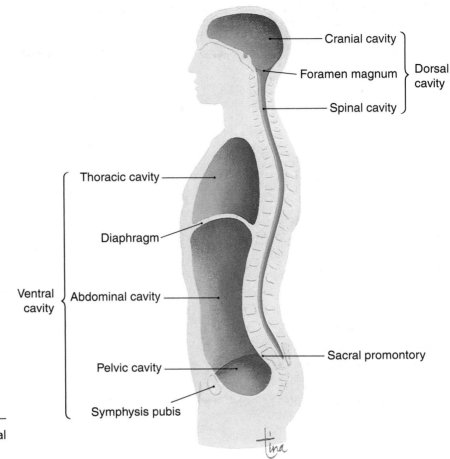

Cranial cavity

Foramen magnum

Spinal cavity

Dorsal cavity

Thoracic cavity

Diaphragm

Ventral cavity

Abdominal cavity

Sacral promontory

Pelvic cavity

Symphysis pubis

Figure 1–4 Body cavities (lateral view from the left side).

membrane, folded around and covering the outer surfaces of the abdominal organs.

The **pelvic cavity** is inferior to the abdominal cavity. Although the peritoneum does not line the pelvic cavity, it covers the free surfaces of several pelvic organs. Within the pelvic cavity are the urinary bladder and reproductive organs such as the uterus in women and the prostate gland in men.

PLANES AND SECTIONS

When internal anatomy is described, the body or an organ is often cut or **sectioned** in a specific way so as to make particular structures easily visible. A **plane** is an imaginary flat surface that separates two portions of the body or an organ. These planes and sections are shown in Fig. 1–5 (see Box 1–2: Visualizing the Interior of the Body).

Frontal (coronal) section—a plane from side to side separates the body into front and back portions.

Sagittal section—a plane from front to back separates the body into right and left portions. A midsagittal section creates equal right and left halves.

Transverse section—a horizontal plane separates the body into upper and lower portions.

Cross-section—a plane perpendicular to the long axis of an organ. A cross-section of the small intestine (which is a tube) would look like a circle with the cavity of the intestine in the center.

Longitudinal section—a plane along the long axis of an organ. A longitudinal section of the intestine is shown in Fig. 1–5, and a frontal section of the femur (thigh bone) would also be a longitudinal section (see Fig. 6–1 in Chapter 6).

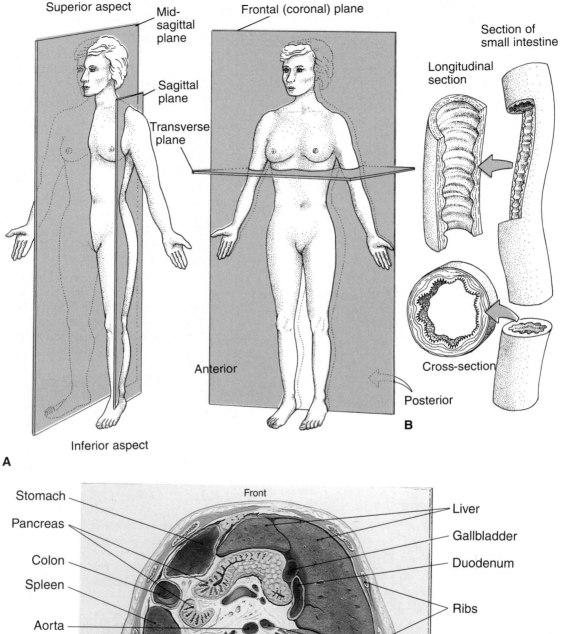

Figure 1–5 **(A)** Planes and sections of the body. **(B)** Cross-section and longitudinal section of the small intestine. **(C)** Transverse section through the upper abdomen.

Box 1–2   VISUALIZING THE INTERIOR OF THE BODY

In the past, the need for exploratory surgery brought with it hospitalization, risk of infection, and discomfort and pain for the patient. Today, however, new technologies and the extensive use of computers permit us to see the interior of the body without surgery.

Computed tomography (CT) scanning uses a narrowly focused x-ray beam that circles rapidly around the body. A detector then measures how much radiation passes through different tissues, and a computer constructs an image of a thin slice through the body. Several images may be made at different levels—each takes only a few seconds—to provide a more complete picture of an organ or part of the body. The images are much more detailed than are those produced by conventional x-rays.

Magnetic resonance imaging (MRI) is another diagnostic tool that is especially useful for visualizing soft tissues, including the brain and spinal cord. Recent refinements have produced images of individual nerve bundles, which had not been possible using any other technique. The patient is placed inside a strong magnetic field, and the tissues are pulsed with radio waves. Because each tissue has different proportions of various atoms, which resonate or respond differently, each tissue emits a characteristic signal. A computer then translates these signals into an image; the entire procedure takes 30 to 45 minutes.

Positron emission tomography (PET) scanning creates images that depict the rates of physiological processes such as blood flow, oxygen usage, or glucose metabolism. The comparative rates are depicted by colors: Red represents the highest rate, followed by yellow, then green, and finally blue representing the lowest rate.

One drawback of the new technologies is their cost; they are expensive. However, the benefits to patients are great: highly detailed images of the body are obtained without the risks of surgery and with virtually no discomfort in the procedures themselves.

A   B   C

Box Figure 1–A   Imaging techniques. **(A)** CT scan of eye in lateral view showing a tumor (*arrow*) below the optic nerve. **(B)** MRI of midsagittal section of head (compare with Figs. 8–6 and 15–1). **(C)** PET scan of brain in transverse section (frontal lobes at top) showing glucose metabolism. (From Mazziotta, JC, and Gilman, S: Clinical Brain Imaging: Principles and Applications. FA Davis, Philadelphia, 1992, pp 27 and 298, with permission.)

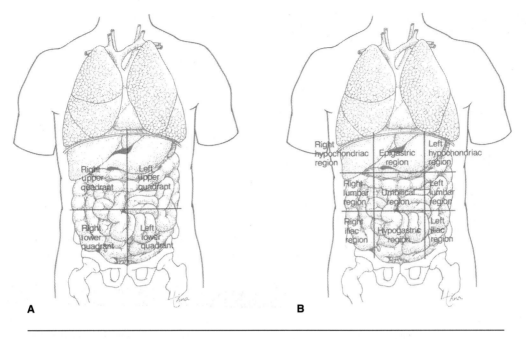

A   B

Figure 1–6 Areas of the abdomen. **(A)** Four quadrants. **(B)** Nine regions.

AREAS OF THE ABDOMEN

The abdomen is a large area of the lower trunk of the body. If a patient reported abdominal pain, the physician or nurse would want to know more precisely where the pain was. In order to determine this, the abdomen may be divided into smaller regions or areas, which are shown in Fig. 1–6.

Quadrants—a transverse plane and a midsagittal plane that cross at the umbilicus will divide the abdomen into four quadrants. Clinically, this is probably the division used more frequently. The pain of gallstones might then be described as in the right upper quadrant.

Nine areas—two transverse planes and two sagittal planes divide the abdomen into nine areas.

   Upper areas—above the level of the rib cartilages are the left hypochondriac, epigastric, and right hypochondriac.

   Middle areas—the left lumbar, umbilical, and right lumbar.

   Lower areas—below the level of the top of the pelvic bone are the left iliac, hypogastric, and

right iliac. This division is often used in anatomic studies to describe the location of organs. The liver, for example, is located in the epigastric and right hypochondriac areas.

SUMMARY

As you will see, the terminology presented in this chapter is used throughout the text to describe the anatomy of organs and the names of their parts. All organs of the body contribute to homeostasis, the healthy state of the body that is maintained by constant and appropriate responses to internal and external changes. In the chapters that follow, you will find detailed descriptions of the physiology of each organ and organ system, and how each is necessary to homeostasis. We will now return to a consideration of the structural organization of the body and to more extensive descriptions of its levels of organization. The first of these, the chemical level, is the subject of the next chapter.

STUDY OUTLINE

Introduction
1. Anatomy—the study of structure.
2. Physiology—the study of function.
3. Pathophysiology—the study of disorders of functioning.

Levels of Organization
1. Chemical—inorganic and organic chemicals make up all matter, both living and non-living.
2. Cells—the smallest living units of the body.
3. Tissues—groups of cells with similar structure and function.
4. Organs—groups of tissues that contribute to specific functions.
5. Organ systems—groups of organs that work together to perform specific functions (see Table 1–1 and Fig. 1–2).
6. Person—all the organ systems functioning properly.

Homeostasis
1. A state of good health maintained by the normal functioning of the organ systems.
2. The body constantly responds to internal and external changes, yet remains stable, its many aspects are kept within normal limits.
3. Negative feedback mechanism—a control system in which a stimulus initiates a response that reverses or reduces the stimulus, thereby stopping the response until the stimulus occurs again and there is a need for the response.
4. Positive feedback mechanism—a control system that requires an external interruption. Has the potential for harm, therefore is rare in the body.

Terminology and General Plan of the Body
1. Body parts and areas—see Table 1–2 and Fig. 1–3.

2. Terms of location and position—used to describe relationships of position (see Table 1–3 and Figs. 1–3 and 1–4).
3. Body cavities and their membranes (see Fig. 1–4).
   - Dorsal cavity—lined with membranes called meninges; consists of the cranial and vertebral cavities.
     - Cranial cavity contains the brain.
     - Vertebral cavity contains the spinal cord.
   - Ventral cavity—the diaphragm separates the thoracic and abdominal cavities; the pelvic cavity is inferior to the abdominal cavity.
     - Thoracic cavity—contains the lungs and heart.
       - Pleural membranes line the chest wall and cover the lungs.
       - Pericardial membranes surround the heart.
     - Abdominal cavity—contains many organs including the stomach, liver, and intestines.
       - The peritoneum lines the abdominal cavity; the mesentery covers the abdominal organs.
     - Pelvic cavity—contains the urinary bladder and reproductive organs.
4. Planes and sections—cutting the body or an organ in a specific way (see Fig. 1–5).
   - Frontal or coronal—separates front and back parts.
   - Sagittal—separates right and left parts.
   - Transverse—separates upper and lower parts.
   - Cross—a section perpendicular to the long axis.
   - Longitudinal—a section along the long axis.
5. Areas of the abdomen—permits easier description of locations:
   - Quadrants—see Fig. 1–6.
   - Nine areas—see Fig. 1–6.

REVIEW QUESTIONS

1. Explain how the physiology of a bone is related to its anatomy. Explain how the physiology of the hand is related to its anatomy. (p. 4)

2. Describe anatomic position. Why is this knowledge important? (p. 11)

3. Name the organ system with each of the following functions: (p. 7)
   a. Moves the skeleton
   b. Regulates body functions by means of hormones

c. Covers the body and prevents entry of pathogens
d. Destroys pathogens that enter the body
e. Exchanges oxygen and carbon dioxide between the air and blood

4. Name the two major body cavities and their subdivisions. Name the cavity lined by the peritoneum, meninges, and parietal pleura. (pp. 12–13)

5. Name the four quadrants of the abdomen. Name at least one organ in each quadrant. (p. 16)

6. Name the section through the body that would result in each of the following: equal right and left halves, anterior and posterior parts, superior and inferior parts. (pp. 13–14)

7. Review Table 1–2, and try to find each external area on your own body. (pp. 10–11)

8. Define cell. When similar cells work together, what name are they given? (p. 4)

9. Define organ. When a group of organs works together, what name is it given? (p. 6)

10. Define homeostasis. (pp. 7, 10)
    a. Give an example of an external change and explain how the body responds to maintain homeostasis.
    b. Give an example of an internal change and explain how the body responds to maintain homeostasis.
    c. Briefly explain how a negative feedback mechanism works.

FOR FURTHER THOUGHT

1. The human foot is similar to the human hand, but does have anatomic differences. Describe two of these differences, and explain how they are related to the physiology of the hand and the foot.

2. Complete each statement using the everyday term for the body part.
    a. The distal femoral area is immediately superior to the ____.
    b. The proximal brachial area is immediately inferior to the ____.
    c. The patellar area is directly proximal to the ____.
    d. The volar area is directly distal to the ____.

3. Name a structure or organ that is both superior and inferior to the brain. Name one that is both anterior and posterior.

4. If a person has appendicitis (inflammation of the appendix caused by bacteria), pain is felt in which abdominal quadrant? (If not sure, take a look at Fig. 16–1 in Chapter 16.) Surgery is usually necessary to remove an inflamed appendix before it ruptures and causes peritonitis. Using your knowledge of the location of the peritoneum, explain why peritonitis is a very serious condition.

5. Keep in mind your answer to Question 4, and explain why bacterial meningitis can be a very serious infection.

6. Use a mental picture to cut the following sections. Then describe in simple words what each section looks like, and give each a proper anatomic name.

First: a tree trunk cut top to bottom, then cut side to side.

Second: a grapefruit cut top to bottom (straight down from where the stem was attached), then sliced through its equator.

CHAPTER 2

Some Basic Chemistry

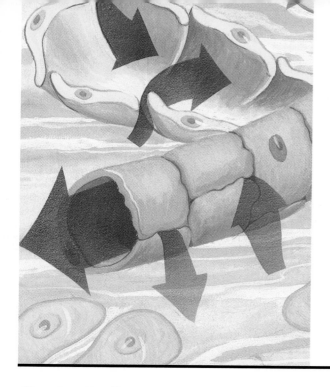

CHAPTER 2

Student Objectives

- Define the terms *element, atom, proton, neutron,* and *electron.*
- Describe the formation and purpose of ionic bonds, covalent bonds, disulfide bonds, and hydrogen bonds.
- Describe what happens in synthesis and decomposition reactions.
- Explain the importance of water to the functioning of the human body.
- Name and describe the water compartments.
- Explain the roles of oxygen and carbon dioxide in cell respiration.
- State what trace elements are, and name some, with their functions.
- Explain the pH scale. State the normal pH ranges of body fluids.
- Explain how a buffer system limits great changes in pH.
- Describe the functions of monosaccharides, disaccharides, oligosaccharides, and polysaccharides.
- Describe the functions of true fats, phospholipids, and steroids.
- Describe the functions of proteins, and explain how enzymes function as catalysts.
- Describe the functions of DNA, RNA, and ATP.

Some Basic Chemistry

New Terminology

Acid (**ASS**-sid)
Amino acid (ah-**MEE**-noh **ASS**-sid)
Atom (**A**-tum)
Base (**BAYSE**)
Buffer system (**BUFF**-er **SIS**-tem)
Carbohydrates (KAR-boh-**HIGH**-drayts)
Catalyst (**KAT**-ah-list)
Cell respiration (SELL RES-pi-**RAY**-shun)
Covalent bond (ko-**VAY**-lent)
Dissociation/ionization (dih-SEW-see-**AY**-shun/EYE-
    uh-nih-**ZAY**-shun)
Element (**EL**-uh-ment)
Enzyme (**EN**-zime)
Extracellular fluid (EX-trah-**SELL**-yoo-ler)
Intracellular fluid (IN-trah-**SELL**-yoo-ler)
Ion (**EYE**-on)
Ionic bond (eye-**ON**-ik)
Lipids (**LIP**-ids)
Matter (**MAT**-ter)
Molecule (**MAHL**-e-kuhl)
Nucleic acids (new-**KLEE**-ik **ASS**-sids)
pH and pH scale (Pee-H SKALE)
Protein (**PRO**-teen)
Salt (**SAWLT**)
Solvent/solution (**SAHL**-vent/suh-**LOO**-shun)
Steroid (**STEER**-oyd)
Trace elements (TRAYSE **EL**-uh-ments)

Related Clinical Terminology

Acidosis (ASS-i-**DOH**-sis)
Atherosclerosis (ATH-er-oh-skle-**ROH**-sis)
Hypoxia (high-**POCK**-see-ah)
Saturated (**SAT**-uhr-ay-ted) fats
Unsaturated (un-**SAT**-uhr-ay-ted) fats

*Terms that appear in **bold type** in the chapter text are defined in the glossary that begins on page 521.*

When you hear or see the word chemistry, you may think of test tubes and Bunsen burners in a laboratory experiment. However, literally everything in our physical world is made of chemicals. The paper used for this book, which was once the wood of a tree, is made of chemicals. The air we breathe is a mixture of chemicals in the form of gases. Water, gasoline, and diet soda are chemicals in liquid form. Our foods are chemicals, and our bodies are complex arrangements of thousands of chemicals. Recall from Chapter 1 that the simplest level of organization of the body is the chemical level.

This chapter covers some very basic aspects of chemistry as they are related to living organisms, and most especially as they are related to our understanding of the human body.

ELEMENTS

All matter, both living and not living, is made of elements, the simplest chemicals. An element is a substance made of only one type of atom (therefore, an atom is the smallest part of an element). There are 92 naturally occurring elements in the world around

us. Examples are hydrogen (H), iron (Fe), oxygen (O), calcium (Ca), nitrogen (N), and carbon (C). In nature, an element does not usually exist by itself but rather combines with the atoms of other elements to form compounds. Examples of some compounds important to our study of the human body are water (H_2O), in which two atoms of hydrogen combine with one atom of oxygen; carbon dioxide (CO_2), in which an atom of carbon combines with two atoms of oxygen; and glucose ($C_6H_{12}O_6$), in which six carbon atoms and six oxygen atoms combine with 12 hydrogen atoms.

The elements carbon, hydrogen, oxygen, nitrogen, phosphorus, and sulfur are found in all living things. If calcium is included, these seven elements make up approximately 99% of the human body (weight).

More than 20 different elements are found, in varying amounts, in the human body. Some of these are listed in Table 2–1. As you can see, each element has a standard chemical symbol. This is simply the first (and sometimes the second) letter of the element's English or Latin name. You should know the symbols of the elements in this table, since they are used in textbooks, articles, hospital lab reports, and so on. Notice that if a two-letter symbol is used for an element, the second letter is always lowercase, not a

Table 2–1 ELEMENTS IN THE HUMAN BODY			
Elements	**Symbol**	**Atomic Number***	**Percent of the Body by Weight**
Hydrogen	H	1	9.5
Carbon	C	6	18.5
Nitrogen	N	7	3.3
Oxygen	O	8	65.0
Fluorine	F	9	Trace
Sodium	Na	11	0.2
Magnesium	Mg	12	0.1
Phosphorus	P	15	1.0
Sulfur	S	16	0.3
Chlorine	Cl	17	0.2
Potassium	K	19	0.4
Calcium	Ca	20	1.5
Manganese	Mn	25	Trace
Iron	Fe	26	Trace
Cobalt	Co	27	Trace
Copper	Cu	29	Trace
Zinc	Zn	30	Trace
Iodine	1	53	Trace

* Atomic number is the number of protons in the nucleus of the atom. It also represents the number of electrons that orbit the nucleus.

capital. For example, the symbol for calcium is Ca, not CA. CA is an abbreviation often used for cancer.

ATOMS

Atoms are the smallest parts of an element that have the characteristics of that element. An atom consists of three major subunits or particles: protons, neutrons, and electrons (Fig. 2–1). A **proton** has a positive electrical charge and is found in the nucleus (or center) of the atom. A **neutron** is electrically neutral (has no charge) and is also found in the nucleus. An **electron** has a negative electrical charge and is found outside the nucleus orbiting in what may be called an electron cloud or shell around the nucleus.

The number of protons in an atom gives it its **atomic number**. Protons and neutrons have mass and weight; they give an atom its **atomic weight**. In an atom, the number of protons (+) equals the number of electrons (–); therefore, an atom is electrically neutral. The electrons, however, are important in that they may enable an atom to connect or **bond** to other atoms to form **molecules**. A molecule is a combination of atoms (usually of more than one element) that are so tightly bound together that the molecule behaves as a single unit.

Each atom is capable of bonding in only very specific ways. This capability depends on the number

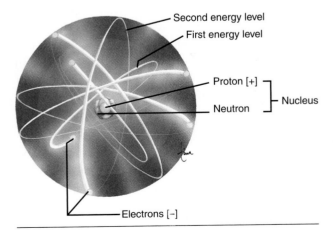

Figure 2–1 An atom of carbon. The nucleus contains six protons and six neutrons (not all are visible here). Six electrons orbit the nucleus, two in the first energy level and four in the second energy level.

Second energy level
First energy level
Proton [+]
Neutron
Nucleus
Electrons [–]

and the arrangement of the electrons of the atom. Electrons orbit the nucleus of an atom in shells or **energy levels**. The first, or innermost, energy level can contain a maximum of two electrons and is then considered stable. The second energy level is stable when it contains its maximum of eight electrons. The remaining energy levels, more distant from the nucleus, are also most stable when they contain eight electrons, or a multiple of eight.

A few atoms (elements) are naturally stable, or uninterested in reacting, because their outermost energy level already contains the maximum number of electrons. The gases helium and neon are examples of these stable atoms, which do not usually react with other atoms. Most atoms are not stable, however, and tend to gain, lose, or share electrons in order to fill their outermost shell. By doing so, an atom is capable of forming one or more chemical bonds with other atoms. In this way, the atom becomes stable, because its outermost shell of electrons has been filled. It is these reactive atoms that are of interest in our study of anatomy and physiology.

CHEMICAL BONDS

A chemical bond is not a structure, but rather a force or attraction between positive and negative electrical charges that keeps two or more atoms closely associated with each other to form a molecule. By way of comparison, think of gravity. We know that gravity is not a "thing," but rather the force that keeps our feet on the floor and allows us to pour coffee with consistent success. Molecules formed by chemical bonding often have physical characteristics different from those of the atoms of the original elements. For example, the elements hydrogen and oxygen are gases, but atoms of each may chemically bond to form molecules of water, which is a liquid.

The type of chemical bonding depends upon the tendencies of the electrons of atoms involved, as you will see. Four kinds of bonds are very important to the chemistry of the body: ionic bonds, covalent bonds, disulfide bonds, and hydrogen bonds.

IONIC BONDS

An **ionic bond** involves the loss of one or more electrons by one atom and the gain of the electron(s) by another atom or atoms. Refer to Fig. 2–2 as you read the following.

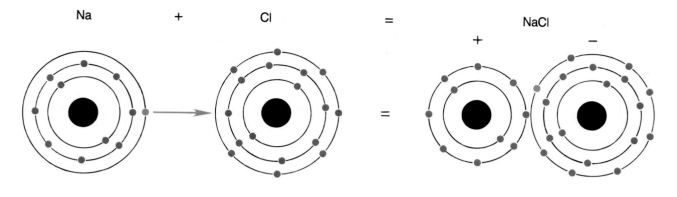

Figure 2–2 Formation of an ionic bond. An atom of sodium loses an electron to an atom of chlorine. The two ions formed have unlike charges, are attracted to one another, and form a molecule of sodium chloride.

An atom of sodium (Na) has one electron in its outermost shell, and in order to become stable, it tends to lose that electron. When it does so, the sodium atom has one more proton than it has electrons. Therefore, it now has an electrical charge (or **valence**) of +1 and is called a sodium **ion** (Na^+). An atom of chlorine has seven electrons in its outermost shell, and in order to become stable tends to gain one electron. When it does so, the chlorine atom has one more electron than it has protons, and now has a charge (valence) of –1. It is called a chloride ion (Cl^-).

When an atom of sodium loses an electron to an atom of chlorine, their ions have unlike charges (positive and negative) and are thus attracted to one another. The result is the formation of a molecule of sodium chloride: NaCl, or common table salt. The bond that holds these ions together is called an ionic bond.

Another example is the bonding of chlorine to calcium. An atom of calcium has two electrons in its outermost shell and tends to lose those electrons in order to become stable. If two atoms of chlorine each gain one of those electrons, they become chloride ions. The positive and negative ions are then attracted to one another, forming a molecule of calcium chloride, $CaCl_2$, which is also a salt. A **salt** is a molecule made of ions other than hydrogen (H^+) ions or hydroxyl (OH^-) ions.

Ions with positive charges are called **cations**. These include Na^+, Ca^{+2}, K^+, Fe^{+2}, and Mg^{+2}. Ions with negative charges are called **anions**, which include Cl^-, SO_4^{-2} (sulfate), and HCO_3^- (bicarbonate). The types of compounds formed by ionic bonding are salts, acids, and bases. (Acids and bases are discussed later in this chapter.)

In the solid state, ionic bonds are relatively strong. Our bones, for example, contain the salt calcium carbonate ($CaCO_3$), which helps give bone its strength. However, in an **aqueous** (water) **solution**, many ionic bonds are weakened. The bonds may become so weak that the bound ions of a molecule separate, creating a solution of free positive and negative ions. For example, if sodium chloride is put in water, it dissolves, then **ionizes**. The water now contains Na^+ ions and Cl^- ions. Ionization, also called **dissociation**, is important to living organisms because once dissociated, the ions are free to take part in other chemical reactions within the body. Cells in the stomach lining produce hydrochloric acid (HCl) and must have Cl^- ions to do so. The chloride in NaCl would not be free to take part in another reaction since it is tightly bound to the sodium atom. However, the Cl^- ions available from ionized NaCl in the cellular water can be used for the **synthesis**, or chemical manufacture, of HCl in the stomach.

COVALENT BONDS

Covalent bonds involve the sharing of electrons between atoms. As shown in Fig. 2–3, an atom of oxygen needs two electrons to become stable. It may share two of its electrons with another atom of oxygen, also sharing two electrons. Together they

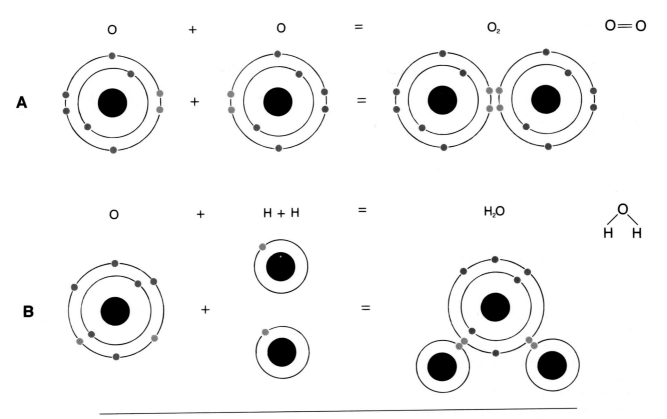

Figure 2–3 Formation of covalent bonds. **(A)** Two atoms of oxygen share two electrons each, forming a molecule of oxygen gas. **(B)** An atom of oxygen shares one electron with each of two hydrogen atoms, each sharing its electron. A molecule of water is formed.

form a molecule of oxygen gas (O_2), which is the form in which oxygen exists in the atmosphere.

An atom of oxygen may also share two of its electrons with two atoms of hydrogen, each sharing its single electron (see Fig. 2–3). Together they form a molecule of water (H_2O). When writing structural formulas for chemical molecules, a pair of shared electrons is indicated by a single line, as shown in the formula for water; this is a single covalent bond. A double covalent bond is indicated by two lines, as in the formula for oxygen; this represents two pairs of shared electrons.

The element carbon always forms covalent bonds; an atom of carbon has four electrons to share with other atoms. If these four electrons are shared with four atoms of hydrogen, each sharing its one electron, a molecule of methane gas (CH_4) is formed. Carbon may form covalent bonds with other carbons, hydrogen, oxygen, nitrogen, or other elements.

Organic compounds such as proteins and carbohydrates are complex and precise arrangements of these atoms covalently bonded to one another. Covalent bonds are relatively strong and are not weakened in an aqueous solution. This is important because the proteins produced by the body, for example, must remain intact in order to function properly in the water of our cells and blood. The functions of organic compounds will be considered later in this chapter.

DISULFIDE BONDS AND HYDROGEN BONDS

Two other types of bonds that are important to the chemistry of the body are disulfide bonds and hydrogen bonds. Disulfide bonds are found in some proteins. Hydrogen bonds are part of many different molecules.

A **disulfide bond** (also called a disulfide bridge) is a covalent bond formed between two atoms of sulfur, usually within the same large protein molecule. The hormone insulin, for example, is a protein that must have a very specific three-dimensional shape in order to function properly to regulate the blood glucose level. Each molecule of insulin has two disulfide bonds that help maintain its proper shape and function (see Box Fig. 10–A). Other proteins with shapes that depend upon disulfide bonds are antibodies of the immune system (see Fig. 14-6) and keratin of the skin.

A **hydrogen bond** does not involve the sharing or exchange of electrons, but rather results because of a property of hydrogen atoms. When a hydrogen atom shares its one electron in a covalent bond with another atom, its proton has a slight positive charge and may then be attracted to a nearby oxygen or nitrogen atom, which has a slight negative charge.

Although they are weak bonds, hydrogen bonds are important in several ways. Large organic molecules such as proteins and DNA have very specific functions that depend upon their three-dimensional shapes. The shapes of these molecules, so crucial to their proper functioning, are often maintained by hydrogen bonds.

Hydrogen bonds also make water cohesive; that is, each water molecule is attracted to nearby water molecules. Such cohesiveness can be seen if water is dropped onto clean glass; the surface tension created by the hydrogen bonds makes the water form three-dimensional beads. Within the body, the cohesiveness of water helps keep blood a continuous stream as it flows within the blood vessels, and keeps tissue fluid continuous around cells. These hydrogen bonds are also responsible for the other important characteristics of water, which are discussed in a later section.

CHEMICAL REACTIONS

A chemical reaction is a change brought about by the formation or breaking of chemical bonds. Two general types of reactions are synthesis reactions and decomposition reactions.

In a synthesis reaction, bonds are formed to join two or more atoms or molecules to make a new compound. The production of the protein hemoglobin in potential red blood cells is an example of a synthesis reaction. Proteins are synthesized by the bonding of many amino acids, their smaller subunits. Synthesis reactions require energy for the formation of bonds.

In a decomposition reaction, bonds are broken, and a large molecule is changed to two or more smaller ones. One example is the digestion of large molecules of starch to many smaller glucose molecules. Some decomposition reactions release energy; this is described in a later section on cell respiration.

In this and future chapters, keep in mind that the term *reaction* refers to the making or breaking of chemical bonds and thus to changes in the physical and chemical characteristics of the molecules involved.

INORGANIC COMPOUNDS OF IMPORTANCE

Inorganic compounds are usually simple molecules that often consist of only one or two different elements. Despite their simplicity, however, some inorganic compounds are essential to normal structure and functioning of the body.

WATER

Water makes up 60% to 75% of the human body, and is essential to life for several reasons:

1. *Water is a **solvent**,* that is, many substances (called solutes) can dissolve in water. Nutrients such as glucose are dissolved in blood plasma (which is largely water) to be transported to cells throughout the body. The sense of taste depends upon the solvent ability of saliva; dissolved food stimulates the receptors in taste buds. The excretion of waste products is possible because they are dissolved in the water of urine.

2. *Water is a lubricant,* which prevents friction where surfaces meet and move. In the digestive tract, swallowing depends upon the presence of saliva, and mucus is a slippery fluid that permits the smooth passage of food through the intestines. Synovial fluid within joint cavities prevents friction as bones move.

3. *Water changes temperature slowly.* Water has a high heat capacity, which means that it will absorb a great deal of heat before its temperature rises significantly, or it must lose a great deal of heat before its temperature drops significantly. This is one of

Intracellular fluid

Cell

Fluid movement

Lymph

Interstitial (tissue) fluid

Plasma

Capillary

Lymph capillary

Figure 2–4 Water compartments, showing the names water is given in its different locations and the ways in which water moves between compartments.

the factors that helps the body maintain a constant temperature. Water also has a high heat of vaporization, which is important for the process of sweating. Excess body heat evaporates sweat on the skin surfaces, rather than overheating the body's cells.

WATER COMPARTMENTS

All water within the body is continually moving, but water is given different names when it is in specific body locations, which are called compartments (Fig. 2–4).

Intracellular fluid (ICF)—the water within cells; about 65% of the total body water

Extracellular fluid (ECF)—all the rest of the water in the body; about 35% of the total. More specific compartments of extracellular fluid include:

    Plasma—water found in blood vessels

    Lymph—water found in lymphatic vessels

    Tissue fluid or interstitial fluid—water found in the small spaces between cells

    Specialized fluids—synovial fluid, cerebrospinal fluid, aqueous humor in the eye, and others

The movement of water between compartments in the body and the functions of the specialized fluids will be discussed in later chapters.

OXYGEN

Oxygen in the form of a gas (O_2) is approximately 21% of the atmosphere, which we inhale. We all know that without oxygen we wouldn't survive very long, but exactly what does it do? Oxygen is important to us because it is essential for a process called cell respiration, in which cells break down simple nutrients such as glucose in order to release energy. The reason we breathe is to obtain oxygen for cell respiration and to exhale the carbon dioxide produced in cell respiration (this will be discussed in the next section). Biologically useful energy that is released by the reactions of cell respiration is trapped in a molecule called ATP (adenosine triphosphate).

ATP can then be used for cellular processes that require energy.

CARBON DIOXIDE

Carbon dioxide (CO_2) is produced by cells as a waste product of cell respiration. You may ask why a waste product is considered important. Keep in mind that "important" does not always mean "beneficial," but it does mean "significant." If the amount of carbon dioxide in the body fluids increases, it causes these fluids to become too acidic. Therefore, carbon dioxide must be exhaled as rapidly as it is formed to keep the amount in the body within normal limits. Normally this is just what happens, but severe pulmonary diseases such as pneumonia or emphysema decrease gas exchange in the lungs and permit carbon dioxide to accumulate in the blood. When this happens, a person is said to be in a state of **acidosis**, which may seriously disrupt body functioning (see the sections on pH and enzymes later in this chapter; see also Box 2–1: Blood Gases).

CELL RESPIRATION

Cell respiration is the name for energy production within cells and involves both respiratory gases, oxygen, and carbon dioxide. Many chemical reactions are involved, but in its simplest form, cell respiration may be summarized by the following equation:

$$\text{Glucose (C}_6\text{H}_{12}\text{O}_6) + 6O_2 \rightarrow 6CO_2 + 6H_2O + \text{ATP} + \text{heat}$$

This reaction shows us that glucose and oxygen combine to yield carbon dioxide, water, ATP, and heat. Food, represented here by glucose, in the presence of oxygen is broken down into the simpler molecules carbon dioxide and water. The potential energy in the glucose molecule is released in two forms: ATP and heat. Each of the four products of this process has a purpose or significance in the body. The carbon dioxide is a waste product that moves from the cells into the blood to be carried to the lungs and eventually exhaled. The water formed is useful and becomes part of the intracellular fluid. The heat produced contributes to normal body temperature. ATP is used for cell processes such as mitosis, protein synthesis, and muscle contraction, all of which require energy and will be discussed a bit further on in the text.

We will also return to cell respiration in later chapters. For now, the brief description above will suffice to show that eating and breathing are interrelated; both are essential for energy production.

Box 2–1   BLOOD GASES

A patient is admitted to the emergency room with a possible heart attack, and the doctor in charge orders "blood gases." Another patient hospitalized with pneumonia has "blood gases" monitored at frequent intervals. What are blood gases, and what does measurement of them tell us? The blood gases are oxygen and carbon dioxide, and their levels in arterial blood provide information about the functioning of the respiratory and circulatory systems. Arterial blood normally has a high concentration of oxygen and a low concentration of carbon dioxide. These levels are maintained by gas exchange in the lungs and by the proper circulation of blood.

A pulmonary disease such as pneumonia interferes with efficient gas exchange in the lungs. As a result, blood oxygen concentration may decrease, and blood carbon dioxide concentration may increase. Either of these changes in blood gases may become lifethreatening for the patient, so monitoring of blood gases is important. If blood oxygen falls below the normal range, oxygen will be administered; if blood carbon dioxide rises above the normal range, blood pH will be corrected to prevent serious acidosis.

Damage to the heart may also bring about a change in blood gases, especially oxygen. Oxygen is picked up by red blood cells as they circulate through lung capillaries; as red blood cells circulate through the body, they release oxygen to tissues. What keeps the blood circulating or moving? The pumping of the heart.

A mild heart attack, when heart failure is unlikely, is often characterized by a blood oxygen level that is low but still within normal limits. A more severe heart attack that seriously impairs the pumping of the heart will decrease the blood oxygen level to less than normal. This condition is called **hypoxia**, which means that too little oxygen is reaching tissues. When this is determined by measurement of blood gases, appropriate oxygen therapy can be started to correct the hypoxia.

TRACE ELEMENTS

Trace elements are those that are needed by the body in very small amounts. Although they may not be as abundant in the body as are carbon, hydrogen, or oxygen, they are nonetheless essential. Table 2–2 lists some of these trace elements and their functions (see also Box 2–2: Nitric Oxide).

ACIDS, BASES, AND PH

An **acid** may be defined as a substance that increases the concentration of hydrogen ions (H^+) in a water solution. A **base** is a substance that decreases the concentration of H^+ ions, which in the case of water, has the same effect as increasing the concentration of hydroxyl ions (OH^-).

The acidity or alkalinity (basicity) of a solution is measured on a scale of values called **pH** (parts hydrogen). The values on the **pH scale** range from 0 to 14, with 0 indicating the most acidic level and 14 the most alkaline. A solution with a pH of 7 is neutral because it contains the same number of H^+ ions and OH^- ions. Pure water has a pH of 7. A solution with a higher concentration of H^+ ions than OH^- ions is an acidic solution with a pH below 7. An alkaline solution, therefore, has a higher concentration of OH^- ions than H^+ ions and has a pH above 7.

The pH scale, with the relative concentrations of H^+ ions, and OH^- ions, is shown in Fig. 2–5. A change of one pH unit is a 10-fold change in H^+ ion concentration. This means that a solution with a pH of 4 has 10 times as many H^+ ions as a solution with a pH of 5, and 100 times as many H^+ ions as a solution with a pH of 6. Figure 2–5 also shows the pH of some body fluids and other familiar solutions. Notice that gastric juice has a pH of 1 and coffee has a pH of 5. This means that gastric juice has 10,000 times as many H^+

Table 2–2	TRACE ELEMENTS
Element	**Function**
Calcium	• Provides strength in bones and teeth • Necessary for blood clotting • Necessary for muscle contraction
Phosphorus	• Provides strength in bones and teeth • Part of DNA and RNA • Part of cell membranes
Iron	• Part of hemoglobin in red blood cells; transports oxygen • Part of myoglobin in muscles; stores oxygen • Necessary for cell respiration
Copper	• Necessary for cell respiration • Necessary for hemoglobin synthesis
Sodium and potassium	• Necessary for muscle contraction • Necessary for nerve impulse transmission
Sulfur	• Part of some proteins such as insulin and keratin
Cobalt	• Part of vitamin B12
Iodine	• Part of thyroid hormones—thyroxine

Box 2–2	NITRIC OXIDE

Nitric oxide is a gas with the molecular formula NO. You have probably heard of it as a component of air pollution and cigarette smoke, but it is produced by certain human tissues, and research has discovered several functions for this deceptively simple molecule.

Nitric oxide promotes vasodilation of arterioles, permitting greater blood flow and oxygen delivery to tissues. It is involved in nerve impulse transmission in the brain, and may contribute to memory storage. Some immune system cells produce nitric oxide as a cytotoxic (cell-poisoning) agent to help destroy foreign cells such as bacteria.

Investigations are under way to determine if nitric oxide can be used therapeutically. It has already been found useful in the treatment of pulmonary hypertension, to relax abnormally constricted arteries in the lungs to permit normal gas exchange. Another possible therapy is for sickle-cell anemia. Nitric oxide bonds to hemoglobin and may prevent the change of shape characteristic of sickle-cell hemoglobin (see Box 3–2).

Much more research is needed, including a determination of possible harmful side effects of greater than normal amounts of nitric oxide, but the results of clinical trials thus far are very promising.

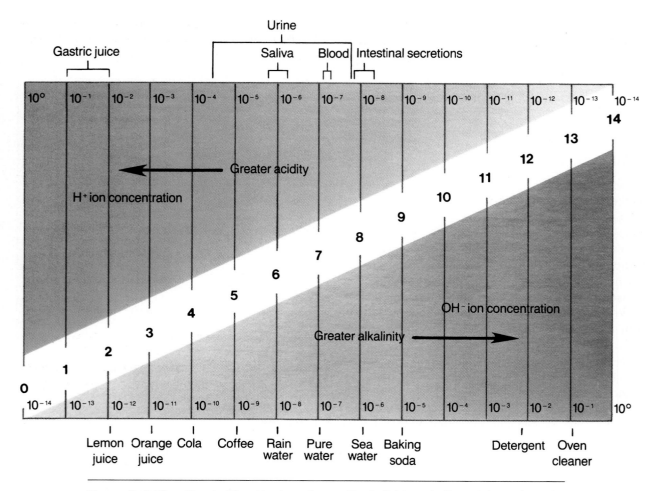

Figure 2–5 The pH scale. The pH values of several body fluids are indicated above the scale. The pH values of some familiar solutions are indicated below the scale.

ions as does coffee. Although coffee is acidic, it is a weak acid and does not have the corrosive effect of gastric juice, a strong acid.

The cells and internal fluids of the human body have a pH close to neutral. The pH of intracellular fluid is around 6.8, and the normal pH range of blood is 7.35 to 7.45. Fluids such as gastric juice and urine are technically external fluids, since they are in body tracts that open to the environment. The pH of these fluids may be more strongly acidic or alkaline without harm to the body.

The pH of blood, however, must be maintained within its very narrow, slightly alkaline range. A decrease of only one pH unit, which is 10 times as many H^+ ions, would disrupt the chemical reactions of the blood and cause the death of the individual. Normal metabolism tends to make body fluids more

acidic, and this tendency to acidosis must be continually corrected. Normal pH of internal fluids is maintained by the kidneys, respiratory system, and buffer systems. Although acid–base balance will be a major topic of Chapter 19, we will briefly mention buffer systems here.

Buffer Systems

A **buffer system** is a chemical or pair of chemicals that minimizes changes in pH by reacting with strong acids or strong bases to transform them into substances that will not drastically change pH. Expressed in another way, a buffer may bond to H^+ ions when a body fluid is becoming too acidic, or release H^+ ions when a fluid is becoming too alkaline.

As a specific example, we will use the bicarbonate buffer system, which consists of carbonic acid (H_2CO_3), a weak acid, and sodium bicarbonate ($NaHCO_3$), a weak base. This pair of chemicals is present in all body fluids but is especially important to buffer blood and tissue fluid.

Carbonic acid ionizes as follows (but remember, because it is a weak acid it does not contribute many H^+ ions to a solution):

$$H_2CO_3 \rightarrow H^+ + HCO_3^-$$

Sodium bicarbonate ionizes as follows:

$$NaHCO_3 \rightarrow Na^+ + HCO_3^-$$

If a strong acid, such as HCl, is added to extracellular fluid, this reaction will occur:

$$HCl + NaHCO_3 \rightarrow NaCl + H_2CO_3$$

What has happened here? Hydrochloric acid, a strong acid that would greatly lower pH, has reacted with sodium bicarbonate. The products of this reaction are NaCl, a salt which has no effect on pH, and H_2CO_3, a weak acid that lowers pH only slightly. This prevents a drastic change in the pH of the extracellular fluid.

If a strong base, such as sodium hydroxide, is added to the extracellular fluid, this reaction will occur:

$$NaOH + H_2CO_3 \rightarrow H_2O + NaHCO_3$$

Sodium hydroxide, a strong base that would greatly raise pH, has reacted with carbonic acid. The products of this reaction are water, which has no effect on pH, and sodium bicarbonate, a weak base that raises pH only slightly. Again, this prevents a drastic change in the pH of the extracellular fluid.

In the body, such reactions take place in less than a second whenever acids or bases are formed that would greatly change pH. Because of the body's tendency to become more acidic, the need to correct acidosis is more frequent. With respect to the bicarbonate buffer system, this means that more $NaHCO_3$ than H_2CO_3 is needed. For this reason, the usual ratio of these buffers is 20:1 ($NaHCO_3:H_2CO_3$).

ORGANIC COMPOUNDS OF IMPORTANCE

Organic compounds all contain covalently bonded carbon and hydrogen atoms and perhaps other elements as well. In the human body there are four major groups of organic compounds: carbohydrates, lipids, proteins, and nucleic acids.

CARBOHYDRATES

A primary function of **carbohydrates** is to serve as sources of energy. All carbohydrates contain carbon, hydrogen, and oxygen and are classified as monosaccharides, disaccharides, oligosaccharides, and polysaccharides. Saccharide means sugar, and the prefix indicates how many are present.

Monosaccharides or single-sugar compounds are the simplest sugars. Glucose is a **hexose**, or 6-carbon, sugar with the formula $C_6H_{12}O_6$ (Fig. 2–6). Fructose and galactose also have the same formula, but the physical arrangement of the carbon, hydrogen, and oxygen atoms in each differs from that of glucose. This gives each hexose sugar a different three-dimensional shape. The liver is able to change fructose and galactose to glucose, which is then used by cells in the process of cell respiration to produce ATP.

Another type of monosaccharide is the **pentose**, or 5-carbon, sugar. These are not involved in energy

Figure 2–6 Carbohydrates. **(A)** Glucose, depicting its structural formula. **(B)** A disaccharide such as maltose. **(C)** Cellulose, a polysaccharide. **(D)** Starch, a polysaccharide. **(E)** Glycogen, a polysaccharide. Each hexagon represents a hexose sugar such as glucose.

production but rather are structural components of the nucleic acids. Deoxyribose ($C_5H_{10}O_4$) is part of DNA, which is the genetic material of chromosomes. Ribose ($C_5H_{10}O_5$) is part of RNA, which is essential for protein synthesis. We will return to the nucleic acids later in this chapter.

Disaccharides are double sugars, made of two monosaccharides linked by covalent bonds. Examples are sucrose, lactose, and maltose, which are present in food. They are digested into monosaccharides and then used for energy production.

The prefix *oligo* means "few"; **oligosaccharides** consist of from 3 to 20 monosaccharides. In human cells, oligosaccharides are found on the outer surface of cell membranes. Here they serve as **antigens**, which are chemical markers (or "signposts") that identify cells. The A, B, and AB blood types, for example, are the result of oligosaccharide antigens on the outer surface of red blood cell membranes. All of our cells have "self" antigens, which identify the cells that belong in an individual. The presence of "self" antigens on our own cells enables the immune system to recognize antigens that are "non-self." Such foreign antigens include bacteria and viruses, and immunity will be a major topic of Chapter 14.

Polysaccharides are made of thousands of glucose molecules, bonded in different ways, resulting in different shapes (see Fig. 2–6). **Starches** are branched chains of glucose and are produced by plant cells to store energy. We have digestive enzymes that split the bonds of starch molecules, releasing glucose. The glucose is then absorbed and used by cells to produce ATP.

Glycogen, a highly branched chain of glucose molecules, is our own storage form for glucose. After a meal high in carbohydrates, the blood glucose level rises. Excess glucose is then changed to glycogen and stored in the liver and skeletal muscles. When the blood glucose level decreases between meals, the glycogen is converted back to glucose, which is released into the blood. The blood glucose level is kept within normal limits, and cells can take in this glucose to produce energy.

Cellulose is a nearly straight chain of glucose molecules produced by plant cells as part of their cell walls. We have no enzyme to digest the cellulose we consume as part of vegetables and grains, and it passes through the digestive tract unchanged. Another name for dietary cellulose is "fiber," and although we cannot use its glucose for energy, it does have a function.

Fiber provides bulk within the cavity of the large intestine. This promotes efficient **peristalsis**, the waves of contraction that propel undigested material through the colon. A diet low in fiber does not give the colon much exercise, and the muscle tissue of the colon will contract weakly, just as our skeletal muscles will become flabby without exercise. A diet high in fiber provides exercise for the colon muscle and may help prevent chronic constipation.

The structure and functions of the carbohydrates are summarized in Table 2–3.

LIPIDS

Lipids contain the elements carbon, hydrogen, and oxygen; some also contain phosphorus. In this group of organic compounds are different types of substances with very different functions. We will consider three types: true fats, phospholipids, and steroids (Fig. 2–7).

True fats are made of one molecule of glycerol and one, two, or three fatty acid molecules. If three fatty acid molecules are bonded to a single glycerol, a **triglyceride** is formed. (You can usually find this term on the nutrition labels of some highly processed foods; it means that fat has been added.) You have undoubtedly heard of saturated and unsaturated fats; the differences between them are discussed in Box 2–3. True fats are a storage form for excess food, that is, they are stored energy. Any type of food consumed in excess of the body's caloric needs will be converted to fat and stored in adipose tissue. Most adipose tissue is subcutaneous, between the skin and muscles. Some organs, however, such as the eyes and kidneys, are enclosed in a layer of fat that acts as a cushion to absorb shock.

Phospholipids are diglycerides with a phosphate group (PO_4) in the third bonding site of glycerol. Although similar in structure to the true fats, phospholipids are not stored energy but rather structural components of cells. Lecithin is a phospholipid that is part of our **cell membranes**. Another example is **myelin**, which forms the myelin sheath around nerve cells and provides electrical insulation for nerve impulse transmission.

The structure of **steroids** is very different from that of the other lipids. **Cholesterol** is an important steroid; it is made of four rings of carbon and hydrogen (not fatty acids and glycerol) and is shown in Fig. 2–7. The liver synthesizes cholesterol, in addition to

Table 2–3   CARBOHYDRATES

Name	Structure	Function
Monosaccharides—"Single" Sugars		
Glucose	Hexose sugar	• Most important energy source for cells
Fructose and galactose	Hexose sugars	• Converted to glucose by the liver, then used for energy production
Deoxyribose	Pentose sugar	• Part of DNA, the genetic code in the chromosomes of cells
Ribose	Pentose sugar	• Part of RNA, needed for protein synthesis within cells
Disaccharides—"Double" Sugars		
Sucrose, lactose and maltose	Two hexose sugars	• Present in food; digested to monosaccharides, which are then used for energy production
Oligosaccharides—"Few" Sugars (3–20)		
		• Form "self" antigens on cell membranes; important to permit the immune system to distinguish "self" from foreign antigens (pathogens)
Polysaccharides—"Many" Sugars (Thousands)		
Starches	Branched chains of glucose molecules	• Found in plant foods; digested to monosaccharides and used for energy production
Glycogen	Highly branched chains of glucose molecules	• Storage form for excess glucose in the liver and skeletal muscles
Cellulose	Straight chains of glucose molecules	• Part of plant cell walls; provides fiber to promote peristalsis, especially by the colon

Figure 2–7 Lipids. **(A)** A triglyceride made of one glycerol and three fatty acids. **(B)** The steroid cholesterol. The hexagons represent rings of carbon and hydrogen.

the cholesterol we eat in food as part of our diet. Cholesterol is another component of cell membranes and is the precursor (raw material) for the synthesis of other steroids. In the ovaries or testes, cholesterol is used to synthesize the steroid hormones estrogen or testosterone, respectively. A form of cholesterol in the skin is changed to vitamin D on exposure to sunlight. Liver cells use cholesterol for the synthesis of bile salts, which emulsify fats in digestion. Despite its link to coronary artery disease and heart attacks, cholesterol is an essential substance for human beings.

The structure and functions of lipids are summarized in Table 2–4.

PROTEINS

Proteins are made of smaller subunits or building blocks called **amino acids**, which all contain the elements carbon, hydrogen, oxygen, and nitrogen. Some amino acids contain sulfur, which permits the formation of disulfide bonds. There are about 20 amino acids that make up human proteins. The struc-

Box 2–3   SATURATED AND UNSATURATED FATS

You have probably heard or read that eating foods high in **unsaturated fats** may help prevent heart disease and that a diet high in **saturated fats** may contribute to heart disease. "Heart disease" actually refers to **atherosclerosis** of the coronary arteries, those that supply the heart muscle with oxygen. Atherosclerosis is the deposition of cholesterol and other substances in the walls of these arteries, leading to obstruction or clot formation and a heart attack. These abnormal deposits of cholesterol are more likely to occur when blood cholesterol levels are high, and diet does have an effect on blood cholesterol.

The true fats may be divided into saturated and unsaturated fats. Refer to Fig. 2–7 and notice that one of the fatty acids has single covalent bonds between all its carbon atoms. Each of these carbons is then bonded to the maximum number of hydrogens; this is a saturated fatty acid. The other fatty acids shown have one or more (poly) double covalent bonds between their carbons and less than the maximum number of hydrogens; these are unsaturated fatty acids. At room temperature, saturated fats are often in solid form, while unsaturated fats are often (not always) in liquid form.

Saturated fats tend to be found in animal foods such as beef, pork, eggs, and cheese, but palm oil and coconut oil are also saturated. Unsaturated fats are found in other plant oils such as corn oil, sunflower oil, and safflower oil, but certain fish oils are also unsaturated.

The breakdown products of saturated fats are used by the liver to synthesize cholesterol, which raises the blood cholesterol level. This is not true for the unsaturated fats; they do not contribute to cholesterol formation. This is why a diet high in unsaturated fats may help prevent atherosclerosis. Unsaturated fats, especially polyunsaturated fats, may actually help lower blood cholesterol by decreasing the formation of cholesterol by the liver.

There are other contributing factors to coronary artery disease, such as heredity, smoking, being overweight, and lack of exercise. Diet alone cannot prevent atherosclerosis. However, a diet low in total fat and high in polyunsaturated fats is a good start.

ture of amino acids is shown in Fig. 2–8. Each amino acid has a central carbon atom covalently bonded to an atom of hydrogen, an amino group (NH_2), and a carboxyl group (COOH). At the fourth bond of the central carbon is the variable portion of the amino acid, represented by R. The R group may be a single hydrogen atom, or a CH_3 group, or a more complex configuration of carbon and hydrogen. This gives each of the 20 amino acids a slightly different physical shape. A bond between two amino acids is called a **peptide bond**, and a short chain of amino acids linked by peptide bonds is a **polypeptide**.

Table 2–4   LIPIDS

Name	Structure	Function
True fats	A triglyceride consists of three fatty acid molecules bonded to a glycerol molecule (some are monoglycerides or diglycerides)	• Storage form for excess food molecules in subcutaneous tissue • Cushion organs such as the eyes and kidneys
Phospholipids	Diglycerides with a phosphate group bonded to the glycerol molecule	• Part of cell membranes (lecithin) • Form the myelin sheath to provide electrical insulation for neurons
Steroids (cholesterol)	Four carbon–hydrogen rings	• Part of cell membranes • Converted to vitamin D in the skin on exposure to UV rays of the sun • Converted by the liver to bile salts, which emulsify fats during digestion • Precursor for the steroid hormones such as estrogen in women (ovaries) or testosterone in men (testes)

Figure 2–8 Amino acids. **(A)** The structural formula of an amino acid. The "R" represents the variable portion of the molecule. **(B)** A polypeptide. Several amino acids, represented by different shapes, are linked by peptide bonds.

Table 2–5	FUNCTIONS OF PROTEINS
Type of Protein	**Function**
Structural proteins	• Form pores and receptor sites in cell membranes • Keratin—part of skin and hair • Collagen—part of tendons and ligaments
Hormones	• Insulin—enables cells to take in glucose; lowers blood glucose level • Growth hormone—increases protein synthesis and cell division
Hemoglobin	• Enables red blood cells to carry oxygen
Antibodies	• Produced by lymphocytes (white blood cells); label pathogens for destruction
Myosin and actin	• Muscle structure and contraction
Enzymes	• Catalyze reactions

A protein may consist of from 50 to thousands of amino acids. The sequence of the amino acids is specific and unique for each protein. This unique sequence, and the hydrogen bonds and disulfide bonds formed within the amino acid chain, determines the protein's characteristic three-dimensional shape, which in turn determines its function. Some proteins consist of more than one amino acid chain. Hemoglobin, for example, has four amino acid chains. Our body proteins have many functions; some of these are listed in Table 2–5 and will be mentioned again in later chapters. And though we usually do not think of protein as an energy food, if our diet includes more amino acids than are necessary for our protein synthesis, those excess amino acids will be converted to simple carbohydrates or even to fat, to be stored as potential energy. (See Box 2–4: A Protein Mystery: Prions, for a discussion of disease-causing proteins.) One very important function of proteins will be discussed further here: the role of proteins as enzymes.

Enzymes

Enzymes are **catalysts**, which means that they speed up chemical reactions without the need for an external source of energy such as heat. The many reactions that take place within the body are catalyzed by specific enzymes; all of these reactions must take place at body temperature.

The way in which enzymes function as catalysts is called the **Active Site Theory**, which is based on the shape of the enzyme and the shapes of the reacting molecules, called **substrates**. A simple reaction is depicted in Fig. 2–9. Notice that the enzyme has a specific shape, as do the substrate molecules. The active site of the enzyme is the part that matches the shapes of the substrates. The substrates must "fit" into the active site of the enzyme, and temporary bonds may form between the enzyme and the substrate. This is called the enzyme–substrate complex. In this case, two substrate molecules are thus brought close together so that chemical bonds are formed between them, creating a new compound. The product of the reaction, the new compound, is then released, leaving the enzyme itself unchanged and able to catalyze another reaction of the same type.

Each enzyme is specific in that it will catalyze only one type of reaction. An enzyme that digests the protein in food, for example, has the proper shape for that reaction but cannot digest starches. For starch digestion, another enzyme with a differently shaped active site is needed. Thousands of chemical reactions take place within the body, and therefore we have

Box 2–4   A PROTEIN MYSTERY: PRIONS

Prions are proteinaceous infectious particles, the cause of lethal diseases of the nervous system in people and animals. Mad-cow disease is perhaps the best known; its formal name is bovine spongiform encephalopathy (BSE). The name tells us about the disease: Encephalopathy means that the brain is affected, and spongiform indicates that brain tissue becomes spongy, full of holes. Unfortunately, people may acquire BSE by eating beef contaminated with infected cow brain tissue. They develop what is called variant Creutzfeldt-Jakob disease (CJD). CJD is characterized by loss of coordination, loss of memory and personality, and death within a few months. There is no treatment.

How do prions cause this disease? We do not yet have the entire answer. We do know that prions change the structure of other brain proteins, which brings about deterioration of brain tissue. We do not know how to destroy prions. Prions are not living; they do not contain genetic material or carry out processes that might be disrupted by antibiotics or antiviral medications. Standard sterilization practices that kill bacteria and viruses do not seem to inactivate prions, nor are they destroyed by cooking.

Prevention of prion disease depends upon keeping animal brain tissue from contaminating meat destined for human or animal consumption. In Great Britain, where the human form of mad-cow disease has killed nearly 100 people (as of 2001), butchering practices are now stringently regulated. The first cases of mad-cow disease in Canada and the United States were found in 2003.

---

thousands of enzymes, each with its own shape and active site.

The ability of enzymes to function may be limited or destroyed by changes in the intracellular or extracellular fluids in which they are found. Changes in pH and temperature are especially crucial. Recall that the pH of intracellular fluid is approximately 6.8, and that a decrease in pH means that more H^+ ions are present. If pH decreases significantly, the excess H^+ ions will react with the active sites of cellular enzymes, change their shapes, and prevent them from catalyzing reactions. This is why a state of acidosis may cause the death of cells—the cells' enzymes are unable to function properly.

With respect to temperature, most human enzymes have their optimum functioning in the normal range of body temperature: 97° to 99°F (36° to 38°C). A temperature of 106°F, a high fever, may break the chemical bonds that maintain the shapes of enzymes. If an enzyme loses its shape, it is said to be **dentured**, and a denatured enzyme is unable to function as a catalyst.

NUCLEIC ACIDS

DNA and RNA

The **nucleic acids, DNA** (deoxyribonucleic acid) and **RNA** (ribonucleic acid), are large molecules made of smaller subunits called nucleotides. A **nucleotide**

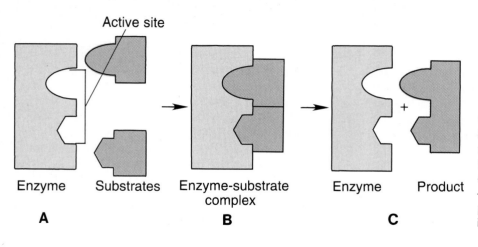

Figure 2–9 Active Site Theory, as shown in a synthesis reaction. **(A)** The enzyme and substrates of this reaction. **(B)** The enzyme –substrate complex. **(C)** The product of the reaction and the intact enzyme.

Active site

Enzyme   Substrates   Enzyme-substrate complex   Enzyme   Product

A   B   C

consists of a pentose sugar, a phosphate group, and one of several nitrogenous bases. In DNA nucleotides, the sugar is deoxyribose, and the bases are adenine, guanine, cytosine, or thymine. In RNA nucleotides, the sugar is ribose, and the bases are adenine, guanine, cytosine, or uracil. Small segments of DNA and RNA molecules are shown in Fig. 2–10.

Notice that DNA looks somewhat like a twisted ladder; this ladder is two strands of nucleotides called a double helix (coil or twist). Alternating phosphate and sugar molecules form the uprights of the ladder, and pairs of nitrogenous bases form the rungs. The size of the bases and the number of hydrogen bonds each can form create the complementary base pairing of the nucleic acids. In DNA, adenine is always paired with thymine, and guanine is always paired with cytosine.

DNA makes up the chromosomes of cells and is, therefore, the **genetic code** for hereditary characteristics. The sequence of bases in the DNA strands is actually a code for the many kinds of proteins living things produce; the code is the same in plants, other animals, and microbes. The sequence of bases for one protein is called a gene. Human genes are the codes for the proteins produced by human cells (though many of these genes are also found in all other forms of life—we are all very much related). The functioning of DNA will be covered in more detail in the next chapter.

RNA is a single strand of nucleotides (see Fig. 2–10), with uracil nucleotides in place of thymine nucleotides. RNA is synthesized from DNA in the nucleus of a cell but carries out its function in the cyto-plasm. This function is protein synthesis, which will also be discussed in the following chapter.

ATP

ATP (adenosine triphosphate) is a specialized nu-cleotide that consists of the base adenine, the sugar ribose, and three phosphate groups. Mention has already been made of ATP as a product of cell res-piration that contains biologically useful energy. ATP is one of several "energy transfer" molecules within cells, transferring the potential energy in food mole-cules to cell processes. When a molecule of glucose is broken down into carbon dioxide and water with the release of energy, the cell uses some of this energy to synthesize ATP. Present in cells are mole-cules of ADP (adenosine diphosphate) and phos-phate. The energy released from glucose is used to loosely bond a third phosphate to ADP, forming ATP. When the bond of this third phosphate is again broken and energy is released, ATP then be-comes the energy source for cell processes such as mitosis.

All cells have enzymes that can remove the third phosphate group from ATP to release its energy, form-ing ADP and phosphate. As cell respiration continues, ATP is resynthesized from ADP and phosphate. ATP formation to trap energy from food and breakdown to release energy for cell processes is a continuing cycle in cells.

The structure and functions of the nucleic acids are summarized in Table 2–6.

Table 2–6	NUCLEIC ACIDS	
Name	**Structure**	**Function**
DNA (deoxyribonucleic acid)	A double helix of nucleotides; adenine paired with thymine, and guanine paired with cytosine	• Found in the chromosomes in the nucleus of a cell • Is the genetic code for hereditary characteristics
RNA (ribonucleic acid)	A single strand of nucleotides; adenine, guanine, cytosine, and uracil	• Copies the genetic code of DNA to direct protein synthesis in the cytoplasm of cells
ATP (adenosine triphosphate)	A single adenine nucleotide with three phosphate groups	• An energy-transferring molecule • Formed when cell respiration releases energy from food molecules • Used for energy-requiring cellular processes

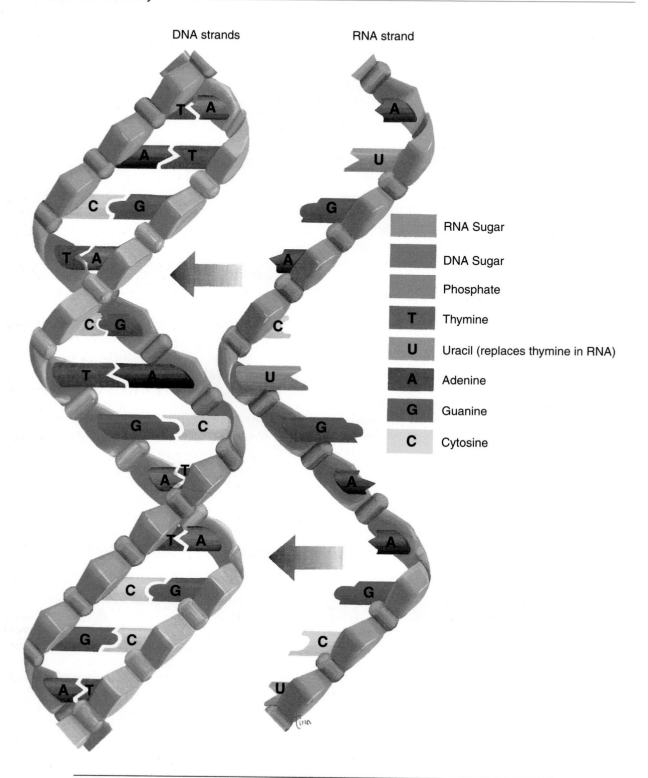

DNA strands

RNA strand

RNA Sugar

DNA Sugar

Phosphate

T　Thymine

U　Uracil (replaces thymine in RNA)

A　Adenine

G　Guanine

C　Cytosine

Figure 2–10 DNA and RNA. A small portion of each molecule is shown, with each part of a nucleotide represented by a different color. Note the complementary base pairing of DNA (A–T and G–C). When RNA is synthesized, it is a complementary copy of half the DNA molecule (with U in place of T).

SUMMARY

All of the chemicals we have just described are considered to be non-living, even though they are essential parts of all living organisms. The cells of our bodies are precise arrangements of these non-living chemicals and yet are considered living matter. The cellular level, therefore, is the next level of organization we will examine.

STUDY OUTLINE

Elements
1. Elements are the simplest chemicals, which make up all matter.
2. Carbon, hydrogen, oxygen, nitrogen, phosphorus, sulfur, and calcium make up 99% of the human body.
3. Elements combine in many ways to form molecules.

Atoms (see Fig. 2–1)
1. Atoms are the smallest part of an element that still retains the characteristics of the element.
2. Atoms consist of positively and negatively charged particles and neutral (or uncharged) particles.
   - Protons have a positive charge and are found in the nucleus of the atom.
   - Neutrons have no charge and are found in the nucleus of the atom.
   - Electrons have a negative charge and orbit the nucleus.
3. The number and arrangement of electrons give an atom its bonding capabilities.

Chemical Bonds
1. An ionic bond involves the loss of electrons by one atom and the gain of these electrons by another atom: Ions are formed that attract one another (see Fig. 2–2).
   - Cations are ions with positive charges: Na^+, Ca^{+2}.
   - Anions are ions with negative charges: Cl^-, HCO_3^-.
   - Salts, acids, and bases are formed by ionic bonding.
   - In water, many ionic bonds break; dissociation releases ions for other reactions.
2. A covalent bond involves the sharing of electrons between two atoms (see Fig. 2–3).
   - Oxygen gas (O_2) and water (H_2O) are covalently bonded molecules.
   - Carbon always forms covalent bonds; these are the basis for the organic compounds.
   - Covalent bonds are not weakened in an aqueous solution.
3. A disulfide bond is a covalent bond between two sulfur atoms in a protein; it helps maintain the three-dimensional shape of some proteins.
4. A hydrogen bond is the attraction of a covalently bonded hydrogen to a nearby oxygen or nitrogen atom.
   - The three-dimensional shape of proteins and nucleic acids is maintained by hydrogen bonds.
   - Water is cohesive because of hydrogen bonds.

Chemical Reactions
1. A change brought about by the formation or breaking of chemical bonds.
2. Synthesis—bonds are formed to join two or more molecules.
3. Decomposition—bonds are broken within a molecule.

Inorganic Compounds of Importance
1. Water—makes up 60% to 75% of the body.
   - Solvent—for transport of nutrients in the blood and excretion of wastes in urine.
   - Lubricant—mucus in the digestive tract.
   - Changes temperature slowly, and prevents sudden changes in body temperature; absorbs body heat in evaporation of sweat.
   - Water compartments—the locations of water within the body (see Fig. 2–4).
     ○ Intracellular—within cells; 65% of total body water.
     ○ Extracellular—35% of total body water.
       - Plasma—in blood vessels.
       - Lymph—in lymphatic vessels.
       - Tissue fluid—in tissue spaces between cells.
2. Oxygen—21% of the atmosphere.
   - Essential for cell respiration: the breakdown of food molecules to release energy.

3. Carbon dioxide
   - Produced as a waste product of cell respiration.
   - Must be exhaled; excess CO_2 causes acidosis.
4. Cell respiration—the energy-producing processes of cells.
   - Glucose + $O_2 \rightarrow CO_2 + H_2O$ + ATP + heat
   - This is why we breathe: to take in oxygen to break down food; to exhale the CO_2 produced.
5. Trace elements—needed in small amounts (see Table 2–2).
6. Acids, bases, and pH
   - The pH scale ranges from 0 to 14; 7 is neutral; below 7 is acidic; above 7 is alkaline.
   - An acid increases the H^+ ion concentration of a solution; a base decreases the H^+ ion concentration (or increases the OH^- ion concentration) (see Fig. 2–5).
   - The pH of cells is about 6.8. The pH range of blood is 7.35 to 7.45.
   - Buffer systems maintain normal pH by reacting with strong acids or strong bases to change them to substances that do not greatly change pH.
   - The bicarbonate buffer system consists of H_2CO_3 and $NaHCO_3$.

Organic Compounds of Importance

1. Carbohydrates (see Table 2–3 and Fig. 2–6).
   - Monosaccharides are simple sugars. Glucose, a hexose sugar ($C_6H_{12}O_6$), is the primary energy source for cell respiration.
     - Pentose sugars are part of the nucleic acids DNA and RNA.
   - Disaccharides are made of two hexose sugars. Sucrose, lactose, and maltose are digested to monosaccharides and used for cell respiration.
   - Oligosaccharides consist of from 3 to 20 monosaccharides; they are antigens on the cell membrane that identify cells as "self."
   - Polysaccharides are made of thousands of glucose molecules.
     - Starches are plant products broken down in digestion to glucose.
     - Glycogen is the form in which our bodies store glucose in the liver and muscles.
     - Cellulose, the fiber portion of plant cells, cannot be digested but promotes efficient peristalsis in the colon.
2. Lipids (see Table 2–4 and Fig. 2–7).
   - True fats are made of fatty acids and glycerol; a storage form for energy in adipose tissue. The eyes and kidneys are cushioned by fat.

- Phospholipids are part of cell membranes. An example is myelin, which provides electrical insulation for nerve cells.
- Steroids consist of four rings of carbon and hydrogen. Cholesterol, produced by the liver and consumed in food, is the basic steroid from which the body manufactures others: steroid hormones, vitamin D, and bile salts.

3. Proteins
   - Amino acids are the subunits of proteins; 20 amino acids make up human proteins. Peptide bonds join amino acids to one another (see Fig. 2–8).
   - A protein consists of from 50 to thousands of amino acids in a specific sequence. Some proteins are made of two or more amino acid chains.
   - Protein functions—see Table 2–5.
   - Amino acids in excess of the need for protein synthesis are converted to simple carbohydrates or to fat, for energy production.
   - Enzymes are catalysts, which speed up reactions without additional energy. The Active Site Theory is based on the shapes of the enzyme and the substrate molecules: These must "fit" (see Fig. 2–9). The enzyme remains unchanged after the product of the reaction is released. Each enzyme is specific for one type of reaction. The functioning of enzymes may be disrupted by changes in pH or body temperature, which change the shape of the active sites of enzymes.
4. Nucleic acids (see Table 2–6 and Fig. 2–10).
   - Nucleotides are the subunits of nucleic acids. A nucleotide consists of a pentose sugar, a phosphate group, and a nitrogenous base.
   - DNA is a double strand of nucleotides, coiled into a double helix, with complementary base pairing: A–T and G–C. DNA makes up the chromosomes of cells and is the genetic code for the synthesis of proteins.
   - RNA is a single strand of nucleotides, synthesized from DNA, with U in place of T. RNA functions in protein synthesis.
   - ATP is a nucleotide that is specialized to trap and release energy. Energy released from food in cell respiration is used to synthesize ATP from ADP + P. When cells need energy, ATP is broken down to ADP + P and the energy is released for cell processes.

REVIEW QUESTIONS

1. State the chemical symbol for each of the following elements: sodium, potassium, iron, calcium, oxygen, carbon, hydrogen, copper, and chlorine. (p. 22)

2. Explain, in terms of their electrons, how an atom of sodium and an atom of chlorine form a molecule of sodium chloride. (p. 24)

3. a. Explain, in terms of their electrons, how an atom of carbon and two atoms of oxygen form a molecule of carbon dioxide. (pp. 25–26)
   b. Explain the functions of hydrogen bonds.
   c. Explain the function of disulfide bonds.

4. Name the subunits (smaller molecules) of which each of the following is made: DNA, glycogen, a true fat, and a protein. (pp. 32, 33, 37)

5. State precisely where in the body each of these fluids is found: plasma, intracellular water, lymph, and tissue fluid. (p. 27)

6. Explain the importance of the fact that water changes temperature slowly. (pp. 26–27)

7. Describe two ways in which the solvent ability of water is important to the body. (p. 26)

8. Name the organic molecule with each of the following functions: (pp. 31–33, 37)
   a. The genetic code in chromosomes
   b. "Self" antigens in our cell membranes
   c. The storage form for glucose in the liver
   d. The storage form for excess food in adipose tissue
   e. The precursor molecule for the steroid hormones
   f. The undigested part of food that promotes peristalsis
   g. The sugars that are part of the nucleic acids

9. State the summary equation of cell respiration. (p. 28)

10. State the role or function of each of the following in cell respiration: CO_2, glucose, O_2, heat, and ATP. (p. 28)

11. State a specific function of each of the following in the human body: Ca, Fe, Na, I, and Co. (p. 29)

12. Explain, in terms of relative concentrations of H^+ ions and OH^- ions, each of the following: acid, base, and neutral substance. (p. 29)

13. State the normal pH range of blood. (p. 30)

14. Complete the following equation, and state how each of the products affects pH: (p. 31)

    $HCl + NaHCO_3 \rightarrow$ _____ + _____.

15. Explain the Active Site Theory of enzyme functioning. (p. 35)

16. Explain the difference between a synthesis reaction and a decomposition reaction. (p. 26)

FOR FURTHER THOUGHT

1. Orange juice usually has a pH of around 4. How does this compare with the pH of the blood? Why is it possible for us to drink orange juice without disrupting the pH of our blood?

2. Estrela, age seven, has cereal with milk and sugar for breakfast, then walks to school. Explain the relationship between eating and walking, and remember that Estrela is breathing.

3. The body is able to store certain nutrients. Name the storage forms, and state an advantage and a disadvantage.

4. Many "vitamin pills" also contain minerals. Which minerals are likely to be found in such dietary supplements? What purpose do they have, that is, what are their functions?

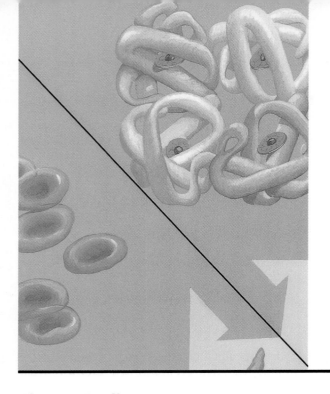

CHAPTER 3

Student Objectives

- Name the organic molecules that make up cell membranes and state their functions.
- State the function of the nucleus and chromosomes.
- Describe the functions of the cell organelles.
- Define each of these cellular transport mechanisms and give an example of the role of each in the body: diffusion, osmosis, facilitated diffusion, active transport, filtration, phagocytosis, pinocytosis.
- Describe the triplet code of DNA.
- Explain how the triplet code of DNA is translated in the synthesis of proteins.
- Describe what happens in mitosis and in meiosis.
- Use examples to explain the importance of mitosis.
- Explain the importance of meiosis.

Cells

New Terminology

Absorption (ab-**ZORB**-shun)
Active transport (**AK**-tiv **TRANS**-port)
Aerobic (air-**ROH**-bik)
Cell membrane (SELL **MEM**-brayn)
Chromosomes (**KROH**-muh-sohms)
Cytoplasm (**SIGH**-toh-plazm)
Diffusion (di-**FEW**-zhun)
Diploid number (**DIH**-ployd)
Filtration (fill-**TRAY**-shun)
Gametes (**GAM**-eets)
Gene (JEEN)
Haploid number (**HA**-ployd)
Meiosis (my-**OH**-sis)
Microvilli (MY-kro-**VILL**-eye)
Mitochondria (MY-toh-**KAHN**-dree-ah)
Mitosis (my-**TOH**-sis)
Nucleus (**NEW**-klee-us)
Organelles (OR-gan-**ELLS**)
Osmosis (ahs-**MOH**-sis)
Pinocytosis (PIN-oh-sigh-**TOH**-sis)
Phagocytosis (FAG-oh-sigh-**TOH**-sis)
Selectively permeable (se-**LEK**-tiv-lee
    PER-me-uh-buhl)
Theory (**THEER**-ree)

Related Clinical Terminology

Benign (bee-**NINE**)
Carcinogen (kar-**SIN**-oh-jen)
Chemotherapy (KEE-moh-**THER**-uh-pee)
Genetic disease (je-**NET**-ik di-**ZEEZ**)
Hypertonic (HIGH-per-**TAHN**-ik)
Hypotonic (HIGH-po-**TAHN**-ik)
Isotonic (EYE-so-**TAHN**-ik)
Malignant (muh-**LIG**-nunt)
Metastasis (muh-**TASS**-tuh-sis)
Mutation (mew-**TAY**-shun)

*Terms that appear in **bold type** in the chapter text are defined in the glossary, which begins on page 521.*

All living organisms are made of cells and cell products. This simple statement, called the Cell Theory, was first proposed over 150 years ago. You may think of a **theory** as a guess or hypothesis, and sometimes this is so. A scientific theory, however, is actually the best explanation of all available evidence. All of the evidence science has gathered so far supports the validity of the Cell Theory.

Cells are the smallest living subunits of a multicellular organism such as a human being. A cell is a complex arrangement of the chemicals discussed in the previous chapter, is living, and carries out specific activities. Microorganisms, such as amoebas and bacteria, are single cells that function independently. Human cells, however, must work together and function interdependently. Homeostasis depends upon the contributions of all of the different kinds of cells.

Human cells vary in size, shape, and function. Most human cells are so small they can only be seen with the aid of a microscope and are measured in units called **microns** (1 micron = 1/25,000 of an inch—see Appendix A: Units of Measure). One exception is the human ovum or egg cell, which is about 1 millimeter in diameter, just visible to the unaided eye. Some nerve cells, although microscopic in diameter, may be quite long. Those in our arms and legs, for example, are at least 2 feet (60 cm) long.

With respect to shape, human cells vary greatly. Some are round or spherical, others rectangular, still others irregular. White blood cells even change shape as they move.

Cell functions also vary, and since our cells do not act independently, we will cover specialized cell functions as part of tissue functions in Chapter 4. Based on function, there are more than 200 different kinds of human cells. This chapter is concerned with the basic structure of cells and the cellular activities common to all our cells.

CELL STRUCTURE

Despite their many differences, human cells have several similar structural features: a cell membrane, cytoplasm and cell organelles, and a nucleus. Red blood cells are an exception because they have no nuclei when mature. The cell membrane forms the outer boundary of the cell and surrounds the cytoplasm, organelles, and nucleus.

CELL MEMBRANE

Also called the **plasma membrane**, the **cell membrane** is made of phospholipids, cholesterol, and proteins. The arrangement of these organic molecules is shown in Fig. 3–1. The phospholipids form a bilayer, or double layer, which makes up most of the membrane. Phospholipids permit lipid-soluble materials to easily enter or leave the cell by diffusion through the cell membrane. The presence of cholesterol decreases the fluidity of the membrane, thus making it more stable. The proteins have several functions: Some form **pores** or channels to permit passage of materials; others are carrier **enzymes** that also help substances enter the cell. Still other proteins, with oligosaccharides on their outer surface, are **antigens**, markers that identify the cells of an individual as "self." Yet another group of proteins serves as **receptor sites** for hormones. Many hormones bring about their specific effects by first bonding to a particular receptor on the cell membrane, a receptor with the proper shape. This bonding, or fit, then triggers chemical reactions within the cell membrane or the interior of the cell (see Box 10–3 for an illustration involving the hormone insulin).

Many receptors for other molecules are also part of cell membranes. These molecules are part of the chemical communication networks our cells have. An unavoidable consequence of having so many receptors for chemical communication is that some pathogens have evolved shapes to match certain receptors. HIV, for example, the virus that causes AIDS, just happens to fit a particular surface receptor on our white blood cells. When the virus fits in, the receptor becomes a gateway into the cell, which begins the takeover of the cell by the virus.

Most often, however, the cell membrane is a beneficial structure. Although the cell membrane is the outer boundary of the cell, it should already be apparent to you that it is not a static or wall-like boundary, but rather an active, dynamic one. The cell membrane is **selectively permeable**, that is, certain substances are permitted to pass through and others are not. These mechanisms of cellular transport will be covered later in this chapter. The cell membrane is of particular importance for muscle cells and nerve cells

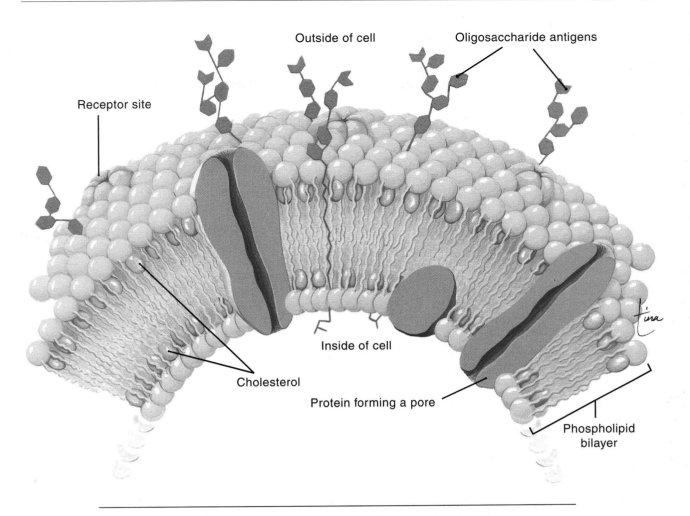

Figure 3–1 The cell (plasma) membrane depicting the types of molecules present.

because it carries electrical impulses. This will be covered in Chapters 7 and 8.

NUCLEUS

With the exception of mature red blood cells, all human cells have a nucleus. The **nucleus** is within the cytoplasm and is bounded by a double-layered **nuclear membrane** with many pores. It contains one or more nucleoli and the chromosomes of the cell (Fig. 3–2).

A **nucleolus** is a small sphere made of DNA, RNA, and protein. The nucleoli form a type of RNA called ribosomal RNA, which becomes part of ribosomes (a cell organelle) and is involved in protein synthesis.

The nucleus is the control center of the cell because it contains the chromosomes. The 46 **chromosomes** of a human cell are usually not visible; they are long threads called **chromatin**. When a cell divides, however, the chromatin coils extensively into visible chromosomes. Chromosomes are made of DNA and protein. Remember from our earlier discussion that the DNA is the genetic code for the characteristics and activities of the cell. Although the DNA in the nucleus of each cell contains all of the genetic information for all human traits, only a small number of genes (a **gene**

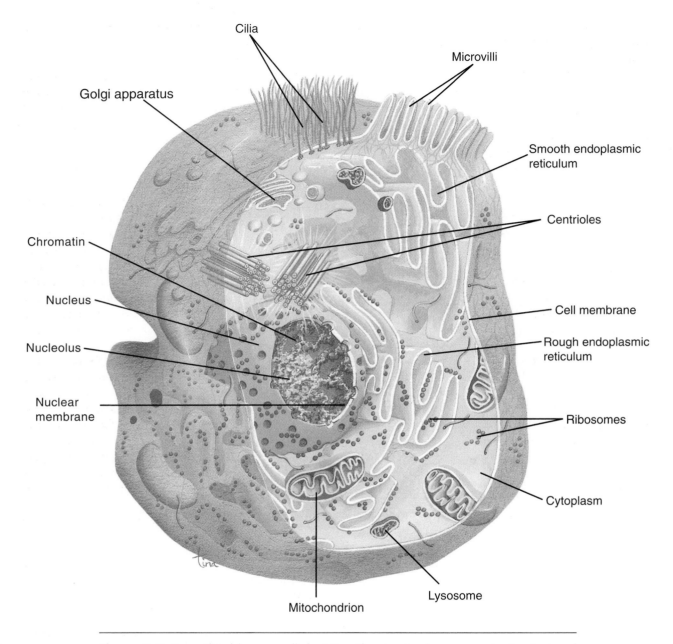

Figure 3–2 Generalized human cell depicting the structural components. See text and Table 3–1 for descriptions.

is the genetic code for one protein) are actually active, or "switched on," in a particular cell. These active genes are the codes for the proteins necessary for the specific cell type and its functions. For example, the gene for insulin is present in all human cells, but only in certain islet cells of the pancreas is the gene active or switched on. Only in these cells is insulin produced.

How the genetic code in chromosomes is translated into proteins will be covered in a later section.

CYTOPLASM AND CELL ORGANELLES

Cytoplasm is a watery solution of minerals, gases, and organic molecules that is found between the cell membrane and the nucleus. Chemical reactions take place within the cytoplasm, and many of the cell organelles are found here. Cell **organelles** are intracellular structures, often bounded by their own membranes, that have specific roles in cellular functioning. They are also shown in Fig. 3–2.

The **endoplasmic reticulum** (ER) is an extensive network of membranous tubules that extend from the nuclear membrane to the cell membrane. Rough ER has numerous ribosomes on its surface, whereas smooth ER has no ribosomes at all. As a network of interconnected tunnels, the ER serves as a passageway for the transport of the materials necessary for cell function within the cell. These include proteins synthesized by the ribosomes on the rough ER, and lipids synthesized by the smooth ER.

Ribosomes are very small structures made of protein and ribosomal RNA. Some are found on the surface of rough ER, while others float freely within the cytoplasm. Ribosomes are the site of protein synthesis.

The **Golgi apparatus** is a series of flat, membranous sacs, somewhat like a stack of saucers. Carbohydrates are synthesized within the Golgi apparatus, and are packaged, along with other materials, for secretion from the cell. To secrete a substance, small sacs of the Golgi membrane break off and fuse with the cell membrane, releasing the substance to the exterior of the cell.

Mitochondria are oval or spherical organelles within the cytoplasm, bounded by a double membrane. The inner membrane has folds called cristae. Within the mitochondria, the **aerobic** (oxygen-requiring) reactions of cell respiration take place. Therefore, mitochondria are the site of ATP (and hence energy) production. Cells that require large amounts of ATP, such as muscle cells, have many mitochondria to meet their need for energy. Mitochondria contain their own genes (an estimated 37 genes in a single DNA molecule) and duplicate themselves when a cell divides.

Lysosomes are single-membrane structures within the cytoplasm that contain digestive enzymes. When certain white blood cells engulf bacteria, the bacteria are digested and destroyed by these lysosomal enzymes. Worn-out cell parts and dead cells are also digested by these enzymes. This is a beneficial process, and is necessary before tissue repair can begin. But it does have a disadvantage in that lysosomal digestion contributes to inflammation in damaged tissues. An excess of inflammation can start a vicious cycle, actually a positive feedback mechanism, that results in extensive tissue damage.

Centrioles are a pair of rod-shaped structures perpendicular to one another, located just outside the nucleus. Their function is to organize the spindle fibers during cell division. The spindle fibers are contracting proteins that pull the two sets of chromosomes apart, toward the ends of the original cell as it divides into two new cells. Each new cell then has a full set of chromosomes.

Cilia and **flagella** are mobile thread-like projections through the cell membrane. **Cilia** are usually shorter than flagella, and an individual cell has many of them on its free surface. The cilia of a cell beat in unison and sweep materials across the cell surface. Cells lining the fallopian tubes, for example, have cilia to sweep the egg cell toward the uterus. The only human cell with a **flagellum** is the sperm cell. The flagellum provides **motility**, or movement, for the sperm cell.

Microvilli are folds of the cell membrane on the free surface of a cell. These folds greatly increase the surface area of the membrane, and are part of the cells lining organs that absorb materials. The small intestine, for example, requires a large surface area for the absorption of nutrients, and many of its lining cells have microvilli. Some cells of the kidney tubules also have microvilli (see Fig. 1–1) that provide for the efficient reabsorption of useful materials back to the blood.

The functions of the cell organelles are summarized in Table 3–1.

CELLULAR TRANSPORT MECHANISMS

Living cells constantly interact with the blood or tissue fluid around them, taking in some substances and secreting or excreting others. There are several mechanisms of transport that enable cells to move materials into or out of the cell: diffusion, osmosis, facilitated diffusion, active transport, filtration, phagocytosis, and pinocytosis. Some of these take place without the expenditure of energy by the cells. But others *do* require energy, often in the form of ATP. Each of these mechanisms is described in the following sections and an example is included to show how each is important to the body.

Table 3-1	FUNCTIONS OF CELL ORGANELLES
Organelle	**Function(s)**
Endoplasmic reticulum (ER)	• Passageway for transport of materials within the cell • Synthesis of lipids
Ribosomes	• Site of protein synthesis
Golgi apparatus	• Synthesis of carbohydrates • Packaging of materials for secretion from the cell
Mitochondria	• Site of aerobic cell respiration—ATP production
Lysosomes	• Contain enzymes to digest ingested material or damaged tissue
Centrioles	• Organize the spindle fibers during cell division
Cilia	• Sweep materials across the cell surface
Flagellum	• Enables a cell to move
Microvilli	• Increase a cell's surface area for absorption

DIFFUSION

Diffusion is the movement of molecules from an area of greater concentration to an area of lesser concentration (that is, with or along a **concentration gradient**). Diffusion occurs because molecules have free energy, that is, they are always in motion. The molecules in a solid move very slowly; those in a liquid move faster, and those in a gas move faster still, such as when ice absorbs heat energy, melts, and then evaporates. In Fig. 3–3, a sugar cube in a glass of water is shown. As the sugar dissolves, the sugar molecules collide with one another. These collisions spread out the sugar molecules until they are evenly dispersed among the water molecules (this would take a very long time). The molecules are still moving, but as some go to the top, others go to the bottom, and so on. Thus, an equilibrium (or steady state) is reached.

Diffusion is a very slow process, but may be an effective transport mechanism across microscopic distances. Within the body, the gases oxygen and carbon dioxide move by diffusion. In the lungs, for example, there is a high concentration of oxygen in the alveoli (air sacs) and a low concentration of oxygen in the blood in the surrounding pulmonary capillaries. The opposite is true for carbon dioxide: a low concentration in the air in the alveoli and a high concentration in the blood in the pulmonary capillaries. These gases diffuse in opposite directions, each moving from where there is more to where there is less. Oxygen diffuses from the air to the blood to be circulated throughout the body. Carbon dioxide diffuses from the blood to the air to be exhaled.

Sugar cube in water   Sugar dissolving   Equilibrium

A   B   C

Figure 3–3 Diffusion of sugar in water. **(A)** Sugar cube. **(B)** Partial dissolving and diffusion of sugar molecules. **(C)** Sugar molecules distributed evenly throughout the water (such an equilibrium would take a very long time).

OSMOSIS

Osmosis may be simply defined as the diffusion of water through a selectively permeable membrane or barrier. That is, water will move from an area with more water present to an area with less water. Another way to say this is that water will naturally tend to move to an area where there is more dissolved material, such as salt or sugar. If a 2% salt solution and a 6% salt solution are separated by a membrane allowing water but not salt to pass through it, water will diffuse from the 2% salt solution to the 6% salt solution. The result is that the 2% solution will become more concentrated, and the 6% solution will become more dilute.

In the body, the cells lining the small intestine absorb water from digested food by osmosis. These cells have first absorbed salts, have become more "salty," and water follows salt into the cells. The process of osmosis also takes place in the kidneys, which reabsorb large amounts of water (many gallons each day) to prevent its loss in urine. Box 3–1: Terminology of Solutions lists some terminology we use when discussing solutions and the effects of various solutions on cells.

FACILITATED DIFFUSION

The word *facilitate* means to help or assist. In **facilitated diffusion**, molecules move through a membrane from an area of greater concentration to an area of lesser concentration, but they need some help to do this.

In the body, our cells must take in glucose to use for ATP production. Glucose, however, will not diffuse through most cell membranes by itself, even if there is more outside the cell than inside. Diffusion of glucose into most cells requires **carrier enzymes**, which may also be called **transporters.** These are proteins that are part of the cell membrane. Glucose bonds to the carrier enzyme, and by doing so changes the shape of the carrier. This physical change propels the glucose into the interior of the cell. Other transporters are specific for other organic molecules such as amino acids.

ACTIVE TRANSPORT

Active transport requires the energy of ATP to move molecules from an area of lesser concentration to an area of greater concentration. Notice that this is the opposite of diffusion, in which the free energy of molecules causes them to move to where there are fewer of them. Active transport is therefore said to be movement against a concentration gradient.

In the body, nerve cells and muscle cells have "sodium pumps" to move sodium ions (Na^+) out of the cells. Sodium ions are more abundant outside the cells, and they constantly diffuse into the cell, their area of lesser concentration. Without the sodium pumps to return them outside, the incoming sodium ions would bring about an unwanted nerve impulse or muscle contraction. Nerve and muscle cells constantly produce ATP to keep their sodium pumps working and prevent spontaneous impulses.

Another example of active transport is the absorption of glucose and amino acids by the cells lining the small intestine. The cells use ATP to absorb these nutrients from digested food, even when their intracellular concentration becomes greater than their extracellular concentration.

FILTRATION

The process of **filtration** also requires energy, but the energy needed does not come directly from ATP. It is the energy of mechanical pressure. Filtration means that water and dissolved materials are forced through a membrane from an area of higher pressure to an area of lower pressure.

In the body, **blood pressure** is created by the pumping of the heart. Filtration occurs when blood flows through capillaries, whose walls are only one cell thick and very permeable. The blood pressure in capillaries is higher than the pressure of the surrounding tissue fluid. In capillaries throughout the body, blood pressure forces plasma and dissolved materials through the capillary membranes into the surrounding tissue spaces. This creates more tissue fluid and is how cells receive glucose, amino acids, and other nutrients. Blood pressure in the capillaries of the kidneys also brings about filtration, which is the first step in the formation of urine.

PHAGOCYTOSIS AND PINOCYTOSIS

These two processes are similar in that both involve a cell engulfing something. An example of **phagocytosis** is a white blood cell engulfing bacteria. The white blood cell flows around the bacterium, taking it in and eventually digesting it. Digestion is accomplished by the enzymes in the cell's lysosomes.

Box 3–1   TERMINOLOGY OF SOLUTIONS

Human cells or other body fluids contain many dissolved substances (called **solutes**) such as salts, sugars, acids, and bases. The concentration of solutes in a fluid creates the **osmotic pressure** of the solution, which in turn determines the movement of water through membranes.

As an example here, we will use sodium chloride (NaCl). Human cells have an NaCl concentration of 0.9%. With human cells as a reference point, the relative NaCl concentrations of other solutions may be described with the following terms:

Isotonic—a solution with the same salt concentration as in cells.

  The blood plasma is isotonic to red blood cells.

Hypotonic—a solution with a lower salt concentration than in cells.

  Distilled water (0% salt) is hypotonic to human cells.

Hypertonic—a solution with a higher salt concentration than in cells.

  Sea water (3% salt) is hypertonic to human cells.

Refer now to the diagrams below of red blood cells (RBCs) in each of these different types of solutions, and note the effect of each on osmosis:

- When RBCs are in plasma, water moves into and out of them at equal rates, and the cells remain normal in size and water content.
- If RBCs are placed in distilled water, more water will enter the cells than leave, and the cells will swell and eventually burst.
- If RBCs are placed in seawater, more water will leave the cells than enter, and the cells will shrivel and die.

This knowledge of osmotic pressure is used when replacement fluids are needed for a patient who has become dehydrated. Isotonic solutions are usually used; normal saline and Ringer's solution are examples. These will provide rehydration without causing osmotic damage to cells or extensive shifts of fluid between the blood and tissues.

Normal (isotonic) solution   Hypotonic solution   Hypertonic solution

Box Figure 3–A   Red blood cells in different solutions and the effect of osmosis in each.

Other cells that are stationary may take in small molecules that become adsorbed or attached to their membranes. The cells of the kidney tubules reabsorb small proteins by **pinocytosis**, so that the protein is not lost in urine.

Table 3–2 summarizes the cellular transport mechanisms.

THE GENETIC CODE AND PROTEIN SYNTHESIS

The structure of DNA, RNA, and protein was described in Chapter 2 but will be reviewed briefly here.

Table 3–2 CELLULAR TRANSPORT MECHANISMS

Mechanism	Definition	Example in the Body
Diffusion	Movement of molecules from an area of greater concentration to an area of lesser concentration.	Exchange of gases in the lungs or body tissues.
Osmosis	The diffusion of water.	Absorption of water by the small intestine or kidneys.
Facilitated diffusion	Carrier and transporter enzymes move molecules across cell membranes.	Intake of glucose by most cells.
Active transport	Movement of molecules from an area of lesser concentration to an area of greater concentration (requires ATP).	Absorption of amino acids and glucose from food by the cells of the small intestine.
Filtration	Movement of water and dissolved substances from an area of higher pressure to an area of lower pressure (blood pressure).	Formation of tissue fluid; the first step in the formation of urine.
Phagocytosis	A moving cell engulfs something.	White blood cells engulf bacteria.
Pinocytosis	A stationary cell engulfs something.	Cells of the kidney tubules reabsorb small proteins.

DNA AND THE GENETIC CODE

DNA is a double strand of nucleotides in the form of a **double helix**, very much like a spiral ladder. The rungs of the ladder are made of the four nitrogenous bases, always found in complementary pairs: adenine with thymine (A–T) and guanine with cytosine (G–C). Although DNA contains just these four bases, the bases may be arranged in many different sequences (reading up or down the ladder). It is the sequence of bases, the sequence of A, T, C, and G, that is the **genetic code**. The DNA of our 46 chromosomes may also be called our **genome,** which is the term for the total genetic information in a particular species. The human genome is believed to contain about 6 billion base pairs, which make up our estimated 30,000 (and perhaps as many as 40,000) genes.

Recall that in Chapter 2 you read that a **gene** is the genetic code for one protein. This is a simplification, and the functioning of genes is often much more complex. We have genes with segments that may be shuffled or associated in many combinations, with the potential for coding for many more proteins. A full explanation is beyond the scope of this book, so for the sake of simplicity, and in the following discussion, we will say that a gene is the code for one protein. Recall too that a protein is a specific sequence of amino acids. Therefore, a gene, or segment of DNA, is the code for the sequence of amino acids in a particular protein.

The code for a single amino acid consists of three bases in the DNA molecule; this **triplet** of bases may be called a **codon** (Fig. 3–4). There is a triplet of bases in the DNA for each amino acid in the protein. If a protein consists of 100 amino acids, the gene for that protein would consist of 100 triplets, or 300 bases. Some of the triplets will be the same, since the same amino acid may be present in several places within the protein. Also part of the gene are other triplets that start and stop the process of making the protein, rather like punctuation marks start and stop sentences.

RNA AND PROTEIN SYNTHESIS

The transcription of the genetic code in DNA into proteins requires the other nucleic acid, **RNA**. DNA is found in the chromosomes in the nucleus of the cell, but protein synthesis takes place on the ribosomes in the cytoplasm. **Messenger RNA (mRNA)** is the intermediary molecule between these two sites.

When a protein is to be made, the segment of DNA that is its gene uncoils, and the hydrogen bonds between the base pairs break (see Fig. 3–4). Within the nucleus are RNA nucleotides (A, C, G, U) and enzymes to construct a single strand of nucleotides that is a complementary copy of half the DNA gene (with uracil in place of thymine). This copy of the gene is mRNA, which then separates from the DNA. The gene coils back into the double helix, and the mRNA

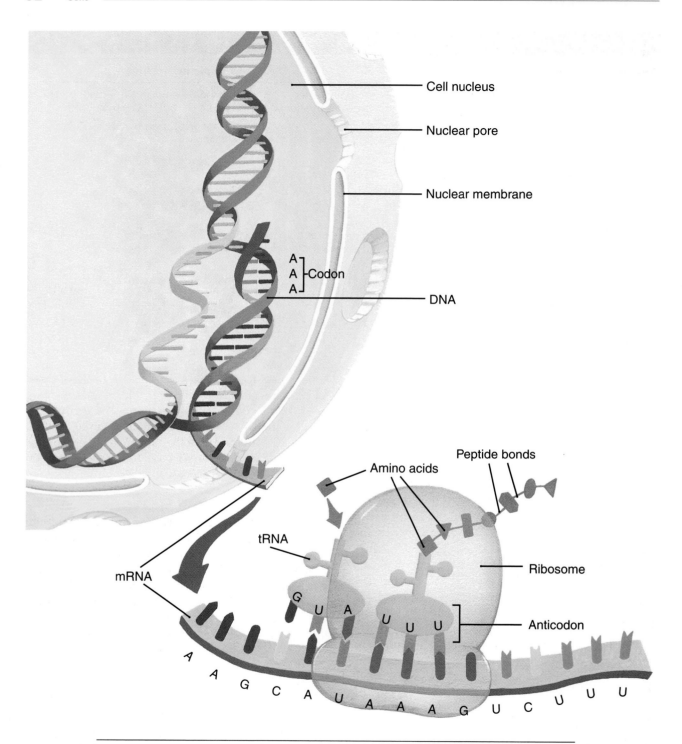

Figure 3–4 Protein synthesis. The mRNA is formed as a copy of a portion of the DNA in the nucleus of a cell. In the cytoplasm, the mRNA becomes attached to ribosomes. See text for further description.

Table 3–3   PROTEIN SYNTHESIS

Molecule or Organelle	Functions
DNA	• A double strand (helix) of nucleotides that is the genetic code in the chromosomes of cells • A gene is the sequence of bases (segment of DNA) that is the code for one protein
mRNA (messenger RNA)	• A single strand of nucleotides formed as a complementary copy of a gene in the DNA • Now contains the triplet code: three bases is the code for one amino acid • Leaves the DNA in the nucleus, enters the cytoplasm of the cell, and becomes attached to ribosomes
Ribosomes	• The cell organelles that are the site of protein synthesis • Attach the mRNA molecule • Contain enzymes to form peptide bonds between amino acids
tRNA (transfer RNA)	• Picks up amino acids (from food) in the cytoplasm and transports them to their proper sites (triplets) along the mRNA molecule

leaves the nucleus, enters the cytoplasm, and becomes attached to ribosomes.

As the copy of the gene, mRNA is a series of triplets of bases; each triplet is the code for one amino acid. Another type of RNA, called **transfer RNA (tRNA)**, is also found in the cytoplasm. Each tRNA molecule has an **anticodon**, a triplet complementary to a triplet on the mRNA. The tRNA molecules pick up specific amino acids (which have come from protein in our food) and bring them to their proper triplets on the mRNA. The ribosomes contain enzymes to catalyze the formation of **peptide bonds** between the amino acids. When an amino acid has been brought to each triplet on the mRNA, and all peptide bonds have been formed, the protein is finished.

The protein then leaves the ribosomes and may be transported by the ER to wherever it is needed in the cell, or it may be packaged by the Golgi apparatus for secretion from the cell. A summary of the process of protein synthesis is found in Table 3–3.

Thus, the expression of the genetic code may be described by the following sequence:

Each of us is the sum total of our genetic characteristics. Blood type, hair color, muscle proteins, nerve cells, and thousands of other aspects of our structure and functioning have their basis in the genetic code of DNA.

If there is a "mistake" in the DNA, that is, incorrect bases or triplets of bases, this mistake will be copied by the mRNA. The result is the formation of a malfunctioning or nonfunctioning protein. This is called a **genetic** or **hereditary disease**, and a specific example is described in Box 3–2: Genetic Disease—Sickle-Cell Anemia.

CELL DIVISION

Cell division is the process by which a cell reproduces itself. There are two types of cell division, mitosis and meiosis. Although both types involve cell reproduction, their purposes are very different.

MITOSIS

Each of us began life as one cell, a fertilized egg. Each of us now consists of billions of cells produced by the process of mitosis. In **mitosis**, one cell with the **diploid number** of chromosomes (the usual number, 46 for people) divides into two identical cells, each with the diploid number of chromosomes. This production of identical cells is necessary for the growth of the organism and for repair of tissues (see also Box 3–3: Abnormal Cellular Functioning—Cancer).

Before mitosis can take place, a cell must have two complete sets of chromosomes, because each new cell must have the diploid number. The process of **DNA replication** enables each chromosome to make a copy of itself. The time during which this takes place is called **interphase**, the time between mitotic divisions. Although interphase is sometimes referred to as the resting stage, resting means "not dividing," not "inactive." The cell is quite actively producing a second set of chromosomes and storing energy in ATP.

The stages of mitosis are **prophase, metaphase, anaphase,** and **telophase.** What happens in each of

Box 3–2   GENETIC DISEASE—SICKLE-CELL ANEMIA

A **genetic disease** is a hereditary disorder, one that may be passed from generation to generation. Although there are hundreds of genetic diseases, they all have the same basis: a mistake in DNA. Because DNA makes up the chromosomes that are found in egg and sperm, this mistake may be passed from parents to children.

Sickle-cell anemia is the most common genetic disorder among people of African descent and affects the hemoglobin in red blood cells. Normal hemoglobin, called hemoglobin A (HbA), is a protein made of two identical alpha chains (141 amino acids each) and two identical beta chains (146 amino acids each). In sickle-cell hemoglobin (HbS), the 6th amino acid in each beta chain is incorrect; valine is present instead of the glutamic acid found in HbA.

This difference seems minor—only two incorrect amino acids out of a total of over 500—but the consequences for the person are very serious.

HbS has a great tendency to crystallize when oxygen levels are low, as is true in capillaries. When HbS crystallizes, the red blood cells are deformed into crescents (sickles) and other irregular shapes. These irregular, rigid red blood cells clog and rupture capillaries, causing internal bleeding and severe pain. These red blood cells are also fragile, have a short life span, and break up easily, leading to anemia and hypoxia (lack of oxygen). In the past, children with sickle-cell anemia often died before the age of 20 years. Treatment of this disease has improved greatly, but it is still incurable.

(Continued)

these stages is described in Table 3–4. As you read the events of each stage, refer to Fig. 3–5, which depicts mitosis in a cell with a diploid number of four.

As mentioned previously, mitosis is essential for repair of tissues, to replace damaged or dead cells. Some examples may help illustrate this. In several areas of the body, mitosis takes place constantly. These sites include the epidermis of the skin, the stomach lining, and the red bone marrow. For each of these sites, there is a specific reason why this constant mitosis is necessary.

What happens to the surface of the skin? The dead, outer cells are worn off by contact with the environment. Mitosis of the epidermal cells in the lower living layer replaces these cells, and the epidermis maintains its normal thickness.

The stomach lining, although internal, is also constantly worn away. Gastric juice, especially hydrochloric acid, is very damaging to cells. Rapid mitosis of the several kinds of lining cells replaces damaged cells and keeps the stomach lining intact.

One of the functions of red bone marrow is the production of red blood cells. Because red blood cells have a life span of only about 120 days, new ones are needed to replace the older ones that die. Very rapid mitosis in the red bone marrow produces approximately 2 million new red blood cells every second. These dividing cells in the red bone marrow are among the stem cells present in the body. A **stem cell** is an unspecialized cell that may develop into several different kinds of cells. Those in the red bone marrow may become red blood cells, white blood cells, or platelets. (These marrow stem cells are often called adult stem cells. Embryonic stem cells will be described in a later chapter; these are cells in which all of the DNA still has the potential to be active. They may become any of the more than 200 different kinds of human cells.)

It is also important to be aware of the areas of the body where mitosis does not take place. In an adult, most muscle cells and neurons (nerve cells) do not reproduce themselves. If they die, their functions are also lost. Someone whose spinal cord has been severed will have paralysis and loss of sensation below the level of the injury. The spinal cord neurons do not undergo mitosis to replace the ones that were lost, and such an injury is permanent.

Skeletal muscle cells are capable of limited mitosis for repair. The heart is made of cardiac muscle cells, which, like neurons, seem to be incapable of mitosis. A heart attack (myocardial infarction) means that a portion of cardiac muscle dies because of lack of oxygen. These cells are not replaced, and the heart will be a less effective pump. If a large enough area of the heart muscle dies, the heart attack may be fatal.

Recent research has found evidence for the potential for mitosis after damage in both the central nervous system and the heart. Such cell division may be

Box 3–2   GENETIC DISEASE—SICKLE-CELL ANEMIA (Continued)

What has happened to cause the formation of HbS rather than HbA? Because hemoglobin is a protein, the genetic code for it is in the DNA (of chromosome 11). One amino acid in the beta chains is incorrect, therefore, one triplet in the DNA gene for the beta chain must be, and is, incorrect. This mistake is copied by mRNA in the cells of the red bone marrow, and HbS is synthesized in red blood cells.

Sickle-cell anemia is a recessive genetic disease, which means that a person with one gene for HbS and one gene for HbA will have "sickle-cell trait." Such a person, sometimes called a carrier, usually will not have the severe effects of sickle-cell anemia, but may pass the gene for HbS to children. It is estimated that 9% of African-Americans have sickle-cell trait and about 1% have sickle-cell anemia.

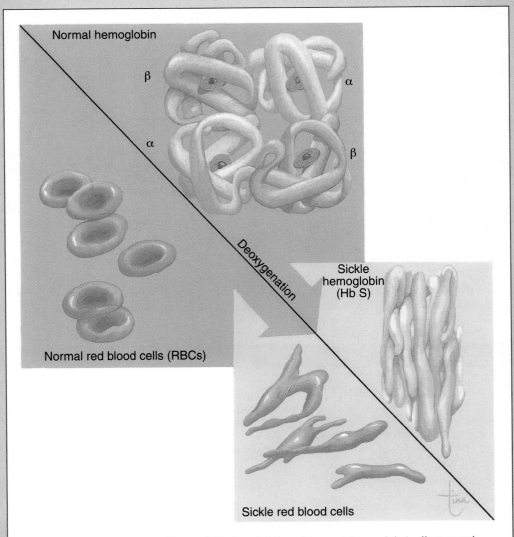

Box Figure 3–B   Structure of hemoglobin A and sickle-cell hemoglobin and their effect on red blood cells.

Box 3–3   ABNORMAL CELLULAR FUNCTIONING—CANCER

There are more than 100 different types of **cancer**, all of which are characterized by abnormal cellular functioning. Normally, our cells undergo mitosis only when necessary and stop when appropriate. A cut in the skin, for example, is repaired by mitosis, usually without formation of excess tissue. The new cells fill in the damaged area, and mitosis slows when the cells make contact with surrounding cells. This is called contact inhibition, which limits the new tissue to just what is needed. **Malignant** (cancer) cells, however, are characterized by uncontrolled cell division. Our cells are genetically programmed to have particular life spans and to divide or die. One gene is known to act as a brake on cell division; another gene enables cells to live indefinitely, beyond their normal life spans, and to keep dividing. Any imbalance in the activity of these genes may lead to abnormal cells division. Such cells are not inhibited by contact with other cells, keep dividing, and tend to spread.

A malignant tumor begins in a primary site such as the colon, then may spread or metastasize. Often the malignant cells are carried by the lymph or blood to other organs such as the liver, where secondary tumors develop. **Metastasis** is characteristic only of malignant cells; **benign** tumors do not metastasize but remain localized in their primary site.

What causes normal cells to become malignant? At present, we have only partial answers. A malignant cell is created by a **mutation**, a genetic change that brings about abnormal cell functions or responses. Environmental substances that cause mutations are called **carcinogens**. One example is the tar found in cigarette smoke, which is definitely linked to lung cancer. Ultraviolet light may also cause mutations, especially in skin that is over exposed to sunlight. For a few specific kinds of cancer, the trigger is believed to be infection with certain viruses that cause cellular mutations. Carriers of hepatitis B virus, for example, are more likely to develop primary liver cancer than are people who have never been exposed to this virus. Research has discovered two genes, one on chromosome 2 and the other on chromosome 3, that contribute to a certain form of colon cancer. Both of these genes are the codes for proteins that correct the "mistakes" that may occur when the new DNA is synthesized. When these proteins do not function properly, the mistakes (mutations) in the DNA lead to the synthesis of yet other faulty proteins that impair the functioning of the cell and predispose it to becoming malignant.

Once cells have become malignant, their functioning cannot return to normal. Therefore, the treatments for cancer are directed at removing or destroying the abnormal cells. Surgery to remove tumors, radiation to destroy cells, and **chemotherapy** to stop cell division or interfere with other aspects of cell metabolism are all aspects of cancer treatment.

Table 3–4   STAGES OF MITOSIS

Stage	Events
Prophase	1. The chromosomes coil up and become visible as short rods. Each chromosome is really 2 chromatids (original DNA plus its copy) still attached at a region called the centromere. 2. The nuclear membrane disappears. 3. The centrioles move toward opposite poles of the cell and organize the spindle fibers, which extend across the equator of the cell.
Metaphase	1. The pairs of chromatids line up along the equator of the cell. The centromere of each pair is attached to a spindle fiber. 2. The centromeres now divide.
Anaphase	1. Each chromatid is now considered a separate chromosome; there are two complete and separate sets. 2. The spindle fibers contract and pull the chromosomes, one set toward each pole of the cell.
Telophase	1. The sets of chromosomes reach the poles of the cell and become indistinct as their DNA uncoils to form chromatin. 2. A nuclear membrane re-forms around each set of chromosomes.
Cytokinesis	1. The cytoplasm divides; new cell membrane is formed.

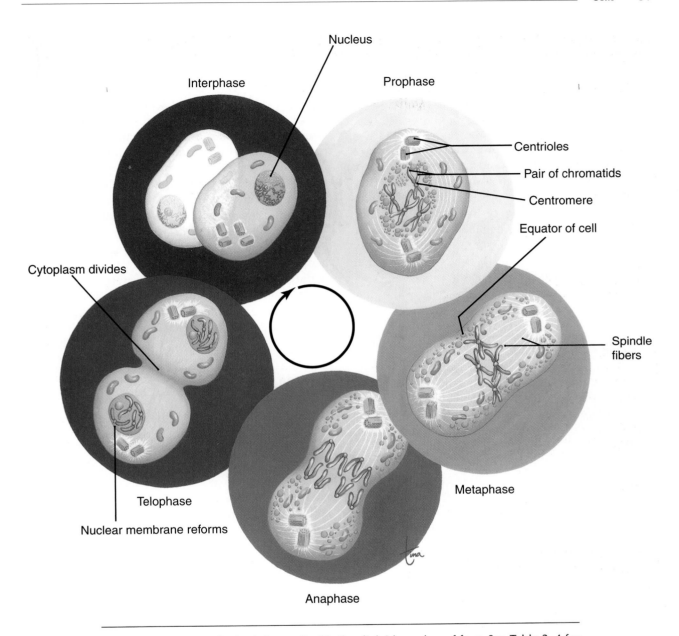

Figure 3–5 Stages of mitosis in a cell with the diploid number of four. See Table 3–4 for description.

that of neurons or muscle cells that were stimulated to divide by chemicals from the adjacent damaged tissue. Or the dividing cells may be stem cells that are among the specialized cells. At present, we know that for most people with heart damage or central nervous system injury, mitosis does not take place, or not sufficiently enough to replace the cells that have died and preserve or restore normal functioning of the organ. Research is continuing, and researchers may eventu-ally find the stimulus necessary to provoke extended mitosis that would bring about true tissue repair.

MEIOSIS

Meiosis is a more complex process of cell division that results in the formation of **gametes**, which are egg and sperm cells. In meiosis, one cell with the diploid number of chromosomes divides twice to form four cells, each with the **haploid number** (half the usual number) of chromosomes. In women, meiosis takes place in the ovaries and is called **oogenesis**. In men, meiosis takes place in the testes and is called **spermatogenesis**. The differences between oogenesis and spermatogenesis will be discussed in Chapter 20, The Reproductive Systems.

The egg and sperm cells produced by meiosis have the haploid number of chromosomes, which is 23 for humans. Meiosis is sometimes called reduction division because the division process reduces the chromosome number in egg or sperm. Then, during **fertilization** in which the egg unites with the sperm, the 23 chromosomes of the sperm plus the 23 chromosomes of the egg will restore the diploid number of 46 in the fertilized egg. Thus the proper chromosome number is maintained in the cells of the new individual.

AGING AND CELLS

Multicellular organisms, including people, age and eventually die; our cells do not have infinite life spans. It has been proposed that some cells capable of mitosis are limited to a certain number of divisions, that is, every division is sort of a tick-tock off a biological clock. At present, it is not known exactly what this cellular biological clock is. There is evidence that the ends of chromosomes, called telomeres, may be an aspect of it. With each cell division, part of the telomeres is lost (rather like a piece of rope fraying at both ends), and eventually the telomeres are gone. With the next division, the ends of the chromosomes, actual genes, begin to be lost. This may be one signal that a cell's life span has come to an end (there are probably many different kinds of signals).

Cellular aging also involves the inevitable deterioration of membranes and cell organelles. Just as the parts of a car break down in time, so too will cells. Unlike cars or machines, however, cells can often repair themselves, but they do have limits. As cells age, structural proteins break down and are not replaced, or necessary enzymes are not synthesized.

Much about the chemistry of the aging process remains a mystery, though we can describe what happens to organs and to the body as a whole. Each of the following chapters on body systems provides a brief discussion of how aging affects the system. Keep in mind that a system is the sum of its cells, in tissues and organs, and that all aging is ultimately at the cellular level.

SUMMARY

As mentioned at the beginning of this chapter, human cells work closely together and function interdependently. Each type of human cell makes a contribution to the body as a whole. Usually, however, cells do not function as individuals, but rather in groups. Groups of cells with similar structure and function form a tissue, which is the next level of organization.

STUDY OUTLINE

Human cells vary in size, shape, and function. Our cells function interdependently to maintain homeostasis.

Cell Structure—the major parts of a cell are the cell membrane, nucleus (except mature RBCs), cytoplasm, and cell organelles
1. Cell membrane—the selectively permeable boundary of the cell (see Fig. 3–1).
   • Phospholipids permit diffusion of lipid-soluble materials.
   • Cholesterol provides stability.
   • Proteins form pores, carrier enzymes, "self" antigens, and receptor sites for hormones.
2. Nucleus—the control center of the cell; has a double-layer membrane.
   • Nucleolus—forms ribosomal RNA.
   • Chromosomes—made of DNA and protein; DNA is the genetic code for the structure and functioning of the cell. A gene is a segment of DNA that is the code for one protein. Human cells have 46 chromosomes, and their genetic information is called the genome.
3. Cytoplasm—a watery solution of minerals, gases, and organic molecules; contains the cell organelles; site for many chemical reactions.
4. Cell organelles—intracellular structures with specific functions (see Table 3–1 and Fig. 3–2).

Cellular Transport Mechanisms—the processes by which cells take in or secrete or excrete materials through the selectively permeable cell membrane

1. Diffusion—movement of molecules from an area of greater concentration to an area of lesser concentration; occurs because molecules have free energy: They are constantly in motion. Oxygen and carbon dioxide are exchanged by diffusion in the lungs.
2. Osmosis—the diffusion of water. Water diffuses to an area of less water, that is, to an area of more dissolved material. The small intestine absorbs water from digested food by osmosis. Isotonic, hypertonic, and hypotonic (see Box 3–1).
3. Facilitated diffusion—carrier enzymes (transporters) that are part of the cell membrane permit cells to take in materials that would not diffuse by themselves. Most cells take in glucose by facilitated diffusion.
4. Active transport—a cell uses ATP to move substances from an area of lesser concentration to an area of greater concentration. Nerve cells and muscle cells have sodium pumps to return Na^+ ions to the exterior of the cells; this prevents spontaneous impulses. Cells of the small intestine absorb glucose and amino acids from digested food by active transport.
5. Filtration—pressure forces water and dissolved materials through a membrane from an area of higher pressure to an area of lower pressure. Tissue fluid is formed by filtration: Blood pressure forces plasma and dissolved nutrients out of capillaries and into tissues. Blood pressure in the kidney capillaries creates filtration that is the first step in the formation of urine.
6. Phagocytosis—a moving cell engulfs something; white blood cells phagocytize bacteria to destroy them.
7. Pinocytosis—a stationary cell engulfs small molecules; kidney tubule cells reabsorb small proteins by pinocytosis.

The Genetic Code and Protein Synthesis (see Fig. 3–4 and Table 3–3)

1. DNA and the genetic code
   - DNA is a double helix with complementary base pairing: A–T and G–C.
   - The sequence of bases in the DNA is the genetic code for proteins.
   - The triplet code: three bases (a codon) is the code for one amino acid.
   - A gene consists of all the triplets that code for a single protein.
2. RNA and Protein Synthesis
   - mRNA is a complementary copy of the sequence of bases in a gene (DNA).
   - mRNA moves from the nucleus to the ribosomes in the cytoplasm.
   - tRNA molecules (in the cytoplasm) have anticodons for the triplets on the mRNA.
   - tRNA molecules bring amino acids to their proper triplets on the mRNA.
   - Ribosomes contain enzymes to form peptide bonds between the amino acids.
3. Expression of the genetic code
   - DNA $\rightarrow$ RNA $\rightarrow$ Proteins (structural and enzymes) $\rightarrow$ Hereditary characteristics.
   - A genetic disease is a "mistake" in the DNA, which is copied by mRNA and results in a malfunctioning protein.

Cell Division

1. Mitosis—one cell with the diploid number of chromosomes divides once to form two cells, each with the diploid number of chromosomes (46 for humans).
   - DNA replication forms two sets of chromosomes during interphase.
   - Stages of mitosis (see Fig. 3–5 and Table 3–4): prophase, metaphase, anaphase, and telophase. Cytokinesis is the division of the cytoplasm following telophase.
   - Mitosis is essential for growth and for repair and replacement of damaged cells.
   - Most adult nerve and muscle cells seem unable to divide; their loss may involve permanent loss of function.
2. Meiosis—one cell with the diploid number of chromosomes divides twice to form four cells, each with the haploid number of chromosomes (23 for humans).
   - Oogenesis in the ovaries forms egg cells.
   - Spermatogenesis in the testes forms sperm cells.
   - Fertilization of an egg by a sperm restores the diploid number in the fertilized egg.

REVIEW QUESTIONS

1. State the functions of the organic molecules of cell membranes: cholesterol, proteins, and phospholipids. (p. 44)

2. Describe the function of each of these cell organelles: mitochondria, lysosomes, Golgi apparatus, ribosomes, and endoplasmic reticulum. (p. 47)

3. Explain why the nucleus is the control center of the cell. (p. 45)

4. What part of the cell membrane is necessary for facilitated diffusion? Describe one way this process is important within the body. (p. 49)

5. What provides the energy for filtration? Describe one way this process is important within the body. (p. 49)

6. What provides the energy for diffusion? Describe one way this process is important within the body. (p. 48)

7. What provides the energy for active transport? Describe one way this process is important within the body. (p. 49)

8. Define osmosis, and describe one way this process is important within the body. (p. 49)

9. Explain the difference between hypertonic and hypotonic, using human cells as a reference point. (p. 50)

10. In what way are phagocytosis and pinocytosis similar? Describe one way each process is important within the body. (pp. 49–50)

11. How many chromosomes does a human cell have? What are these chromosomes made of? (p. 45)

12. Name the stage of mitosis in which each of the following takes place: (p. 56)
    a. The two sets of chromosomes are pulled toward opposite poles of the cell.
    b. The chromosomes become visible as short rods.
    c. A nuclear membrane re-forms around each complete set of chromosomes.
    d. The pairs of chromatids line up along the equator of the cell.
    e. The centrioles organize the spindle fibers.
    f. Cytokinesis takes place after this stage.

13. Describe two specific ways mitosis is important within the body. Explain why meiosis is important. (pp. 53, 57)

14. Compare mitosis and meiosis in terms of: (pp. 53, 57–58)
    a. Number of divisions
    b. Number of cells formed
    c. Chromosome number of the cells formed

15. Explain the triplet code of DNA. Name the molecule that copies the triplet code of DNA. Name the organelle that is the site of protein synthesis. What other function does this organelle have in protein formation? (pp. 51–53)

FOR FURTHER THOUGHT

1. Antibiotics are drugs used to treat bacterial infections. Some antibiotics disrupt the process of protein synthesis within bacteria. Others block DNA synthesis and cell division by the bacteria. Still others inhibit cell wall synthesis by the bacteria. If all antibiotics worked equally well against bacteria, would any of those mentioned above be better than the others, from the patient's perspective? Explain your answer.

2. A new lab instructor wants his students to see living cells. He puts a drop of his own blood on a glass slide, adds two drops of distilled water "so the cells will be spread out and easier to see," puts on a cover glass, and places the slide under a microscope on high power. He invites his students to see living red blood cells. The students claim that they cannot see any red blood cells. Explain what has happened. How could this have been prevented?

3. A friend asks you how DNA can be used to identify someone, and why it is called a "DNA fingerprint." What simple explanation can you give?

4. A cell has extensive rough ER and Golgi apparatus. Give a brief explanation of its function. A second cell has microvilli and many mitochondria. Give a brief explanation of its function.

5. A bacterial toxin is found to cause harm by first fitting into a receptor on human cell membranes; once the toxin fits, the cell will be destroyed. A medication is going to be made to stop this toxin, and can work in one of two ways: The drug can block the receptors to prevent the toxin from fitting in, or the drug can act as decoy molecules shaped like the receptors. Which one of these might be better, and why?

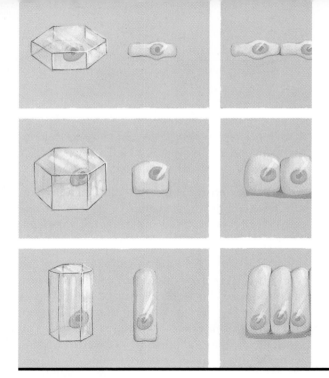

CHAPTER 4

Box 4–1	CYSTIC FIBROSIS
Box 4–2	VITAMIN C AND COLLAGEN
Box 4–3	COSMETIC COLLAGEN

Student Objectives
- Describe the general characteristics of each of the four major categories of tissues.
- Describe the functions of the types of epithelial tissues with respect to the organs in which they are found.
- Describe the functions of the connective tissues, and relate them to the functioning of the body or a specific organ system.
- Explain the differences, in terms of location and function, among skeletal muscle, smooth muscle, and cardiac muscle.
- Name the three parts of a neuron and state the function of each. Name the organs made of nerve tissue.
- Describe the locations of the pleural membranes, the pericardial membranes, and the peritoneum-mesentery. State the function of serous fluid in each of these locations.
- State the locations of mucous membranes and the functions of mucus.
- Name some membranes made of connective tissue.
- Explain the difference between exocrine and endocrine glands, and give an example of each.

Tissues and Membranes

New Terminology

Bone (BOWNE)
Cartilage (**KAR**-ti-lidj)
Chondrocyte (**KON**-droh-sight)
Collagen (**KAH**-lah-jen)
Connective tissue (kah-**NEK**-tiv **TISH**-yoo)
Elastin (eh-**LAS**-tin)
Endocrine gland (**EN**-doh-krin GLAND)
Epithelial tissue (EP-i-**THEE**-lee-uhl **TISH**-yoo)
Exocrine gland (**EK**-so-krin GLAND)
Hemopoietic (HEE-moh-poy-**ET**-ik)
Matrix (**MAY**-tricks)
Mucous membrane (**MEW**-kuss **MEM**-brayn)
Muscle tissue (**MUSS**-uhl **TISH**-yoo)
Myocardium (MY-oh-**KAR**-dee-um)
Nerve tissue (NERV **TISH**-yoo)
Neuron (**NYOOR**-on)
Neurotransmitter (NYOOR-oh-**TRANS**-mih-ter)
Osteocyte (**AHS**-tee-oh-sight)
Plasma (**PLAZ**-mah)
Secretion (see-**KREE**-shun)
Serous membrane (**SEER**-us **MEM**-brayn)
Synapse (**SIN**-aps)

*Terms that appear in **bold type** in the chapter text are defined in the glossary, which begins on page 521.*

A **tissue** is a group of cells with similar structure and function. The tissue contributes to the functioning of the organs in which it is found. You may recall that in Chapter 1 the four major groups of tissues were named and very briefly described. These four groups are epithelial, connective, muscle, and nerve tissue.

This chapter presents more detailed descriptions of the tissues in these four categories. For each tissue, its functions are related to the organs of which it is a part. Also in this chapter is a discussion of **membranes**, which are sheets of tissues. As you might expect, each type of membrane has its specific locations and functions.

EPITHELIAL TISSUE

Epithelial tissues are found on surfaces as either coverings (outer surfaces) or linings (inner surfaces). Because they have no capillaries of their own, epithelial tissues receive oxygen and nutrients from the blood supply of the connective tissue beneath them. Many epithelial tissues are capable of secretion and may be called glandular epithelium, or more simply, **glands**.

Classification of the epithelial tissues is based on the type of cell of which the tissue is made, its characteristic shape, and the number of layers of cells.

There are three distinctive shapes: **squamous** cells are flat, **cuboidal** cells are cube shaped, and **columnar** cells are tall and narrow. "**Simple**" is the term for a single layer of cells, and "**stratified**" means that many layers of cells are present (Fig. 4–1 and Table 4–1).

SIMPLE SQUAMOUS EPITHELIUM

Simple squamous epithelium is a single layer of flat cells (Fig. 4–2). These cells are very thin and very smooth—these are important physical characteristics. The alveoli (air sacs) of the lungs are simple squamous epithelium. The thinness of the cells permits the diffusion of gases between the air and blood.

Another location of this tissue is capillaries, the smallest blood vessels. Capillary walls are only one cell thick, which permits the exchange of gases, nutrients, and waste products between the blood and tissue fluid. The interior surface of capillaries is also very smooth (and these cells continue as the lining of the arteries, veins, and heart); this is important because it prevents abnormal blood clotting within blood vessels.

STRATIFIED SQUAMOUS EPITHELIUM

Stratified squamous epithelium consists of many layers of mostly flat cells, although lower cells are

Shapes — Squamous, Cuboidal, Columnar

Simple — Simple squamous, Simple cuboidal, Simple columnar

Stratified — Stratified squamous

FIGURE 4–1 Classification of epithelial tissues based on the shape of the cells and the number of layers of cells.

Table 4–1   TYPES OF EPITHELIAL TISSUE

Type	Structure	Location and Function
Simple squamous	One layer of flat cells	• Alveoli of the lungs—thin to permit diffusion of gases • Capillaries—thin to permit exchanges of materials; smooth to prevent abnormal blood clotting
Stratified squamous	Many layers of cells; surface cells flat; lower cells rounded; lower layer undergoes mitosis	• Epidermis—surface cells are dead; a barrier to pathogens • Lining of esophagus, vagina—surface cells are living; a barrier to pathogens
Transitional	Many layers of cells; surface cells change from rounded to flat	• Lining of urinary bladder—permits expansion without tearing the lining
Cuboidal	One layer of cube-shaped cells	• Thyroid gland—secretes thyroxine • Salivary glands—secrete saliva • Kidney tubules—permits reabsorption of useful materials back to the blood
Columnar	One layer of column-shaped cells	• Lining of stomach—secretes gastric juice • Lining of small intestine—secretes enzymes and absorbs end products of digestion (microvilli present)
Ciliated	One layer of columnar cells with cilia on their free surfaces	• Lining of trachea—sweeps mucus and dust to the pharynx • Lining of fallopian tube—sweeps ovum toward uterus

rounded. Mitosis takes place in the lowest layer to continually produce new cells to replace those worn off the surface (see Fig. 4–2). This type of epithelium makes up the epidermis of the skin, where it is called "keratinizing" because the protein keratin is produced, and the surface cells are dead. Stratified squamous epithelium of the nonkeratinizing type lines the oral cavity, esophagus, and, in women, the vagina. In these locations the surface cells are living and make up the mucous membranes of these organs. In all of its body locations, this tissue is a barrier to microorganisms because the cells of which it is made are very close together. The more specialized functions of the epidermis will be covered in the next chapter.

TRANSITIONAL EPITHELIUM

Transitional epithelium is a type of stratified epithelium in which the surface cells change shape from round to squamous. The urinary bladder is lined with transitional epithelium. When the bladder is empty, the surface cells are rounded (see Fig. 4–2). As the bladder fills, these cells become flattened. Transitional epithelium enables the bladder to fill and stretch without tearing the lining.

SIMPLE CUBOIDAL EPITHELIUM

Simple cuboidal epithelium is a single layer of cube-shaped cells (Fig. 4–3). This type of tissue makes up the functional units of the thyroid gland and salivary glands. These are examples of **glandular epithelium**; their function is **secretion**. In these glands the cuboidal cells are arranged in small spheres and secrete into the cavity formed by the sphere. In the thyroid gland, the cuboidal epithelium secretes the thyroid hormones; thyroxine is an example. In the salivary glands the cuboidal cells secrete saliva. Cuboidal epithelium also makes up portions of the kidney tubules. Here the cells have microvilli (see Fig. 1–1), and their function is the reabsorption of useful materials back to the blood.

SIMPLE COLUMNAR EPITHELIUM

Columnar cells are taller than they are wide and are specialized for secretion and **absorption**. The stom-

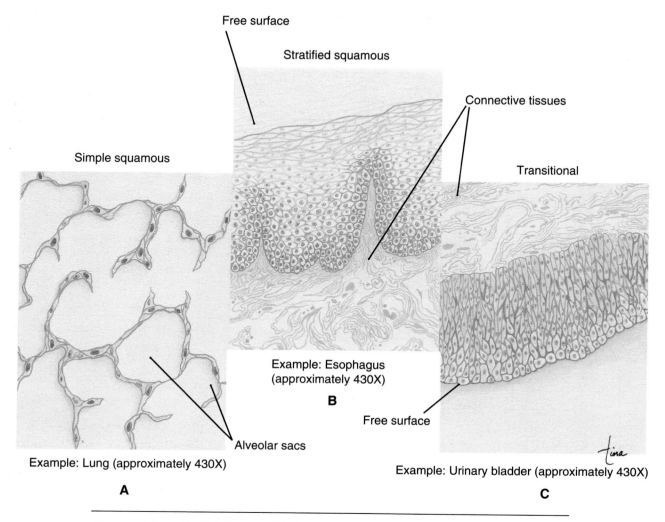

Figure 4–2 Epithelial tissues. **(A)** Simple squamous. **(B)** Stratified squamous. **(C)** Transitional.

ach lining is made of **columnar epithelium** that secretes gastric juice for digestion. The lining of the small intestine (see Fig. 4–3) secretes digestive enzymes, but these cells also absorb the end products of digestion from the cavity of the intestine into the blood and lymph. In order to absorb efficiently, the columnar cells of the small intestine have **microvilli**, which you may recall are folds of the cell membrane on their free surfaces (see Fig. 3–2). These microscopic folds greatly increase the surface area for absorption.

Yet another type of columnar cell is the **goblet cell**, which is a unicellular gland. Goblet cells secrete **mucus** and are found in the lining of the intestines and the lining of parts of the respiratory tract such as

the trachea. Mucous membranes will be described in a later section.

CILIATED EPITHELIUM

Ciliated epithelium consists of columnar cells that have **cilia** on their free surfaces (see Fig. 4–3). Recall from Chapter 3 that the function of cilia is to sweep materials across the cell surface. Ciliated epithelium lines the nasal cavities, larynx, trachea, and large bronchial tubes. The cilia sweep mucus, with trapped dust and bacteria from the inhaled air, toward the pharynx to be swallowed. Bacteria are then destroyed by the hydrochloric acid in the stomach. The air that

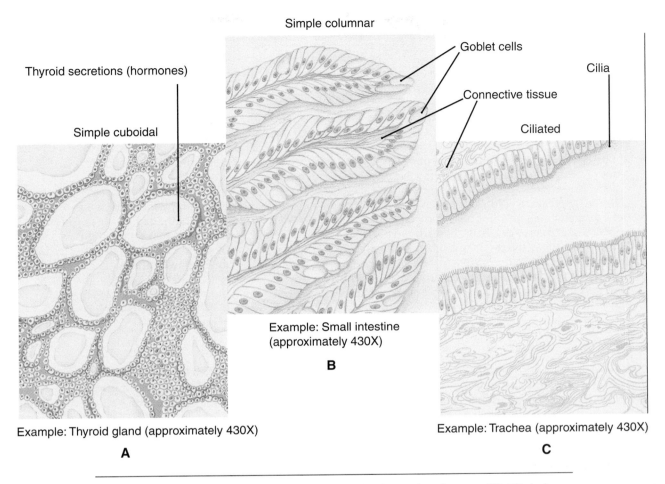

Figure 4–3 Epithelial tissues. **(A)** Simple cuboidal. **(B)** Simple columnar. **(C)** Ciliated.

reaches the lungs is almost entirely free of pathogens and particulate pollution.

Another location of ciliated epithelium in women is the lining of the fallopian tubes. The cilia here sweep the ovum, which has no means of self-locomotion, toward the uterus.

GLANDS

Glands are cells or organs that secrete something, that is, they produce a substance that has a function either at that site or at a more distant site.

Unicellular Glands

Unicellular means "one cell." Goblet cells are an example of unicellular glands. As mentioned earlier, goblet cells are found in the lining of the respiratory

and digestive tracts. Their secretion is mucus (see also Box 4–1: Cystic Fibrosis).

Multicellular Glands

Most glands are made of many similar cells, or of a variety of cells with their secretions mingled into a collective secretion. **Multicellular** glands may be divided into two major groups: exocrine glands and endocrine glands.

Exocrine glands have **ducts** (tubes) to take the secretion away from the gland to the site of its function. Salivary glands, for example, secrete saliva that is carried by ducts to the oral cavity. Sweat glands secrete sweat that is transported by ducts to the skin surface, where it can be evaporated by excess body heat. The gastric glands of the stomach lining contain different kinds of cells (see Fig. 16–5), which produce

---

Box 4–1   CYSTIC FIBROSIS

Cystic fibrosis (CF) is a genetic disorder of certain exocrine glands including the salivary glands, sweat glands, the pancreas, and the mucous glands of the respiratory tract.

In the pancreas, thick mucus clogs the ducts and prevents pancreatic enzymes from reaching the small intestine, thus impairing digestion, especially of fats. But the most serious effects of CF are in the lungs. The genetic mistake in CF involves a gene called CFTR, which codes for protein channels called chloride gateways in epithelial cells. In the lungs, the defective channels prevent salt from entering the cells, creating a very salty tissue fluid around the cells. This salty fluid inactivates defensin, a natural antibiotic produced by lung tissue. In the absence of defensin, a bacterium called *Pseudomonas aeruginosa* stimulates the lung cells to produce copious

thick mucus, an ideal growth environment for bacteria. Defensive white blood cells cannot get through the thick mucus, and their activity mistakenly destroys lung tissue. A person with CF has clogged bronchial tubes, frequent episodes of pneumonia, and ultimately, lungs that cannot carry out gas exchange. CF is a chronic, progressive disease that is eventually fatal unless a lung transplant is performed.

CF is one of several disorders believed to be correctable by gene therapy. Current research trials involve the use of non-pathogenic viruses to transfer a normal gene into the cells that line the respiratory airways. Because it involves human subjects, this kind of work proceeds slowly, and it may be several years before conclusive results are obtained as to whether gene therapy offers a cure for CF.

---

hydrochloric acid and the enzyme pepsin. Both of these secretions are part of gastric juice.

Endocrine glands are ductless glands. The secretions of endocrine glands are a group of chemicals called **hormones**, which enter capillaries and are circulated throughout the body. Hormones then bring about specific effects in their target organs. These effects include aspects of growth, use of minerals and other nutrients, and regulation of blood pressure, and will be covered in more detail in Chapter 10. Examples of endocrine glands are the thyroid gland, adrenal glands, and pituitary gland.

The pancreas is an organ that functions as both an exocrine and an endocrine gland. The exocrine portions secrete digestive enzymes that are carried by ducts to the duodenum of the small intestine, their site of action. The endocrine portions of the pancreas, called islets of Langerhans, secrete the hormones insulin and glucagon directly into the blood.

CONNECTIVE TISSUE

There are several kinds of **connective tissue**, some of which may at first seem more different than alike. The types of connective tissue include areolar, adipose, fibrous, and elastic tissue as well as blood, bone, and cartilage (Table 4–2). A characteristic that

all connective tissues have in common is the presence of a matrix in addition to cells. The **matrix** is a structural network or solution of non-living intercellular material. Each connective tissue has its own specific kind of matrix. The matrix of blood, for example, is blood plasma, which is mostly water. The matrix of bone is made primarily of calcium salts, which are hard and strong. As each type of connective tissue is described in the following sections, mention will be made of the types of cells present as well as the kind of matrix.

BLOOD

Although **blood** is the subject of Chapter 11, a brief description will be given here. Blood consists of cells and plasma; cells are the living portion. The matrix of blood is **plasma**, which is about 52% to 62% of the total blood volume in the body. The water of plasma contains dissolved salts, nutrients, and waste products. As you might expect, one of the primary functions of plasma is transport of these materials within the body.

The cells of blood are red blood cells, white blood cells, and platelets, which are actually fragments of cells. These are shown in Fig. 4–4. The blood-forming or **hemopoietic tissues** are the red bone marrow and lymphatic tissue, which includes the spleen and the lymph nodes. Red bone marrow produces red

Table 4–2	TYPES OF CONNECTIVE TISSUE	

Type	Structure	Location and Function
Blood	Plasma (matrix) and red blood cells, white blood cells, and platelets	Within blood vessels: • *Plasma*—transports materials • *RBCs*—carry oxygen • *WBCs*—destroy pathogens • *Platelets*—prevent blood loss
Areolar (loose)	Fibroblasts and a matrix of tissue fluid, collagen, and elastin fibers	Subcutaneous • Connects skin to muscles; WBCs destroy pathogens Mucous membranes (digestive, respiratory, urinary, reproductive tracts) • WBCs destroy pathogens
Adipose	Adipocytes that store fat (little matrix)	Subcutaneous • Stores excess energy Around eyes and kidneys • Cushions
Fibrous	Mostly collagen fibers (matrix) with few fibroblasts	Tendons and ligaments (regular) • Strong to withstand forces of movement of joints Dermis (irregular) • The strong inner layer of the skin
Elastic	Mostly elastin fibers (matrix) with few fibroblasts	Walls of large arteries • Helps maintain blood pressure Around alveoli in lungs • Promotes normal exhalation
Bone	Osteocytes in a matrix of calcium salts and collagen	Bones • Support the body • Protect internal organs from mechanical injury • Store excess calcium • Contain and protect red bone marrow
Cartilage	Chondrocytes in a flexible protein matrix	Wall of trachea • Keeps airway open On joint surfaces of bones • Smooth to prevent friction Tip of nose and outer ear • Support Between vertebrae • Absorb shock

blood cells, the five kinds of white blood cells, and the platelets. Two kinds of white blood cells are also produced in lymphatic tissue.

The blood cells make up 38% to 48% of the total blood, and each type of cell has its specific function. **Red blood cells** (RBCs) carry oxygen bonded to their hemoglobin. **White blood cells** (WBCs) destroy pathogens and provide us with immunity to some diseases. **Platelets** prevent blood loss; the process of blood clotting involves platelets.

AREOLAR CONNECTIVE TISSUE

The cells of **areolar** (or **loose**) **connective tissue** are called **fibroblasts**, which produce protein fibers. **Collagen** fibers are very strong; **elastin** fibers are elastic, that is, able to return to their original length, or recoil, after being stretched. These protein fibers and tissue fluid make up the matrix, or non-living portion, of areolar connective tissue (see Fig. 4–4). Also within the matrix are many white blood cells,

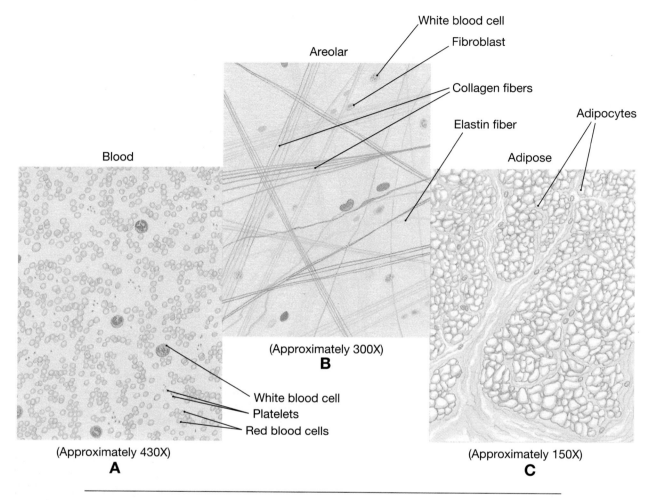

Figure 4–4 Connective tissues. **(A)** Blood. **(B)** Areolar. **(C)** Adipose.

which are capable of self-locomotion. Their importance here is related to the locations of areolar connective tissue.

Areolar tissue is found beneath the dermis of the skin and beneath the epithelial tissue of all the body systems that have openings to the environment. Recall that one function of white blood cells is to destroy pathogens. How do pathogens enter the body? Many do so through breaks in the skin. Bacteria and viruses also enter with the air we breathe and the food we eat, and some may get through the epithelial linings of the respiratory and digestive tracts. Areolar connective tissue with its many white blood cells is strategically placed to intercept pathogens before they get to the blood and circulate throughout the body.

ADIPOSE TISSUE

The cells of **adipose tissue** are called **adipocytes** and are specialized to store fat in microscopic droplets. True fats are the chemical form of long-term energy storage. Excess nutrients have calories that are not wasted but are converted to fat to be stored for use when food intake decreases. Any form of excess calories, whether in the form of fats, carbohydrates, or amino acids from protein, may be changed to triglycerides and stored. The amount of matrix in adipose tissue is small and consists of tissue fluid and a few collagen fibers (see Fig. 4–4).

Most fat is stored subcutaneously in the areolar connective tissue between the dermis and the

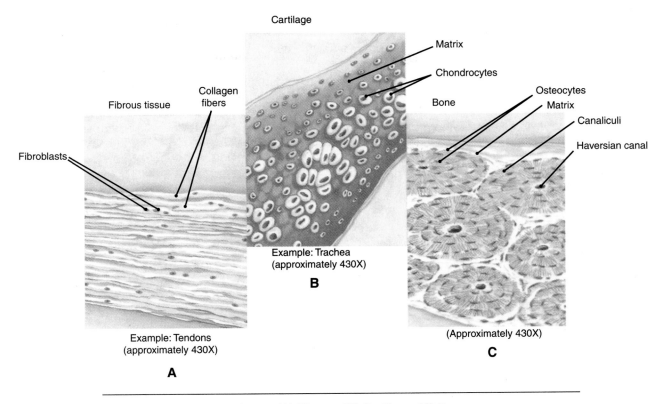

Figure 4–5 Connective tissues. **(A)** Fibrous. **(B)** Cartilage. **(C)** Bone.

muscles. This layer varies in thickness among individuals; the more excess calories consumed, the thicker the layer. As was mentioned in Chapter 2, adipose tissue also cushions organs such as the eyes and kidneys.

FIBROUS CONNECTIVE TISSUE

Fibrous connective tissue consists mainly of parallel (regular) collagen fibers with few fibroblasts scattered among them (Fig. 4–5). This parallel arrangement of collagen provides great strength, yet is flexible. The locations of this tissue are related to the need for flexible strength. The outer walls of arteries are reinforced with fibrous connective tissue, because the blood in these vessels is under high pressure. The strong outer wall prevents rupture of the artery (see also Box 4–2: Vitamin C and Collagen). Tendons and ligaments are made of fibrous connective tissue. Tendons connect muscle to bone; ligaments connect bone to bone. When the skeleton is moved, these structures must be able to withstand the great mechanical forces exerted upon them.

Fibrous connective tissue has a relatively poor blood supply, which makes repair a slow process. If you have ever had a severely sprained ankle (which means the ligaments have been overly stretched), you know that complete healing may take several months.

An irregular type of fibrous connective tissue forms the dermis of the skin and the fascia (membranes) around muscles. Although the collagen fibers here are not parallel to one another, the tissue is still strong. The dermis is different from other fibrous connective tissue in that it has a good blood supply (see also Box 4–3: Cosmetic Collagen).

ELASTIC CONNECTIVE TISSUE

As its name tells us, **elastic connective tissue** is primarily elastin fibers. One of its locations is in the walls of large arteries. These vessels are stretched when the heart contracts and pumps blood, then they recoil, or snap back, when the heart relaxes. This recoil helps keep the blood moving away from the heart, and is important to maintain normal blood pressure.

Box 4–2   VITAMIN C AND COLLAGEN

In the last two decades, many claims have been made for the effectiveness of vitamin C in preventing or treating the common cold and even cancer. There is no conclusive evidence for these claims, but one function of vitamin C is known with certainty, and that is its role in the synthesis of collagen.

Imagine the protein collagen as a ladder with three uprights and rungs that connect adjacent uprights. Vitamin C is essential for forming the "rungs," without which the uprights will not stay together as a strong unit. Collagen formed in the absence of vitamin C is weak, and the effects of weak collagen are dramatically seen in the disease called scurvy.

In 1753 James Lind, a Scottish Surgeon, recommended to the British Navy that lime juice be taken on long voyages to prevent scurvy among the sailors. Scurvy is characterized by bleeding gums and loss of teeth, poor healing of wounds, fractures, and bleeding in the skin, joints, and elsewhere in the body. The lime juice did prevent this potentially fatal disease, as did consumption of fresh fruits and vegetables, although at the time no one knew why. Vitamin C was finally isolated in the laboratory in 1928.

Box 4–3   COSMETIC COLLAGEN

Collagen is the protein that makes tendons, ligaments, and other connective tissues strong. In 1981, the Food and Drug Administration (FDA) approved the use of cattle collagen by injection for cosmetic purposes, to minimize wrinkles and scars. Indeed, collagen injected below the skin will flatten out deep facial wrinkles and make them less prominent, and millions of people in the United States have had this seemingly simple cosmetic surgery.

There are, however, drawbacks. Injected collagen lasts only a few months; the injections must be repeated several times a year, and they are expensive. Some people experience allergic reactions to the cattle collagen, which is perceived by the immune system as foreign tissue. More seriously, an autoimmune response may be triggered in some individuals, and the immune system may begin to destroy the person's own connective tissue.

In an effort to avoid these problems, some cosmetic surgeons now use the person's own collagen and fat, which may be extracted from the thigh, hip, or abdomen. The long-term consequences and outcomes of such procedures have yet to be evaluated. We might remember that for many years the use of silicone injections had been considered safe. Silicone injections are now banned by the FDA, since we now know that they carry significant risk of serious tissue damage.

Elastic connective tissue is also found surrounding the alveoli of the lungs. The elastic fibers are stretched during inhalation, then recoil during exhalation to squeeze air out of the lungs. If you pay attention to your breathing for a few moments, you will notice that normal exhalation does not require "work" or energy. This is because of the normal elasticity of the lungs.

BONE

The prefix that designates bone is "osteo," so bone cells are called **osteocytes**. The matrix of **bone** is made of calcium salts and collagen and is strong, hard, and not flexible. In the shafts of long bones such as the femur, the osteocytes, matrix, and blood vessels are in very precise arrangements called **haversian systems** (see Fig. 4–5). Bone has a good blood supply, which enables it to serve as a storage site for calcium and to repair itself relatively rapidly after a simple fracture. Some bones, such as the sternum (breastbone) and pelvic bone, contain red bone marrow, one of the hemopoietic tissues that produces blood cells.

Other functions of bone tissue are related to the strength of bone matrix. The skeleton supports the body, and some bones protect internal organs from mechanical injury. A more complete discussion of bone is found in Chapter 6.

CARTILAGE

The protein matrix of **cartilage** does not contain calcium salts, and also differs from that of bone in that it contains more water, which makes it resilient. It is firm, yet smooth and flexible. Cartilage is found on the joint surfaces of bones, where its smooth surface helps prevent friction. The tip of the nose and external ear are supported by flexible cartilage. The wall of the trachea, the airway to the lungs, contains firm rings of cartilage to maintain an open air passageway. Discs of cartilage are found between the vertebrae of the spine. Here the cartilage is a firm cushion; it absorbs shock and permits movement.

Within the cartilage matrix are the **chondrocytes**, or cartilage cells (see Fig. 4–5). There are no capillaries within the cartilage matrix, so these cells are nourished by diffusion through the matrix, a slow process. This becomes clinically important when cartilage is damaged, for repair will take place very slowly or not at all. Athletes sometimes damage cartilage within the knee joint. Such damaged cartilage is usually surgically removed in order to preserve as much joint mobility as possible.

MUSCLE TISSUE

Muscle tissue is specialized for contraction. When muscle cells contract, they shorten and bring about some type of movement. There are three types of muscle tissue: skeletal, smooth, and cardiac (Table 4–3). The movements each can produce have very different purposes.

SKELETAL MUSCLE

Skeletal muscle may also be called **striated** muscle or **voluntary** muscle. Each name describes a partic-

ular aspect of this tissue, as you will see. The skeletal muscle cells are cylindrical, have several nuclei each, and appear striated, or striped (Fig. 4–6). The striations are the result of the precise arrangement of the contracting proteins within the cells.

Skeletal muscle tissue makes up the muscles that are attached to bones. These muscles are supplied with motor nerves, and thus move the skeleton. They also produce a significant amount of heat, which is important to help maintain the body's constant temperature. Each muscle cell has its own motor nerve ending. The nerve impulses that can then travel to the muscles are essential to cause contraction. Although we do not have to consciously plan all our movements, the nerve impulses for them originate in the cerebrum, the "thinking" part of the brain.

Let us return to the three names for this tissue: "skeletal" describes its location, "striated" describes its appearance, and "voluntary" describes how it functions. The skeletal muscles and their functioning are the subject of Chapter 7.

SMOOTH MUSCLE

Smooth muscle may also be called **involuntary** muscle or **visceral** muscle. The cells of smooth muscle have tapered ends, a single nucleus, and no striations (see Fig. 4–6). Although nerve impulses do bring about contractions, this is not something most of us can control, hence the name *involuntary*. The term *visceral* refers to internal organs, many of which contain smooth muscle. The functions of smooth muscle are actually functions of the organs in which the muscle is found.

Table 4–3	TYPES OF MUSCLE TISSUE		
Type	Structure	Location and Function	Effect of Nerve Impulses
Skeletal	Large cylindrical cells with striations and several nuclei each	Attached to bones • Moves the skeleton and produces heat	Essential to cause contraction (voluntary)
Smooth	Small tapered cells with no striations and one nucleus each	Walls of arteries • Maintains blood pressure Walls of stomach and intestines • Peristalsis Iris of eye • Regulates size of pupil	Bring about contraction or regulate the rate of contration (involuntary)
Cardiac	Branched cells with faint striations and one nucleus each	Walls of the chambers of the heart • Pumps blood	Regulate only the rate of contraction

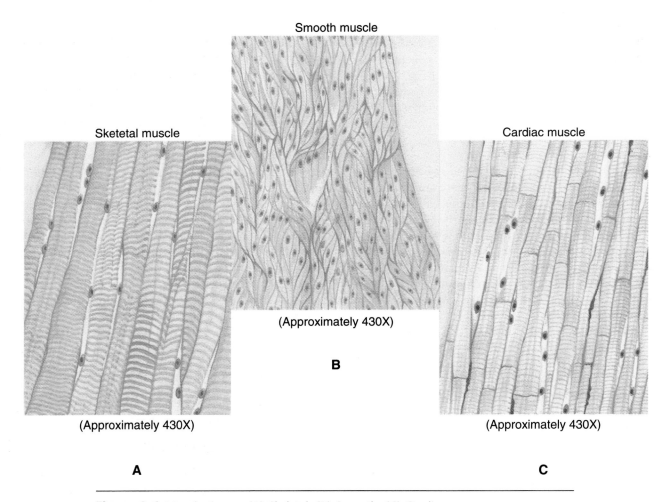

Smooth muscle

Sketetal muscle

Cardiac muscle

(Approximately 430X)

B

(Approximately 430X)

(Approximately 430X)

A

C

Figure 4–6 Muscle tissues. **(A)** Skeletal. **(B)** Smooth. **(C)** Cardiac.

In the stomach and intestines, smooth muscle contracts in waves called peristalsis to propel food through the digestive tract.

In the walls of arteries and veins, smooth muscle constricts or dilates the vessels to maintain normal blood pressure. The iris of the eye has two sets of smooth muscle fibers to constrict or dilate the pupil, which regulates the amount of light that strikes the retina.

Other functions of smooth muscle are mentioned in later chapters. This is an important tissue that you will come across again and again in our study of the human body.

CARDIAC MUSCLE

The cells of **cardiac muscle** are shown in Fig. 4–6. They are branched, have one nucleus each, and have faint striations. Cardiac muscle, called the **myocardium**, forms the walls of the chambers of the heart. Its function, therefore, is the function of the heart, to pump blood. The contractions of the myocardium create blood pressure and keep blood circulating throughout the body, so that the blood can carry out its many functions.

Cardiac muscle cells have the ability to contract by themselves. Thus the heart maintains its own beat. The role of nerve impulses is to increase or decrease the heart rate, depending upon whatever is needed by the body in a particular situation. We will return to the heart in Chapter 12.

NERVE TISSUE

Nerve tissue consists of nerve cells called **neurons** and some specialized cells found only in the nervous system. The nervous system has two divisions: the central nervous system (CNS) and the peripheral nervous system (PNS). The brain and spinal cord are the organs of the CNS. They are made of neurons and specialized cells called neuroglia. The CNS and the neuroglia are discussed in detail in Chapter 8. The PNS consists of all of the nerves that emerge from the CNS and supply the rest of the body. These nerves are made of neurons and specialized cells called Schwann cells. The Schwann cells form the myelin sheath to electrically insulate neurons (Table 4–4).

Neurons are capable of generating and transmitting electrochemical impulses. There are many different kinds of neurons, but they all have the same basic structure (Fig. 4–7). The **cell body** contains the nucleus and is essential for the continuing life of the neuron. An **axon** is a process (the term *process* here means "a thing," a cellular extension) that carries impulses away from the cell body; a neuron has only one axon. **Dendrites** are processes that carry impulses toward the cell body; a neuron may have several dendrites. A nerve impulse travels along the cell membrane of a neuron, and is electrical, but where neurons meet there is a small space called a **synapse**, which an electrical impulse cannot cross. At a synapse, between the axon of one neuron and the dendrite or cell body of the next neuron, impulse transmission depends upon chemicals called **neurotransmitters**. Each of these aspects of nerve tissue is covered in more detail in Chapter 8.

Nerve tissue makes up the brain, spinal cord, and peripheral nerves. As you can imagine, each of these organs has very specific functions. For now, we will just summarize the functions of nerve tissue. These functions include sensation, movement, the rapid regulation of body functions such as heart rate and breathing, and the organization of information for learning and memory.

MEMBRANES

Membranes are sheets of tissue that cover or line surfaces or that separate organs or parts (lobes) of organs from one another. Many membranes produce secretions that have specific functions. The two major categories of membranes are epithelial membranes and connective tissue membranes.

EPITHELIAL MEMBRANES

There are two types of epithelial membranes, serous and mucous. Each type is found in specific locations within the body and secretes a fluid. These fluids are called serous fluid and mucus.

Table 4–4	NERVE TISSUE	
Part	**Structure**	**Function**
Neuron (nerve cell)		
Cell body	• Contains the nucleus	• Regulates the functioning of the neuron
Axon	• Cellular process (extension)	• Carries impulses away from the cell body
Dendrites	• Cellular process (extension)	• Carry impulses toward the cell body
Synapse	• Space between axon of one neuron and the dendrite or cell body of the next neuron	• Transmits impulses from one neuron to others
Neurotransmitters	• Chemicals released by axons	• Transmit impulses across synapses
Neuroglia	• Specialized cells in the central nervous system	• Form myelin sheaths and other functions
Schwann cells	• Specialized cells in the peripheral nervous system	• Form the myelin sheaths around neurons

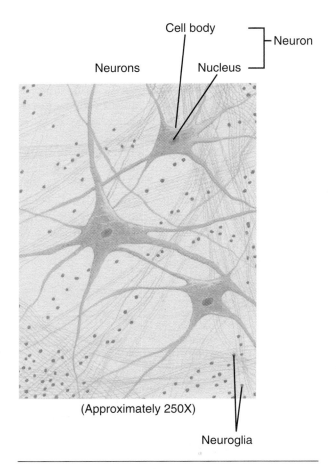

Cell body

Neurons

Nucleus

Neuron

(Approximately 250X)

Neuroglia

Figure 4–7 Nerve tissue of the central nervous system (CNS).

Serous Membranes

Serous membranes are sheets of simple squamous epithelium that line some closed body cavities and cover the organs in these cavities (Fig. 4–8). The **pleural membranes** are the serous membranes of the thoracic cavity. The parietal pleura lines the chest wall and the visceral pleura covers the lungs. (Notice that *line* means "on the inside" and *cover* means "on the outside." These terms cannot be used interchangeably, because each indicates a different location.) The pleural membranes secrete **serous fluid**, which prevents friction between them as the lungs expand and recoil during breathing.

The heart, in the thoracic cavity between the lungs, has its own set of serous membranes. The parietal

pericardium lines the fibrous pericardium (a connective tissue membrane), and the visceral **pericardium**, or epicardium, is on the surface of the heart muscle (see also Fig. 12–1). Serous fluid is produced to prevent friction as the heart beats.

In the abdominal cavity, the **peritoneum** is the serous membrane that lines the cavity. The **mesentery**, or visceral peritoneum, is folded over and covers the abdominal organs. Here, the serous fluid prevents friction as the stomach and intestines contract and slide against other organs (see also Fig. 16–4).

Mucous Membranes

Mucous membranes line the body tracts (systems) that have openings to the environment. These are the respiratory, digestive, urinary, and reproductive tracts. The epithelium of a mucous membrane (**mucosa**) varies with the different organs involved. The mucosa of the esophagus and of the vagina is stratified squamous epithelium; the mucosa of the trachea is ciliated epithelium; the mucosa of the stomach is columnar epithelium.

The **mucus** secreted by these membranes keeps the lining epithelial cells wet. Remember that these are living cells, and if they dry out, they will die. In the digestive tract, mucus also lubricates the surface to permit the smooth passage of food. In the respiratory tract the mucus traps dust and bacteria, which are then swept to the pharynx by ciliated epithelium.

CONNECTIVE TISSUE MEMBRANES

Many membranes are made of connective tissue. Because these will be covered with the organ systems of which they are a part, their locations and functions are summarized in Table 4–5.

AGING AND TISSUES

As mentioned in the previous chapter, aging takes place at the cellular level, but of course is apparent in the groups of cells we call tissues. In muscle tissue, for example, the proteins that bring about contraction deteriorate and are not repaired or replaced. The same is true of collagen and elastin, the proteins of connective tissue such as the dermis of the skin. Other aspects of the aging of tissues will be more meaningful to you

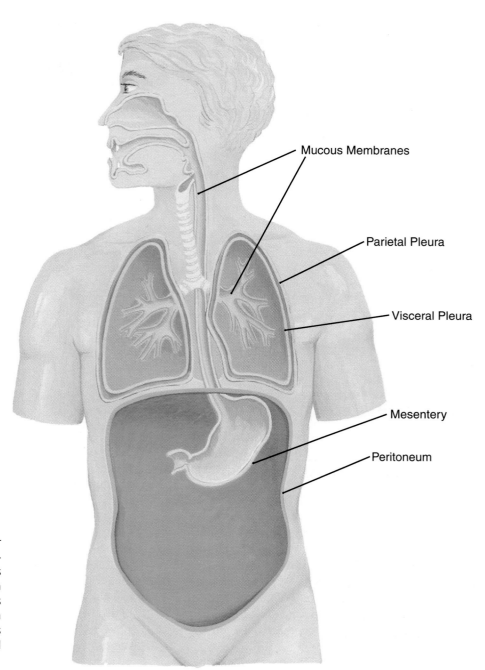

Mucous Membranes

Parietal Pleura

Visceral Pleura

Mesentery

Peritoneum

Figure 4–8 Epithelial membranes. Mucous membranes line body tracts that open to the environment. Serous membranes are found within closed body cavities such as the thoracic and abdominal cavities.

Table 4–5	CONNECTIVE TISSUE MEMBRANES
Membrane	**Location and Function**
Superficial fascia	• Between the skin and muscles; adipose tissue stores fat
Periosteum	• Covers each bone; contains blood vessels that enter the bone • Anchors tendons and ligaments
Perichondrium	• Covers cartilage; contains capillaries, the only blood supply for cartilage
Synovial	• Lines joint cavities; secretes synovial fluid to prevent friction when joints move
Deep fascia	• Covers each skeletal muscle; anchors tendons
Meninges	• Cover the brain and spinal cord; contain cerebrospinal fluid
Fibrous pericardium	• Forms a sac around the heart; lined by the serous parietal pericardium

in the context of the functions of organs and systems, so we will save those for the following chapters.

SUMMARY

The tissues and membranes described in this chapter are more complex than the individual cells of which they are made. However, we have only reached an intermediate level with respect to the structural and functional complexity of the body as a whole. The following chapters are concerned with the organ systems, the most complex level. In the descriptions of the organs of these systems, you will find mention of the tissues and their contributions to each organ and organ system.

STUDY OUTLINE

A tissue is a group of cells with similar structure and function. The four main groups of tissues are epithelial, connective, muscle, and nerve.

Epithelial Tissue—found on surfaces; have no capillaries; some are capable of secretion; classified as to shape of cells and number of layers of cells (see Table 4–1 and Figs. 4–1, 4–2, and 4–3)

1. Simple squamous—one layer of flat cells; thin and smooth. Sites: alveoli (to permit diffusion of gases); capillaries (to permit exchanges between blood and tissues).
2. Stratified squamous—many layers of mostly flat cells; mitosis takes place in lowest layer. Sites: epidermis, where surface cells are dead (a barrier to pathogens); lining of mouth; esophagus; and vagina (a barrier to pathogens).
3. Transitional—stratified, yet surface cells are rounded and flatten when stretched. Site: urinary bladder (to permit expansion without tearing the lining).

4. Simple cuboidal—one layer of cube-shaped cells. Sites: thyroid gland (to secrete thyroid hormones); salivary glands (to secrete saliva); kidney tubules (to reabsorb useful materials back to the blood).
5. Simple columnar—one layer of column-shaped cells. Sites: stomach lining (to secrete gastric juice); small intestinal lining (to secrete digestive enzymes and absorb nutrients—microvilli increase surface area for absorption).
6. Ciliated—columnar cells with cilia on free surfaces. Sites: trachea (to sweep mucus and bacteria to the pharynx); fallopian tubes (to sweep ovum to uterus).
7. Glands—Epithelial tissues that produce secretions.
   • Unicellular—one-celled glands. Goblet cells secrete mucus in the respiratory and digestive tracts.
   • Multicellular—many-celled glands.
     ○ Exocrine glands have ducts; salivary glands secrete saliva into ducts that carry it to the oral cavity.
     ○ Endocrine glands secrete hormones directly

into capillaries (no ducts); thyroid gland secretes thyroxine.

Connective Tissue—all have a non-living intercellular matrix and specialized cells (see Table 4–2 and Figs. 4–4 and 4–5)

1. Blood—the matrix is plasma, mostly water; transports materials in the blood. Red blood cells carry oxygen; white blood cells destroy pathogens and provide immunity; platelets prevent blood loss, as in clotting.
2. Areolar (loose)—cells are fibroblasts, which produce protein fibers: collagen is strong, elastin is elastic; the matrix is collagen, elastin, and tissue fluid. White blood cells are also present. Sites: below the dermis and below the epithelium of tracts that open to the environment (to destroy pathogens that enter the body).
3. Adipose—cells are adipocytes that store fat; little matrix. Sites: between the skin and muscles (to store energy); around the eyes and kidneys (to cushion).
4. Fibrous—mostly matrix, strong collagen fibers; cells are fibroblasts. Regular fibrous sites: tendons (to connect muscle to bone); ligaments (to connect bone to bone). Irregular fibrous sites: dermis of the skin and the fascia around muscles.
5. Elastic—mostly matrix, elastin fibers. Sites: walls of large arteries (to maintain blood pressure); around alveoli (to promote normal exhalation).
6. Bone—cells are osteocytes; matrix is calcium salts and collagen, strong and not flexible. Sites: bones of the skeleton (to support the body and protect internal organs from mechanical injury).
7. Cartilage—cells are chondrocytes; protein matrix is firm yet flexible; no capillaries in matrix. Sites: joint surfaces of bones (to prevent friction); tip of nose and external ear (to support); wall of trachea (to keep air passage open); discs between vertebrae (to absorb shock).

Muscle Tissue—specialized to contract and bring about movement (see Table 4–3 and Fig.4–6)

1. Skeletal—also called striated or voluntary muscle. Cells are cylindrical, have several nuclei, and have striations. Each cell has a motor nerve ending; nerve impulses are essential to cause contraction. Site: skeletal muscles attached to bones (to move the skeleton and produce heat).
2. Smooth—also called visceral or involuntary muscle. Cells have tapered ends, one nucleus each, and no striations. Contraction is not under voluntary control. Sites: stomach and intestines (peristalsis); walls of arteries and veins (to maintain blood pressure); iris (to constrict or dilate pupil).
3. Cardiac—cells are branched, have one nucleus each, and faint striations. Site: walls of chambers of the heart (to pump blood; nerve impulses regulate the rate of contraction).

Nerve Tissue—neurons are specialized to generate and transmit impulses (see Table 4–4 and Fig. 4–7)

1. Cell body contains the nucleus; axon carries impulses away from the cell body; dendrites carry impulses toward the cell body.
2. A synapse is the space between two neurons; a neurotransmitter carries the impulse across a synapse.
3. Specialized cells in nerve tissue are neuroglia in the CNS and Schwann cells in the PNS.
4. Sites: brain; spinal cord; and peripheral nerves (to provide sensation, movement, regulation of body functions, learning, and memory).

Membranes—sheets of tissue on surfaces, or separating organs or lobes

1. Epithelial membranes (see Fig. 4–8)
   - Serous membranes—in closed body cavities; the serous fluid prevents friction between the two layers of the serous membrane.
     ○ Thoracic cavity—partial pleura lines chest wall; visceral pleura covers the lungs.
     ○ Pericardial sac—parietal pericardium lines fibrous pericardium; visceral pericardium (epicardium) covers the heart muscle.
     ○ Abdominal cavity—peritoneum lines the abdominal cavity; mesentery covers the abdominal organs.
   - Mucous membranes—line body tracts that open to the environment: respiratory, digestive, urinary, and reproductive. Mucus keeps the living epithelium wet; provides lubrication in the digestive tract; traps dust and bacteria in the respiratory tract.
2. Connective tissue membranes—see Table 4–5.

REVIEW QUESTIONS

1. Explain the importance of each tissue in its location: (pp. 64, 66, 73)
   a. Simple squamous epithelium in the alveoli of the lungs
   b. Ciliated epithelium in the trachea
   c. Cartilage in the trachea

2. Explain the importance of each tissue in its location: (pp. 71–73)
   a. Bone tissue in bones
   b. Cartilage on the joint surfaces of bones
   c. Fibrous connective tissue in ligaments

3. State the functions of red blood cells, white blood cells, and platelets. (p. 69)

4. Name two organs made primarily of nerve tissue, and state the general functions of nerve tissue. (p. 75)

5. State the location and function of cardiac muscle. (p. 74)

6. Explain the importance of each of these tissues in the small intestine: smooth muscle and columnar epithelium. (pp. 66, 74)

7. State the precise location of each of the following membranes: (p. 76)
   a. Peritoneum
   b. Visceral pericardium
   c. Parietal pleura

8. State the function of: (pp. 68, 76)
   a. Serous fluid
   b. Mucus
   c. Blood plasma

9. State two functions of skeletal muscles. (p. 73)

10. Name three body tracts lined with mucous membranes. (p. 76)

11. Explain how endocrine glands differ from exocrine glands. (pp. 67–68)

12. State the function of adipose tissue: (pp. 70–71)
    a. Around the eyes
    b. Between the skin and muscles

13. State the location of: (p. 78)
    a. Meninges
    b. Synovial membranes

14. State the important physical characteristics of collagen and elastin, and name the cells that produce these protein fibers (p. 69).

FOR FURTHER THOUGHT

1. A friend suffers a knee injury involving damage to bone, cartilage, and ligaments. What can you tell your friend about the healing of these tissues?

2. Stratified squamous keratinizing epithelium is an excellent barrier to pathogens in the epidermis of the skin. Despite the fact that it is such a good barrier, this tissue would not be suitable for the lining of the trachea or small intestine. Explain why.

3. Many tissues have protective functions, but it is important to be specific about the kind of protection provided. Name at least three tissues with a protective function, and state what each protects the body (or parts of the body) against.

4. Why is blood classified as a connective tissue? What does it connect? What kinds of connections does it make?

CHAPTER 5

The Integumentary System

CHAPTER 5

Chapter Outline

The Skin

Epidermis

    Stratum germinativum

    Stratum corneum

    Langerhans cells

    Melanocytes

Dermis

    Hair follicles

    Nail follicles

    Receptors

    Glands

    Blood vessels

Other Functions of the Skin

Subcutaneous Tissue

Aging and the Integumentary System

Box 5–1	BURNS
Box 5–2	PREVENTING SKIN CANCER: COMMON SENSE AND SUNSCREENS
Box 5–3	COMMON SKIN DISORDERS
Box 5–4	ADMINISTERING MEDICATIONS

Student Objectives

- Name the two major layers of the skin and the tissue of which each is made.
- State the locations and describe the functions of the stratum corneum and stratum germinativum.
- Describe the function of Langerhans' cells.
- Describe the function of melanocytes and melanin.
- Describe the functions of hair and nails.
- Name the cutaneous senses and explain their importance.
- Describe the functions of the secretions of sebaceous glands, ceruminous glands, and eccrine sweat glands.
- Describe how the arterioles in the dermis respond to heat, cold, and stress.
- Name the tissues that make up the subcutaneous tissue, and describe their functions.

The Integumentary System

New Terminology

Arterioles (ar-**TEER**-ee-ohls)
Ceruminous gland/Cerumen (suh-**ROO**-mi-nus GLAND/suh-**ROO**-men)
Dermis (**DER**-miss)
Eccrine sweat gland (**EK**-rin SWET GLAND)
Epidermis (EP-i-**DER**-miss)
Hair follicle (HAIR **FAH**-li-kull)
Keratin (**KER**-uh-tin)
Melanin (**MEL**-uh-nin)
Melanocyte (muh-**LAN**-oh-sight)
Nail follicle (NAIL **FAH**-li-kull)
Papillary layer (**PAP**-i-LAR-ee **LAY**-er)
Receptors (ree-**SEP**-turs)
Sebaceous gland/sebum (suh-**BAY**-shus GLAND/ **SEE**-bum)
Stratum corneum (**STRA**-tum **KOR**-nee-um)
Stratum germinativum (**STRA**-tum JER-min-ah-**TEE**-vum)
Subcutaneous tissue (SUB-kew-**TAY**-nee-us **TISH**-yoo)
Vasoconstriction (VAY-zoh-kon-**STRIK**-shun)
Vasodilation (VAY-zoh-dye-**LAY**-shun)

Related Clinical Terminology

Acne (**AK**-nee)
Alopecia (AL-oh-**PEE**-she-ah)
Biopsy (**BYE**-op-see)
Carcinoma (KAR-sin-**OH**-mah)
Circulatory shock (**SIR**-kew-lah-TOR-ee SHAHK)
Contusion (kon-**TOO**-zhun)
Decubitus ulcer (dee-**KEW**-bi-tuss **UL**-ser)
Dehydration (DEE-high-**DRAY**-shun)
Dermatology (DER-muh-**TAH**-luh-gee)
Eczema (**EK**-zuh-mah)
Erythema (ER-i-**THEE**-mah)
Histamine (**HISS**-tah-meen)
Hives (**HIGH**-VZ)
Inflammation (IN-fluh-**MAY**-shun)
Melanoma (MEL-ah-**NO**-mah)
Nevus (**NEE**-vus)
Pruritus (proo-**RYE**-tus)

*Terms that appear in **bold type** in the chapter text are defined in the glossary, which begins on page 521.*

The integumentary system consists of the skin, its accessory structures such as hair and sweat glands, and the subcutaneous tissue below the skin. The skin is made of several different tissue types and is considered an organ. Because the skin covers the surface of the body, one of its functions is readily apparent: It separates the body from the external environment and prevents the entry of many harmful substances. The subcutaneous tissue directly underneath the skin connects it to the muscles and has other functions as well.

◉ THE SKIN

The two major layers of the skin are the outer **epidermis** and the inner **dermis.** Each of these layers is made of different tissues and has very different functions.

EPIDERMIS

The **epidermis** is made of stratified squamous keratinizing epithelial tissue and is thickest on the palms and soles. The cells that are most abundant are called **keratinocytes,** and there are no capillaries present between them. Although the epidermis may be further subdivided into four or five sublayers, two of these are of greatest importance: the innermost layer, the stratum germinativum, and the outermost layer, the stratum corneum (Fig. 5–1).

Stratum Germinativum

The **stratum germinativum** may also be called the stratum basale. Each name tells us something about this layer. To *germinate* means "to sprout" or "to grow." *Basal* means the "base" or "lowest part." The stratum germinativum is the base of the epidermis, the innermost layer in which **mitosis** takes place. New cells are continually being produced, pushing the older cells toward the skin surface. These cells produce the protein **keratin,** and as they get farther away from the capillaries in the dermis, they die. As dead cells are worn off the skin's surface, they are replaced by cells from the lower layers. Scattered among the keratinocytes of the stratum germinativum are very different cells called Merkel cells (or Merkel discs); these are receptors for the sense of touch (Fig. 5–2).

Stratum Corneum

The **stratum corneum,** the outermost epidermal layer, consists of many layers of dead cells; all that is left is their **keratin.** The protein keratin is relatively waterproof, and though the stratum corneum should not be thought of as a plastic bag encasing the body, it does prevent most evaporation of body water. Also of importance, keratin prevents the entry of water. Without a waterproof stratum corneum, it would be impossible to swim in a pool or even take a shower without damaging our cells.

The stratum corneum is also a barrier to pathogens and chemicals. Most bacteria and other microorganisms cannot penetrate unbroken skin. The flaking of dead cells from the skin surface helps remove microorganisms, and the fatty acids in sebum help inhibit their growth. Most chemicals, unless they are corrosive, will not get through unbroken skin to the living tissue within. One painful exception is the sap of poison ivy. This resin does penetrate the skin and initiates an allergic reaction in susceptible people. The inflammatory response that characterizes allergies causes blisters and severe itching. The importance of the stratum corneum becomes especially apparent when it is lost (see Box 5–1: Burns).

Certain minor changes in the epidermis are undoubtedly familiar to you. When first wearing new shoes, for example, the skin of the foot may be subjected to friction. This will separate layers of the epidermis, or separate the epidermis from the dermis, and tissue fluid may collect, causing a **blister.** If the skin is subjected to pressure, the rate of mitosis in the stratum germinativum will increase and create a thicker epidermis; we call this a **callus.** Although calluses are more common on the palms and soles, they may occur on any part of the skin.

Langerhans Cells

Within the epidermis are **Langerhans cells,** which are also called dendritic cells because of their branched appearance (see Fig. 5–2). These cells originate in the bone marrow, and are quite mobile. They are able to phagocytize foreign material, such as bacteria that enter the body through breaks in the skin. With such ingested pathogens, the Langerhans cells migrate to lymph nodes and present the pathogen to lymphocytes, a type of white blood cell. This triggers an immune response such as the

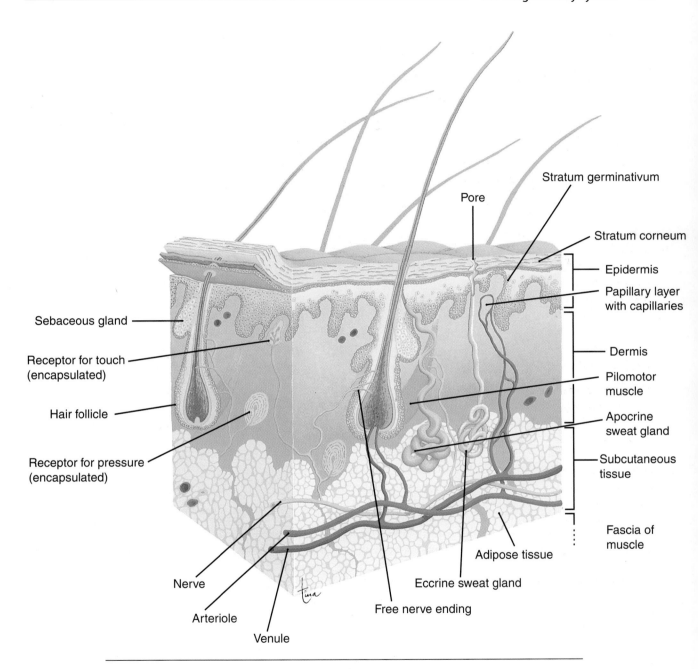

Figure 5–1 Skin. Structure of the skin and subcutaneous tissue.

production of antibodies. We now know that the skin is much more active in immunity than was previously believed, though many of the exact aspects of this have yet to be determined. Immunity is covered in Chapter 14.

Melanocytes

Another type of cell found in the lower epidermis is the melanocyte, which is also shown in Fig. 5–2. **Melanocytes** produce another protein, a pigment

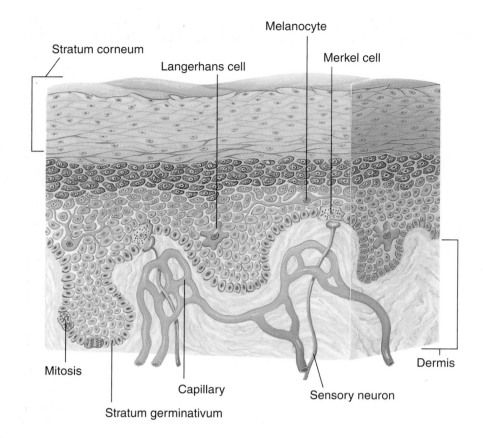

Stratum corneum

Langerhans cell

Melanocyte

Merkel cell

Mitosis

Capillary

Stratum germinativum

Sensory neuron

Dermis

Figure 5–2 The epidermis, showing the different kinds of cells present and the blood supply in the upper dermis.

called **melanin.** People of the same size have approximately the same number of melanocytes, though these cells may differ in their level of activity. In people with dark skin, the melanocytes continuously produce large amounts of melanin. The melanocytes of light-skinned people produce less melanin. The activity of melanocytes is genetically regulated; skin color is one of our hereditary characteristics.

In all people, melanin production is increased by exposure of the skin to ultraviolet rays, which are part of sunlight and are damaging to living cells. As more melanin is produced, it is taken in by the epidermal cells as they are pushed toward the surface. This gives the skin a darker color, which prevents further exposure of the living stratum germinativum to ultraviolet rays. People with dark skin already have good protection against the damaging effects of ultraviolet rays; people with light skin do not (see Box 5–2: Preventing Skin Cancer: Common Sense and Sunscreens).

Melanin also gives color to hair, though its protective function is confined to the hair of the head. Two parts of the eye obtain their color from melanin: the iris and the interior choroid layer of the eyeball (the eye is discussed in Chapter 9). The functions of the epidermis and its cells are summarized in Table 5–1.

DERMIS

The **dermis** is made of an irregular type of fibrous connective tissue. Fibroblasts produce both collagen and elastin fibers. Recall that **collagen** fibers are strong, and **elastin** fibers are able to recoil after being stretched. Strength and elasticity are two characteristics of the dermis. With increasing age, however, the deterioration of the elastin fibers causes the skin to lose its elasticity. We can all look forward to at least a few wrinkles as we get older.

The uneven junction of the dermis with the epidermis is called the **papillary layer** (see Fig. 5–1). Capil-

Box 5–1   BURNS

Burns of the skin may be caused by flames, hot water or steam, sunlight, electricity, or corrosive chemicals. The severity of burns ranges from minor to fatal, and the classification of burns is based on the extent of damage.

   First-Degree Burn—only the superficial epidermis is burned, and is painful but not blistered. Light-colored skin will appear red due to localized **vasodilation** in the damaged area. Vasodilation is part of the inflammatory response that brings more blood to the injured site.

   Second-Degree Burn—deeper layers of the epidermis are affected. Another aspect of **inflammation** is that damaged cells release

(Continued)

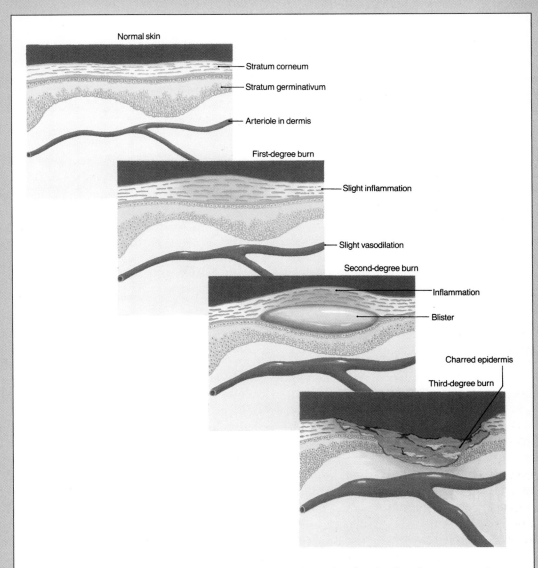

Box Figure 5–A   Normal skin section and representative section showing first-degree, second-degree, and third-degree burns.

Box 5–1   BURNS (Continued)

histamine, which makes capillaries more permeable. More plasma leaves these capillaries and becomes tissue fluid, which collects at the burn site, creating blisters. The burned skin is often very painful.

Third-Degree Burn—the entire epidermis is charred or burned away, and the burn may extend into the dermis or subcutaneous tissue. Often such a burn is not painful at first, if the receptors in the dermis have been destroyed.

Extensive third-degree burns are potentially life-threatening because of the loss of the stratum corneum. Without this natural barrier, living tissue is exposed to the environment and is susceptible to infection and dehydration.

Bacterial infection is a serious problem for burn patients; the pathogens may get into the blood **(septicemia)** and quickly spread throughout the body. Dehydration may also be fatal if medical intervention does not interrupt and correct the following sequence: Tissue fluid evaporates from the burned surface, and more plasma is pulled out of capillaries into the tissue spaces. As more plasma is lost, blood volume and blood pressure decrease. This is called **circulatory shock;** eventually the heart simply does not have enough blood to pump, and heart failure is the cause of death. To prevent these serious consequences, third-degree burns are covered with donor skin or artificial skin until skin grafts of the patients's own skin can be put in place.

---

laries are abundant here to nourish not only the dermis but also the stratum germinativum. The epidermis has no capillaries of its own, and the lower, living cells depend on the blood supply in the dermis for oxygen and nutrients.

Within the dermis are the accessory skin structures: hair and nail follicles, sensory receptors, and several types of glands. Some of these project through the epidermis to the skin surface, but their active portions are in the dermis.

Hair Follicles

Hair follicles are made of epidermal tissue, and the growth process of hair is very similar to growth of the epidermis. At the base of a follicle is the **hair root,** which contains cells called the **matrix,** where mitosis takes place (Fig. 5–3). The new cells produce keratin, get their color from melanin, then die and become incorporated into the **hair shaft,** which is pushed toward the surface of the skin. The hair that we comb and brush every day consists of dead, keratinized cells.

Compared to some other mammals, humans do not have very much hair. The actual functions of human hair are quite few. Eyelashes and eyebrows help to keep dust and perspiration out of the eyes, and the hairs just inside the nostrils help to keep dust out of the nasal cavities. Hair of the scalp does provide insulation from cold for the head. The hair on our bodies, however, no longer serves this function, but we have

the evolutionary remnants of it. Attached to each hair follicle is a small, smooth muscle called the **pilomotor** or arrector pili muscle. When stimulated by cold or emotions such as fear, these muscles pull the hair follicles upright. For an animal with fur, this would provide greater insulation. Because people do not have thick fur, all this does for us is give us "goose bumps."

Nail Follicles

Found on the ends of fingers and toes, **nail follicles** produce nails just as hair follicles produce hair. Mitosis takes place in the **nail root** (Fig. 5–4), and the new cells produce keratin (a stronger form of this protein than is found in hair) and then die. Although the nail itself consists of keratinized dead cells, the flat nail bed is living tissue. This is why cutting a nail too short can be quite painful. Nails protect the ends of the fingers and toes from mechanical injury, and give the fingers greater ability to pick up small objects. Fingernails are also good for scratching. This is more important than it may seem at first. An itch might mean the presence of an arthropod parasite, a mosquito, tick, flea, or louse. These parasites (all but the tick are insects) feed on blood, and all are potential vectors of diseases caused by bacteria, viruses, or protozoa. A quick and vigorous scratch may kill or at least dislodge the arthropod, and prevent the transmission of the disease.

Box 5–2 PREVENTING SKIN CANCER : COMMON SENSE AND SUNSCREENS

Anyone can get skin cancer, and the most important factor is exposure to sunlight. Light-skinned people are, of course, more susceptible to the effects of ultraviolet (UV) rays, which may trigger **mutations** in living epidermal cells.

Squamous cell **carcinoma** and basal cell carcinoma (see A below) are the most common forms of skin cancer. The lesions are visible as changes in the normal appearance of the skin, and a **biopsy** (microscopic examination of a tissue specimen) is used to confirm the diagnosis. These lesions usually do not metastasize rapidly, and can be completely removed using simple procedures.

Malignant melanoma (see B below) is a more serious form of skin cancer, which begins in melanocytes. Any change in a pigmented spot or mole **(nevus)** should prompt a person to see a doctor. Melanoma is serious not because of its growth in the skin, but because it may **metastasize** very rapidly to the lungs, liver, or other vital organ. Researchers are currently testing a vaccine for people who have had melanoma. The purpose of the vaccine is to stimulate the immune system strongly enough to prevent a second case, for such recurrences are often fatal.

Although the most common forms of skin cancer are readily curable, prevention is a much better strategy. We cannot, and we would not want to, stay out of the sun altogether, but we may be able to do so when sunlight is most damaging. During the summer months, UV rays are especially intense between 10 A.M. and 2 P.M.. If we are or must be outdoors during this time, use of a sunscreen is recommended by dermatologists.

Sunscreens contain chemicals such as PABA (para-amino benzoic acid) that block UV rays and prevent them from damaging the epidermis. An SPF (sun protection factor) of 15 or higher is considered good protection. Use of a sunscreen on exposed skin not only helps prevent skin cancer but prevents sunburn and its painful effects. It is especially important to prevent children from getting severely sunburned, because such burns have been linked to the development of skin cancer years later.

Box Figure 5–B **(A)** Classic basal cell carcinoma on face. **(B)** Melanoma in finger web. (From Goldsmith, LA, Lazarus, GS, and Tharp, MD: Adult and Pediatric Dermatology: A Color Guide to Diagnosis and Treatment. FA Davis, 1997, pp 137 and 144, with permission.)

Receptors

Most sensory **receptors** for the cutaneous senses are found in the dermis (Merkel cells are in the stratum germinativum, as are some nerve endings). The cutaneous senses are touch, pressure, heat, cold, and pain. For each sensation there is a specific type of receptor, which is a structure that will detect a particular change. For pain, heat, and cold, the receptors are **free nerve endings.** For touch and pressure, the receptors are called **encapsulated nerve endings,** which means there is a cellular structure around the sensory nerve ending (see Fig. 5–1). The purpose of these receptors and sensations is to provide the central nervous system with information about the external environment and its effect on the skin. This information may stimulate responses, such as washing a painful cut finger, scratching an insect bite, or responding to a feeling of cold by putting on a sweater.

The sensitivity of an area of skin is determined by how many receptors are present. The skin of the fingertips, for example, is very sensitive to touch

Table 5–1	EPIDERMIS
Part	**Function**
Stratum corneum (keratin)	• Prevents loss or entry of water • If unbroken, prevents entry of pathogens and most chemicals
Stratum germinativum (stratum basale)	• Continuous mitosis produces new cells to replace worn-off surface cells
Langerhans cells	• Phagocytize foreign material and stimulate an immune response by lymphocytes
Merkel cells	• Receptors for sense of touch
Melanocytes	• Produce melanin on exposure to ultraviolet (UV) rays
Melanin	• Protects living skin layers from further exposure to UV rays

Free edge of nail
Nail body
Lunula
Nail bed
Cuticle
Nail root

Figure 5–4 Structure of a fingernail shown in longitudinal section.

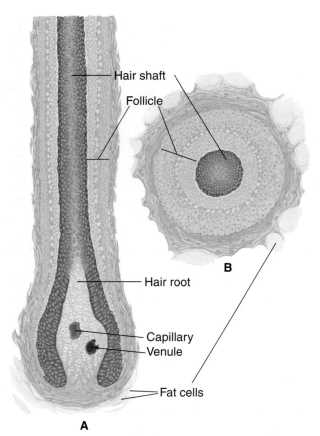

Hair shaft
Follicle
B
Hair root
Capillary
Venule
Fat cells
A

Figure 5–3 Structure of a hair follicle. **(A)** Longitudinal section. **(B)** Cross-section.

because there are many receptors per square inch. The skin of the upper arm, with few touch receptors per square inch, is less sensitive.

When receptors detect changes, they generate nerve impulses that are carried to the brain, which interprets the impulses as a particular sensation. Sensation, therefore, is actually a function of the brain (we will return to this in Chapters 8 and 9).

Glands

Glands are made of epithelial tissue. The exocrine glands of the skin have their secretory portions in the dermis. Some of these are shown in Fig. 5–1.

Sebaceous Glands   The ducts of **sebaceous glands** open into hair follicles or directly to the skin surface. Their secretion is **sebum,** a lipid substance that we commonly refer to as oil. As mentioned previously, sebum inhibits the growth of bacteria on the skin surface. Another function of sebum is to prevent drying of skin and hair. The importance of this may not be readily apparent, but skin that is dry tends to crack more easily. Even very small breaks in the skin are potential entryways for bacteria. Decreased sebum production is another consequence of getting older, and elderly people often have dry and more fragile skin.

Adolescents may have the problem of overactive sebaceous glands. Too much sebum may trap bacteria within hair follicles and create small infections.

Because sebaceous glands are more numerous around the nose and mouth, these are common sites of pimples in young people (see also Box 5–3: Common Skin Disorders).

Ceruminous Glands   These glands are located in the dermis of the ear canals. Their secretion is called **cerumen** or ear wax (which includes the sebum secreted in the ear canals). Cerumen keeps the outer surface of the eardrum pliable and prevents drying. However, if excess cerumen accumulates in the ear canal, it may become impacted against the eardrum. This might diminish the acuity of hearing by preventing the eardrum from vibrating properly.

Sweat Glands   There are two types of sweat glands, apocrine and eccrine. **Apocrine glands** are most numerous in the axillae (underarm) and genital areas and are most active in stress and emotional situations. Although their secretion does have an odor, it is barely perceptible to other people. However, animals, such as dogs, can tell people apart by their individual scents. If the apocrine secretions are allowed to accumulate on the skin, bacteria metabolize the chemicals in the sweat and produce waste products that have distinct odors that many people find unpleasant.

Eccrine glands are found all over the body but are especially numerous on the forehead, upper lip, palms, and soles. The secretory portion of these glands is simply a coiled tube in the dermis. The duct of this tube extends to the skin's surface, where it opens into a **pore**.

The sweat produced by eccrine glands is important in the maintenance of normal body temperature. In a warm environment, or during exercise, more sweat is secreted onto the skin surface, where it is then evaporated by excess body heat. Although this is a very effective mechanism of heat loss, it has a potentially serious disadvantage. Loss of too much body water in sweat may lead to **dehydration,** as in heat exhaustion. Increased sweating during exercise or on a hot day should always be accompanied by increased fluid intake.

Blood Vessels

Besides the capillaries in the dermis, the other blood vessels of great importance are the arterioles. **Arterioles** are small arteries, and the smooth muscle in their walls permits them to constrict (close) or dilate (open). This is important in the maintenance of body temper-

ature, because blood carries heat, which is a form of energy.

In a warm environment the arterioles dilate **(vasodilation)**, which increases blood flow through the dermis, and brings excess heat close to the body surface to be radiated to the environment. In a cold environment, however, body heat must be conserved if possible, so the arterioles constrict. The **vasoconstriction** decreases the flow of blood through the dermis and keeps heat within the core of the body. This adjusting mechanism is essential for maintaining homeostasis. Regulation of the diameter of the arterioles in response to external temperature changes is controlled by the nervous system. These changes can often be seen in light-skinned people. Flushing, especially in the face, may be observed in hot weather. In cold, the skin of the extremities may become even paler as blood flow through the dermis decreases. In people with dark skin, such changes are not as readily apparent because they are masked by melanin in the epidermis.

Vasoconstriction in the dermis may also occur during stressful situations. For our ancestors, stress usually demanded a physical response: Either stand and fight or run away to safety. This is called the "fight or flight response." Our nervous systems are still programmed to respond as if physical activity were necessary to cope with the stress situation. Vasoconstriction in the dermis will shunt, or redirect, blood to more vital organs such as the muscles, heart, and brain. In times of stress, the skin is a relatively unimportant organ and can function temporarily with a minimal blood flow. You have probably heard the expression "broke out in a cold sweat," and may even have felt it in a stressful situation. Such sweating feels cold because vasoconstriction in the dermis makes the skin relatively cool.

Blood flow in the dermis may be interrupted by prolonged pressure on the skin. For example, a hospital patient who cannot turn over by herself may develop a **decubitus ulcer,** also called a pressure ulcer. The skin is compressed between the object outside, such as a bed, and a bony prominence within, such as the heel bone or the sacrum in the lower back. Without its blood supply the skin dies, and the dead tissue is a potential site for bacterial infection.

OTHER FUNCTIONS OF THE SKIN

Excretion—small amounts of **urea** (a waste product of protein metabolism) and sodium chloride are

Box 5–3 COMMON SKIN DISORDER

Impetigo—a bacterial infection often caused by *streptococci* or *staphylococci*. The characteristic pustules (pus-containing lesions) crust as they heal; the infection is contagious to other children.

Eczema—a symptom of what is more properly called atopic dermatitis. This may be an allergic reaction, and is more common in children than adults; the rash is itchy (pruritus), and may blister or ooze. Eczema may be related to foods such as fish, eggs, or milk products, or to inhaled allergens such as dust, pollens, or animal dander. Prevention depends upon determining what the child is allergic to and eliminating or at least limiting exposure.

Warts—caused by a virus that makes epidermal cells divide abnormally, producing a growth on the skin that is often raised and has a rough or pitted surface. Warts are probably most common on the hands, but they may be anywhere on the skin. Plantar warts on the sole of the foot may become quite painful because of the constant pressure of standing and walking.

Fever blisters (cold sores)—caused by the Herpes simplex virus, to which most people are exposed as children. An active lesion, usually at the edge of the lip, (but may be anywhere on the skin) is painful and oozes. If not destroyed by the immune system, the virus "hides out" and becomes dormant in nerves of the face. Another lesion, weeks or months later, may be triggered by stress or another illness.

Box Figure 5–C **(A)** Impetigo. **(B)** Eczema of atopic dermatitis. **(C)** Warts on back of hands. **(D)** Fever blister on finger, localized but severe. (From Goldsmith, LA, Lazarus, GS, and Tharp, MD: Adult and Pediatric Dermatology: A Color Guide to Diagnosis and Treatment. FA Davis, 1997, pp 80, 241, 306, and 317, with permission.)

Table 5–2	DERMIS
Part	**Function**
Papillary layer	• Contains capillaries that nourish the stratum germinativum
Hair (follicles)	• Eyelashes and nasal hair keep dust out of eyes and nasal cavities • Scalp hair provides insulation from cold for the head
Nails (follicles)	• Protect ends of fingers and toes from mechanical injury
Receptors	• Detect changes that are felt as the cutaneous senses: touch, pressure, heat, cold, and pain
Sebaceous glands	• Produce sebum, which prevents drying of skin and hair and inhibits growth of bacteria
Ceruminous glands	• Produce cerumen, which prevents drying of the eardrum
Eccrine sweat glands	• Produce watery sweat that is evaporated by excess body heat to cool the body
Arterioles	• Dilate in response to warmth to increase heat loss • Constrict in response to cold to conserve body heat • Constrict in stressful situations to shunt blood to more vital organs
Cholesterol	• Converted to vitamin D on exposure to UV rays

Table 5–3	SUBCUTANEOUS TISSUE
Part	**Function**
Areolar connective tissue	• Connects skin to muscles • Contains many WBCs to destroy pathogens that enter breaks in the skin
Adipose tissue	• Contains stored energy in the form of true fats • Cushions bony prominences • Provides some insulation from cold

excreted in sweat. This is a very minor function of the skin; the kidneys are primarily responsible for removing waste products from the blood.

Formation of **vitamin D**—there is a form of cholesterol in the skin that, on exposure to ultraviolet light, is changed to vitamin D. This is why vitamin D is sometimes referred to as the "sunshine vitamin." People who do not get much sunlight depend more on nutritional sources of vitamin D, such as fortified milk. Vitamin D is important for the absorption of calcium and phosphorus from food in the small intestine. The functions of dermal structures are summarized in Table 5–2.

SUBCUTANEOUS TISSUE

The **subcutaneous tissue** may also be called the **superficial fascia,** one of the connective tissue membranes. Made of areolar connective tissue and adipose tissue, the superficial fascia connects the dermis to the underlying muscles. Its other functions are those of its tissues, as you may recall from Chapter 4.

Areolar connective tissue contains collagen and elastin fibers and many white blood cells that have left capillaries to wander around in the tissue fluid between skin and muscles. These migrating white blood cells destroy pathogens that enter the body through breaks in the skin.

The cells (adipocytes) of adipose tissue are specialized to store fat, and our subcutaneous layer of fat stores excess nutrients as a potential energy source. This layer also cushions bony prominences, such as when sitting, and provides some insulation from cold. For people, this last function is relatively minor, because we do not have a thick layer of fat, as do animals such as whales and seals. The functions of subcutaneous tissue are summarized in Table 5–3. Box 5–4, Administering Medications, describes ways in which we give medications through the skin.

AGING AND THE INTEGUMENTARY SYSTEM

The effects of age on the integumentary system are often quite visible. Both layers of skin become thinner and more fragile as mitosis in the epidermis slows and fibroblasts in the dermis die and are not replaced. The skin becomes wrinkled as collagen and elastin fibers in the dermis deteriorate. Sebaceous glands and sweat glands become less active; the skin becomes dry, and temperature regulation in hot weather becomes more difficult. Hair follicles become inactive

Box 5–4   ADMINISTERING MEDICATIONS

You have probably seen television or print advertisements for skin patches that supply nicotine, and you know that their purpose is to help smokers give up cigarettes. This method of supplying a medication is called *transdermal administration.* The name is a little misleading because the most difficult part of cutaneous absorption of a drug is absorption through the stratum corneum of the epidermis. Because such absorption is slow, skin patches are useful for medications needed in small but continuous amounts, and over a prolonged period of time.

You would expect that such patches should be worn where the epidermis is thin. These sites include the upper arm and the chest. The recommended site for a patch to prevent motion sickness is the skin behind the ear. A skin patch for birth control for women has also been developed. It contains the hormones estrogen and progesterone, and is similar to birth control pills in that its purpose is to prevent ovulation.

Medications may also be injected through the skin. Some injections are given subcutaneously, that is, into subcutaneous tissue (see Box Fig. 5–D). Subcutaneous adipose tissue has a moderate blood supply, so the rate of absorption of the drug will be moderate, but is predictable. Insulin is given subcutaneously. Other injections are intramuscular, and absorption into the blood is rapid because muscle tissue has a very good blood supply. Most injectable vaccines are given intramuscularly, to promote rapid absorption to stimulate antibody production.

Box Figure 5–D   The skin, subcutaneous tissue, and muscle sites for the delivery of medications.

and hair on the scalp and body thins. Melanocytes die and the hair that remains becomes white. There is often less fat in the subcutaneous tissue, which may make an elderly person more sensitive to cold. It is important for elderly people (and those who care for them) to realize that extremes of temperature may be harmful and to take special precautions in very hot or very cold weather.

SUMMARY

The integumentary system is the outermost organ system of the body. You have probably noticed that many of its functions are related to this location. The skin protects the body against pathogens and chemicals, minimizes loss or entry of water, and blocks the harmful effects of sunlight. Sensory receptors in the skin provide information about the external environment, and the skin helps regulate body temperature in response to environmental changes.

STUDY OUTLINE

The integumentary system consists of the skin and its accessory structures and the subcutaneous tissue. The two major layers of the skin are the outer epidermis and the inner dermis.

Epidermis—made of stratified squamous epithelium; no capillaries; cells called keratinocytes (see Figs. 5–1 and 5–2 and Table 5–1)
1. Stratum germinativum—the innermost layer where mitosis takes place; new cells produce keratin and die as they are pushed toward the surface.
2. Stratum corneum—the outermost layers of dead cells; keratin prevents loss and entry of water and resists entry of pathogens and chemicals.
3. Langerhans cells—phagocytize foreign material and stimulate an immune response by lymphocytes.
4. Melanocytes—in the lower epidermis, produce melanin. UV rays stimulate melanin production; melanin prevents further exposure of the stratum germinativum to UV rays by darkening the skin.

Dermis—made of irregular fibrous connective tissue; collagen provides strength, and elastin provides elasticity; capillaries in the papillary layer nourish the stratum germinativum (see Table 5–2 and Fig. 5–1)
1. Hair follicles—mitosis takes place in the hair root; new cells produce keratin, die, and become the hair shaft. Hair of the scalp provides insulation from cold for the head; eyelashes keep dust out of eyes; nostril hairs keep dust out of nasal cavities (see Figs. 5–1 and 5–3).
2. Nail follicles—at the ends of fingers and toes; mitosis takes place in the nail root; the nail itself is dead, keratinized cells. Nails protect the ends of the fingers and toes, enable the fingers to pick up small objects, and provide for efficient scratching (see Fig. 5–4).
3. Receptors—detect changes in the skin: touch, pressure, heat, cold, and pain; provide information about the external environment that initiates appropriate responses; sensitivity of the skin depends on the number of receptors present.
4. Sebaceous glands—secrete sebum into hair follicles or to the skin surface; sebum inhibits the growth of bacteria and prevents drying of skin and hair.
5. Ceruminous glands—secrete cerumen in the ear canals; cerumen prevents drying of the eardrum.
6. Apocrine sweat glands—modified scent glands in axillae and genital area; activated by stress and emotions.
7. Eccrine sweat glands—most numerous on face, palms, soles. Activated by high external temperature or exercise; sweat on skin surface is evaporated by excess body heat; potential disadvantage is dehydration.
8. Arterioles—smooth muscle permits constriction or dilation. Vasoconstriction in cold temperatures decreases dermal blood flow to conserve heat in the body core. Vasodilation in warm temperatures increases dermal blood flow to bring heat to the surface to be lost. Vasoconstriction during stress shunts blood away from the skin to more vital organs, such as muscles, to permit a physical response, if necessary.

Other Functions of the Skin
1. Excretion of small amounts of urea and NaCl (minor function).
2. Formation of vitamin D from cholesterol on exposure to UV rays of sunlight.

Subcutaneous Tissue—also called the superficial fascia; connects skin to muscles (see Fig. 5–1 and Table 5–3)

1. Areolar tissue—contains WBCs that destroy pathogens that get through breaks in the skin.

2. Adipose tissue—stores fat as potential energy; cushions bony prominences; provides some insulation from cold.

REVIEW QUESTIONS

1. Name the parts of the integumentary system. (p. 84)

2. Name the two major layers of skin, the location of each, and the tissue of which each is made. (pp. 84, 86)

3. In the epidermis: (p. 84)
   a. Where does mitosis take place?
   b. What protein do the new cells produce?
   c. What happens to these cells?
   d. What is the function of Langerhans cells?

4. Describe the functions of the stratum corneum. (p. 84)

5. Name the cells that produce melanin. What is the stimulus? Describe the function of melanin (p. 86)

6. Where, on the body, does human hair have important functions? Describe these functions. (p. 88)

7. Describe the functions of nails. (p. 88)

8. Name the cutaneous senses. Describe the importance of these senses. (p. 89–90)

9. Explain the functions of sebum and cerumen. (pp. 90–91)

10. Explain how sweating helps maintain normal body temperature. (p. 91)

11. Explain how the arterioles in the dermis respond to cold or warm external temperatures and to stress situations. (p. 91)

12. What vitamin is produced in the skin? What is the stimulus for the production of this vitamin? (p. 93)

13. Name the tissues of which the superficial fascia is made. Describe the functions of these tissues. (p. 93)

FOR FURTHER THOUGHT

1. The epidermis has no capillaries of its own; the stratum corneum is made of dead cells and doesn't need a blood supply at all. Explain why the epidermis is affected by a decubitus ulcer. Name another group of people, besides hospital or nursing home patients, that is especially susceptible to developing pressure ulcers.

2. Going out in the sun stimulates quite a bit of activity in the skin, especially on a hot summer day. Describe what is happening in the skin in response to sunlight.

3. Ringworm is a skin condition characterized by scaly red patches, often circular or oval in shape. It is not caused by a worm, but rather by certain fungi. What is the food of these fungi, that is, what are they digesting?

4. There are several kinds of cells in the epidermis. Which cells exert their functions when they are dead? Which cells must be living in order to function?

5. Wearing a hat in winter is a good idea. What happens to the arterioles in the dermis in a cold environment? How does this affect heat loss? Is the head an exception? Explain.

CHAPTER 6

The Skeletal System

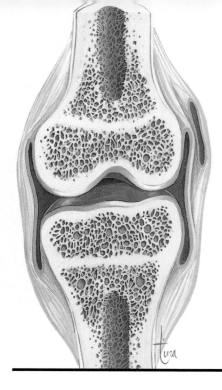

CHAPTER 6

Student Objectives

- Describe the functions of the skeleton.
- Explain how bones are classified, and give an example of each type.
- Describe how the embryonic skeleton model is replaced by bone.
- Name the nutrients necessary for bone growth, and explain their functions.
- Name the hormones involved in bone growth and maintenance, and explain their functions.
- Explain what is meant by "exercise" for bones, and explain its importance.
- Name all the bones of the human skeleton (be able to point to each on diagrams, skeleton models, or yourself).
- Describe the functions of the skull, vertebral column, rib cage, scapula, and pelvic bone.
- Explain how joints are classified. For each type, give an example, and describe the movement possible.
- Describe the parts of a synovial joint, and explain their functions.

The Skeletal System

New Terminology

Appendicular (AP-en-**DIK**-yoo-lar)
Articulation (ar-TIK-yoo-**LAY**-shun)
Axial (**AK**-see-uhl)
Bursa (**BURR**-sah)
Diaphysis (dye-**AFF**-i-sis)
Epiphyseal disc (e-**PIFF**-i-SEE-al DISK)
Epiphysis (e-**PIFF**-i-sis)
Fontanel (FON-tah-**NELL**)
Haversian system (ha-**VER**-zhun **SIS**-tem)
Ligament (**LIG**-uh-ment)
Ossification (AHS-i-fi-**KAY**-shun)
Osteoblast (**AHS**-tee-oh-BLAST)
Osteoclast (**AHS**-tee-oh-KLAST)
Paranasal sinus (PAR-uh-**NAY**-zuhl **SIGH**-nus)
Periosteum (PER-ee-**AHS**-tee-um)
Suture (**SOO**-cher)
Symphysis (**SIM**-fi-sis)
Synovial fluid (sin-**OH**-vee-al **FLOO**-id)

Related Clinical Terminology

Autoimmune disease (AW-toh-im-**YOON** di-**ZEEZ**)
Bursitis (burr-**SIGH**-tiss)
Cleft palate (KLEFT **PAL**-uht)
Fracture (**FRAK**-chur)
Herniated disc (**HER**-nee-ay-ted DISK)
Kyphosis (kye-**FOH**-sis)
Lordosis (lor-**DOH**-sis)
Osteoarthritis (AHS-tee-oh-ar-**THRY**-tiss)
Osteomyelitis (AHS-tee-oh-my-uh-**LYE**-tiss)
Osteoporosis (AHS-tee-oh-por-**OH**-sis)
Rheumatoid arthritis (**ROO**-muh-toyd ar-**THRY**-tiss)
Rickets (**RIK**-ets)
Scoliosis (SKOH-lee-**OH**-sis)

*Terms that appear in **bold type** in the chapter text are defined in the glossary, which begins on page 521.*

Imagine for a moment that people did not have skeletons. What comes to mind? Probably that each of us would be a little heap on the floor, much like a jellyfish out of water. Such an image is accurate and reflects the most obvious function of the skeleton: to support the body. Although it is a framework for the body, the skeleton is not at all like the wooden beams that support a house. Bones are living organs that actively contribute to the maintenance of the internal environment of the body.

The **skeletal system** consists of bones and other structures that make up the joints of the skeleton. The types of tissue present are bone tissue, cartilage, and fibrous connective tissue, which forms the ligaments that connect bone to bone.

FUNCTIONS OF THE SKELETON

1. Provides a framework that supports the body; the muscles that are attached to bones move the skeleton.
2. Protects some internal organs from mechanical injury; the rib cage protects the heart and lungs, for example.
3. Contains and protects the red bone marrow, one of the hemopoietic (blood-forming) tissues.
4. Provides a storage site for excess calcium. Calcium may be removed from bone to maintain a normal blood calcium level, which is essential for blood clotting and proper functioning of muscles and nerves.

TYPES OF BONE TISSUE

Bone was described as a tissue in Chapter 4. Recall that bone cells are called **osteocytes**, and the **matrix** of bone is made of calcium salts and collagen. The **calcium salts** are calcium carbonate ($CaCO_3$) and calcium phosphate ($Ca_3(PO_4)_2$), which give bone the strength for its supportive and protective functions. Bone matrix is non-living, but it changes constantly, with calcium that is taken from bone into the blood replaced by calcium from the diet. In normal circumstances, the amount of calcium that is removed is replaced by an equal amount of calcium deposited. This is the function of osteocytes, to regulate the amount of calcium that is deposited in, or removed from, the bone matrix.

In bone as an organ, two types of bone tissue are present (Fig. 6–1). **Compact bone** looks solid but is very precisely structured. Compact bone is made of **haversian systems**: microscopic cylinders of bone matrix with osteocytes in concentric rings around central **haversian canals**. In the haversian canals are blood vessels; the osteocytes are in contact with these blood vessels and with one another through microscopic channels (**canaliculi**) in the matrix.

The second type of bone tissue is **spongy bone**, which does look rather like a sponge with its visible holes or cavities. Osteocytes, matrix, and blood vessels are present but are not arranged in haversian systems. The cavities in spongy bone often contain **red bone marrow**, which produces red blood cells, platelets, and the five types of white blood cells.

CLASSIFICATION OF BONES

1. **Long bones**—the bones of the arms, legs, hands, and feet (but not the wrists and ankles). The shaft of a long bone is the **diaphysis**, and the ends are called **epiphyses** (see Fig. 6–1). The diaphysis is made of compact bone and is hollow, forming a canal within the shaft. This **marrow canal** (or medullary cavity) contains **yellow bone marrow**, which is mostly adipose tissue. The epiphyses are made of spongy bone covered with a thin layer of compact bone. Although red bone marrow is present in the epiphyses of children's bones, it is largely replaced by yellow bone marrow in adult bones.
2. **Short bones**—the bones of the wrists and ankles.
3. **Flat bones**—the ribs, shoulder blades, hip bones, and cranial bones.
4. **Irregular bones**—the vertebrae and facial bones.

Short, flat, and irregular bones are all made of spongy bone covered with a thin layer of compact bone. Red bone marrow is found within the spongy bone.

The joint surfaces of bones are covered with **articular cartilage**, which provides a smooth surface. Covering the rest of the bone is the **periosteum**, a fibrous connective tissue membrane whose collagen fibers merge with those of the tendons and ligaments that are attached to the bone. The periosteum anchors these structures, contains the blood vessels that enter the bone itself, and contains osteoblasts that will become active if the bone is damaged.

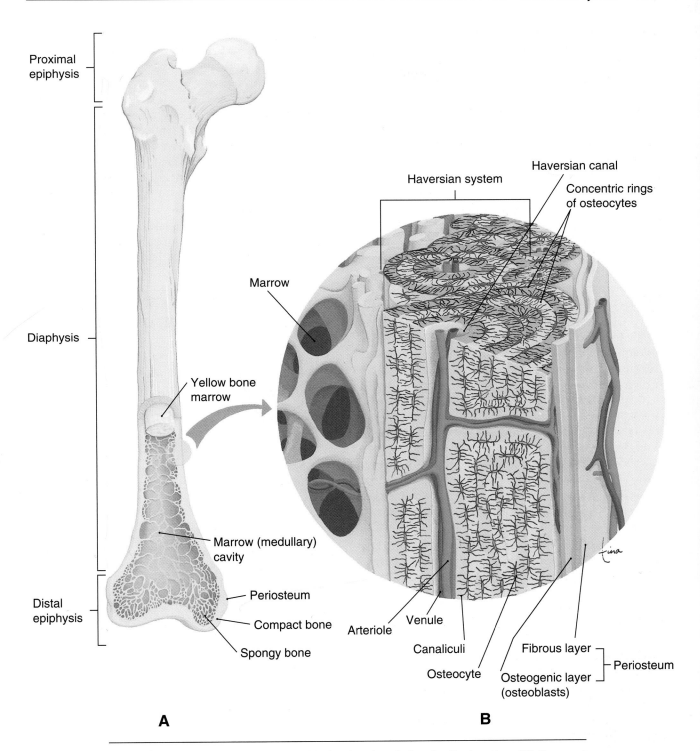

Figure 6–1 Bone tissue. **(A)** Femur with distal end cut in longitudinal section. **(B)** Compact bone showing haversian systems.

EMBRYONIC GROWTH OF BONE

During embryonic development, the skeleton is first made of cartilage and fibrous connective tissue, which are gradually replaced by bone. Bone matrix is produced by cells called **osteoblasts** (a *blast* cell is a "producing" cell, and *osteo* means "bone"). In the embryonic model of the skeleton, osteoblasts differentiate from the fibroblasts that are present. The production of bone matrix, called **ossification**, begins in a **center of ossification** in each bone.

The cranial and facial bones are first made of fibrous connective tissue. In the third month of fetal development, fibroblasts (spindle-shaped connective tissue cells) become more specialized and differentiate into osteoblasts, which produce bone matrix. From each center of ossification, bone growth radiates outward as calcium salts are deposited in the collagen of the model of the bone. This process is not complete at birth; a baby has areas of fibrous connective tissue remaining between the bones of the skull. These are called **fontanels** (Fig. 6–2), which permit compression of the baby's head during birth without breaking the still thin cranial bones. The fontanels also permit the growth of the brain after birth. You may have heard fontanels referred to as "soft spots," and indeed they are. A baby's skull is still quite fragile and must be protected from trauma. By the age of 2 years, all the fontanels have become ossified, and the skull becomes a more effective protective covering for the brain.

The rest of the embryonic skeleton is first made of cartilage, and ossification begins in the third month of gestation in the long bones. Osteoblasts produce bone matrix in the center of the diaphyses of the long bones and in the center of short, flat, and irregular bones. Bone matrix gradually replaces the original cartilage (Fig. 6–3).

The long bones also develop centers of ossification in their epiphyses. At birth, ossification is not yet complete and continues throughout childhood. In long bones, growth occurs in the **epiphyseal discs** at the junction of the diaphysis with each epiphysis. An epiphyseal disc is still cartilage, and the bone grows in length as more cartilage is produced on the epiphysis side (see Fig. 6–3). On the diaphysis side, osteoblasts produce bone matrix to replace the cartilage. Between the ages of 16 and 25 years (influenced by estrogen or testosterone), all of the cartilage of the epiphyseal discs is replaced by bone. This is called closure of the epiphyseal discs, and the bone lengthening process stops.

Also in bones are specialized cells called **osteoclasts**. These cells are very active in embryonic long bones, and reabsorb bone matrix in the center of the diaphysis to form the **marrow canal**. Blood vessels grow into the marrow canals of embryonic long bones, and red bone marrow is established. After birth, the red bone marrow is replaced by yellow bone marrow. Red bone marrow remains in the spongy bone of short, flat, and irregular bones. For other functions of osteoclasts and osteoblasts, see Box 6–1: Fractures and Their Repair.

FACTORS THAT AFFECT BONE GROWTH AND MAINTENANCE

1. Heredity—each person has a genetic potential for height, that is, a maximum height, with genes inherited from both parents. Many genes are involved, and their interactions are not well understood. Some of these genes are probably those for the enzymes involved in cartilage and bone production, for this is how bones grow.
2. Nutrition—nutrients are the raw materials of which bones are made. Calcium, phosphorus, and protein become part of the bone matrix itself. Vitamin D is needed for the efficient absorption of calcium and phosphorus by the small intestine. Vitamins A and C do not become part of bone but are necessary for the process of bone matrix formation (ossification).

   Without these and other nutrients, bones cannot grow properly. Children who are malnourished grow very slowly and may not reach their genetic potential for height.
3. Hormones—endocrine glands produce hormones that stimulate specific effects in certain cells. Several hormones have important roles in bone growth and maintenance. These include growth hormone, thyroxine, parathyroid hormone, and insulin, which help regulate cell division, protein synthesis, calcium metabolism, and energy production. The hormones and their specific functions are listed in Table 6–1.
4. Exercise or "stress"—for bones, exercise means bearing weight, which is just what bones are

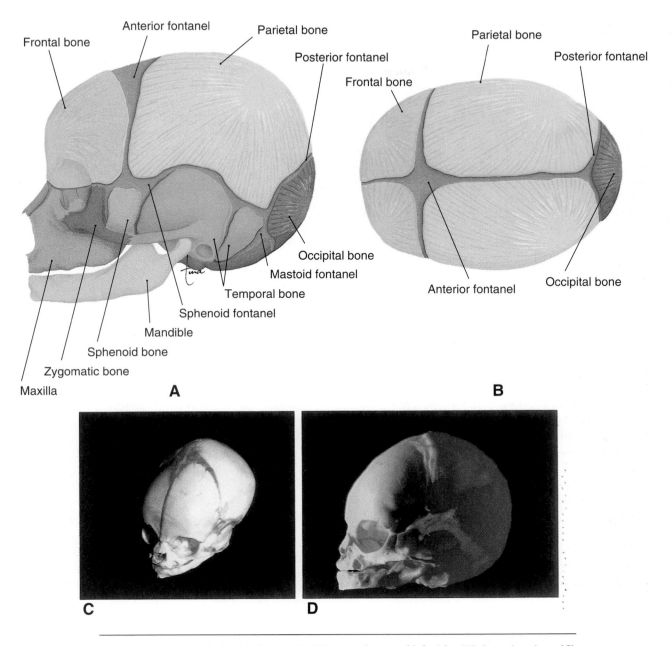

Figure 6–2 Infant skull with fontanels. **(A)** Lateral view of left side. **(B)** Superior view. **(C)** Fetal skull in anterior superior view. **(D)** Fetal skull in left lateral view. Try to name the bones; use part A as a guide. The fontanels are translucent connective tissue. (C and D photographs by Dan Kaufman.)

B Epiphyseal disc

Chondrocytes producing cartilage

Osteoblasts producing bone

Bone

Epiphyseal disc

Cartilage

Compact bone

Secondary ossification center

Medullary cavity containing marrow

Compact bone

Cartilaginous model

Bone collar and calcifying cartilage in ossification center

Medullary cavity and development of secondary ossification centers

Spongy bone

Articular cartilage

A

Figure 6–3 The ossification process in a long bone. **(A)** Progression of ossification from the cartilage model of the embryo to the bone of a young adult. **(B)** Microscopic view of an epiphyseal disc showing cartilage production and bone replacement.

Box 6–1   FRACTURES AND THEIR REPAIR

A fracture means that a bone has been broken. There are different types of fractures classified as to extent of damage.

Simple (closed)—the broken parts are still in normal anatomic position; surrounding tissue damage is minimal (skin is not pierced).

Compound (open)—the broken end of a bone has been moved, and it pierces the skin; there may be extensive damage to surrounding blood vessels, nerves, and muscles.

Greenstick—the bone splits longitudinally. The bones of children contain more collagen than do adult bones and tend to splinter rather than break completely.

Comminuted—two or more intersecting breaks create several bone fragments.

Impacted—the broken ends of a bone are forced into one another; many bone fragments may be created.

Pathologic spontaneous—a bone breaks without apparent trauma; may accompany bone disorders such as osteoporosis.

The Repair Process

Even a simple fracture involves significant bone damage that must be repaired if the bone is to resume its normal function. Fragments of dead or damaged bone must first be removed. This is accomplished by osteoclasts, which dissolve and reabsorb the calcium salts of bone matrix. Imagine a building that has just collapsed; the rubble must be removed before reconstruction can take place. This is what the osteoclasts do. Then, new bone must be produced. The inner layer of the periosteum contains osteoblasts that are activated when bone is damaged. The osteoblasts produce bone matrix to knit the broken ends of the bone together.

Because most bone has a good blood supply, the repair process is usually relatively rapid, and a simple fracture often heals within 6 weeks. Some parts of bones, however, have a poor blood supply, and repair of fractures takes longer. These areas are the neck of the femur (the site of a "fractured hip") and the lower third of the tibia.

Other factors that influence repair include the age of the person, general state of health, and nutri-tion. The elderly and those in poor health often have slow healing of fractures. A diet with sufficient calcium, phosphorus, vitamin D, and protein is also important. If any of these nutrients is lacking, bone repair will be a slower process.

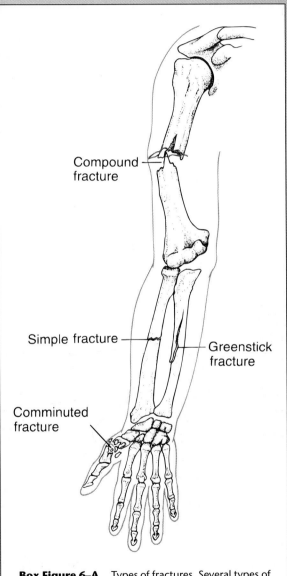

Box Figure 6–A   Types of fractures. Several types of fractures are depicted in the right arm.

Table 6–1	**HORMONES INVOLVED IN BONE GROWTH AND MAINTENANCE**
Growth hormone (anterior pituitary gland)	• Increases the rate of mitosis of chondrocytes and osteoblasts • Increases the rate of protein synthesis (collagen, cartilage matrix, and enzymes for cartilage and bone formation)
Thyroxine (thyroid gland)	• Increases the rate of protein synthesis • Increases energy production from all food types
Insulin (pancreas)	• Increases energy production from glucose
Parathyroid hormone (parathyroid glands)	• Increases the reabsorption of calcium from bones to the blood (raises blood calcium level) • Increases the absorption of calcium by the small intestine and kidneys (to the blood)
Calcitonin (thyroid gland)	• Decreases the reabsorption of calcium from bones (lowers blood calcium level)
Estrogen (ovaries) or Testosterone (testes)	• Promotes closure of the epiphyses of long bones (growth stops) • Helps retain calcium in bones to maintain a strong bone matrix

specialized to do. Without this stress (which is normal), bones will lose calcium faster than it is replaced. Exercise need not be strenuous; it can be as simple as the walking involved in everyday activities. Bones that do not get this exercise, such as those of bed-ridden patients, will become thinner and more fragile. This condition is discussed further in Box 6–2: Osteoporosis.

THE SKELETON

The human skeleton has two divisions: the **axial skeleton**, which forms the axis of the body, and the **appendicular skeleton**, which supports the appendages or limbs. The axial skeleton consists of the skull, vertebral column, and rib cage. The bones of the arms and legs and the shoulder and pelvic girdles make up the appendicular skeleton. There are 206 bones in total, and the complete skeleton is shown in Fig. 6–4.

SKULL

The **skull** consists of 8 cranial bones and 14 facial bones. Also in the head are three small bones in each middle ear cavity and the hyoid bone that supports the base of the tongue. The **cranial bones** form the braincase (lined with the meninges) that encloses and protects the brain, eyes, and ears. The names of some of these bones will be familiar to you; they are the

same as the terminology used (see Chapter 1) to describe areas of the head. These are the **frontal bone, parietal bones** (two), **temporal bones** (two), and **occipital bone**. The **sphenoid bone** and **ethmoid bone** are part of the floor of the braincase and the orbits (sockets) for the eyes. The sphenoid bone also encloses the pituitary gland, in a depression called the sella turcica. The ethmoid bone also forms the roof and upper walls of the nasal cavities, and the upper part of the nasal septum.

All of the joints between cranial bones are immovable joints called **sutures**. It may seem strange to refer to a joint without movement, but the term *joint* is used for any junction of two bones. The classification of joints will be covered later in this chapter. All the bones of the skull, as well as the large sutures, are shown in Figs. 6–5 through 6–8. Their anatomically important parts are described in Table 6–2.

Of the 14 **facial bones**, only the **mandible** (lower jaw) is movable; it forms a **condyloid joint** with each temporal bone. The other joints between facial bones are all sutures. The **maxillae** are the upper jaw bones, which also form the anterior portion of the hard palate (roof of the mouth). Sockets for the roots of the teeth are found in the maxillae and the mandible. The other facial bones are described in Table 6–2.

Paranasal sinuses are air cavities located in the maxillae, and frontal, sphenoid, and ethmoid bones (Fig. 6–9). As the name *paranasal* suggests, they open into the nasal cavities and are lined with **cili-**

Box 6–2 OSTEOPOROSIS

Bone is an active tissue; calcium is constantly being removed to maintain normal blood calcium levels. Usually, however, calcium is replaced in bones at a rate equal to its removal, and the bone matrix remains strong.

Osteoporosis is characterized by excessive loss of calcium from bones without sufficient replacement. Research has suggested that a certain gene for bone buildup in youth is an important factor; less buildup would mean earlier bone thinning. Contributing environmental factors include smoking, insufficient dietary intake of calcium, inactivity, and lack of the sex hormones. Osteoporosis is most common among elderly women, because estrogen secretion decreases sharply at menopause (in older men, testosterone is still secreted in significant amounts). Factors such as bed rest or inability to get even minimal exercise will make calcium loss even more rapid.

As bones lose calcium and become thin and brittle, fractures are much more likely to occur. Among elderly women, a fractured hip (the neck of the femur) is an all-too-common consequence of this degenerative bone disorder. Such a serious injury is not inevitable, however, and neither is the thinning of the vertebrae that bows the spines of some elderly people. After menopause, women may wish to have a bone density test to determine the strength of their bone matrix. Several medications are available that diminish the rate of bone loss. A diet high in calcium and vitamin D is essential for both men and women, as is moderate exercise. Also an option for women is estrogen replacement therapy, which slows bone loss (but is not without risks). Young women and teenagers should make sure they get adequate dietary calcium to form strong bone matrix, because this will delay the serious effects of osteoporosis later in life.

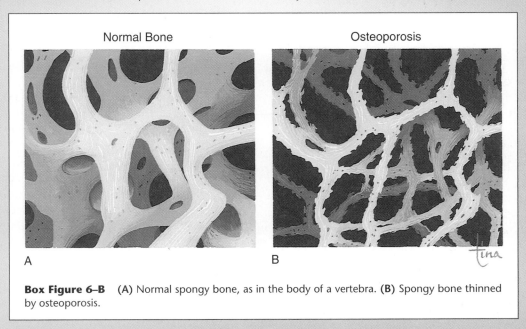

Normal Bone   Osteoporosis

A   B

Box Figure 6–B (A) Normal spongy bone, as in the body of a vertebra. (B) Spongy bone thinned by osteoporosis.

ated epithelium continuous with the mucosa of the nasal cavities. We are aware of our sinuses only when they become "stuffed up," which means that the mucus they produce cannot drain into the nasal cavities. This may happen during upper respiratory infections such as colds, or with allergies such as hay fever. These sinuses, however, do have functions: They make the skull lighter in weight, because air is lighter than bone, and they provide resonance for the voice.

The **mastoid sinuses** are air cavities in the mastoid process of each temporal bone; they open into the middle ear. Before the availability of antibiotics, middle ear infections often caused mastoiditis, infection of these sinuses.

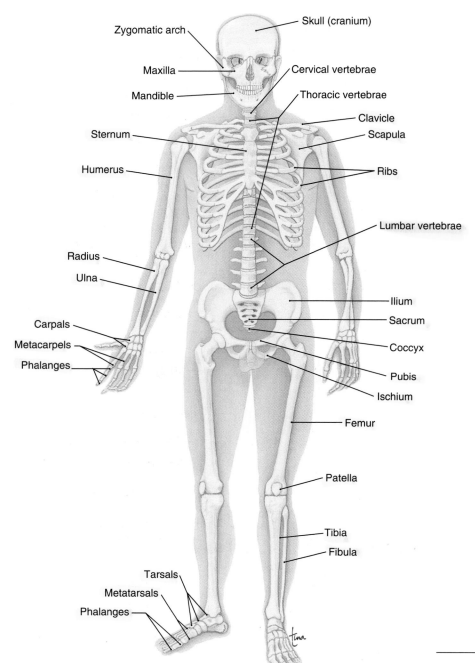

Zygomatic arch

Skull (cranium)

Maxilla

Mandible

Cervical vertebrae

Thoracic vertebrae

Sternum

Clavicle

Scapula

Humerus

Ribs

Lumbar vertebrae

Radius

Ulna

Carpals

Metacarpels

Phalanges

Ilium

Sacrum

Coccyx

Pubis

Ischium

Femur

Patella

Tibia

Fibula

Tarsals

Metatarsals

Phalanges

Figure 6–4 Skeleton. Anterior view.

Within each middle ear cavity are three **auditory bones:** the malleus, incus, and stapes. As part of the hearing process (discussed in Chapter 9), these bones transmit vibrations from the eardrum to the receptors in the inner ear (see Fig. 9–7).

VERTEBRAL COLUMN

The **vertebral column** (spinal column or backbone) is made of individual bones called **vertebrae**. The names of vertebrae indicate their location along the

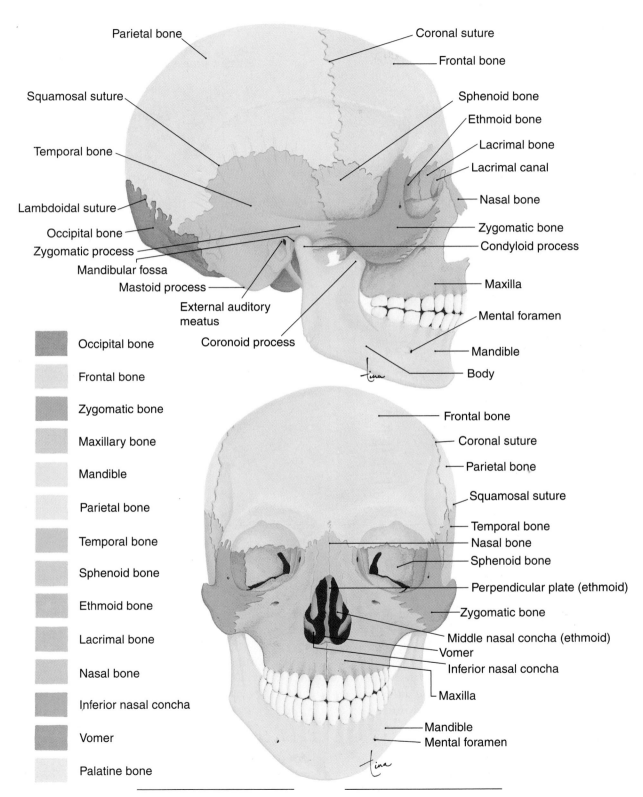

Figure 6–5 Skull. Lateral view of right side.

Figure 6–6 Skull. Anterior view.

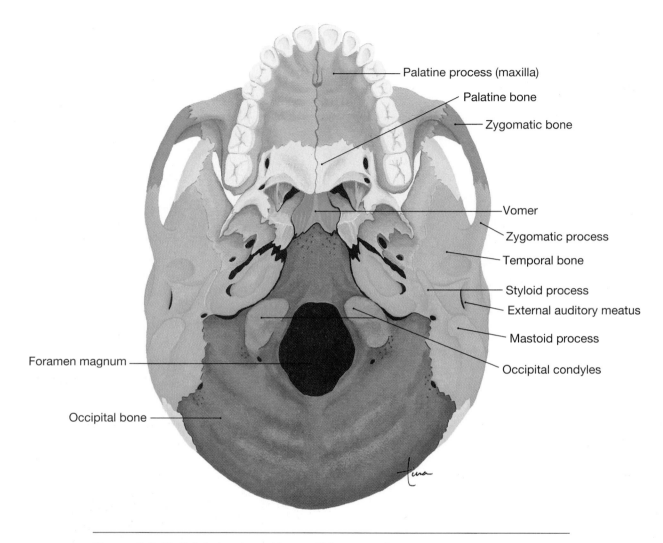

Figure 6–7 Skull. Inferior view with mandible removed.

length of the spinal column. There are 7 cervical vertebrae, 12 thoracic, 5 lumbar, 5 sacral fused into 1 sacrum, and 4 to 5 small coccygeal vertebrae fused into 1 coccyx (Fig. 6–10).

The seven **cervical vertebrae** are those within the neck. The first vertebra is called the **atlas**, which supports the skull and forms a **pivot joint** with the odontoid process of the **axis**, the second cervical vertebra. This pivot joint allows us to turn our heads from side to side. The remaining five cervical vertebrae do not have individual names.

The **thoracic vertebrae** articulate (form joints) with the ribs on the posterior side of the trunk. The **lumbar vertebrae**, the largest and strongest bones of the spine, are found in the small of the back. The **sacrum** permits the articulation of the two hip bones: the **sacroiliac joints**. The **coccyx** is the remnant of tail vertebrae, and some muscles of the perineum (pelvic floor) are anchored to it.

All of the vertebrae articulate with one another in sequence to form a flexible backbone that supports the trunk and head. They also form the **vertebral canal**, a continuous tunnel (lined with the meninges) within the bones that contains the spinal cord and protects it from mechanical injury. The spinous and transverse processes are projections for the

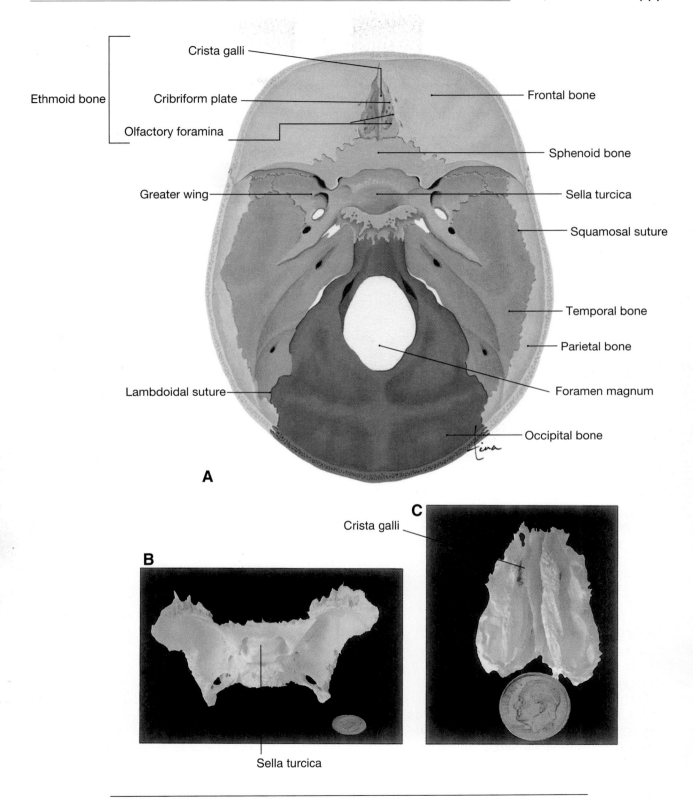

Figure 6–8 **(A)** Skull. Superior view with the top of cranium removed. **(B)** Sphenoid bone in superior view. **(C)** Ethmoid bone in superior view. (B and C photographs by Dan Kaufman.)

Table 6–2   **BONES OF THE SKULL—IMPORTANT PARTS**

Terminology of Bone Markings
Foramen—a hole or opening   Meatus—a tunnel-like cavity   Condyle—a rounded projection
Fossa—a depression   Process—a projection   Plate—a flat projection

Bone	Part	Description
Frontal	• Frontal sinus • Coronal suture	• Air cavity that opens into nasal cavity • Joint between frontal and parietal bones
Parietal (2)	• Sagittal suture	• Joint between the 2 parietal bones
Temporal (2)	• Squamosal suture • External auditory meatus • Mastoid process • Mastoid sinus • Mandibular fossa • Zygomatic process	• Joint between temporal and parietal bone • The tunnel-like ear canal • Oval projection behind the ear canal • Air cavity that opens into middle ear • Oval depression anterior to the ear canal; articulates with mandible • Anterior projection that articulates with the zygomatic bone
Occipital	• Foramen magnum • Condyles • Lambdoidal suture	• Large opening for the spinal cord • Oval projections on either side of the foramen magnum; articulate with the atlas • Joint between occipital and parietal bones
Sphenoid	• Greater wing • Sella turcica • Sphenoid sinus	• Flat, lateral portion between the frontal and temporal bones • Central depression that encloses the pituitary gland • Air cavity that opens into nasal cavity
Ethmoid	• Ethmoid sinus • Crista galli • Cribriform plate and Olfactory foramina • Perpendicular plate • Conchae (4 are part of ethmoid; 2 inferior are separate bones)	• Air cavity that opens into nasal cavity • Superior projection for attachment of meninges • On either side of base of crista galli; olfactory nerves pass through foramina • Upper part of nasal septum • Shelf-like projections into nasal cavities which increase surface area of nasal mucosa
Mandible	• Body • Condyles • Sockets	• U-shaped portion with lower teeth • Oval projections that articulate with the temporal bones • Conical depressions that hold roots of lower teeth
Maxilla (2)	• Maxillary sinus • Palatine process • Sockets	• Air cavity that opens into nasal cavity • Projection that forms anterior part of hard palate • Conical depressions that hold roots of upper teeth
Nasal (2)	—	• Forms the bridge of the nose
Lacrimal (2)	Lacrimal canal	• Opening for nasolacrimal duct to take tears to nasal cavity
Zygomatic (2)	—	• Form point of cheek; articulate with frontal, temporal, and maxillae
Palatine (2)	—	• Forms the posterior part of hard palate
Vomer	—	• Lower part of nasal septum

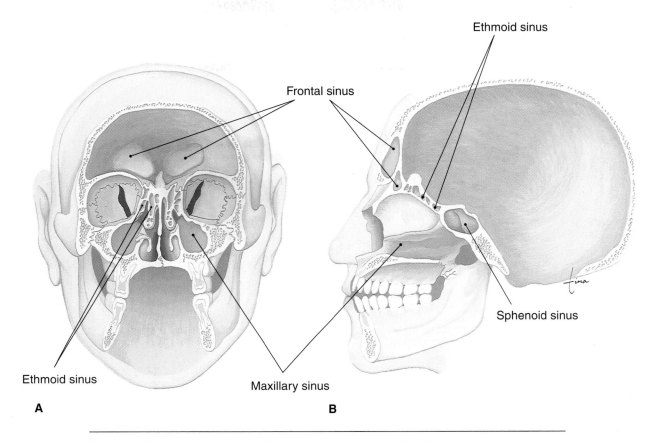

Figure 6–9 Paranasal sinuses. **(A)** Anterior view of the skull. **(B)** Left lateral view of skull.

attachment of the muscles that bend the vertebral column.

The supporting part of a vertebra is its body; the bodies of adjacent vertebrae are separated by **discs** of fibrous cartilage. These discs cushion and absorb shock and permit some movement between vertebrae **(symphysis joints)**. Since there are so many joints, the backbone as a whole is quite flexible (see also Box 6–3: Herniated Disc).

The normal spine in anatomic position has four natural curves, which are named after the vertebrae that form them. Refer to Fig. 6–10, and notice that the cervical curve is forward, the thoracic curve backward, the lumbar curve forward, and the sacral curve backward. These curves center the skull over the rest of the body, which enables a person to more easily walk upright (see Box 6–4: Abnormalities of the Curves of the Spine).

RIB CAGE

The **rib cage** consists of the 12 pairs of ribs and the sternum, or breast bone. The three parts of the **sternum** are the upper **manubrium**, the central **body**, and the lower **xiphoid process** (Fig. 6–11).

All of the **ribs** articulate posteriorly with the thoracic vertebrae. The first seven pairs of ribs are called **true ribs**; they articulate directly with the manubrium and body of the sternum by means of costal cartilages. The next three pairs are called **false ribs**; their cartilages join the 7th rib cartilage. The last two pairs are called **floating ribs** because they do not articulate with the sternum at all (see Fig. 6–10).

An obvious function of the rib cage is that it encloses and protects the heart and lungs. Keep in mind, though, that the rib cage also protects organs in the upper abdominal cavity, such as the liver and

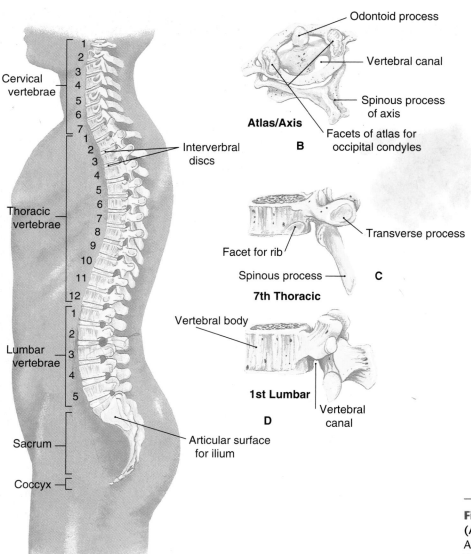

Figure 6–10 Vertebral column. **(A)** Lateral view of left side. **(B)** Atlas and axis, superior view. **(C)** 7th thoracic vertebra, left lateral view. **(D)** 1st lumbar vertebra, left lateral view.

spleen. The other important function of the rib cage depends upon its flexibility: The ribs are pulled upward and outward by the external intercostal muscles. This enlarges the chest cavity, which expands the lungs and contributes to inhalation.

THE SHOULDER AND ARM

The shoulder girdles attach the arms to the axial skeleton. Each consists of a scapula (shoulder blade) and

clavicle (collarbone). The **scapula** is a large, flat bone that anchors some of the muscles that move the upper arm. A shallow depression called the glenoid fossa forms a **ball-and-socket joint** with the humerus, the bone of the upper arm (Fig. 6–12).

Each **clavicle** articulates laterally with a scapula and medially with the manubrium of the sternum. In this position the clavicles act as braces for the scapulae and prevent the shoulders from coming too far forward. Although the shoulder joint is capable of a wide range

Box 6–3   HERNIATED DISC

The vertebrae are separated by discs of fibrous cartilage that act as cushions to absorb shock. An intervertebral disc has a tough outer covering and a soft center called the nucleus pulposus. Extreme pressure on a disc may rupture the outer layer and force the nucleus pulposus out. This may occur when a person lifts a heavy object improperly, that is, using the back rather than the legs and jerking upward, which puts sudden, intense pressure on the spine. Most often this affects discs in the lumbar region.

Although often called a "slipped disc," the affected disc is usually not moved out of position.

The terms **"herniated"** or **"ruptured" disc** more accurately describe what happens. The nucleus pulposus is forced out, usually posteriorly, where it puts pressure on a spinal nerve. For this reason a herniated disc may be very painful or impair function in the muscles supplied by the nerve.

Healing of a herniated disc may occur naturally if the damage is not severe and the person rests and avoids activities that would further compress the disc. Surgery may be required, however, to remove the portion of the nucleus pulposus that is out of place and disrupting nerve functioning.

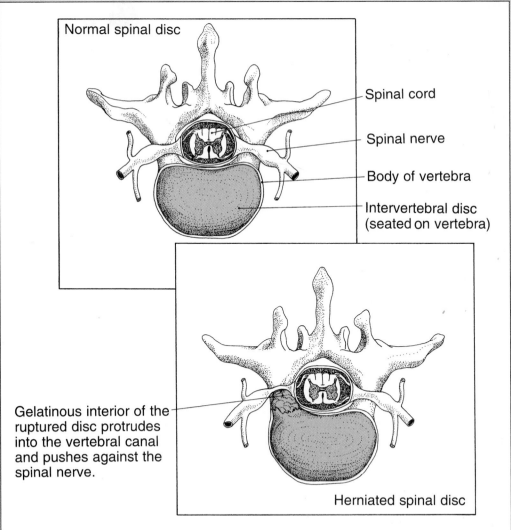

Normal spinal disc

Spinal cord

Spinal nerve

Body of vertebra

Intervertebral disc (seated on vertebra)

Gelatinous interior of the ruptured disc protrudes into the vertebral canal and pushes against the spinal nerve.

Herniated spinal disc

Box Figure 6–C Herniated disc. As a result of compression, a ruptured intervertebral disc puts pressure on a spinal nerve.

Box 6–4   ABNORMALITIES OF THE CURVES OF THE SPINE

Scoliosis—an abnormal lateral curvature, which may be congenital, the result of having one leg longer than the other, or the result of chronic poor posture during childhood while the vertebrae are still growing. Usually the thoracic vertebrae are affected, which displaces the rib cage to one side. In severe cases, the abdominal organs may be compressed, and the expansion of the rib cage during inhalation may be impaired.

Kyphosis*—an exaggerated thoracic curve; sometimes referred to as hunchback.

Lordosis*—an exaggerated lumbar curve; sometimes referred to as swayback.

These abnormal curves are usually the result of degenerative bone diseases such as osteoporosis or tuberculosis of the spine. If osteoporosis, for example, causes the bodies of the thoracic vertebrae to collapse, the normal thoracic curve will be increased. Most often the vertebral body "settles" slowly (rather than collapses suddenly) and there is little, if any, damage to the spinal nerves. The damage to the vertebrae, however, cannot be corrected, so these conditions should be though of in terms of prevention rather than cure.

---

* Although descriptive of normal anatomy, the terms *kyphosis* and *lordosis*, respectively, are commonly used to describe the abnormal condition associated with each.

Figure 6–11 Rib cage. Anterior view.

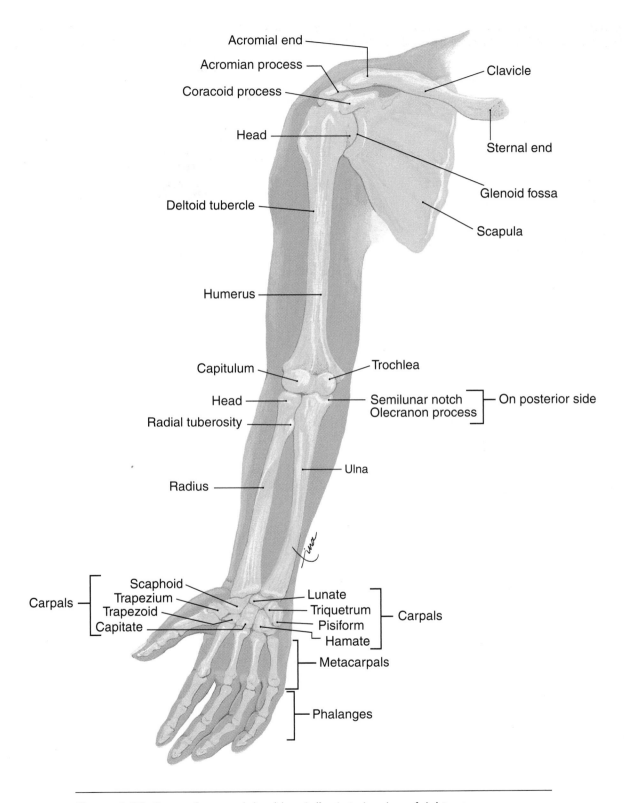

Figure 6–12 Bones of arm and shoulder girdle. Anterior view of right arm.

Table 6–3   BONES OF THE SHOULDER AND ARM—IMPORTANT PARTS

Bone	Part	Description
Scapula	• Glenoid fossa • Spine • Acromion process	• Depression that articulates with humerus • Long, posterior process for muscle attachment • Articulates with clavicle
Clavicle	• Acromial end • Sternal end	• Articulates with scapula • Articulates with manubrium of sternum
Humerus	• Head • Olecranon fossa • Capitulum • Trochlea	• Round process that articulates with scapula • Posterior, oval depression for the olecranon process of the ulna • Round process superior to radius • Concave surface that articulates with ulna
Radius	• Head	• Articulates with the ulna
Ulna	• Olecranon process • Semilunar notch	• Fits into olecranon fossa of humerus • "Half-moon" depression that articulates with the trochlea of ulna
Carpals (8)	• Scaphoid • Lunate • Triquetrum • Pisiform • Trapezium • Trapezoid • Capitate • Hamate	• Proximal row • Distal row

of movement, the shoulder itself must be relatively stable if these movements are to be effective.

The **humerus** is the long bone of the upper arm. Proximally, the humerus forms a **ball-and-socket joint** with the scapula. Distally, the humerus forms a **hinge joint** with the ulna of the forearm. This hinge joint, the elbow, permits movement in one plane, that is, back and forth with no lateral movement.

The forearm bones are the **ulna** on the little finger side and the **radius** on the thumb side. The radius and ulna articulate proximally to form a **pivot joint**, which permits turning the hand palm up to palm down. You can demonstrate this yourself by holding your arm palm up in front of you, and noting that the radius and ulna are parallel to each other. Then turn your hand palm down, and notice that your upper arm does not move. The radius crosses over the ulna, which permits the hand to perform a great variety of movements without moving the entire arm.

The **carpals** are eight small bones in the wrist; **gliding joints** between them permit a sliding movement. The carpals also articulate with the distal ends of the ulna and radius, and with the proximal ends of the **metacarpals**, the five bones of the hand.

The **phalanges** are the bones of the fingers. There are two phalanges in each thumb and three in each of the fingers. Between phalanges are **hinge joints**, which permit movement in one plane. The thumb, however, is more movable than the fingers because of its carpometacarpal joint. This is a **saddle joint**, which enables the thumb to cross over the palm, and permits gripping. Important parts of these bones are described in Table 6–3.

THE HIP AND LEG

The pelvic girdle consists of the two **hip bones** (coxae or innominate bones), which articulate with the axial skeleton at the sacrum. Each hip bone has three major parts (Fig. 6–13): the ilium, ischium, and pubis. The **ilium** is the flared, upper portion that forms the sacroiliac joint. The **ischium** is the lower, posterior part that we sit on. The **pubis** is the lower, most anterior part. The two **pubic bones** articulate with one another at the **pubic symphysis**, with a disc of fibrous cartilage between them.

The **acetabulum** is the socket in the hip bone that forms a **ball-and-socket joint** with the femur. Compared to the glenoid fossa of the scapula, the acetabulum is a much deeper socket. This has great functional importance because the hip is a weight-bearing joint, whereas the shoulder is not. Because

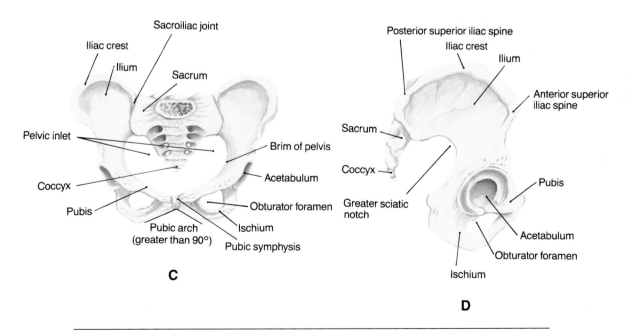

Figure 6–13 Hip bones and sacrum. **(A)** Male pelvis, anterior view. **(B)** Male pelvis, lateral view of right side. **(C)** Female pelvis, anterior view. **(D)** Female pelvis, lateral view of right side.

Table 6–4	BONES OF THE HIP AND LEG—IMPORTANT PARTS	

Bone	Part	Description
Pelvic (2 hip bones)	• Ilium	Flared, upper portion
	• Iliac crest	Upper edge of ilium
	• Posterior superior iliac spine	Posterior continuation of iliac crest
	• Ischium	Lower, posterior portion
	• Pubis	Anterior, medial portion
	• Pubic symphysis	Joint between the 2 pubic bones
	• Acetabulum	Deep depression that articulates with femur
Femur	• Head	Round process that articulates with hip bone
	• Neck	Constricted portion distal to head
	• Greater trochanter	Large lateral process for muscle attachment
	• Lesser trochanter	Medial process for muscle attachment
	• Condyles	Rounded processes that articulate with tibia
Tibia	• Condyles	Articulate with the femur
	• Medial malleolus	Distal process; medial "ankle bone"
Fibula	• Head	Articulates with tibia
	• Lateral malleolus	Distal process; lateral "ankle bone"
Tarsals (7)	• Calcaneus	Heel bone
	• Talus	Articulates with calcaneus and tibia
	• Cuboid, navicular	—
	• Cuneiform: 1st, 2nd, 3rd	—

the acetabulum is deep, the hip joint is not easily dislocated, even by activities such as running and jumping (landing), which put great stress on the joint.

The **femur** is the long bone of the thigh. As mentioned, the femur forms a very movable ball-and-socket joint with the hip bone. At its distal end, the femur forms a **hinge joint**, the knee, with the tibia of the lower leg. The **patella**, or kneecap, is anterior to the knee joint, enclosed in the tendon of the quadriceps femoris, a large muscle group of the thigh.

The **tibia** is the weight-bearing bone of the lower leg. Notice in Fig. 6–14 that the **fibula** is not part of the knee joint and does not bear weight. The fibula is important, however, in that leg muscles are attached and anchored to it, and it helps stabilize the ankle. The tibia and fibula do not form a pivot joint as do the radius and ulna in the arm. This makes the lower leg and foot more stable, and thus able to support the body.

The **tarsals** are the seven bones in the ankle. The largest is the **calcaneus**, or heel bone; the **talus** transmits weight between the calcaneus and the tibia. **Metatarsals** are the five long bones of each foot, and

phalanges are the bones of the toes. There are two phalanges in the big toe and three in each of the other toes. The phalanges of the toes form hinge joints with each other. Because there is no saddle joint in the foot, the big toe is not as movable as is the thumb. Important parts of these bones are described in Table 6–4.

JOINTS—ARTICULATIONS

A joint is where two bones meet, or **articulate**.

THE CLASSIFICATION OF JOINTS

The classification of joints is based on the amount of movement possible. A **synarthrosis** is an immovable joint, such as a suture between two cranial bones. An **amphiarthrosis** is a slightly movable joint, such as the symphysis joint between adjacent vertebrae. A **diarthrosis** is a freely movable joint. This is the largest category of joints and includes the ball-and-socket joint, the pivot, hinge, and others. Examples of each type of joint are described in Table 6–5, and many of these are illustrated in Fig. 6–15.

Figure 6–14 **(A)** Bones of the leg and portion of hip bone, anterior view of left leg. **(B)** Lateral view of left foot.

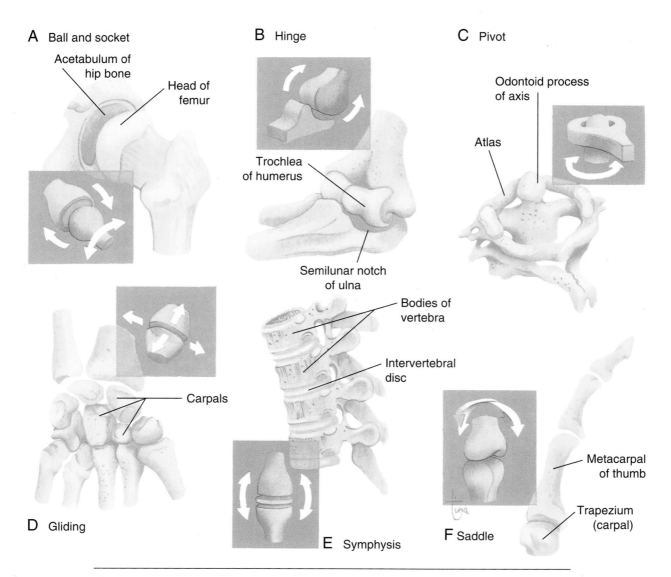

A Ball and socket

Acetabulum of hip bone

Head of femur

B Hinge

Trochlea of humerus

Semilunar notch of ulna

C Pivot

Odontoid process of axis

Atlas

Bodies of vertebra

Intervertebral disc

Carpals

D Gliding

Metacarpal of thumb

Trapezium (carpal)

E Symphysis

F Saddle

Figure 6–15 Types of joints. For each type, a specific joint is depicted, and a simple diagram shows the position of the joint surfaces. **(A)** Ball and socket. **(B)** Hinge. **(C)** Pivot. **(D)** Gliding. **(E)** Symphysis. **(F)** Saddle.

Table 6–5	TYPES OF JOINTS	
Category	**Type and Description**	**Examples**
Synarthrosis (immovable)	Suture—fibrous connective tissue between bone surfaces	• Between cranial bones; between facial bones
Amphiarthrosis (slightly movable)	Symphysis—disc of fibrous cartilage between bones	• Between vertebrae; between pubic bones
Diarthrosis (freely movable)	Ball and socket—movement in all planes	• Scapula and humerus; pelvic bone and femur
	Hinge—movement in one plane	• Humerus and ulna; femur and tibia; between phalanges
	Condyloid—movement in one plane with some lateral movement	• Temporal bone and mandible
	Pivot—rotation	• Atlas and axis; radius and ulna
	Gliding—side to side movement	• Between carpals
	Saddle—movement in several planes	• Carpometacarpal of thumb

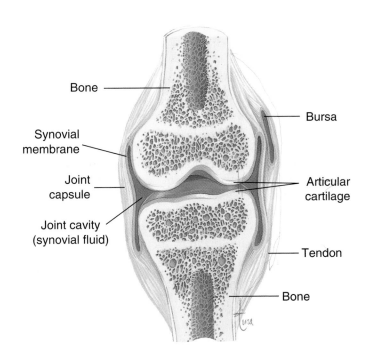

Figure 6–16 Structure of a synovial joint. See text for description.

Box 6-5   ARTHRITIS

The term **arthritis** means inflammation of a joint. Of the many types of arthritis, we will consider two: osteoarthritis and rheumatoid arthritis.

Osteoarthritis is a natural consequence of getting older. In joints that have borne weight for many years, the articular cartilage is gradually worn away. The once smooth joint surface becomes rough, and the affected joint is stiff and painful. As you might guess, the large, weight-bearing joints are most often subjected to this form of arthritis. If we live long enough, most of us can expect some osteoarthritis in knees, hips, or ankles.

Rheumatoid arthritis can be a truly crippling disease that may begin in early middle age or, less commonly, during adolescence. It is an **autoimmune disease**, which means that the immune system mistakenly directs its destructive capability against part of the body. Exactly what triggers this abnormal response by the immune system is not known with certainty, but certain bacterial and viral infections have been suggested as possibilities.

Rheumatoid arthritis often begins in joints of the extremities, such as those of the fingers. The autoimmune activity seems to affect the synovial membrane, and joints become painful and stiff. Sometimes the disease progresses to total destruction of the synovial membrane and calcification of the joint. Such a joint is then fused and has no mobility at all.

Treatment of rheumatoid arthritis is directed at reducing inflammation as much as possible, for it is the inflammatory process that causes the damage. Therapies being investigated involve selectively blocking specific aspects of the immune response, and limiting this blockage only to joints. At present there is no cure for autoimmune diseases.

SYNOVIAL JOINTS

All diarthroses, or freely movable joints, are **synovial joints** because they share similarities of structure. A typical synovial joint is shown in Fig. 6–16. On the joint surface of each bone is the **articular cartilage**, which provides a smooth surface. The **joint capsule**, made of fibrous connective tissue, encloses the joint in a strong sheath, like a sleeve. Lining the joint capsule is the **synovial membrane**, which secretes synovial fluid into the joint cavity. **Synovial fluid** is thick and slippery and prevents friction as the bones move.

Many synovial joints also have **bursae** (or bursas), which are small sacs of synovial fluid between the joint and the tendons that cross over the joint. Bursae permit the tendons to slide easily as the bones are moved. If a joint is used excessively, the bursae may become inflamed and painful; this condition is called **bursitis**. Some other disorders of joints are described in Box 6–5: Arthritis.

AGING AND THE SKELETAL SYSTEM

With age, bone tissue tends to lose more calcium than is replaced. Bone matrix becomes thinner, the bones themselves more brittle, and spontaneous fractures are more likely to occur.

Erosion of the articular cartilages of joints is also a common consequence of aging. Joints affected include weight-bearing joints such as the knees, and active, small joints such as those of the fingers.

Although the normal wear and tear of joints cannot be prevented, elderly people can preserve their bone matrix with exercise and diets high in calcium and vitamin D.

SUMMARY

Your knowledge of the bones and joints will be useful in the next chapter as you learn the actions of the muscles that move the skeleton. It is important to remember, however, that bones have other functions as well. As a storage site for excess calcium, bones contribute to the maintenance of a normal blood calcium level. The red bone marrow found in flat and irregular bones produces the blood cells: red blood cells, white blood cells, and platelets. Some bones protect vital organs such as the brain, heart, and lungs. As you can see, bones themselves may also be considered vital organs.

STUDY OUTLINE

The skeleton is made of bone and cartilage and has these functions:
1. Is a framework for support, moved by muscles.
2. Protects internal organs from mechanical injury.
3. Contains and protects red bone marrow.
4. Stores excess calcium; important to regulate blood calcium level.

Bone Tissue (see Fig. 6–1)
1. Osteocytes (cells) are found in the matrix of calcium phosphate, calcium carbonate, and collagen.
2. Compact bone—haversian systems are present.
3. Spongy bone—no haversian systems; red bone marrow present.
4. Articular cartilage—smooth, on joint surfaces.
5. Periosteum—fibrous connective tissue membrane; anchors tendons and ligaments; has blood vessels that enter the bone.

Classification of Bones
1. Long—arms, legs; shaft is the diaphysis (compact bone) with a marrow cavity containing yellow bone marrow (fat); ends are epiphyses (spongy bone) (see Fig. 6–1).
2. Short—wrists, ankles (spongy bone covered with compact bone).
3. Flat—ribs, pelvic bone, cranial bones (spongy bone covered with compact bone).
4. Irregular—vertebrae, facial bones (spongy bone covered with compact bone).

Embryonic Growth of Bone
1. The embryonic skeleton is first made of other tissues that are gradually replaced by bone. Ossification begins in the third month of gestation; osteoblasts differentiate from fibroblasts and produce bone matrix.
2. Cranial and facial bones are first made of fibrous connective tissue; osteoblasts produce bone matrix in a center of ossification in each bone; bone growth radiates outward; fontanels remain at birth, permit compression of infant skull during birth; fontanels are calcified by age 2 (see Fig. 6–2).
3. All other bones are first made of cartilage; in a long bone the first center of ossification is in the diaphysis, other centers develop in the epiphyses. After

birth a long bone grows at the epiphyseal discs: Cartilage is produced on the epiphysis side, and bone replaces cartilage on the diaphysis side. Osteoclasts form the marrow cavity by reabsorbing bone matrix in the center of the diaphysis (see Fig. 6–3).

Factors That Affect Bone Growth and Maintenance
1. Heredity—many pairs of genes contribute to genetic potential for height.
2. Nutrition—calcium, phosphorus, and protein become part of the bone matrix; vitamin D is needed for absorption of calcium in the small intestine; vitamins C and A are needed for bone matrix production (calcification).
3. Hormones—produced by endocrine glands; concerned with cell division, protein synthesis, calcium metabolism, and energy production (see Table 6–1).
4. Exercise or stress—weight-bearing bones must bear weight or they will lose calcium and become brittle.

The Skeleton—206 bones in total (see Fig. 6–4)
1. Axial—skull, vertebrae, rib cage.
   - Skull—see Figs. 6–5 through 6–8 and Table 6–2.
     - Eight cranial bones form the braincase, which also protects the eyes and ears; 14 facial bones make up the face; the immovable joints between these bones are called sutures.
     - Paranasal sinuses are air cavities in the maxillae, frontal, sphenoid, and ethmoid bones; lighten the skull and provide resonance for voice (see Fig. 6–9).
     - Three auditory bones in each middle ear cavity transmit vibrations for the hearing process.
   - Vertebral column—see Fig. 6–10.
     - Individual bones are called vertebrae: 7 cervical, 12 thoracic, 5 lumbar, 5 sacral (fused into one sacrum), 4 to 5 coccygeal (fused into one coccyx). Supports trunk and head, encloses and protects the spinal cord in the vertebral canal. Discs of fibrous cartilage absorb shock between the bodies of adjacent vertebrae, also

permit slight movement. Four natural curves center head over body for walking upright (see Table 6–5 for joints).
- Rib cage—see Fig. 6–11.
  ○ Sternum and 12 pairs of ribs; protects thoracic and upper abdominal organs from mechanical injury and is expanded to contribute to inhalation. Sternum consists of manubrium, body, and xiphoid process. All ribs articulate with thoracic vertebrae; true ribs (first seven pairs) articulate directly with sternum by means of costal cartilages; false ribs (next three pairs) articulate with 7th costal cartilage; floating ribs (last two pairs) do not articulate with the sternum.
2. Appendicular—bones of the arms and legs and the shoulder and pelvic girdles.
- Shoulder and arm—see Fig. 6–12 and Table 6–3.
  ○ Scapula—shoulder muscles are attached; glenoid fossa articulates with humerus.
  ○ Clavicle—braces the scapula.
  ○ Humerus—upper arm; articulates with the scapula and the ulna (elbow).
  ○ Radius and ulna—forearm—articulate with one another and with carpals.
  ○ Carpals—eight—wrist; metacarpals—five—hand; phalanges—14—fingers (for joints, see Table 6–5).
- Hip and leg—see Figs. 6–13 and 6–14 and Table 6–4.
  ○ Pelvic bone—two hip bones; ilium, ischium, pubis; acetabulum articulates with femur.
  ○ Femur—thigh; articulates with pelvic bone and tibia (knee).
  ○ Patella—kneecap; in tendon of quadriceps femoris muscle.
  ○ Tibia and fibula—lower leg; tibia bears weight; fibula does not bear weight, but does anchor muscles and stabilizes ankle.
  ○ Tarsals—seven—ankle; calcaneus is heel bone.
  ○ Metatarsals—five—foot; phalanges—14—toes (see Table 6–5 for joints).

Joints—Articulations
1. Classification based on amount of movement:
- Synarthrosis—immovable.
- Amphiarthrosis—slightly movable.
- Diarthrosis—freely movable (see Table 6–5 for examples; see also Fig. 6–15).
2. Synovial Joints—all diarthroses have similar structure (see Fig. 6–16):
- Articular cartilage—smooth on joint surfaces.
- Joint capsule—strong fibrous connective tissue sheath that encloses the joint.
- Synovial membrane—lines the joint capsule; secretes synovial fluid that prevents friction.
- Bursae—sacs of synovial fluid that permit tendons to slide easily across joints.

REVIEW QUESTIONS

1. Explain the differences between compact bone and spongy bone, and state where each type is found. (p. 100)

2. State the locations of red bone marrow, and name the blood cells it produces. (p. 100)

3. Name the tissue of which the embryonic skull is first made. Explain how ossification of cranial bones occurs. (p. 102)

4. State what fontanels are, and explain their function. (p. 102)

5. Name the tissue of which the embryonic femur is first made. Explain how ossification of this bone occurs. Describe what happens in epiphyseal discs to produce growth of long bones. (p. 102)

6. Explain what is meant by "genetic potential" for height, and name the nutrients a child must have in order to attain genetic potential. (p. 102)

7. Explain the functions of calcitonin and parathyroid hormone with respect to bone matrix and to blood calcium level. (p. 106)

8. Explain how estrogen or testosterone affects bone growth, and when. (p. 106)

9. State one way each of the following hormones helps promote bone growth: insulin, thyroxine, growth hormone. (p. 106)

10. Name the bones that make up the braincase. (p. 106)

11. Name the bones that contain paranasal sinuses and explain the functions of these sinuses. (pp. 106–107)

12. Name the bones that make up the rib cage, and describe two functions of the rib cage. (pp. 113–114)

13. Describe the functions of the vertebral column. State the number of each type of vertebra. (p. 110)

14. Explain how the shoulder and hip joints are similar and how they differ. (pp. 114, 118)

15. Give a specific example (name two bones) for each of the following types of joints: (p. 123)
    a. Hinge
    b. Symphysis

  c. Pivot
  d. Saddle
  e. Suture
  f. Ball and socket

16. Name the part of a synovial joint with each of the following functions: (p. 124)
    a. Fluid within the joint cavity that prevents friction
    b. Encloses the joint in a strong sheath
    c. Provides a smooth surface on bone surfaces
    d. Lines the joint capsule and secretes synovial fluid

17. Refer to the diagram (Fig. 6–4) of the full skeleton, and point to each bone on yourself. (p. 108)

FOR FURTHER THOUGHT

1. Following a severe spinal cord injury in the lumbar region, the voluntary muscles of the legs and hips will be paralyzed. Describe the effects of paralysis on the skeleton.

2. The sutures of the adult skull are joints that do not allow movement. Why have joints at all if no movement is permitted? Explain.

3. Without looking at any of the illustrations, try to name all the bones that form the orbits, the sockets for the eyes. Check your list with Figs. 6–5 and 6–6.

4. In an effort to prevent sudden infant death syndrome (SIDS), parents were advised to put their infants to sleep lying on their backs, not their stomachs. Since then (1994), the number of SIDS deaths has decreased markedly. What do you think has happened to the skulls of many of those infants? Explain.

5. A five-month-old infant is brought to a clinic after having diarrhea for two days. The nurse checks the baby's anterior fontanel and notices that it appears sunken. What has caused this?

6. Look at the lateral view of the adult skull in Fig. 6–5 and notice the size of the face part in proportion to the braincase part. Compare the infant skull in Fig. 6–2, and notice how small the infant face is, relative to the size of the braincase. There is a very good reason for this. What do you think it is?

7. Look at the photograph below, Question Fig. 6–A. Name the bone and the type of section in which it is cut. What are the large arrows indicating? What are the smaller arrows indicating? Look carefully at this site, describe it, and explain possible consequences.

Question Figure 6–A (Photograph by Dan Kaufman.)

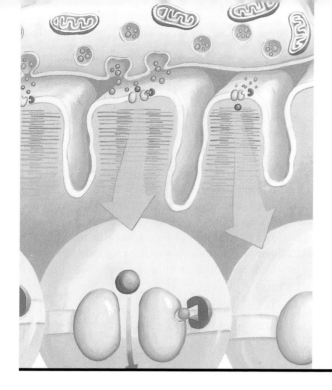

CHAPTER 7

Student Objectives

- Name the organ systems directly involved in movement, and state how they are involved.
- Describe muscle structure in terms of muscle cells, tendons, and bones.
- Describe the difference between antagonistic and synergistic muscles, and explain why such arrangements are necessary.
- Explain the role of the brain with respect to skeletal muscle.
- Define muscle tone and explain its importance.
- Explain the difference between isotonic and isometric exercise.
- Define muscle sense and explain its importance.
- Name the energy sources for muscle contraction, and state the simple equation for cell respiration.
- Explain the importance of hemoglobin and myoglobin, oxygen debt, and lactic acid.
- Describe the neuromuscular junction and state the function of each part.
- Describe the structure of a sarcomere.
- Explain the following in terms of ions and charges: polarization, depolarization, and repolarization.
- Describe the Sliding Filament Theory of muscle contraction.
- Describe some of the body's responses to exercise and explain how each maintains homeostasis.
- Learn the major muscles of the body and their functions.

The Muscular System

*Terms that appear in **bold type** in the chapter text are defined in the glossary, which begins on page 521.*

Do you like to dance? Most of us do, or we may simply enjoy watching good dancers. The grace and coordination involved in dancing result from the inter-action of many of the organ systems, but the one you think of first is probably the muscular system.

There are more than 600 muscles in the human body. Most of these muscles are attached to the bones of the skeleton by tendons, although a few muscles are attached to the undersurface of the skin. The primary function of the **muscular system** is to move the skeleton. The muscle contractions required for movement also produce heat, which contributes to the maintenance of a constant body temperature. The other body systems directly involved in movement are the nervous, respiratory, and circulatory systems. The nervous system transmits the electrochemical impulses that cause muscle cells to contract. The respiratory system exchanges oxygen and carbon dioxide between the air and blood. The circulatory system brings oxygen to the muscles and takes carbon dioxide away.

These interactions of body systems are covered in this chapter, which focuses on the **skeletal muscles**. You may recall from Chapter 4 that there are two other types of muscle tissue: smooth muscle and cardiac muscle. These types of muscle tissue will be discussed in other chapters in relation to the organs of which they are part. Before you continue, you may find it helpful to go back to Chapter 4 and review the structure and characteristics of skeletal muscle tissue. In this chapter we will begin with the gross (large) anatomy and physiology of muscles, then discuss the microscopic structure of muscle cells and the biochemistry of muscle contraction.

MUSCLE STRUCTURE

All muscle cells are specialized for contraction. When these cells contract, they shorten and pull a bone in order to produce movement. Each skeletal muscle is made of thousands of individual muscle cells, which also may be called **muscle fibers** (see Fig. 7–3 later in this chapter). Depending on the work a muscle is required to do, variable numbers of muscle fibers contract. When picking up a pencil, for example, only a small portion of the muscle fibers in a muscle will contract. If the muscle has more work to do, such as picking up a book, more muscle fibers will contract to accomplish the task.

Muscles are anchored firmly to bones by **tendons**. Tendons are made of fibrous connective tissue, which, you may remember, is very strong and merges with the **fascia** that covers the muscle and with the **periosteum**, the fibrous connective tissue membrane that covers bones. A muscle usually has at least two tendons, each attached to a different bone. The more immobile or stationary attachment of the muscle is its **origin**; the more movable attachment is called the **insertion**. The muscle itself crosses the joint of the two bones to which it is attached, and when the muscle contracts it pulls on its insertion and moves the bone in a specific direction.

MUSCLE ARRANGEMENTS

Muscles are arranged around the skeleton so as to bring about a variety of movements. The two general types of arrangements are the opposing **antagonists** and the cooperative **synergists**.

Antagonistic Muscles

Antagonists are opponents, so we use the term **antagonistic muscles** for muscles that have opposing or opposite functions. An example will be helpful here—refer to Fig. 7–1 as you read the following. The biceps brachii is the muscle on the front of the upper arm. The origin of the biceps is on the scapula (there are actually two tendons, hence the name *biceps*), and the insertion is on the radius. When the biceps contracts it **flexes** the forearm, that is, bends the elbow (see Table 7–2 later in this chapter). Recall that when a muscle contracts, it gets shorter and pulls. Muscles cannot push, for when they relax they exert no force. Therefore, the biceps can bend the elbow but cannot straighten it; another muscle is needed. The triceps brachii is located on the back of the upper arm. Its origins (the prefix *tri* tells you that there are three of them) are on the scapula and humerus, and its insertion is on the ulna. When the triceps contracts and pulls, it **extends** the forearm, that is, straightens the elbow.

Joints that are capable of a variety of movements have several sets of antagonists. Notice how many ways you can move your upper arm at the shoulder, for instance. Abducting (laterally raising) the arm is the function of the deltoid. Adducting the arm is brought about by the pectoralis major and latissimus dorsi. Flexion of the arm (across the chest) is also a function of the pectoralis major, and extension of the

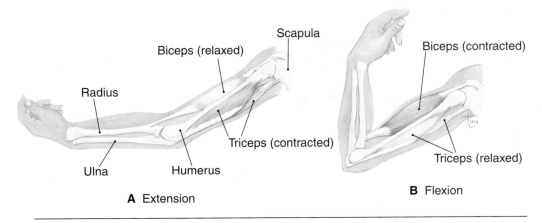

Figure 7–1 Antagonistic muscles. **(A)** Extension of the forearm. **(B)** Flexion of the forearm.

arm (behind the back) is also a function of the latissimus dorsi. All of these muscles are described and depicted in the tables and figures later in the chapter. Without antagonistic muscles, this variety of movements would not be possible.

You may be familiar with **range-of-motion** (or ROM) exercises that are often recommended for patients confined to bed. Such exercises are designed to stretch and contract the antagonistic muscles of a joint to preserve as much muscle function and joint mobility as possible.

Synergistic Muscles

Synergistic muscles are those with the same function, or those that work together to perform a particular function. Recall that the biceps brachii flexes the forearm. The brachioradialis, with its origin on the humerus and insertion on the radius, also flexes the forearm. There is even a third flexor of the forearm, the brachialis. You may wonder why we need three muscles to perform the same function, and the explanation lies in the great mobility of the hand. If the hand is palm up, the biceps does most of the work of flexing and may be called the **prime mover**. When the hand is thumb up, the brachioradialis is in position to be the prime mover, and when the hand is palm down, the brachialis becomes the prime mover. If you have ever tried to do chin-ups, you know that it is much easier with your palms toward you than with palms away from you. This is because the biceps is a larger, and usually much stronger, muscle than is the brachialis.

Muscles may also be called synergists if they help to stabilize or steady a joint to make a more precise movement possible. If you drink a glass of water, the biceps brachii may be the prime mover to flex the forearm. At the same time, the muscles of the shoulder keep that joint stable, so that the water gets to your mouth, not over your shoulder or down your chin. The shoulder muscles are considered synergists for this movement because their contribution makes the movement effective.

THE ROLE OF THE BRAIN

Even our simplest movements require the interaction of many muscles, and the contraction of skeletal muscles depends on the brain. The nerve impulses for movement come from the **frontal lobes** of the **cerebrum**. The cerebrum is the largest part of the brain; the frontal lobes are beneath the frontal bone. The **motor areas** of the frontal lobes generate electrochemical impulses that travel along motor nerves to muscle fibers, causing the muscle fibers to contract.

For a movement to be effective, some muscles must contract while others relax. When walking, for example, antagonistic muscles on the front and back of the thigh or the lower leg will alternate their contractions and relaxations, and our steps will be smooth and efficient. This is what we call coordination, and we do not have to think about making it happen. Coordination takes place below the level of conscious thought, and is regulated by the **cerebellum**, which is located below the occipital lobes of the cerebrum.

MUSCLE TONE

Except during certain stages of sleep, most of our muscles are in a state of slight contraction; this is what is known as **muscle tone**. When sitting upright, for example, the tone of your neck muscles keeps your head up, and the tone of your back muscles keeps your back straight. This is an important function of muscle tone for human beings, because it helps us to maintain an upright posture. In order for a muscle to remain slightly contracted, only a few of the muscle

Box 7–1   ANABOLIC STEROIDS

Anabolic steroids are synthetic drugs very similar in structure and action to the male hormone **testosterone**. Normal secretion of testosterone, beginning in males at puberty, increases muscle size and is the reason men usually have larger muscles than do women.

Some athletes, both male and female, both amateur and professional, take anabolic steroids to build muscle mass and to increase muscle strength. There is no doubt that the use of anabolic steroids will increase muscle size, but there are hazards, some of them very serious. Side effects of such self-medication include liver damage, kidney damage, disruption of reproductive cycles, and mental changes such as irritability and aggressiveness.

Women athletes may develop increased growth of facial and body hair and may become sterile as a result of the effects of a male hormone on their own hormonal cycles.

fibers in that muscle must contract. Alternate fibers contract so that the muscle as a whole does not become fatigued. This is similar to a pianist continuously rippling her fingers over the keys of the piano—some notes are always sounding at any given moment, but the notes that are sounding are always changing. This contraction of alternate fibers, muscle tone, is also regulated by the cerebellum of the brain.

Muscle fibers need the energy of ATP in order to contract. When they produce ATP in the process of cell respiration, muscle fibers also produce heat. The heat generated by normal muscle tone is approximately 25% of the total body heat at rest. During exercise, of course, heat production increases significantly.

EXERCISE

Good muscle tone improves coordination. When muscles are slightly contracted, they can react more rapidly if and when greater exertion is necessary. Muscles with poor tone are usually soft and flabby, but exercise will improve muscle tone.

There are two general types of exercise: isotonic and isometric. In **isotonic exercise**, muscles contract and bring about movement. Jogging, swimming, and weight lifting are examples. Isotonic exercise improves muscle tone, muscle strength, and, if done repetitively against great resistance (as in weight lifting), muscle size. This type of exercise also improves cardiovascular and respiratory efficiency, because movement exerts demands on the heart and respiratory muscles. If done for 30 minutes or longer, such exercise may be called "aerobic," because it strengthens the heart and respiratory muscles as well as the muscles attached to the skeleton.

Isometric exercise involves contraction without movement. If you put your palms together and push

one hand against the other, you can feel your arm muscles contracting. If both hands push equally, there will be no movement; this is isometric contraction. Such exercises will increase muscle tone and muscle strength but are not considered aerobic. When the body is moving, the brain receives sensory information about this movement from the joints involved, and responds with reflexes that increase heart rate and respiration. Without movement, the brain does not get this sensory information, and heart rate and breathing do not increase nearly as much as they would during an equally strenuous isotonic exercise.

Many of our actions involve both isotonic and isometric contractions. Pulling open a door requires isotonic contractions of arm muscles, but if the door is then held open for someone else, those contractions become isometric. Picking up your books is isotonic; holding them in your arm is isometric. Both kinds of contractions are needed for even the simplest activities. (With respect to increasing muscle strength, see Box 7–1: Anabolic Steroids.)

MUSCLE SENSE

When you walk up a flight of stairs, do you have to look at your feet to be sure each will get to the next step? Most of us don't (an occasional stumble doesn't count), and for this freedom we can thank our muscle sense. **Muscle sense** is the brain's ability to know where our muscles are and what they are doing, without our having to consciously look at them.

Within muscles are receptors called **stretch receptors** (proprioceptors or muscle spindles). The general function of all sensory receptors is to detect changes. The function of stretch receptors is to detect changes in the length of a muscle as it is stretched. The sensory impulses generated by these receptors are interpreted by the brain as a mental "picture" of where the muscle is.

We can be aware of muscle sense if we choose to be, but usually we can safely take it for granted. In fact, that is what we are meant to do. Imagine what life would be like if we had to watch every move to be sure that a hand or foot performed its intended action. Even simple activities such as walking or eating would require our constant attention.

At times, we may become aware of our muscle sense. Learning a skill such as typing or playing the guitar involves very precise movements of the fingers, and beginners will often watch their fingers to be sure they are moving properly. With practice, however, the movements simply "feel" right, which means that the brain has formed a very good mental picture of the task. Muscle sense again becomes unconscious, and the experienced typist or guitarist need not watch every movement.

All sensation is a function of brain activity, and muscle sense is no exception. The impulses for muscle sense are integrated in the **parietal lobes** of the cerebrum (conscious muscle sense) and in the cerebellum (unconscious muscle sense) to be used to promote coordination.

ENERGY SOURCES FOR MUSCLE CONTRACTION

Before discussing the contraction process itself, let us look first at how muscle fibers obtain the energy they need to contract. The direct source of energy for muscle contraction is **ATP**. ATP, however, is not stored in large amounts in muscle fibers and is depleted in a few seconds.

The secondary energy sources are creatine phosphate and glycogen. **Creatine phosphate** is, like ATP, an energy-transferring molecule. When it is broken down (by an enzyme) to creatine, phosphate, and energy, the energy is used to synthesize more ATP. Most of the creatine formed is used to resynthesize creatine phosphate, but some is converted to **creatinine**, a waste product that is excreted by the kidneys.

The most abundant energy source in muscle fibers is **glycogen**. When glycogen is needed to provide energy for sustained contractions (more than a few seconds), it is first broken down into the **glucose**

molecules of which it is made. Glucose is then further broken down in the process of cell respiration to produce ATP, and muscle fibers may continue to contract.

Recall from Chapter 2 our simple reaction for cell respiration:

$$Glucose + O_2 \rightarrow CO_2 + H_2O + ATP + heat$$

Look first at the products of this reaction. ATP will be used by the muscle fibers for contraction. The heat produced will contribute to body temperature, and if exercise is strenuous, will increase body temperature. The water becomes part of intracellular water, and the carbon dioxide is a waste product that will be exhaled.

Now look at what is needed to release energy from glucose: oxygen. Muscles have two sources of oxygen. The blood delivers a continuous supply of oxygen from the lungs, which is carried by the **hemoglobin** in red blood cells. Within muscle fibers themselves there is another protein called **myoglobin**, which stores some oxygen within the muscle cells. Both hemoglobin and myoglobin contain the mineral iron, which enables them to bond to oxygen. (Iron also makes both molecules red, and it is myoglobin that gives muscle tissue a red or dark color.)

During strenuous exercise, the oxygen stored in myoglobin is quickly used up, and normal circulation may not deliver oxygen fast enough to permit the completion of cell respiration. Even though the respiratory rate increases, the muscle fibers may literally run out of oxygen. This state is called **oxygen debt**, and in this case, glucose cannot be completely broken down into carbon dioxide and water. If oxygen is not present (or not present in sufficient amounts), glucose is converted to an intermediate molecule called **lactic acid**, which causes **muscle fatigue**.

In a state of fatigue, muscle fibers cannot contract efficiently, and contraction may become painful. To be in oxygen debt means that we owe the body some oxygen. Lactic acid from muscles enters the blood and circulates to the liver, where it is converted into pyruvic acid, a simple carbohydrate (three carbons, about half a glucose molecule). This conversion requires ATP, and oxygen is needed to produce the necessary ATP in the liver. This is why, after strenuous exercise, the respiratory rate and heart rate remain high for a time and only gradually return to normal. Another name proposed for this state is **recovery oxygen uptake,** which is a little longer but also makes sense. Oxygen uptake means a faster and deeper respiratory

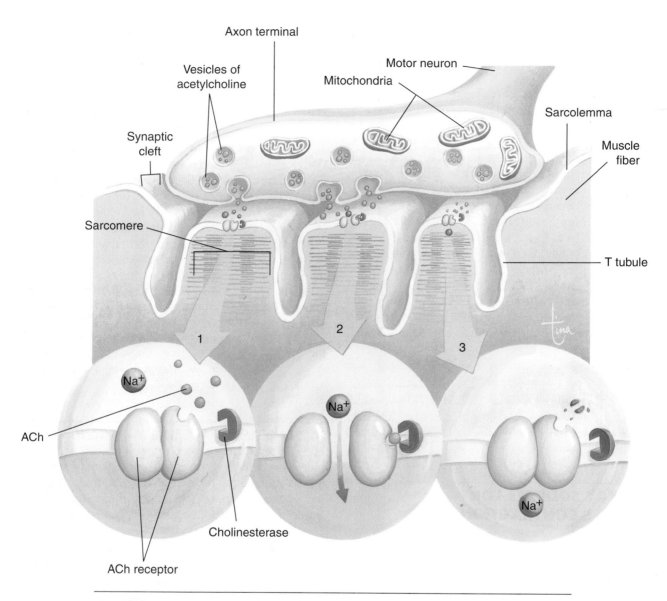

Axon terminal

Vesicles of
acetylcholine

Motor neuron

Mitochondria

Synaptic
cleft

Sarcolemma

Muscle
fiber

Sarcomere

T tubule

1

2

3

Na⁺

ACh

Na⁺

Na⁺

Cholinesterase

ACh receptor

Figure 7–2   Structure of the neuromuscular junction, showing an axon terminal adjacent to the sarcolemma of a muscle fiber. Schematic of events: **(1)** Acetylcholine is about to bond to the ACh receptor in the sarcolemma. **(2)** Channel opens to allow Na⁺ ions into the muscle cell. **(3)** Cholinesterase inactivates acetylcholine.

rate. What is this uptake for? For recovery from strenuous exercise.

MUSCLE FIBER— MICROSCOPIC STRUCTURE

We will now look more closely at a muscle fiber, keeping in mind that there are thousands of these cylindrical cells in one muscle. Each muscle fiber has its own motor nerve ending; the **neuromuscular junction** is where the motor neuron terminates on the muscle fiber (Fig. 7–2). The **axon terminal** is the enlarged tip of the motor neuron; it contains sacs of the neurotransmitter **acetylcholine** (ACh). The membrane of the muscle fiber is the **sarcolemma**, which contains receptor sites for acetylcholine, and an inactivator called **cholinesterase**. The **synapse** (or synaptic cleft) is the small space between the axon terminal and the sarcolemma.

Within the muscle fiber are thousands of individual contracting units called **sarcomeres**, which are arranged end to end in cylinders called **myofibrils**. The structure of a sarcomere is shown in Fig. 7–3: The Z lines are the end boundaries of a sarcomere. Filaments of the protein **myosin** are in the center of the sarcomere, and filaments of the protein **actin** are at the ends, attached to the Z lines. Myosin filaments are anchored to the Z lines by the protein **titin**.

Myosin and actin are the contractile proteins of a muscle fiber. Their interactions produce muscle contraction. Also present are two inhibitory proteins, **troponin** and **tropomyosin**, which are part of the actin filaments and prevent the sliding of actin and myosin when the muscle fiber is relaxed.

Surrounding the sarcomeres is the **sarcoplasmic reticulum**, the endoplasmic reticulum of muscle cells. The sarcoplasmic reticulum is a reservoir for calcium ions (Ca^{+2}), which are essential for the contraction process.

All of these parts of a muscle fiber are involved in the contraction process. Contraction begins when a nerve impulse arrives at the axon terminal and stimulates the release of acetylcholine. Acetylcholine generates electrical changes (the movement of ions) at the sarcolemma of the muscle fiber. These electrical changes initiate a sequence of events within the muscle fiber that is called the **Sliding Filament Theory** of muscle contraction. We will begin our discussion with the sarcolemma.

SARCOLEMMA—POLARIZATION

When a muscle fiber is relaxed, the sarcolemma is polarized (has a resting potential), which refers to a difference in electrical charges between the outside and the inside. During **polarization**, the outside of the sarcolemma has a positive charge relative to the inside, which is said to have a negative charge. Sodium ions (Na^+) are more abundant outside the cell, and potassium ions (K^+) and negative ions are more abundant inside (Fig. 7–4).

The Na^+ ions outside tend to diffuse into the cell, and the **sodium pump** transfers them back out. The K^+ ions inside tend to diffuse outside, and the **potassium pump** returns them inside. Both of these pumps are active transport mechanisms which, you may recall, require ATP. Muscle fibers use ATP to maintain a high concentration of Na^+ ions outside the cell and a high concentration of K^+ inside. The pumps, there-fore, maintain polarization and relaxation until a nerve impulse stimulates a change.

SARCOLEMMA—DEPOLARIZATION

When a nerve impulse arrives at the axon terminal, it causes the release of acetylcholine, which diffuses across the synapse and bonds to **ACh receptors** on the sarcolemma. By doing so, acetylcholine makes the sarcolemma very permeable to Na^+ ions, which rush into the cell. This makes the inside of the sarcolemma positive relative to the outside, which is now considered negative. This reversal of charges is called **depolarization**. The electrical impulse thus generated (called an action potential) then spreads along the entire sarcolemma of a muscle fiber. The sarcolemma has inward folds called **T tubules** (transverse tubules, shown in Fig. 7–3 and Fig. 7–5), which carry the action potential to the interior of the muscle cell. Depolarization initiates changes within the cell that bring about contraction. The electrical changes that take place at the sarcolemma are summarized in Table 7–1 and shown in Fig. 7–4.

MECHANISM OF CONTRACTION— SLIDING FILAMENT THEORY

All of the parts of a muscle fiber and the electrical changes described earlier are involved in the contraction process, which is a precise sequence of events.

In summary, a nerve impulse causes depolarization of a muscle fiber, and this electrical change enables the myosin filaments to pull the actin filaments toward the center of the sarcomere, making the sarcomere shorter. All of the sarcomeres shorten and the muscle fiber contracts. A more detailed description of this process is the following:

1. A nerve impulse arrives at the axon terminal; acetylcholine is released and diffuses across the synapse.
2. Acetylcholine makes the sarcolemma more permeable to Na^+ ions, which rush into the cell.
3. The sarcolemma depolarizes, becoming negative outside and positive inside. The T tubules bring the reversal of charges to the interior of the muscle cell.
4. Depolarization stimulates the release of Ca^{+2} ions from the sarcoplasmic reticulum. Ca^{+2} ions bond

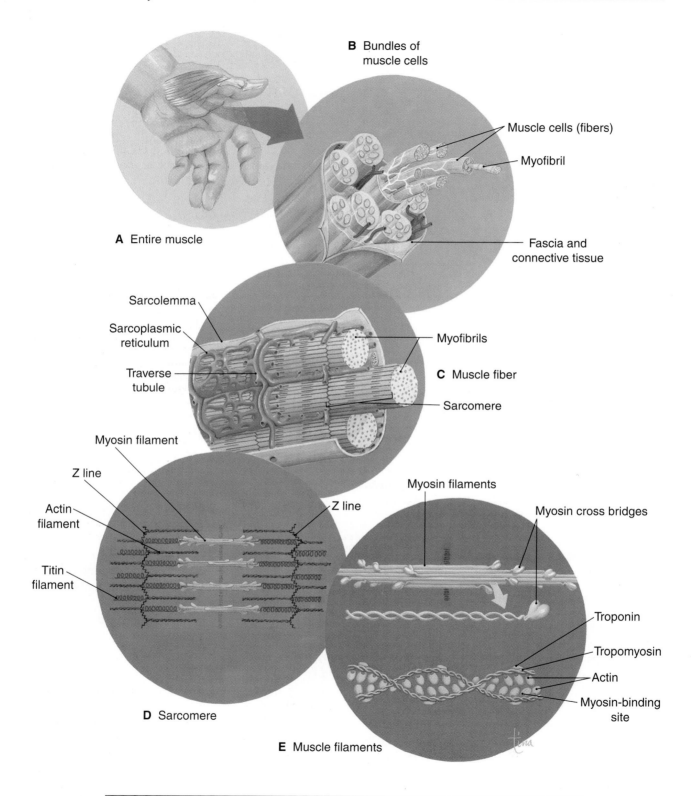

B Bundles of muscle cells

Muscle cells (fibers)

Myofibril

A Entire muscle

Fascia and connective tissue

Sarcolemma

Sarcoplasmic reticulum

Myofibrils

Traverse tubule

C Muscle fiber

Sarcomere

Myosin filament

Z line

Actin filament

Z line

Myosin filaments

Myosin cross bridges

Titin filament

Troponin

Tropomyosin

Actin

Myosin-binding site

D Sarcomere

E Muscle filaments

Figure 7–3   Structure of skeletal muscle. **(A)** Entire muscle. **(B)** Bundles of muscle cells within a muscle. **(C)** Single muscle fiber, microscopic structure. **(D)** A sarcomere. **(E)** Structure of muscle filaments.

A Polarization

B Depolarization   ACh

C Repolarization

Figure 7–4   Electrical charges and ion concentrations at the sarcolemma. **(A)** Polarization, when the muscle fiber is relaxed. **(B)** Wave of depolarization in response to stimulus of acetylcholine. **(C)** Wave of repolarization.

Table 7–1	SARCOLEMMA—ELECTRICAL CHANGES
State or Event	**Description**
Resting Potential	
Polarization	• Sarcolemma has a (+) charge outside and a (–) charge inside. • Na^+ ions are more abundant outside the cell; as they diffuse inward, the sodium pump returns them outside. • K^+ ions are more abundant inside the cell; as they diffuse out the potassium pump returns them inside.
Action Potential	
Depolarization	• ACh makes the sarcolemma very permeable to Na^+ ions, which rush into the cell. • Reversal of charges on the sarcolemma: now (–) outside and (+) inside. • The reversal of charges spreads along the entire sarcolemma. • Cholinesterase at the sarcolemma inactivates ACh.
Repolarization	• Sarcolemma becomes very permeable to K^+ ions, which rush out of the cell. • Restoration of charges on the sarcolemma: (+) outside and (–) inside. • The sodium and potassium pumps return Na^+ ions outside and K^+ ions inside. • The muscle fiber is now able to respond to ACh released by another nerve impulse arriving at the axon terminal.

to the troponin–tropomyosin complex, which shifts it away from the actin filaments.

5. Myosin splits ATP to release its energy; bridges on the myosin attach to the actin filaments and pull them toward the center of the sarcomere, thus making the sarcomere shorter (Fig. 7–5).

6. All of the sarcomeres in a muscle fiber shorten—the entire muscle fiber contracts.

7. The sarcolemma repolarizes: K^+ ions leave the cell, restoring a positive charge outside and a negative charge inside. The pumps then return Na^+ ions outside and K^+ ions inside.

8. Cholinesterase in the sarcolemma inactivates acetylcholine.

9. Subsequent nerve impulses will prolong contraction (more acetylcholine is released).

10. When there are no further impulses, the muscle fiber will relax and return to its original length.

Steps 1–8 of the above sequence describe a single muscle fiber contraction (called a *twitch*) in response to a single nerve impulse. Because all of this takes place in less than a second, useful movements would not be possible if muscle fibers relaxed immediately after contracting. Normally, however, nerve impulses arrive in a continuous stream and produce a sustained contraction called **tetanus**, which is a normal state not to be confused with the disease tetanus (see Box 7–2:

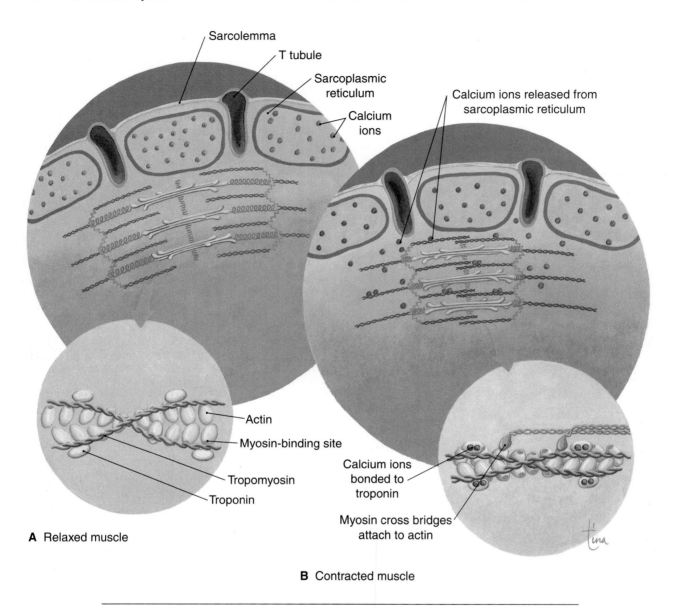

Figure 7–5   Sliding Filament Theory. **(A)** Sarcomere in relaxed muscle fiber. **(B)** Sarcomere in contracted muscle fiber. See text for description.

Tetanus and Botulism). When in tetanus, muscle fibers remain contracted and are capable of effective movements. In a muscle such as the biceps brachii that flexes the forearm, an effective movement means that many of its thousands of muscle fibers are in tetanus, a sustained contraction.

As you might expect with such a complex process, muscle contraction may be impaired in many different ways. Perhaps the most obvious is the loss of nerve impulses to muscle fibers, which can occur when nerves or the spinal cord are severed, or when a **stroke (cerebrovascular accident)** occurs in the frontal lobes of the cerebrum. Without nerve impulses, skeletal muscles become **paralyzed**, unable to contract. Paralyzed muscles eventually **atrophy**, that is, become smaller from lack of use. Other disorders that affect muscle functioning are discussed in Box 7–3: Muscular Dystrophy and Box 7–4: Myasthenia Gravis.

Box 7–2   TETANUS AND BOTULISM

Some bacteria cause disease by producing toxins. A **neurotoxin** is a chemical that in some way disrupts the normal functioning of the nervous system. Because skeletal muscle contraction depends on nerve impulses, the serious consequences for the individual may be seen in the muscular system.

Tetanus is characterized by the inability of muscles to relax. The toxin produced by the tetanus bacteria *(Clostridium tetani)* affects the nervous system in such a way that muscle fibers receive too many impulses, and muscles go into spasms. Lock-jaw, the common name for tetanus, indicates one of the first symptoms, which is difficulty opening the mouth because of spasms of the masseter muscles. Treatment requires the antitoxin (an antibody to the toxin) to neutralize the toxin. In untreated tetanus the cause of death is spasm of the respiratory muscles.

Botulism is usually a type of food poisoning, but it is not characterized by typical food poisoning symptoms such as diarrhea or vomiting. The neuro-toxin produced by the botulism bacteria *(Clostridium botulinum)* prevents the release of acetylcholine at neuromuscular junctions. Without acetylcholine, muscle fibers cannot contract, and muscles become paralyzed. Early symptoms of botulism include blurred or double vision and difficulty speaking or swallowing. Weakness and paralysis spread to other muscle groups, eventually affecting all voluntary muscles. Without rapid treatment with the antitoxin (the specific antibody to this toxin), botulism is fatal because of paralysis of the respiratory muscles.

Box 7–3   MUSCULAR DYSTROPHY

Muscular dystrophy is really a group of genetic diseases in which muscle tissue is replaced by fibrous connective tissue or by fat. Neither of these tissues is capable of contraction, and the result is progressive loss of muscle function. The most common form is Duchenne's muscular dystrophy, in which the loss of muscle function affects not only skeletal muscle but also cardiac muscle. Death usually occurs before the age of 20 due to heart failure, and at present there is no cure.

Duchenne's muscular dystrophy is a **sex-linked** (or x-linked) **trait**, which means that the gene for it is on the X chromosome and is recessive. The female sex chromosomes are XX. If one X chromosome has a gene for muscular dystrophy, and the other X chromosome has a dominant gene for normal muscle function, the woman will not have muscular dystrophy but will be a carrier who may pass the muscular dystrophy gene to her children. The male sex chromosomes are XY, and the Y has no gene at all for muscle function, that is, no gene to prevent the expression of the gene on the X chromosome. If the X chromosome has a gene for muscular dystrophy, the male will have the disease. This is why Duchenne's muscular dystrophy is more common in males; the presence of only one gene means the disease will be present.

The muscular dystrophy gene on the X chromosome has been located, and the protein the gene codes for has been named dystrophin. Dystrophin seems to be necessary for the stability of the sarcolemma and the proper movement of ions. Determining the precise function of dystrophin, and exactly what goes wrong when this protein malfunctions, may provide a basis or starting point for therapy. Treatments being investigated include the injection of normal muscle cells into affected muscles, and the insertion (using viruses) of normal genes for dystrophin into affected muscle cells.

RESPONSES TO EXERCISE— MAINTAINING HOMEOSTASIS

Although entire textbooks are devoted to exercise physiology, we will discuss it only briefly here as an example of the body's ability to maintain homeostasis. Engaging in moderate or strenuous exercise is a physiological stress situation, a change that the body must cope with and still maintain a normal internal environment, that is, homeostasis.

Some of the body's responses to exercise are diagrammed in Fig. 7–6; notice how they are related to cell respiration. As you can see, the respiratory and cardiovascular systems make essential contributions to exercise. The integumentary system also has a role,

Box 7–4   MYASTHENIA GRAVIS

Myasthenia gravis is an **autoimmune** disorder characterized by extreme muscle fatigue even after minimal exertion. Women are affected more often than are men, and symptoms usually begin in middle age. Weakness may first be noticed in the facial or swallowing muscles and may progress to other muscles. Without treatment, the respiratory muscles will eventually be affected, and respiratory failure is the cause of death.

In myasthenia gravis, the autoantibodies (self-antibodies) destroy the **acetylcholine receptors** on the sarcolemma. These receptors are the sites to which acetylcholine bonds and stimulates the entry of Na$^+$ ions. Without these receptors, the acetylcholine released by the axon terminal cannot cause depolarization of a muscle fiber.

Treatment of myasthenia gravis may involve anticholinesterase medications. Recall that cholinesterase is present in the sarcolemma to inactivate acetylcholine and prevent continuous, unwanted impulses. If this action of cholinesterase is inhibited, acetylcholine remains on the sarcolemma for a longer time and may bond to any remaining receptors to stimulate depolarization and contraction.

since it eliminates excess body heat. Although not shown, the nervous system is also directly involved, as we have seen. The brain generates the impulses for muscle contraction, coordinates those contractions, and regulates heart rate, breathing rate, and the diameter of blood vessels. The next time you run up a flight of stairs, hurry to catch a bus, or just go dancing, you might reflect a moment on all of the things that are actually happening to your body . . . after you catch your breath.

AGING AND THE MUSCULAR SYSTEM

With age, muscle cells die and are replaced by fibrous connective tissue or by fat. Regular exercise, however, delays atrophy of muscles. Although muscles become slower to contract and their maximal strength decreases, exercise can maintain muscle functioning at a level that meets whatever a person needs for daily activities. The lifting of small weights is recommended as exercise for elderly people, women as well as men. Such exercise also benefits the cardiovascular, respiratory, and skeletal systems.

MAJOR MUSCLES OF THE BODY

The actions that muscles perform are shown in Fig. 7–7 and are listed in Table 7–2. Most are in pairs as antagonistic functions.

The major muscles are shown in Fig. 7–8. They are listed, according to body area, in Tables 7–3 through

Figure 7–6 Responses of the body during exercise.

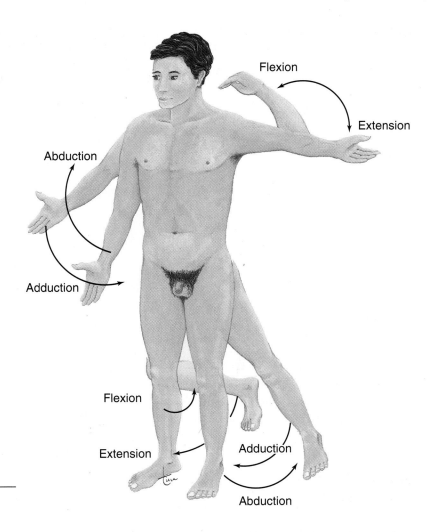

Figure 7–7   Actions of muscles.

7–7, with associated Figs. 7–9 through 7–13, respectively. Learning the muscles and their functions does involve memorization, but the bones you have already learned will help you. For each muscle, note its origin and insertion. If you know the bones to which a muscle is attached, you can determine the joint the muscle affects when it contracts.

The name of the muscle may also be helpful, and again, many of the terms are ones you have already learned. Some examples: "abdominus" refers to an abdominal muscle, "femoris" to a thigh muscle, "brachii" to a muscle of the upper arm, "oculi" to an eye muscle, and so on.

Muscles that are sites for intramuscular injections are shown in Box 7–5.

Table 7–2	ACTIONS OF MUSCLES
Action	**Definition**
Flexion	• To decrease the angle of a joint
Extension	• To increase the angle of a joint
Adduction	• To move closer to the midline
Abduction	• To move away from the midline
Pronation	• To turn the palm down
Supination	• To turn the palm up
Dorsiflexion	• To elevate the foot
Plantar flexion	• To lower the foot (point the toes)
Rotation	• To move a bone around its longitudinal axis

Most are grouped in pairs of antagonistic functions.

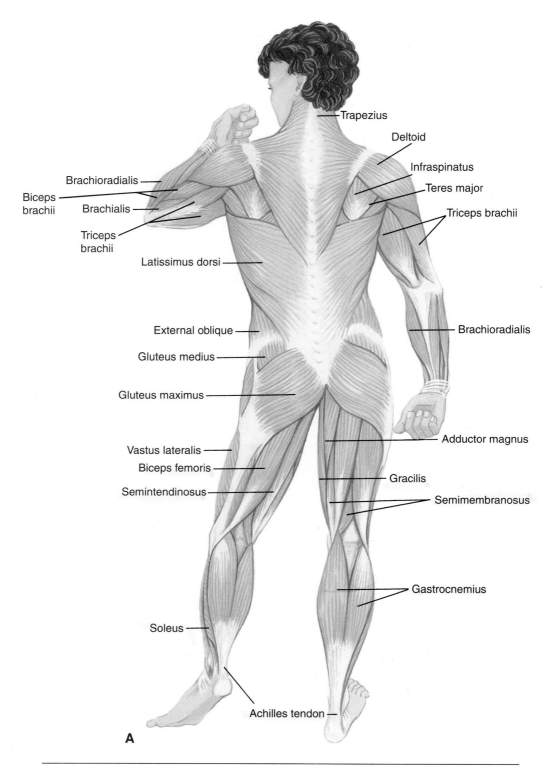

Figure 7–8 Major muscles of the body. **(A)** Posterior view. **(B)** Anterior view.

Masseter

Sternocleidomastoid

Deltoid

Pectoralis major

Brachialis

Biceps
brachii

Brachioradialis

Triceps
brachii

External oblique

Rectus abdominus

Iliopsoas

Pectineus

Sartorius

Adductor longus

Rectus femoris

Gracilis

Vastus lateralis

Vastus medialis

Gastrocnemius

Tibialis anterior

Soleus

B

Figure 7–8   Major muscles of the body. **(A)** Posterior view. **(B)** Anterior view.

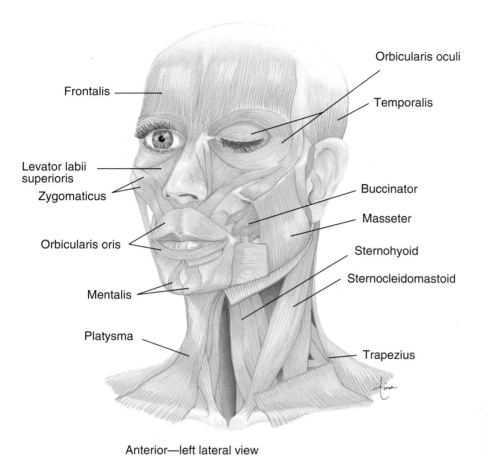

Frontalis

Orbicularis oculi

Temporalis

Levator labii
superioris

Zygomaticus

Buccinator

Masseter

Orbicularis oris

Sternohyoid

Sternocleidomastoid

Mentalis

Platysma

Trapezius

Anterior—left lateral view

Figure 7–9 Muscles of the head and neck in anterior, left-lateral view.

| Table 7–3 | MUSCLES OF THE HEAD AND NECK | | |

Muscle	Function	Origin	Insertion
Orbicularis oculi	Closes eye	• medial side of orbit	• encircles eye
Orbicularis oris	Puckers lips	• encircles mouth	• skin at corners of mouth
Masseter	Closes jaw	• maxilla and zygomatic	• mandible
Buccinator	Pulls corners of mouth laterally	• maxilla and mandible	• orbicularis oris
Sternocleidomastoid	Turns head to opposite side (both—flex head and neck)	• sternum and clavicle	• temporal bone (mastoid process)
Semispinalis capitis (a deep muscle)	Turns head to same side (both—extend head and neck)	• 7th cervical and first 6 thoracic vertebrae	• occipital bone

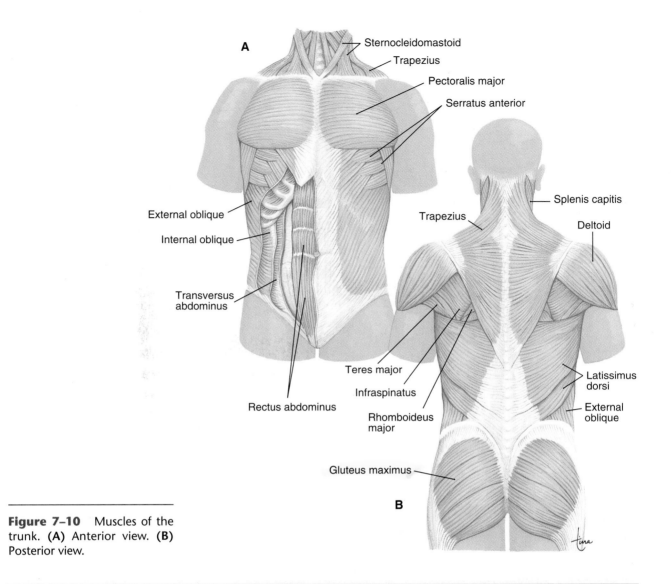

Figure 7–10 Muscles of the trunk. **(A)** Anterior view. **(B)** Posterior view.

Table 7–4	MUSCLES OF THE TRUNK		
Muscle	**Function**	**Origin**	**Insertion**
Trapezius	Raises, lowers, and adducts shoulders	• occipital bone and all thoracic vertebrae	• spine of scapula and clavicle
External intercostals	Pull ribs up and out (inhalation)	• superior rib	• inferior rib
Internal intercostals	Pull ribs down and in (forced exhalation)	• inferior rib	• superior rib
Diaphragm	Flattens (down) to enlarge chest cavity for inhalation	• last 6 costal cartilages and lumbar vertebrae	• central tendon
Rectus abdominus	Flexes vertebral column, compresses abdomen	• pubic bones	• 5th–7th costal cartilages and xiphoid process
External oblique	Rotates and flexes vertebral column, compresses abdomen	• lower 8 ribs	• iliac crest and lines alba
Sacrospinalis group (deep muscles)	Extends vertebral column	• ilium, lumbar, and some thoracic vertebrae	• ribs, cervical, and thoracic vertebrae

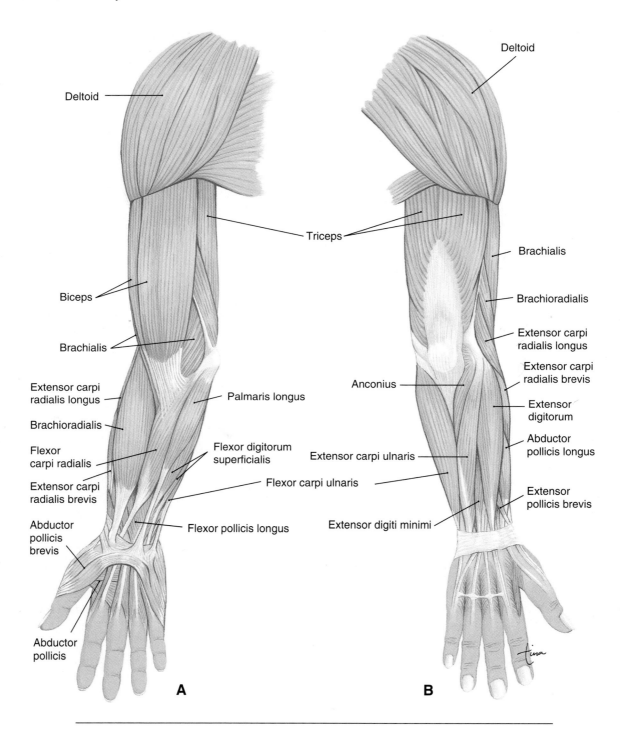

Figure 7–11   Muscles of the arm. **(A)** Anterior view. **(B)** Posterior view.

Table 7–5   MUSCLES OF THE SHOULDER AND ARM

Muscle	Function	Origin	Insertion
Deltoid	Abducts the humerus	• scapula and clavicle	• humerus
Pectoralis major	Flexes and adducts the humerus	• clavicle, sternum, 2nd–6th costal cartilages	• humerus
Latissimus dorsi	Extends and adducts the humerus	• last 6 thoracic vertebrae, all lumbar vertebrae, sacrum, iliac crest	• humerus
Teres major	Extends and adducts the humerus	• scapula	• humerus
Triceps brachii	Extends the forearm	• humerus and scapula	• ulna
Biceps brachii	Flexes the forearm	• scapula	• radius
Brachioradialis	Flexes the forearm	• humerus	• radius

Table 7–6   MUSCLES OF THE HIP AND LEG

Muscle	Function	Origin	Insertion
Iliopsoas	Flexes femur	• ilium, lumbar vertebrae	• femur
Gluteus maximus	Extends femur	• iliac crest, sacrum, coccyx	• femur
Gluteus medius	Abducts femur	• ilium	• femur
Quadriceps femoris group: Rectus femoris Vastus lateralis Vastus medialis Vastus intermedius	Flexes femur and extends lower leg	• ilium and femur	• tibia
Hamstring group: Biceps femoris Semimembranosus Semitendinosus	Extends femur and flexes lower leg	• ischium	• tibia and fibula
Adductor group	Adducts femur	• ischium and pubis	• femur
Sartorius	Flexes femur and lower leg	• ilium	• tibia
Gastrocnemius	Plantar flexes foot	• femur	• calcaneus (Achilles tendon)
Soleus	Plantar flexes foot	• tibia and fibula	• calcaneus (Achilles tendon)
Tibialis anterior	Dorsiflexes foot	• tibia	• metatarsals

Iliopsoas

Pectineus

Gluteus maximus

Sartorius

Adductor
longus

Rectus femoris

Adductor
magnus

Vastus lateralis

Gracilis

Biceps femoris

Vastus lateralis

Semitendinosus

Vastus medialis

Semimembranosus

Plantaris

Peroneus longus

Gastrocnemius

Tibialis anterior

Extensor digitorum longus

Soleus

Peroneus longus

Flexor
digitorum longus

Extensor hallucis longus

Peroneus brevis

Extensor digitorum brevis

Extensor
hallucis brevis

A

B

Figure 7–12   Muscles of the leg. **(A)** Anterior view. **(B)** Posterior view.

| Table 7–7 | MUSCLES OF THE PELVIC FLOOR |

Muscle	Function	Origin	Insertion
Levator ani	Supports pelvic organs, especially during defecation, urination, coughing, and forced exhalation; constricts anus, urethra, and vagina	• pubis and ischium	• coccyx, anal canal, urethra
Coccygeus	Supports pelvic organs, especially during defecation, urination, coughing, and forced exhalation	• ischium	• coccyx and sacrum
Ischiocavernosus	Erection of clitoris in female, penis in male	• ischium and pubis	• clitoris or penis
Bulbospongiosus	Assists urination; erection in female; erection and ejaculation in male	• central tendon of perineum	• fasciae, pubic arch, clitoris, or penis
Transverse perineus (superficial and deep)	Assists urination in female; urination and ejaculation in male	• ischium	• central tendon or perineum
External anal sphincter	Closes anus	• anococcygeal ligament	• central tendon of perineum

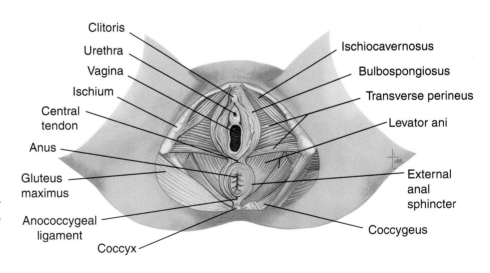

Figure 7–13   Muscles of the female pelvic floor.

Box 7–5 COMMON INJECTION SITES

Intramuscular injections are used when rapid absorption is needed, because muscle has a good blood supply. Common sites are the buttock *(gluteus medius)*, lateral thigh *(vastus lateralis)*, and the shoulder *(deltoid)*. These sites are shown; also shown are the large nerves to be avoided when giving such injections.

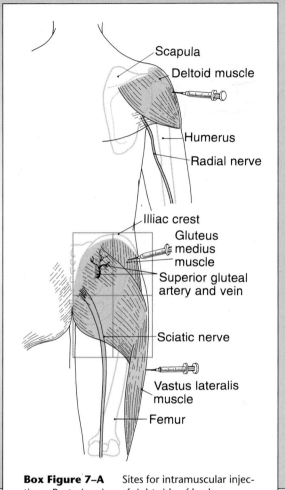

Box Figure 7–A Sites for intramuscular injections. Posterior view of right side of body.

STUDY OUTLINE

Organ Systems Involved in Movement
1. Muscular—moves the bones.
2. Skeletal—bones are moved, at their joints, by muscles.
3. Nervous—transmits impulses to muscles to cause contraction.
4. Respiratory—exchanges O_2 and CO_2 between the air and blood.
5. Circulatory—transports O_2 to muscles and removes CO_2.

Muscle Structure
1. Muscle fibers (cells) are specialized to contract, shorten, and produce movement.
2. A skeletal muscle is made of thousands of muscle fibers. Varying movements require contraction of variable numbers of muscle fibers in a muscle.
3. Tendons attach muscles to bone; the origin is the more stationary bone, the insertion is the more movable bone. A tendon merges with the fascia of a muscle and the periosteum of a bone; all are made of fibrous connective tissue.

Muscle Arrangements
1. Antagonistic muscles have opposite functions. A muscle pulls when it contracts, but exerts no force when it relaxes and cannot push. When one muscle pulls a bone in one direction, another muscle is needed to pull the bone in the other direction (see also Table 7–2 and Fig. 7–1).
2. Synergistic muscles have the same function and alternate as the prime mover depending on the position of the bone to be moved. Synergists also stabilize a joint to make a more precise movement possible.
3. The frontal lobes of the cerebrum generate the impulses necessary for contraction of skeletal muscles. The cerebellum regulates coordination.

Muscle Tone—the state of slight contraction present in muscles
1. Alternate fibers contract to prevent muscle fatigue; regulated by the cerebellum.
2. Good tone helps maintain posture, produces 25% of body heat (at rest), and improves coordination.
3. Isotonic exercise involves contraction with movement; improves tone and strength and improves cardiovascular and respiratory efficiency (aerobic exercise).
4. Isometric exercise involves contraction without movement; improves tone and strength but is not aerobic.

Muscle Sense—knowing where our muscles are without looking at them
1. Permits us to perform everyday activities without having to concentrate on muscle position.
2. Stretch receptors (proprioceptors) in muscles respond to stretching and generate impulses that the brain interprets as a mental "picture" of where the muscles are. Parietal lobes: conscious muscle sense; cerebellum: unconscious muscle sense used to promote coordination.

Energy Sources for Muscle Contraction
1. ATP is the direct source; the ATP stored in muscles lasts only a few seconds.
2. Creatine phosphate is a secondary energy source; is broken down to creatine + phosphate + energy. The energy is used to synthesize more ATP. Some creatine is converted to creatinine, which must be excreted by the kidneys. Most creatine is used for the resynthesis of creatine phosphate.
3. Glycogen is the most abundant energy source and is first broken down to glucose. Glucose is broken down in cell respiration:

$$\text{Glucose} + O_2 \rightarrow CO_2 + H_2O + \text{ATP} + \text{heat}$$

   ATP is used for contraction; heat contributes to body temperature; H_2O becomes part of intracellular fluid; CO_2 is eventually exhaled.
4. Oxygen is essential for the completion of cell respiration. Hemoglobin in RBCs carries oxygen to muscles; myoglobin stores oxygen in muscles; both these proteins contain iron, which enables them to bond to oxygen.
5. Oxygen debt (recovery oxygen uptake): Muscle fibers run out of oxygen during strenuous exercise, and glucose is converted to lactic acid, which causes fatigue. Breathing rate remains high after exercise to deliver more oxygen to the liver, which converts lactic acid to pyruvic acid, a simple carbohydrate (ATP required).

Muscle Fiber—microscopic structure

1. Neuromuscular junction: axon terminal and sarcolemma; the synapse is the space between. The axon terminal contains acetylcholine (a neurotransmitter), and the sarcolemma contains cholinesterase (an inactivator) (see Fig. 7–2).
2. Sarcomeres are the contracting units of a muscle fiber. Myosin and actin filaments are the contracting proteins of sarcomeres. Troponin and tropomyosin are proteins that inhibit the sliding of myosin and actin when the muscle fiber is relaxed (see Fig. 7–3 and Fig. 7–5).
3. The sarcoplasmic reticulum surrounds the sarcomeres and is a reservoir for calcium ions.
4. Polarization (resting potential): When the muscle fiber is relaxed, the sarcolemma has a (+) charge outside and a (−) charge inside. Na^+ ions are more abundant outside the cell and K^+ ions are more abundant inside the cell. The Na^+ and K^+ pumps maintain these relative concentrations on either side of the sarcolemma (see Table 7–1 and Fig. 7–4).
5. Depolarization: This process is started by a nerve impulse. Acetylcholine released by the axon terminal makes the sarcolemma very permeable to Na^+ ions, which enter the cell and cause a reversal of charges to (−) outside and (+) inside. The depolarization spreads along the entire sarcolemma and initiates the contraction process. Folds of the sarcolemma called T tubules carry the depolarization into the interior of the muscle cell.

Mechanism of Contraction—Sliding Filament Theory (see Fig. 7–5)

1. Depolarization stimulates a sequence of events that enables myosin filaments to pull the actin filaments to the center of the sarcomere, which shortens.
2. All of the sarcomeres in a muscle fiber contract in response to a nerve impulse; the entire cell contracts.
3. Tetanus is a sustained contraction brought about by continuous nerve impulses; all our movements involve tetanus.
4. Paralysis: Muscles that do not receive nerve impulses are unable to contract and will atrophy. Paralysis may be the result of nerve damage, spinal cord damage, or brain damage.

Responses to Exercise—maintaining homeostasis

See section in chapter and Fig. 7–6.

Major Muscles

See Tables 7–2 through 7–7 and Figs. 7–7 through 7–13.

REVIEW QUESTIONS

1. Name the organ systems directly involved in movement and for each state how they are involved. (p. 130)

2. State the function of tendons. Name the part of a muscle and a bone to which a tendon is attached. (p. 130)

3. State the term for: (pp. 130–131)
   a. Muscles with the same function
   b. Muscles with opposite functions
   c. The muscle that does most of the work in a movement

4. Explain why antagonistic muscle arrangements are necessary. Give two examples. (p. 130)

5. State three reasons why good muscle tone is important. (pp. 131–132)

6. Explain why muscle sense is important. Name the receptors involved and state what they detect. (pp. 132–133)

7. With respect to muscle contraction, state the functions of the cerebellum and the frontal lobes of the cerebrum. (p. 131)

8. Name the direct energy source for muscle contraction. Name the two secondary energy sources. Which of these is more abundant? (p. 133)

9. State the simple equation of cell respiration and what happens to each of the products of this reaction. (p. 133)

10. Name the two sources of oxygen for muscle fibers. State what the two proteins have in common. (p. 133)

11. Explain what is meant by oxygen debt. What is needed to correct oxygen debt, and where does it come from? (p. 133)

12. Name these parts of the neuromuscular junction: (p. 134)
    a. The membrane of the muscle fiber
    b. The end of the motor neuron
    c. The space between neuron and muscle cell

    State the locations of acetylcholine and cholinesterase.

13. Name the contracting proteins of sarcomeres, and describe their locations in a sarcomere. Where is the sarcoplasmic reticulum and what does it contain? (p. 135)

14. In terms of ions and charges, describe: (p. 137)
    a. Polarization
    b. Depolarization
    c. Repolarization

15. With respect to the Sliding Filament Theory, explain the function of: (pp. 135, 137)
    a. Acetylcholine
    b. Calcium ions
    c. Myosin and actin
    d. Troponin and tropomyosin
    e. Cholinesterase

16. State three of the body's physiological responses to exercise, and explain how each helps maintain homeostasis. (pp. 139–140)

17. Find the major muscles on yourself, and state a function of each muscle.

FOR FURTHER THOUGHT

1. In an accident with farm machinery, Mr. R. had his left arm severed just below the elbow. Mrs. R. stopped the bleeding, called for an ambulance, and packed the severed arm in ice for the EMTs to take to the hospital. Will Mr. R. ever be able to move the fingers of his left hand again? What structures must be reattached, and what has to happen?

2. Name all of the muscles you can think of that move the thigh at the hip. Group them as synergists, if possible. Then pair those groups or individual muscles as antagonists.

3. Muscle contraction is important for posture. Muscles oppose each other, contracting equally to keep us upright. Picture the body in anatomic position, and describe what would happen if each of these muscles *relaxed* completely:
    Semispinalis capitis
    Masseter
    Rectus abdominus
    Sacrospinalis
    Quadriceps femoris
    Gluteus maximus

4. An exercise for skier's involves sitting against a wall as if you were sitting in a chair, but without a chair. Thighs should be parallel to the floor and the knees should make a 90° angle. Try it. What kind of exercise is this? Which muscles are doing most of the work (which ones begin to hurt)? Which do you think would be easier: three minutes of this exercise or three minutes of jogging? Can you think of an explanation?

5. Can you juggle? Don't just say "no"—have you ever tried? Find some old tennis balls and try juggling two balls with one hand, or three balls with two hands. Explain how muscle sense is involved in juggling.

    Now try to imagine what it would be like to be without muscle sense. Some people do not have muscle sense in certain parts of their bodies. Who are these people, and what has happened that cost them their muscle sense (and muscle contraction)?

CHAPTER 8

Box 8–1	MULTIPLE SCLEROSIS
Box 8–2	SHINGLES
Box 8–3	SPINAL CORD INJURIES
Box 8–4	CEREBROVASCULAR ACCIDENTS
Box 8–5	APHASIA
Box 8–6	ALZHEIMER'S DISEASE
Box 8–7	PARKINSON'S DISEASE
Box 8–8	LUMBAR PUNCTURE

Student Objectives

- Name the divisions of the nervous system and the parts of each, and state the general functions of the nervous system.
- Name the parts of a neuron and state the function of each.
- Explain the importance of Schwann cells in the peripheral nervous system and neuroglia in the central nervous system.
- Describe the electrical nerve impulse, and describe impulse transmission at synapses.
- Describe the types of neurons, nerves, and nerve tracts.

The Nervous System

Student Objectives (Continued)

- State the names and numbers of the spinal nerves, and their destinations.
- Explain the importance of stretch reflexes and flexor reflexes.
- State the functions of the parts of the brain; be able to locate each part on a diagram.
- Name the meninges and describe their locations.
- State the locations and functions of cerebrospinal fluid.
- Name the cranial nerves and state their functions.
- Explain how the sympathetic division of the autonomic nervous system enables the body to adapt to a stress situation.
- Explain how the parasympathetic division of the autonomic nervous system promotes normal body functioning in relaxed situations.

New Terminology

Afferent (**AFF**-uh-rent)
Autonomic nervous system (AW-toh-**NOM**-ik)
Cauda equina (**KAW**-dah ee-**KWHY**-nah)
Cerebral cortex (se-**REE**-bruhl **KOR**-teks)
Cerebrospinal fluid (se-**REE**-broh-**SPY**-nuhl)
Choroid plexus (**KOR**-oid **PLEK**-sus)
Corpus callosum (**KOR**-pus kuh-**LOH**-sum)
Cranial nerves (**KRAY**-nee-uhl NERVS)
Efferent (**EFF**-uh-rent)

Gray matter (GRAY **MA**-TUR)
Neuroglia (new-**ROG**-lee-ah)
Neurolemma (NYOO-ro-**LEM**-ah)
Parasympathetic (PAR-uh-SIM-puh-**THET**-ik)
Reflex (**REE**-fleks)
Somatic (soh-**MA**-tik)
Spinal nerves (**SPY**-nuhl NERVS)
Sympathetic (SIM-puh-**THET**-ik)
Ventricles of brain (**VEN**-trick'ls)
Visceral (**VISS**-er-uhl)
White matter (WIGHT **MA**-TUR)

Related Clinical Terminology

Alzheimer's disease (**ALZ**-high-mer's)
Aphasia (ah-**FAY**-zee-ah)
Blood–brain barrier (BLUHD BRAYNE)
Cerebrovascular accident (CVA) (se-**REE**-broh-**VAS**-kyoo-lur)
Lumbar puncture (**LUM**-bar **PUNK**-chur)
Meningitis (MEN-in-**JIGH**-tis)
Multiple sclerosis (MS) (**MULL**-ti-puhl skle-**ROH**-sis)
Neuralgia (new-**RAL**-jee-ah)
Neuritis (new-**RYE**-tis)
Neuropathy (new-**RAH**-puh-thee)
Parkinson's disease (**PAR**-kin-son's)
Remission (ree-**MISH**-uhn)
Spinal shock (**SPY**-nuhl SHAHK)

*Terms that appear in **bold type** in the chapter text are defined in the glossary, which begins on page 521.*

Most of us can probably remember being told, when we were children, not to touch the stove or some other source of potential harm. Because children are curious, such warnings often go unheeded. The result? Touching a hot stove brings about an immediate response of pulling away and a vivid memory of painful fingers. This simple and familiar experience illustrates the functions of the **nervous system**:

1. To detect changes and feel sensations
2. To initiate appropriate responses to changes
3. To organize information for immediate use and store it for future use

The nervous system is one of the regulating systems (the endocrine system is the other and is discussed in Chapter 10). Electrochemical impulses of the nervous system make it possible to obtain information about the external or internal environment and do whatever is necessary to maintain homeostasis. Some of this activity is conscious, but much of it happens without our awareness.

NERVOUS SYSTEM DIVISIONS

The nervous system has two divisions. The **central nervous system (CNS)** consists of the brain and spinal cord. The **peripheral nervous system (PNS)** consists of cranial nerves and spinal nerves. The PNS includes the autonomic nervous system (ANS).

The peripheral nervous system relays information to and from the central nervous system, and the brain is the center of activity that integrates this information, initiates responses, and makes us the individuals we are.

NERVE TISSUE

Nerve tissue was briefly described in Chapter 4, so we will begin by reviewing what you already know and then add to it.

Nerve cells are called **neurons**, or **nerve fibers**. Whatever their specific functions, all neurons have the same physical parts. The **cell body** contains the nucleus (Fig. 8–1) and is essential for the continued life of the neuron. As you will see, neuron cell bodies are found in the central nervous system or close to it in the trunk of the body. In these locations, cell bodies are protected by bone. There are no cell bodies in the arms and legs, which are much more subject to injury.

Dendrites are processes (extensions) that transmit impulses toward the cell body. The one **axon** of a neuron transmits impulses away from the cell body. It is the cell membrane of the dendrites, cell body, and axon that carries the electrical nerve impulse.

In the peripheral nervous system, axons and dendrites are "wrapped" in specialized cells called **Schwann cells** (see Fig. 8–1). During embryonic development, Schwann cells grow to surround the neuron processes, enclosing them in several layers of Schwann cell membrane. These layers are the **myelin sheath**; myelin is a phospholipid that electrically insulates neurons from one another. Without the myelin sheath, neurons would short-circuit, just as electrical wires would if they were not insulated (see Box 8–1: Multiple Sclerosis).

The spaces between adjacent Schwann cells, or segments of the myelin sheath, are called nodes of Ranvier (neurofibril nodes). These nodes are the parts of the neuron cell membrane that depolarize when an electrical impulse is transmitted (see "The Nerve Impulse" section, on pages 161–162).

The nuclei and cytoplasm of the Schwann cells are wrapped around the outside of the myelin sheath and are called the **neurolemma**, which becomes very important if nerves are damaged. If a peripheral nerve is severed and reattached precisely by microsurgery, the axons and dendrites may regenerate through the tunnels formed by the neurolemmas. The Schwann cells are also believed to produce a chemical growth factor that stimulates regeneration. Although this regeneration may take months, the nerves may eventually reestablish their proper connections, and the person may regain some sensation and movement in the once-severed limb.

In the central nervous system, the myelin sheaths are formed by **oligodendrocytes**, one of the **neuroglia**, the specialized cells found only in the brain and spinal cord. Because no Schwann cells are present, however, there is no neurolemma, and regeneration of neurons does not occur. This is why severing of the spinal cord, for example, results in permanent loss of function. Another type of neuroglial cell is the **astrocyte** (literally, "star cell"). In the embryo, these cells provide a framework for the migrating neurons that will form the brain. Thereafter, the extensions of astrocytes are wrapped around brain capillaries and contribute to the **blood–brain**

Afferent (sensory) neuron

Axon terminal

Axon

Nucleus

Cell body

Functional dendrite

Myelin sheath

Receptors

A

Efferent (motor) neuron

Dendrites

Cell body

Nucleus

Axon

Schwann cell nucleus

Myelin sheath

Node of Ranvier

Schwann cell

Axon

Neurolemma

Layers of myelin sheath

Axon terminal

B

C

Figure 8–1   Neuron structure. **(A)** A typical sensory neuron. **(B)** A typical motor neuron. The arrows indicate the direction of impulse transmission. **(C)** Details of the myelin sheath and neurolemma formed by Schwann cells.

barrier, which prevents potentially harmful waste products in the blood from diffusing out into brain tissue. These waste products are normal in the blood and tissue fluid, but brain tissue is much more sensi- tive to even low levels of them than are other tissues such as muscle tissue or connective tissue. The capil- laries of the brain also contribute to this barrier, because they are less permeable than are other capil-

Box 8–1   MULTIPLE SCLEROSIS

Multiple sclerosis (MS) is a demyelinating disease, that is, it involves deterioration of the myelin sheath of neurons in the central nervous system. Without the myelin sheath, the impulses of these neurons are short-circuited and do not reach their proper destinations, and the neuron axons are damaged and gradually die.

There is evidence that multiple sclerosis is an **autoimmune** disorder that is triggered by a virus or bacterial infection. Research has also uncovered a genetic component to some clusters of MS cases in families. Exactly how such genes would increase a person's susceptibility to an autoimmune disease is not yet known. In MS, the autoantibodies destroy the oligodendrocytes, the myelin-producing neuroglia of the central nervous system, which results in the formation of scleroses, or plaques of scar tissue, that do not provide electrical insulation

or protect the axon. Because loss of myelin may occur in many parts of the central nervous system, the symptoms vary, but they usually include muscle weakness or paralysis, numbness or partial loss of sensation, double vision, and loss of spinal cord reflexes, including those for urination and defecation.

The first symptoms usually appear between the ages of 20 and 40 years, and the disease may progress either slowly or rapidly. Some MS patients have **remissions**, periods of time when their symptoms diminish, but remissions and progression of the disease are not predictable. There is still no cure for MS, but therapies include suppression of the immune response, and interferon, which seems to prolong remissions in some patients. The possibility of stimulating remyelination of neurons is also being investigated.

Table 8–1   NEUROGLIA

Name	Function
Oligodendrocytes	• Produce the myelin sheath to electrically insulate neurons of the CNS.
Microglia	• Capable of movement and phagocytosis of pathogens and damaged tissue.
Astrocytes	• Support neurons, help maintain K+ level, contribute to the blood–brain barrier.
Ependyma	• Line the ventricles of the brain; many of the cells have cilia; involved in circulation of cerebrospinal fluid.

laries. A disadvantage of the blood–brain barrier is that some useful medications cannot cross it. This becomes an important consideration when treating brain infections or other diseases or disorders (see Table 8–1 for other functions of the neuroglia).

SYNAPSES

Neurons that transmit impulses to other neurons do not actually touch one another. The small gap or space

between the axon of one neuron and the dendrites or cell body of the next neuron is called the **synapse**. Within the synaptic knob (terminal end) of the presynaptic axon is a chemical **neurotransmitter** that is released into the synapse by the arrival of an electrical nerve impulse (Fig. 8–2). The neurotransmitter diffuses across the synapse, combines with specific receptor sites on the cell membrane of the postsynaptic neuron, and there generates an electrical impulse that in turn is carried by this neuron's axon to the next synapse, and so forth. A chemical **inactivator** at the cell body or dendrite of the postsynaptic neuron quickly inactivates the neurotransmitter. This prevents unwanted, continuous impulses, unless a new impulse from the first neuron releases more neurotransmitter.

Many synapses are termed excitatory, because the neurotransmitter causes the postsynaptic neuron to depolarize and transmit an electrical impulse to another neuron, muscle cell, or gland. Some synapses, however, are inhibitory, meaning that the neurotransmitter causes the postsynaptic neuron to hyperpolarize (become more positive outside as K+ ions leave the cell) and therefore *not* transmit an electrical impulse. Such inhibitory synapses are important, for example, for slowing the heart rate, and for balancing the excitatory impulses transmitted to skeletal muscles. With respect to the skeletal muscles, this inhi-

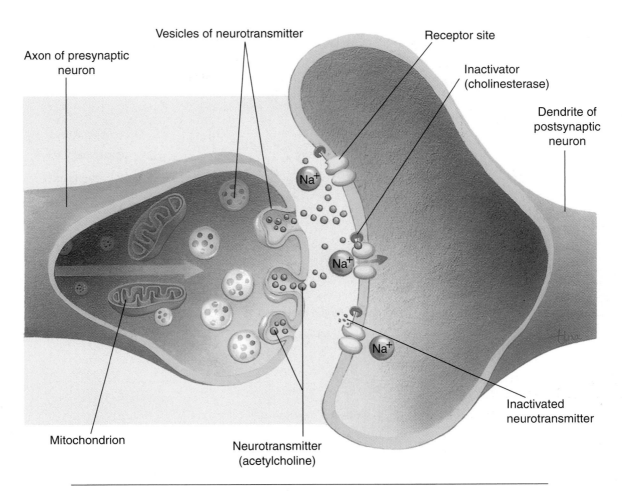

Axon of presynaptic neuron

Vesicles of neurotransmitter

Receptor site

Inactivator (cholinesterase)

Dendrite of postsynaptic neuron

Na⁺

Na⁺

Na⁺

Mitochondrion

Neurotransmitter (acetylcholine)

Inactivated neurotransmitter

Figure 8–2 Impulse transmission at a synapse. The arrow indicates the direction of the electrical impulse.

bition prevents excessive contraction and is important for coordination.

One important consequence of the presence of synapses is that they ensure one-way transmission of impulses in a living person. A nerve impulse cannot go backward across a synapse because there is no neurotransmitter released by the dendrites or cell body. Neurotransmitters can only be released by a neuron's axon, which does not have receptor sites for it, as does the postsynaptic membrane. Keep this in mind when we discuss the types of neurons later in the chapter.

An example of a neurotransmitter is **acetylcholine**, which is found at neuromuscular junctions, in the CNS, and in much of the peripheral nervous system. Acetylcholine usually makes a postsynaptic membrane more permeable to Na⁺ ions, which brings about depolarization of the postsynaptic neuron. **Cholinesterase** is the inactivator of acetylcholine. There are many other neurotransmitters, especially in the central nervous system. These include dopamine, GABA, norepinephrine, glutamate, and serotonin. Each of these neurotransmitters has its own chemical inactivator. Some neurotransmitters are reabsorbed into the neurons that secreted them; this process is called **reuptake** and also terminates the effect of the transmitter.

The complexity and variety of synapses make them frequent targets of medications. For example, drugs that alter mood or behavior often act on

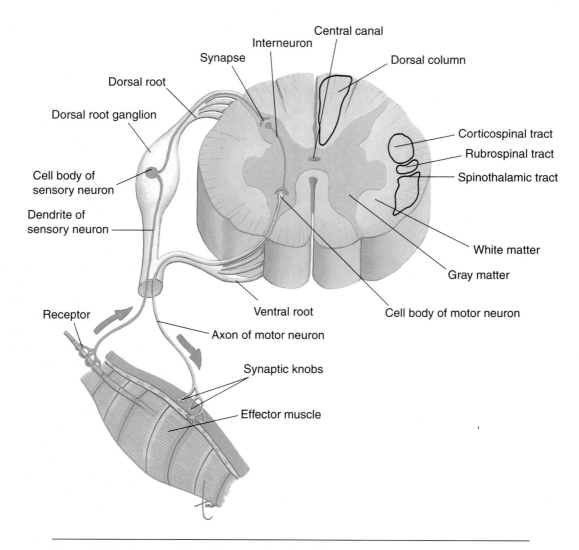

Figure 8–3   Cross-section of the spinal cord and the three types of neurons. Spinal nerve roots and their neurons are shown on the left side. Spinal nerve tracts are shown in the white matter on the right side. All tracts and nerves are bilateral (both sides).

specific neurotransmitters in the brain, and antihypertensive drugs affect synapse transmission at the smooth muscle of blood vessels.

TYPES OF NEURONS

Neurons may be classified into three groups: sensory neurons, motor neurons, and interneurons (Fig. 8–3). **Sensory neurons** (or **afferent neurons**) carry impulses from receptors to the central nervous system.

Receptors detect external or internal changes and send the information to the CNS in the form of impulses by way of the afferent neurons. The central nervous system interprets these impulses as a sensation. Sensory neurons from receptors in skin, skeletal muscles, and joints are called **somatic**; those from receptors in internal organs are called **visceral** sensory neurons.

Motor neurons (or **efferent neurons**) carry impulses from the central nervous system to **effectors**. The two types of effectors are muscles and glands. In response to impulses, muscles contract or relax and glands secrete. Motor neurons linked to skeletal muscle are called somatic; those to smooth muscle, cardiac muscle, and glands are called visceral.

Sensory and motor neurons make up the peripheral nervous system. Visceral motor neurons form the autonomic nervous system, a specialized subdivision of the PNS that will be discussed later in this chapter.

Interneurons are found entirely within the central nervous system. They are arranged so as to carry only sensory or motor impulses, or to integrate these functions. Some interneurons in the brain are concerned with thinking, learning, and memory.

A neuron carries impulses in only one direction. This is the result of the neuron's structure and location, as well as its physical arrangement with other neurons and the resulting pattern of synapses. The functioning nervous system, therefore, is an enormous network of "one-way streets," and there is no danger of impulses running into and canceling one another out.

NERVES AND NERVE TRACTS

A **nerve** is a group of axons and/or dendrites of many neurons, with blood vessels and connective tissue. **Sensory nerves** are made only of sensory neurons. The optic nerves for vision and olfactory nerves for smell are examples of nerves with a purely sensory function. **Motor nerves** are made only of motor neurons; autonomic nerves are motor nerves. A **mixed nerve** contains both sensory and motor neurons. Most of our peripheral nerves, such as the sciatic nerves in the legs, are mixed nerves.

The term **nerve tract** refers to groups of neurons within the central nervous system. All the neurons in a nerve tract are concerned with either sensory or motor activity. These tracts are often referred to as white matter; the myelin sheaths of the neurons give them a white color.

THE NERVE IMPULSE

The events of an electrical nerve impulse are the same as those of the electrical impulse generated in muscle fibers, which is discussed in Chapter 7. Stated simply, a neuron not carrying an impulse is in a state of **polarization**, with Na^+ ions more abundant outside the cell, and K^+ ions and negative ions more abundant inside the cell. The neuron has a positive charge on the outside of the cell membrane and a relative negative charge inside. A stimulus (such as a neurotransmitter) makes the membrane very permeable to Na^+ ions, which rush into the cell. This brings about **depolarization**, a reversal of charges on the membrane. The outside now has a negative charge, and the inside has a positive charge.

As soon as depolarization takes place, the neuron membrane becomes very permeable to K^+ ions, which rush out of the cell. This restores the positive charge outside and the negative charge inside, and is called **repolarization**. (The term *action potential* refers to depolarization followed by repolarization.) Then the sodium and potassium pumps return Na^+ ions outside and K^+ ions inside, and the neuron is ready to respond to another stimulus and transmit another impulse. An action potential in response to a stimulus takes place very rapidly and is measured in milliseconds. An individual neuron is capable of transmitting hundreds of action potentials (impulses) each second. A summary of the events of nerve impulse transmission is given in Table 8–2.

Transmission of electrical impulses is very rapid. The presence of an insulating myelin sheath increases the velocity of impulses, since only the nodes of Ranvier depolarize. This is called **saltatory conduction**. Many of our neurons are capable of transmitting impulses at a speed of many meters per second. Imagine a person 6 feet (about 2 meters) tall who stubs his toe; sensory impulses travel from the toe to the brain in less than a second (crossing a few synapses along the way). You can see how the nervous system can communicate so rapidly with all parts of the body, and why it is such an important regulatory system.

At synapses, nerve impulse transmission changes from electrical to chemical and depends on the release of neurotransmitters. Although diffusion across synapses is slow, the synapses are so small that this does not significantly affect the velocity of impulses in a living person.

THE SPINAL CORD

The **spinal cord** transmits impulses to and from the brain and is the integrating center for the spinal cord reflexes. Although this statement of functions is very

Table 8–2 | THE NERVE IMPULSE

State or Event	Description
Polarization (the neuron is not carrying an electrical impulse)	• Neuron membrane has a (+) charge outside and a (–) charge inside. • Na$^+$ ions are more abundant outside the cell. • K$^+$ ions and negative ions are more abundant inside the cell. Sodium and potassium pumps maintain these ion concentrations.
Depolarization (generated by a stimulus)	• Neuron membrane becomes very permeable to Na$^+$ ions, which rush into the cell. • The neuron membrane then has a (–) charge outside and a (+) charge inside.
Propagation of the impulse from point of stimulus	• Depolarization of part of the membrane makes adjacent membrane very permeable to Na$^+$ ions, and subsequent depolarization, which similarly affects the next part of the membrane, and so on. • The depolarization continues along the membrane of the neuron to the end of the axon.
Repolarization (immediately follows depolarization)	• Neuron membrane becomes very permeable to K$^+$ ions, which rush out of the cell. This restores the (+) charge outside and (–) charge inside the membrane. • The Na$^+$ ions are returned outside and the K$^+$ ions are returned inside by the sodium and potassium pumps. • The neuron is now able to respond to another stimulus and generate another impulse.

interneurons. The external **white matter** is made of myelinated axons and dendrites of interneurons. These nerve fibers are grouped into nerve tracts based on their functions. **Ascending tracts** (such as the dorsal columns and spinothalamic tracts) carry sensory impulses to the brain. **Descending tracts** (such as the corticospinal and rubrospinal tracts) carry motor impulses away from the brain. Lastly, find the **central canal**; this contains **cerebrospinal fluid** and is continuous with cavities in the brain called ventricles.

SPINAL NERVES

There are 31 pairs of **spinal nerves**, those that emerge from the spinal cord. The nerves are named according to their respective vertebrae: 8 cervical pairs, 12 thoracic pairs, 5 lumbar pairs, 5 sacral pairs, and 1 very small coccygeal pair. These are shown in Fig. 8–4; notice that each nerve is designated by a letter and a number. The 8th cervical nerve is C8, the 1st thoracic nerve is T1, and so on.

In general, the cervical nerves supply the back of the head, neck, shoulders, arms, and the diaphragm. The first thoracic nerve also contributes to nerves in the arms. The remaining thoracic nerves supply the trunk of the body. The lumbar and sacral nerves supply the hips, pelvic cavity, and legs. Notice that the lumbar and sacral nerves hang below the end of the spinal cord (in order to reach their proper openings to exit from the vertebral canal); this is called the **cauda equina**, literally, the "horse's tail." Some of the important peripheral nerves and their destinations are listed in Table 8–3.

Each spinal nerve has two roots, which are neurons entering or leaving the spinal cord (see Fig. 8–3). The **dorsal root** is made of sensory neurons that carry impulses into the spinal cord. The **dorsal root ganglion** is an enlarged part of the dorsal root that contains the cell bodies of the sensory neurons. The term **ganglion** means a group of cell bodies outside the CNS. These cell bodies are within the vertebral canal and are thereby protected from injury (see Box 8–2: Shingles).

The **ventral root** is the motor root; it is made of the axons of motor neurons carrying impulses from the spinal cord to muscles or glands. The cell bodies of these motor neurons, as mentioned above, are in the gray matter of the spinal cord. When the two nerve roots merge, the spinal nerve thus formed is a mixed nerve.

brief and sounds very simple, the spinal cord is of great importance to the nervous system and to the body as a whole.

Enclosed in the vertebral canal and the meninges, the spinal cord is well protected from mechanical injury. In length, the spinal cord extends from the foramen magnum of the occipital bone to the disc between the first and second lumbar vertebrae.

A cross-section of the spinal cord is shown in Fig. 8–3; refer to it as you read the following. The internal **gray matter** is shaped like the letter H; gray matter consists of the cell bodies of motor neurons and

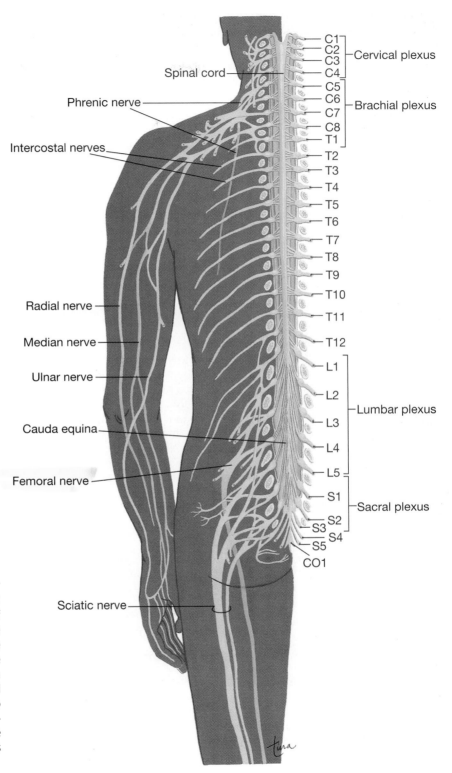

Figure 8–4 The spinal cord and spinal nerves. The distribution of spinal nerves is shown only on the left side. The nerve plexuses are labeled on the right side. A nerve plexus is a network of neurons from several segments of the spinal cord that combine to form nerves to specific parts of the body. For example, the radial and ulnar nerves to the arm emerge from the brachial plexus (see also Table 8–3).

Table 8–3 | MAJOR PERIPHERAL NERVES

Nerve	Spinal Nerves That Contribute	Distribution
Phrenic	C3–C5	• Diaphragm
Radial	C5–C8, T1	• Skin and muscles of posterior arm, forearm, and hand; thumb and first 2 fingers
Median	C5–C8, T1	• Skin and muscles of anterior arm, forearm, and hand
Ulnar	C8, T1	• Skin and muscles of medial arm, forearm, and hand; little finger and ring finger
Intercostal	T2–T12	• Intercostal muscles, abdominal muscles; skin of trunk
Femoral	L2–L4	• Skin and muscles of anterior thigh, medial leg, and foot
Sciatic	L4–S3	• Skin and muscles of posterior thigh, leg and foot

Box 8–2   SHINGLES

Shingles is caused by the same virus that causes chickenpox: the Herpes varicella-zoster virus. Varicella is chickenpox, which most of us probably had as children (there is now a vaccine). When a person recovers from chickenpox, the virus may survive in a dormant (inactive) state in the dorsal root ganglia of some spinal nerves. For most people, the immune system is able to prevent reactivation of the virus. With increasing age, however, the immune system is not as effective, and the virus may become active and cause zoster, or shingles.

The virus is present in sensory neurons, often those of the trunk, but the damage caused by the virus is seen in the skin over the affected nerve. The raised, red lesions of shingles are often very painful and follow the course of the nerve on the skin external to it. Occasionally the virus may affect a cranial nerve and cause facial paralysis called Bell's palsy (7th cranial) or extensive facial lesions, or, rarely, blindness. Although not a cure, some antiviral medications lessen the duration of the illness.

Box Figure 8–A   Lesions of shingles on skin of trunk. (From Goldsmith, LA, Lazarus, GS, and Tharp, MD: Adult and Pediatric Dermatology: A Color Guide to Diagnosis and Treatment. FA Davis, Philadelphia, 1997, p 307, with permission.)

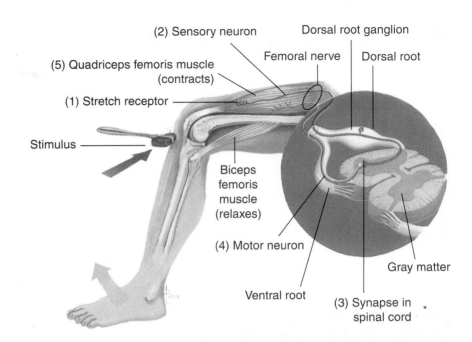

Figure 8–5 Patellar reflex. The reflex arc is shown. See text for description.

SPINAL CORD REFLEXES

When you hear the term *reflex,* you may think of an action that "just happens," and in part this is so. A **reflex** is an involuntary response to a stimulus, that is, an automatic action stimulated by a specific change of some kind. **Spinal cord reflexes** are those that do not depend directly on the brain, although the brain may inhibit or enhance them. We do not have to think about these reflexes, which is very important, as you will see.

Reflex Arc

A **reflex arc** is the pathway nerve impulses travel when a reflex is elicited, and there are five essential parts:

1. **Receptors**—detect a change (the stimulus) and generate impulses.
2. **Sensory neurons**—transmit impulses from receptors to the CNS.
3. **Central nervous system**—contains one or more synapses (interneurons may be part of the pathway).
4. **Motor neurons**—transmit impulses from the CNS to the effector.
5. **Effector**—performs its characteristic action.

Let us now look at the reflex arc of a specific reflex, the **patellar** (or knee-jerk) **reflex**, with which you are probably familiar. In this reflex, a tap on the patellar tendon just below the kneecap causes extension of the lower leg. This is a **stretch reflex**, which means that a muscle that is stretched will automatically contract. Refer now to Fig. 8–5 as you read the following:

In the quadriceps femoris muscle are (1) stretch receptors that detect the stretching produced by striking the patellar tendon. These receptors generate impulses that are carried along (2) sensory neurons in the femoral nerve to (3) the spinal cord. In the spinal cord, the sensory neurons synapse with (4) motor neurons (this is a two-neuron reflex). The motor neurons in the femoral nerve carry impulses back to (5) the quadriceps femoris, the effector, which contracts and extends the lower leg.

The patellar reflex is one of many used clinically to determine whether the nervous system is functioning properly. If the patellar reflex were absent in a patient, the problem could be in the thigh muscle, the femoral nerve, or the spinal cord. Further testing would be needed to determine the precise break in the reflex arc. If the reflex is normal, however, that means that all parts of the reflex arc are intact. So the testing of reflexes may be a first step in the clinical assessment of neurological damage.

Box 8–3   SPINAL CORD INJURIES

Injuries to the spinal cord are most often caused by auto accidents, falls, and gunshot wounds. The most serious injury is transection, or severing, of the spinal cord. If, for example, the spinal cord is severed at the level of the 8th thoracic segment, there will be paralysis and loss of sensation below that level. Another consequence is spinal shock, the at-least-temporary loss of spinal cord reflexes. In this example, the spinal cord reflexes of the lower trunk and legs will not occur. The stretch reflexes and flexor reflexes of the legs will be at least temporarily abolished, as will the urination and defecation reflexes. Although these reflexes do not depend directly on the brain, spinal cord neurons depend on impulses from the brain to enhance their own ability to generate impulses.

As spinal cord neurons below the injury recover their ability to generate impulses, these reflexes, such as the patellar reflex, often return. Urination and defecation reflexes may also be reestablished, but the person will not have an awareness of the need to urinate or defecate. Nor will voluntary control of these reflexes be possible, because inhibiting impulses from the brain can no longer reach the lower segments of the spinal cord.

Potentially less serious injuries are those in which the spinal cord is crushed rather than severed, and treatment is aimed at preserving whatever function remains. Minimizing inflammation and stimulating the production of nerve growth factors are aspects of such treatment.

Perhaps the most challenging research is the attempt to stimulate severed spinal cords to regenerate. Partial success has been achieved in rats, with Schwann cells transplanted from their peripheral nerves, and nerve growth factors produced by genetically engineered cells. The use of stem cells is also being investigated. The researchers caution, however, that it will probably be many years before their procedures will be tested on people.

You may be wondering why we have such reflexes, which are called stretch reflexes. What is their importance in our everyday lives? Imagine a person standing upright—is the body perfectly still? No, it isn't, because gravity exerts a downward pull. However, if the body tilts to the left, the right sides of the leg and trunk are stretched, and these stretched muscles automatically contract and pull the body upright again. This is the purpose of stretch reflexes; they help keep us upright without our having to think about doing so. If the brain had to make a decision every time we swayed a bit, all our concentration would be needed just to remain standing. Since these are spinal cord reflexes, the brain is not directly involved. The brain may become aware that a reflex has taken place, but that involves another set of neurons carrying impulses to the brain.

Flexor reflexes (or **withdrawal reflexes**) are another type of spinal cord reflex. The stimulus is something painful and potentially harmful, and the response is to pull away from it. If you inadvertently touch a hot stove, you automatically pull your hand away. Flexor reflexes are three-neuron reflexes, because sensory neurons synapse with interneurons in the spinal cord, which in turn synapse with motor neurons. Again, however, the brain does not have to make a decision to protect the body; the flexor reflex does that automatically (see Box 8–3: Spinal Cord Injuries). The brain may know that the reflex has taken place, and may even learn from the experience, but that requires different neurons, not the reflex arc.

THE BRAIN

The **brain** consists of many parts that function as an integrated whole. The major parts are the medulla, pons, and midbrain (collectively called the **brain stem**), the cerebellum, the hypothalamus, the thalamus, and the cerebrum. These parts are shown in Fig. 8–6. We will discuss each part separately, but keep in mind that they are all interconnected and work together.

VENTRICLES

The **ventricles** are four cavities within the brain: two lateral ventricles, the third ventricle, and the fourth ventricle (Fig. 8–7). Each ventricle contains a capillary network called a **choroid plexus**, which forms **cerebrospinal fluid** (CSF) from blood plasma. Cerebrospinal fluid is the tissue fluid of the central nervous system; its circulation and functions will be discussed in the section on meninges.

Figure 8–6 **(A)** Midsagittal section of the brain as seen from the left side. This medial plane shows internal anatomy as well as the lobes of the cerebrum. **(B)** Frontal section of the brain in anterior view.

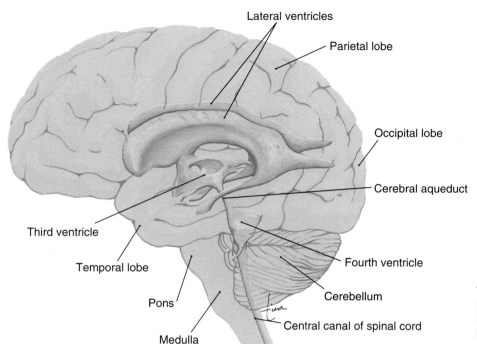

Lateral ventricles

Parietal lobe

Occipital lobe

Cerebral aqueduct

Third ventricle

Temporal lobe

Fourth ventricle

Pons

Cerebellum

Central canal of spinal cord

Medulla

Figure 8–7 Ventricles of the brain as projected into the interior of the brain, which is seen from the left side.

MEDULLA

The **medulla** extends from the spinal cord to the pons and is anterior to the cerebellum. Its functions are those we think of as vital (as in "vital signs"). The medulla contains cardiac centers that regulate heart rate, vasomotor centers that regulate the diameter of blood vessels and, thereby, blood pressure, and respiratory centers that regulate breathing. You can see why a crushing injury to the occipital bone may be rapidly fatal—we cannot survive without the medulla. Also in the medulla are reflex centers for coughing, sneezing, swallowing, and vomiting.

PONS

The **pons** bulges anteriorly from the upper part of the medulla. Within the pons are two respiratory centers that work with those in the medulla to produce a normal breathing rhythm. (The function of all the respiratory centers is discussed in Chapter 15.) The many other neurons in the pons (pons is from the Latin for "bridge") connect the medulla with other parts of the brain.

MIDBRAIN

The **midbrain** extends from the pons to the hypothalamus and encloses the **cerebral aqueduct**, a tunnel that connects the third and fourth ventricles. Several different kinds of reflexes are integrated in the midbrain, including visual and auditory reflexes. If you see a wasp flying toward you, you automatically duck or twist away; this is a visual reflex, as is the coordinated movement of the eyeballs. Turning your head (ear) to a sound is an example of an auditory reflex. The midbrain is also concerned with what are called righting reflexes, those that keep the head upright and maintain balance or equilibrium.

CEREBELLUM

The **cerebellum** is separated from the medulla and pons by the fourth ventricle and is inferior to the occipital lobes of the cerebrum. All of the functions of the cerebellum are concerned with movement. These include coordination, regulation of muscle tone, the appropriate trajectory and endpoint of movements, and the maintenance of posture and equilibrium.

Notice that these are all involuntary, that is, the cerebellum functions below the level of conscious thought. This is important to permit the conscious brain to work without being overburdened. If you decide to pick up a pencil, for example, the impulses for arm movement come from the cerebrum. The cerebellum then modifies these impulses so that your arm and finger movements are coordinated, and you don't reach past the pencil.

In order to regulate equilibrium, the cerebellum (and midbrain) uses information provided by receptors in the inner ears. These receptors are discussed further in Chapter 9.

HYPOTHALAMUS

Located superior to the pituitary gland and inferior to the thalamus, the **hypothalamus** is a small area of the brain with many diverse functions.

1. Production of **antidiuretic hormone** (ADH) and **oxytocin**; these hormones are then stored in the posterior pituitary gland. ADH enables the kidneys to reabsorb water back to the blood and thus helps maintain blood volume. Oxytocin causes contractions of the uterus to bring about labor and delivery.
2. Production of releasing hormones (also called releasing factors) that stimulate the secretion of hormones by the anterior pituitary gland. Because these hormones are covered in Chapter 10, a single example will be given here: The hypothalamus produces **growth hormone releasing hormone** (GHRH), which stimulates the anterior pituitary gland to secrete growth hormone (GH).
3. Regulation of body temperature by promoting responses such as sweating in a warm environment or shivering in a cold environment (see Chapter 17).
4. Regulation of food intake; the hypothalamus is believed to respond to changes in blood nutrient levels, to chemicals secreted by fat cells, and to hormones secreted by the gastrointestinal tract. For example, when blood nutrient levels are low, we experience a sensation of hunger, and eat. This raises blood nutrient levels and brings about a sensation of satiety, or fullness, and eating ceases.
5. Integration of the functioning of the autonomic nervous system, which in turn regulates the activity of organs such as the heart, blood vessels, and intestines. This will be discussed in more detail later in this chapter.
6. Stimulation of visceral responses during emotional situations. When we are angry, heart rate usually increases. Most of us, when embarrassed, will blush, which is vasodilation in the skin of the face. These responses are brought about by the autonomic nervous system when the hypothalamus perceives a change in emotional state. The neurological basis of our emotions is not well understood, and the visceral responses to emotions are not something most of us can control.
7. Regulation of body rhythms such as secretion of hormones, sleep cycles, changes in mood or mental alertness. This is often referred to as our biological clock, the rhythms as circadian rhythms, meaning "about a day." If you have ever had to stay awake for 24 hours, you know how disorienting it can be, until the hypothalamic biological clock has been reset.

THALAMUS

The **thalamus** is superior to the hypothalamus and inferior to the cerebrum. The third ventricle is a narrow cavity that passes through both the thalamus and hypothalamus. The functions of the thalamus are concerned with sensation. Sensory impulses to the brain (except those for the sense of smell) follow neuron pathways that first enter the thalamus, which groups the impulses before relaying them to the cerebrum, where sensations are felt. For example, holding a cup of hot coffee generates impulses for heat, touch and texture, and the shape of the cup (muscle sense), but we do not experience these as separate sensations. The thalamus integrates the impulses, or puts them together, so that the cerebrum feels the whole and is able to interpret the sensation quickly.

Some sensations, especially unpleasant ones such as pain, are believed to be felt by the thalamus. However, the thalamus cannot localize the sensation, that is, it does not know where the painful sensation is. The sensory areas of the cerebrum are required for localization and precise awareness.

The thalamus may also suppress unimportant sensations. If you are reading an enjoyable book, you may not notice someone coming into the room. By temporarily blocking minor sensations, the thalamus permits the cerebrum to concentrate on important tasks.

Motor area

Premotor area

General sensory area

Frontal lobe

Sensory association area

Parietal lobe

Occipital lobe

Visual association area

Visual area

Motor speech area

Auditory association area

Auditory area

Temporal lobe

Figure 8–8 Left cerebral hemisphere showing some of the functional areas that have been mapped.

CEREBRUM

The largest part of the human brain is the **cerebrum**, which consists of two hemispheres separated by the longitudinal fissure. At the base of this deep groove is the **corpus callosum**, a band of 200 million neurons that connects the right and left hemispheres. Within each hemisphere is a lateral ventricle.

The surface of the cerebrum is gray matter called the **cerebral cortex**. Gray matter consists of cell bodies of neurons, which carry out the many functions of the cerebrum. Internal to the gray matter is white matter, made of myelinated axons and dendrites that connect the lobes of the cerebrum to one another and to all other parts of the brain.

In the human brain the cerebral cortex is folded extensively. The folds are called **convolutions** or **gyri** and the grooves between them are **fissures** or **sulci**. This folding permits the presence of millions more neurons in the cerebral cortex. The cerebral cortex of an animal such as a dog or cat does not have this extensive folding. This difference enables us to read, speak, do long division, and so many other "human" things that dogs and cats cannot.

The cerebral cortex is divided into lobes that have the same names as the cranial bones external to them. Therefore, each hemisphere has a frontal lobe, parietal lobe, temporal lobe, and occipital lobe (Fig. 8–8). These lobes have been mapped, that is, certain areas are known to be associated with specific functions. We will discuss the functions of the cerebrum according to these mapped areas.

Frontal Lobes

Within the **frontal lobes** are the **motor areas** that generate the impulses for voluntary movement. The largest portions are for movement of the hands and face, those areas with many muscles capable of very fine or precise movements. It is the large size of the motor area devoted to them that gives these muscles their precision. The left motor area controls movement on the right side of the body, and the right motor area controls the left side of the body. This is why a patient who has had a cerebrovascular accident, or stroke, in the right frontal lobe will have paralysis of muscles on the left side (see Box 8–4: Cerebrovascular Accidents).

Box 8–4   CEREBROVASCULAR ACCIDENTS

A **cerebrovascular accident (CVA)**, or **stroke**, is damage to a blood vessel in the brain, resulting in lack of oxygen to that part of the brain. Possible types of vessel damage are thrombosis or hemorrhage.

A **thrombus** is a blood clot, which most often is a consequence of atherosclerosis, abnormal lipid deposits in cerebral arteries. The rough surface stimulates clot formation, which obstructs the blood flow to the part of the brain supplied by the artery. The symptoms depend on the part of the brain affected and may be gradual in onset if clot formation is slow. Approximately 80% of CVAs are of this type.

A hemorrhage, the result of arteriosclerosis or **aneurysm** of a cerebral artery, allows blood out into brain tissue, which destroys brain neurons by putting excessive pressure on them as well as depriving them of oxygen. Onset of symptoms in this type of CVA is usually rapid.

If, for example, the CVA is in the left frontal lobe, paralysis of the right side of the body will occur. Speech may also be affected if the speech areas are involved. Some CVAs are fatal because the damage they cause is very widespread or affects vital centers in the medulla or pons.

For CVAs of the thrombus type, a clot-dissolving drug may help reestablish blood flow. To be effective, however, the drug must be administered within 3 hours of symptom onset (see also Box 11–7).

Recovery from a CVA depends on its location and the extent of damage, as well as other factors. One of these is the redundancy of the brain. Redundancy means repetition; the cerebral cortex has many more neurons than we actually use in daily activities. These neurons are available for use, especially in younger people (less than 50 years of age). When a patient recovers from a disabling stroke, what has often happened is that the brain has established new pathways, with previously little-used neurons now carrying impulses "full time." Such recovery is highly individual and may take months. Yet another important factor is that CVA patients be started on rehabilitation therapy as soon as their condition permits.

Anterior to the motor areas are the premotor areas, which are concerned with learned motor skills that require a sequence of movements. Tying shoelaces, for example, seems almost automatic to us; we forget having learned it. It is not a reflex, however; rather the premotor cortex has learned the sequence so well that we are able to repeat it without consciously thinking about it.

Also in the frontal lobe, usually only the left lobe for most right-handed people, is **Broca's motor speech** area, which controls the movements of the mouth involved in speaking.

Parietal Lobes

The **general sensory areas** in the **parietal lobes** receive impulses from receptors in the skin and feel and interpret the cutaneous sensations. The left area is for the right side of the body and vice versa. These areas also receive impulses from stretch receptors in muscles for conscious muscle sense. The largest portions of these areas are for sensation in the hands and face, those parts of the body with the most cutaneous receptors and the most muscle receptors. The **taste areas**, which overlap the parietal and temporal lobes, receive impulses from taste buds on the tongue and elsewhere in the oral cavity.

Temporal Lobes

The **olfactory areas** in the **temporal lobes** receive impulses from receptors in the nasal cavities for the sense of smell. The olfactory association area learns the meaning of odors such as the smell of sour milk, or fire, or brownies baking in the oven, and enables the thinking cerebrum to use that information effectively. The **auditory areas**, as their name suggests, receive impulses from receptors in the inner ear for hearing. The auditory association area is quite large. Part of it is concerned with the meanings of words we hear, that is, with speech. Other parts are for the interpretation of sounds such as thunder during a storm, an ambulance siren, or a baby crying. Without proper interpretation, we would hear the sound but would not know what it meant, and could not respond appropriately.

Also in the temporal and parietal lobes in the left hemisphere (for most of us) are other speech areas concerned with the thought that precedes speech. Each of us can probably recall (and regret) times when

Box 8–5   APHASIA

Our use of language sets us apart from other animals and involves speech, reading, and writing. Language is the use of symbols (words) to designate objects and to express ideas. Damage to the speech areas or interpretation areas of the cerebrum may impair one or more aspects of a person's ability to use language; this is called **aphasia.**

Aphasia may be a consequence of a cerebrovascular accident, or of physical trauma to the skull and brain such as a head injury sustained in an automobile accident. If the motor speech (Broca's) area is damaged, the person is still able to understand written and spoken words and knows what he wants to say, but he cannot say it. Without coordination and impulses from the motor speech area, the muscles used for speech cannot contract to form words properly.

Auditory aphasia is **"word deafness,"** caused by damaged to an interpretation area. The person can still hear but cannot comprehend what the words mean. Visual aphasia is **"word blindness"**; the person can still see perfectly well, but cannot make sense of written words (the person retains the ability to understand spoken words). Imagine how you would feel if wms qsbbcljw jmqr rfc yzgjgrw rm pcyb. Frustrating isn't it? You know that those symbols are letters, but you cannot "decode" them right away. Those "words" were formed by shifting the alphabet two letters (A = C, B = D, C = E, etc.), and would normally be read as: "you suddenly lost the ability to read." That may give you a small idea of what word blindness is like.

we have "spoken without thinking," but in actuality that is not possible. The thinking takes place very rapidly and is essential in order to be able to speak (see Box 8–5: Aphasia).

Occipital Lobes

Impulses from the retinas of the eyes travel along the optic nerves to the **visual areas** in the **occipital lobes**. These areas "see." The visual association areas interpret what is seen, and enable the thinking cerebrum to use the information. Imagine looking at a clock. Seeing the clock is far different from being able to interpret it. At one time we learned to interpret the clock face and hands, and now we do not have to consciously decide what time the clock is reading. We can simply use that information, such as hurrying a bit so as not to be late to class. Other parts of the occipital lobes are concerned with spatial relationships; things such as judging distance and seeing in three dimensions, or the ability to read a map and relate it to the physical world.

Association Areas

As you can see in Fig. 8–8, many parts of the cerebral cortex are not concerned with movement or a particular sensation. These may be called **association areas** and perhaps are what truly make us individu-

als. It is probably these areas that give each of us a personality, a sense of humor, and the ability to reason and use logic. Learning and memory are also functions of these areas.

Although much has been learned about the formation of memories, the processes are still incompletely understood and mostly beyond the scope of this book. Briefly, however, we can say that memories of things such as people or what you did last summer involve the hippocampus (from the Greek for "seahorse," because of its shape), part of the temporal lobe on the floor of the lateral ventricle. The hippocampi seem to collect information from many areas of the cerebral cortex. When you meet a friend, for example, the memory emerges as a whole: "Here's Fred," not in pieces. People whose hippocampi are damaged cannot form new memories that last more than a few seconds.

It is believed that most, if not all, of what we have experienced or learned is stored somewhere in the brain. Sometimes a trigger may bring back memories; a certain scent or a song are possible triggers. Then we find ourselves recalling something from the past and wondering where it came from.

The loss of personality due to destruction of brain neurons is perhaps most dramatically seen in Alzheimer's disease (see Box 8–6: Alzheimer's Disease).

Box 8–6   ALZHEIMER'S DISEASE

In the United States, Alzheimer's disease, a progressive, incurable form of mental deterioration, affects approximately 5 million people and is the cause of 100,000 deaths each year. The first symptoms, which usually begin after age 65, are memory lapses and slight personality changes. As the disease progresses, there is total loss of memory, reasoning ability, and personality, and those with advanced disease are unable to perform even the simplest tasks or self-care.

Structural changes in the brains of Alzheimer's patients may be seen at autopsy. Neurofibrillary tangles are abnormal fibrous proteins found in the cerebral cortex in areas important for memory and reasoning. Also present are plaques made of another protein called beta-amyloid. These may be results of the disease rather than causes.

A defective gene has been found in some patients who have late-onset Alzheimer's disease, the most common type. Yet another gene seems to trigger increased synthesis of beta-amyloid. Current research is focused on the interaction of these genes and on inflammation as a contributing factor to this type of brain damage.

Some medications help improve memory by delaying the breakdown of acetylcholine in the brain. It is likely that treatment of Alzheimer's disease will one day mean delaying its onset with a variety of medications, each targeted at a different aspect of this complex disease.

Box 8–7   PARKINSON'S DISEASE

Parkinson's disease is a disorder of the basal ganglia whose cause is unknown, and though there is a genetic component in some families, it is probably not the only factor. The disease usually begins after the age of 60. Neurons in the basal ganglia that produce the neurotransmitter dopamine begin to degenerate and die, and the deficiency of dopamine causes specific kinds of muscular symptoms. Tremor, or involuntary shaking, of the hands is probably the most common symptom. The accessory movements regulated by the basal ganglia gradually diminish, and the affected person walks slowly without swinging the arms. A mask-like face is characteristic of this disease, as the facial muscles become rigid. Eventually all voluntary movements become slower and much more difficult, and balance is seriously impaired.

Dopamine itself cannot be used to treat Parkinson's disease because it does not cross the blood–brain barrier. A substance called L-dopa does cross and can be converted to dopamine by brain neurons. Unfortunately, L-dopa begins to lose its therapeutic effectiveness within a few years.

Other medications in use do not provide a cure. Some researchers suggest that implants of stem cells may offer the best hope of meaningful therapy.

Basal Ganglia

The **basal ganglia** are paired masses of gray matter within the white matter of the cerebral hemispheres (Fig. 8–6). Their functions are certain subconscious aspects of voluntary movement, and they work with the cerebellum. The basal ganglia help regulate muscle tone, and they coordinate accessory movements such as swinging the arms when walking or gesturing while speaking. The most common disorder of the basal ganglia is Parkinson's disease (see Box 8–7: Parkinson's Disease).

Corpus Callosum

As mentioned previously, the **corpus callosum** is a band of nerve fibers that connects the left and right cerebral hemispheres. This enables each hemisphere to know of the activity of the other. This is especially important for people because for most of us, the left hemisphere contains speech areas and the right hemisphere does not. The corpus callosum, therefore, lets the left hemisphere know what the right hemisphere is thinking about, and the right hemisphere know what the left hemisphere is thinking and talking about. A brief example may be helpful. If you put your left hand behind your back and someone places a pencil in your hand (you are not looking at it) and asks you what it is, would you be able to say? Yes, you would. You would feel the shape and weight of the pencil, find the point and the eraser. The sensory impulses from your left hand are interpreted as "pencil" by the general sensory area in your right parietal lobe. Your right hemisphere probably cannot speak, but its thoughts can be conveyed by way of the corpus callosum to the left hemisphere, which does have speech areas. Your left hemisphere can say that you are holding a pencil. Other aspects of the "division of labor" of our cerebral hemispheres are beyond the scope of this book, but it is a fascinating subject that you may wish to explore further.

MENINGES AND CEREBROSPINAL FLUID

The connective tissue membranes that cover the brain and spinal cord are called **meninges**; the three layers are illustrated in Fig. 8–9. The thick outermost layer, made of fibrous connective tissue, is the **dura mater** (Latin for "tough mother"), which lines the skull and vertebral canal. The middle **arachnoid membrane** (arachnids are spiders) is made of web-like strands of connective tissue. The innermost **pia mater** (Latin for "gentle mother") is a very thin membrane on the surface of the spinal cord and brain. Between the arachnoid and the pia mater is the **subarachnoid space**, which contains cerebrospinal fluid (CSF), the tissue fluid of the central nervous system.

Recall the ventricles (cavities) of the brain: two lateral ventricles, the third ventricle, and the fourth ventricle. Each contains a choroid plexus, a capillary network that forms cerebrospinal fluid from blood plasma. This is a continuous process, and the cerebrospinal fluid then circulates in and around the central nervous system (Fig. 8–10).

From the lateral and third ventricles, cerebrospinal fluid flows through the fourth ventricle, then to the central canal of the spinal cord, and to the cranial and spinal subarachnoid spaces. As more cerebrospinal fluid is formed, you might expect that some must be reabsorbed, and that is just what happens. From the cranial subarachnoid space, cerebrospinal fluid is reabsorbed through **arachnoid villi** into the blood in

cranial venous sinuses (large veins within the double-layered cranial dura mater). The cerebrospinal fluid becomes blood plasma again, and the rate of reabsorption normally equals the rate of production.

Since cerebrospinal fluid is tissue fluid, one of its functions is to bring nutrients to CNS neurons and to remove waste products to the blood as the fluid is reabsorbed. The other function of cerebrospinal fluid is to act as a cushion for the central nervous system. The brain and spinal cord are enclosed in fluid-filled membranes that absorb shock. You can, for example, shake your head vigorously without harming your brain. Naturally, this protection has limits; very sharp or heavy blows to the skull will indeed cause damage to the brain.

Examination of cerebrospinal fluid may be used in the diagnosis of certain diseases (see Box 8–8: Lumbar Puncture).

CRANIAL NERVES

The 12 pairs of **cranial nerves** emerge from the brain stem or other parts of the brain—they are shown in Fig. 8–11. The name *cranial* indicates their origin, and many of them do carry impulses for functions involving the head. Some, however, have more far-reaching destinations.

The impulses for the senses of smell, taste, sight, hearing, and equilibrium are all carried by cranial nerves to their respective sensory areas in the brain. Some cranial nerves carry motor impulses to muscles of the face and eyes or to the salivary glands. The vagus nerves (*vagus* means "wanderer") branch extensively to the larynx, heart, stomach and intestines, and the bronchial tubes.

The functions of the cranial nerves are summarized in Table 8–4.

THE AUTONOMIC NERVOUS SYSTEM

The **autonomic nervous system (ANS)** is actually part of the peripheral nervous system in that it consists of motor portions of some cranial and spinal nerves. Because its functioning is so specialized, however, the autonomic nervous system is usually discussed as a separate entity, as we will do here.

involuntarily

A

B

Figure 8–9   Structure of the meninges. **(A)** Meninges of the spinal cord. **(B)** Frontal section through the top of the skull showing the double-layered cranial dura mater and one of the cranial venous sinuses.

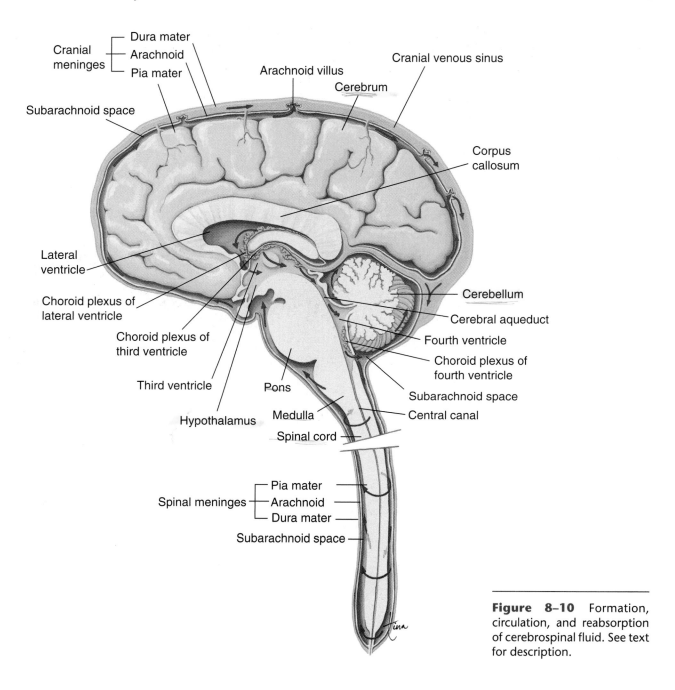

Figure 8–10 Formation, circulation, and reabsorption of cerebrospinal fluid. See text for description.

Making up the autonomic nervous system are **visceral motor neurons** to smooth muscle, cardiac muscle, and glands. These are the **visceral effectors**; muscle will either contract or relax, and glands will either increase or decrease their secretions.

The ANS has two divisions: **sympathetic** and **parasympathetic**. Often, they function in opposition to each other, as you will see. The activity of both divisions is integrated by the hypothalamus, which ensures that the visceral effectors will respond appropriately to the situation.

AUTONOMIC PATHWAYS

An autonomic nerve pathway from the central nervous system to a visceral effector consists of two motor neurons that synapse in a ganglion outside the CNS (Fig. 8–12). The first neuron is called the **pregan-**

Box 8–8   LUMBAR PUNCTURE

A **lumbar puncture** (spinal tap) is a diagnostic procedure that involves the removal of cerebrospinal fluid to determine its pressure and constituents. As the name tells us, the removal, using a syringe, is made in the lumbar area. Because the spinal cord ends between the 1st and 2nd lumbar vertebrae, the needle is usually inserted between the 4th and 5th lumbar vertebrae. The meningeal sac containing cerebrospinal fluid extends to the end of the lumbar vertebrae, permitting access to the cerebrospinal fluid with little chance of damaging the spinal cord.

Cerebrospinal fluid is a circulating fluid and has a normal pressure of 70 to 200 mmH$_2$O. An abnormal pressure usually indicates an obstruction in circulation, which may be caused by infection, a tumor, or mechanical injury. Other diagnostic tests would be needed to determine the precise cause.

Perhaps the most frequent reason for a lumbar puncture is suspected **meningitis**, which may be caused by several kinds of bacteria. If the patient does have meningitis, the cerebrospinal fluid will be cloudy rather than clear and will be examined for the presence of bacteria and many white blood cells. A few WBCs in CSF is normal, because WBCs are found in all tissue fluid.

Another abnormal constituent of cerebrospinal fluid is red blood cells. Their presence indicates bleeding somewhere in the central nervous system. There may be many causes, and again, further testing would be necessary.

Box Figure 8–B   Cerebrospinal fluid from a patient with meningitis. The bacteria are streptococci, found in pairs. The large cells are WBCs. (×500) (From Sacher, RA, and McPherson, RA: Widmann's Clinical Interpretation of Laboratory Tests, ed. 11. FA Davis, Philadelphia, 2000, Plate 52, with permission.)

glionic neuron, from the CNS to the ganglion. The second neuron is called the **postganglionic neuron**, from the ganglion to the visceral effector. The ganglia are actually the cell bodies of the postganglionic neurons.

✳SYMPATHETIC DIVISION

Another name for the sympathetic division is thoracolumbar division, which tells us where the sympathetic preganglionic neurons originate. Their cell bodies are in the thoracic segments and some of the lumbar segments of the spinal cord. Their axons extend to the sympathetic ganglia, most of which are located in two chains just outside the spinal column (see Fig. 8–12). Within the ganglia are the synapses between preganglionic and postganglionic neurons; the postganglionic axons then go to the visceral effectors. One preganglionic neuron often synapses with many postganglionic neurons to many effectors. This anatomic arrangement has physiologic importance: The sympathetic division brings about widespread responses in many organs.

The sympathetic division is dominant in stressful situations, which include anger, fear, or anxiety, as well as exercise. For our prehistoric ancestors, stress-

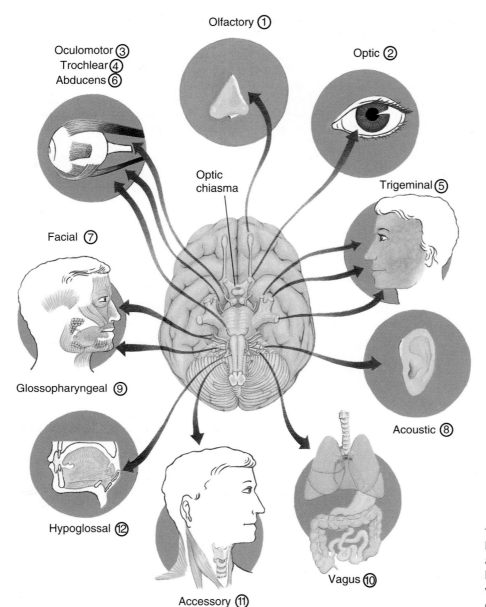

Figure 8–11 Cranial nerves and their distributions. The brain is shown in an inferior view. See Table 8–4 for descriptions.

ful situations often involved the need for intense physical activity—the "fight or flight response." Our nervous systems haven't changed very much in 50,000 years, and if you look at Table 8–5, you will see the kinds of responses the sympathetic division stimulates. The heart rate increases, vasodilation in skeletal muscles supplies them with more oxygen, the bronchioles dilate to take in more air, and the liver changes glycogen to glucose to supply energy. At the same time, digestive secretions decrease and peristalsis slows; these are not important in a stress situation. Vasoconstriction in the skin and viscera shunts blood to more vital organs such as the heart, muscles, and brain. All of these responses enabled our ancestors to stay and fight or to get away from potential danger. Even though we may not always be in life-threaten-

Table 8–4 | CRANIAL NERVES

Number and Name	Function(s)
I Olfactory	• Sense of smell
II Optic	• Sense of sight
III Oculomotor	• Movement of the eyeball; constriction of pupil in bright light or for near vision
IV Trochlear	• Movement of eyeball
V Trigeminal	• Sensation in face, scalp, and teeth; contraction of chewing muscles
VI Abducens	• Movement of the eyeball
VII Facial	• Sense of taste; contraction of facial muscles; secretion of saliva
VIII Acoustic (vestibulocochlear)	• Sense of hearing; sense of equilibrium
IX Glossopharyngeal	• Sense of taste; sensory for cardiac, respiratory, and blood pressure reflexes; contraction of pharynx; secretion of saliva
X Vagus	• Sensory in cardiac, respiratory, and blood pressure reflexes; sensory and motor to larynx (speaking); decreases heart rate; contraction of alimentary tube (peristalsis); increases digestive secretions
XI Accessory	• Contraction of neck and shoulder muscles; motor to larynx (speaking)
XII Hypoglossal	• Movement of the tongue

ing situations during stress (such as figuring out our income taxes), our bodies are prepared for just that.

 PARASYMPATHETIC DIVISION

The other name for the parasympathetic division is the craniosacral division. The cell bodies of parasympathetic preganglionic neurons are in the brain stem and the sacral segments of the spinal cord. Their axons are in cranial nerve pairs 3, 7, 9, and 10 and in some sacral nerves and extend to the parasympathetic ganglia. These ganglia are very close to or actually in the visceral effector (see Fig. 8–12), and contain the postganglionic cell bodies, with very short axons to the cells of the effector.

In the parasympathetic division, one preganglionic neuron synapses with just a few postganglionic neurons to only one effector. With this anatomic arrangement, very localized (one organ) responses are possible.

The parasympathetic division dominates in relaxed (non-stress) situations to promote normal functioning of several organ systems. Digestion will be efficient, with increased secretions and peristalsis; defecation and urination may occur; and the heart will beat at a normal resting rate. Other functions of this division are listed in Table 8–5.

Notice that when an organ receives both sympathetic and parasympathetic impulses, the responses are opposites. Notice also that some visceral effectors receive only sympathetic impulses. In such cases, the opposite response is brought about by a decrease in sympathetic impulses.

NEUROTRANSMITTERS

Recall that neurotransmitters enable nerve impulses to cross synapses. In autonomic pathways there are two synapses: one between preganglionic and postganglionic neurons, and the second between postganglionic neurons and visceral effectors.

Acetylcholine is the transmitter released by all preganglionic neurons, both sympathetic and parasympathetic; it is inactivated by **cholinesterase** in postganglionic neurons. Parasympathetic postganglionic neurons all release acetylcholine at the synapses with their visceral effectors. Most sympathetic postganglionic neurons release the transmitter **norepinephrine** at the synapses with the effector cells. Norepinephrine is inactivated by either catechol-

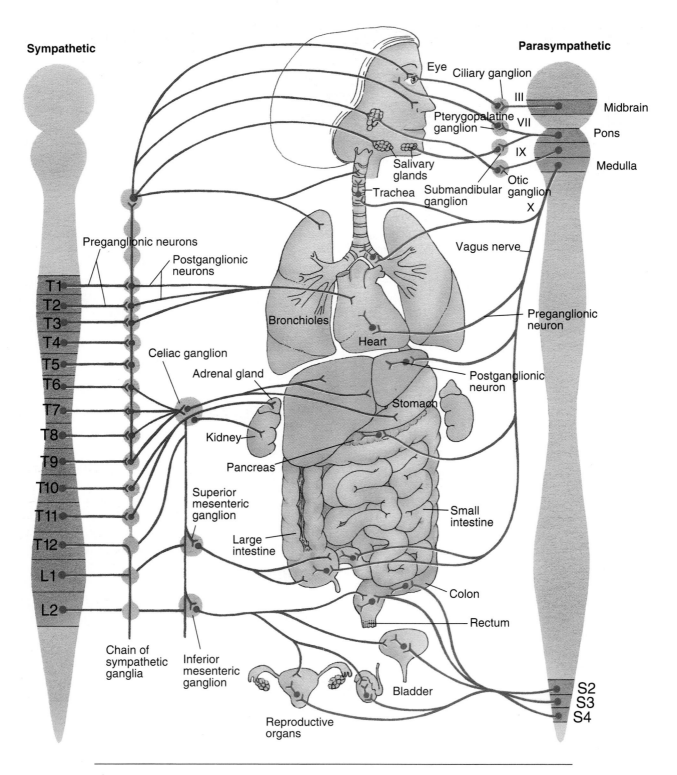

Figure 8–12   The autonomic nervous system. The sympathetic division is shown on the left, and the parasympathetic division is shown on the right (both divisions are bilateral).

Table 8–5	FUNCTIONS OF THE AUTONOMIC NERVOUS SYSTEM	
Organ	Sympathetic Responses	Parasympathetic Response
Heart (cardiac muscle)	• Increase rate	• Decrease rate (to normal)
Bronchioles (smooth muscle)	• Dilate	• Constrict (to normal)
Iris (smooth muscle)	• Pupil dilates	• Pupil constricts (to normal)
Salivary glands	• Decrease secretion	• Increase secretion (to normal)
Stomach and intestines (smooth muscle)	• Decrease peristalsis	• Increase peristalsis for normal digestion
Stomach and intestines (glands)	• Decrease secretion	• Increase secretion for normal digestion
Internal anal sphincter	• Contracts to prevent defecation	• Relaxes to permit defecation
Urinary bladder (smooth muscle)	• Relaxes to prevent urination	• Contracts for normal urination
Internal urethral sphincter	• Contracts to prevent urination	• Relaxes to permit urination
Liver	• Changes glycogen to glucose	• None
Sweat glands	• Increase secretion	• None
Blood vessels in skin and viscera (smooth muscle)	• Constrict	• None
Blood vessels in skeletal muscle (smooth muscle)	• Dilate	• None
Adrenal glands	• Increase secretion of epinephrine and norepinephrine	• None

O-methyl transferase (COMT) or monoamine oxidase (MAO), or it may be removed from the synapse by reuptake.

AGING AND THE NERVOUS SYSTEM

The aging brain does indeed lose neurons, but this is only a small percentage of the total and not the usual cause of mental impairment in elderly people. (Far more common causes are depression, malnutrition, hypotension, and the side effects of medications.) Some forgetfulness is to be expected, however, as is a decreased ability for *rapid* problem solving, but most memory should remain intact. Voluntary movements become slower, as do reflexes and reaction time. Think of driving a car, an ability most of us take for granted. For elderly people, with their slower perceptions and reaction times, greater *consciousness* of driving is necessary.

As the autonomic nervous system ages, dry eyes and constipation may become problems. Transient hypotension may be the result of decreased sympathetic stimulation of vasoconstriction. In most cases, however, elderly people who are aware of these aspects of aging will be able to work with their physicians or nurses to minimize them.

SUMMARY

The nervous system regulates many of our simplest and our most complex activities. The impulses generated and carried by the nervous system are an example of the chemical level of organization of the body. These nerve impulses then regulate the functioning of tissues, organs, and organ systems, which permits us to perceive and respond to the world around us and the changes within us. The detection of such changes is the function of the sense organs, and they are the subject of our next chapter.

STUDY OUTLINE

Functions of the Nervous System
1. Detect changes and feel sensations.
2. Initiate responses to changes.
3. Organize and store information.

Nervous System Divisions
1. Central nervous system (CNS)—brain and spinal cord.
2. Peripheral nervous system (PNS)—cranial nerves and spinal nerves.

Nerve Tissue—neurons (nerve fibers) and specialized cells (Schwann, neuroglia)
1. Neuron cell body contains the nucleus; cell bodies are in the CNS or in the trunk and are protected by bone.
2. Axon carries impulses away from the cell body; dendrites carry impulses toward the cell body.
3. Schwann cells in PNS: Layers of cell membrane form the myelin sheath to electrically insulate neurons; nodes of Ranvier are spaces between adjacent Schwann cells. Nuclei and cytoplasm of Schwann cells form the neurolemma, which is essential for regeneration of damaged axons or dendrites.
4. Oligodendrocytes in CNS form the myelin sheaths; astrocytes contribute to the blood–brain barrier (see Table 8–1).
5. Synapse—the space between the axon of one neuron and the dendrites or cell body of the next neuron. A neurotransmitter carries the impulse across a synapse and is then destroyed by a chemical inactivator. Synapses make impulse transmission one way in the living person.

Types of Neurons—nerve fibers
1. Sensory—carry impulses from receptors to the CNS; may be somatic (from skin, skeletal muscles, joints) or visceral (from internal organs).
2. Motor—carry impulses from the CNS to effectors; may be somatic (to skeletal muscle) or visceral (to smooth muscle, cardiac muscle, or glands). Visceral motor neurons make up the autonomic nervous system.
3. Interneurons—entirely within the CNS.

Nerves and Nerve Tracts
1. Sensory nerve—made only of sensory neurons.

2. Motor nerve—made only of motor neurons.
3. Mixed nerve—made of both sensory and motor neurons.
4. Nerve tract—a nerve within the CNS; also called white matter.

The Nerve Impulse—see Table 8–2
1. Polarization—neuron membrane has a (+) charge outside and a (–) charge inside.
2. Depolarization—entry of Na^+ ions and reversal of charges on either side of the membrane.
3. Impulse transmission is rapid, often several meters per second.
   - Saltatory conduction—in a myelinated neuron only the nodes of Ranvier depolarize; increases speed of impulses.

The Spinal Cord
1. Functions: transmits impulses to and from the brain, and integrates the spinal cord reflexes.
2. Location: within the vertebral canal; extends from the foramen magnum to the disc between the 1st and 2nd lumbar vertebrae.
3. Cross-section: internal H of gray matter contains cell bodies of motor neurons and interneurons; external white matter is the myelinated axons and dendrites of interneurons.
4. Ascending tracts carry sensory impulses to the brain; descending tracts carry motor impulses away from the brain.
5. Central canal contains cerebrospinal fluid and is continuous with the ventricles of the brain.

Spinal Nerves—see Table 8–3 for major peripheral nerves
1. Eight cervical pairs to head, neck, shoulder, arm, and diaphragm; 12 thoracic pairs to trunk; 5 lumbar pairs and 5 sacral pairs to hip, pelvic cavity, and leg; 1 very small coccygeal pair.
2. Cauda equina—the lumbar and sacral nerves that extend below the end of the spinal cord.
3. Each spinal nerve has two roots: dorsal or sensory root; dorsal root ganglion contains cell bodies of sensory neurons; ventral or motor root; the two roots unite to form a mixed spinal nerve.

Spinal Cord Reflexes—do not depend directly on the brain

1. A reflex is an involuntary response to a stimulus.
2. Reflex arc—the pathway of nerve impulses during a reflex: (1) receptors, (2) sensory neurons, (3) CNS with one or more synapses, (4) motor neurons, (5) effector which responds.
3. Stretch reflex—a muscle that is stretched will contract; these reflexes help keep us upright against gravity. The patellar reflex is also used clinically to assess neurological functioning, as are many other reflexes (Fig. 8–5).
4. Flexor reflex—a painful stimulus will cause withdrawal of the body part; these reflexes are protective.

The Brain—many parts that function as an integrated whole; see Figs. 8–6 and 8–8 for locations

1. Ventricles—four cavities: two lateral, 3rd, 4th; each contains a choroid plexus that forms cerebrospinal fluid (Figs. 8–6 and 8–7).
2. Medulla—regulates the vital functions of heart rate, breathing, and blood pressure; regulates reflexes of coughing, sneezing, swallowing, and vomiting.
3. Pons—contains respiratory centers that work with those in the medulla.
4. Midbrain—contains centers for visual reflexes, auditory reflexes, and righting (equilibrium) reflexes.
5. Cerebellum—regulates coordination of voluntary movement, muscle tone, stopping movements, and equilibrium.
6. Hypothalamus—produces antidiuretic hormone (ADH), which increases water reabsorption by the kidneys; produces oxytocin, which promotes uterine contractions for labor and delivery; produces releasing hormones that regulate the secretions of the anterior pituitary gland; regulates body temperature; regulates food intake; integrates the functioning of the autonomic nervous system (ANS); promotes visceral responses to emotional situations; acts as a biological clock that regulates body rhythms.
7. Thalamus—groups sensory impulses as to body part before relaying them to the cerebrum; awareness of pain but inability to localize; suppresses unimportant sensations to permit concentration.
8. Cerebrum—two hemispheres connected by the corpus callosum, which permits communication between the hemispheres. The cerebral cortex is the surface gray matter, which consists of cell bodies of neurons and is folded extensively into convolutions. The internal white matter consists of nerve tracts that connect the lobes of the cerebrum to one another and to other parts of the brain.

- Frontal lobes—motor areas initiate voluntary movement; premotor area regulates sequences of movements for learned skills; Broca's motor speech area (left hemisphere) regulates the movements involved in speech.
- Parietal lobes—general sensory area feels and interprets the cutaneous senses and conscious muscle sense; taste area extends into temporal lobe, for sense of taste; speech areas (left hemisphere) for thought before speech.
- Temporal lobes—auditory areas for hearing and interpretation; olfactory areas for sense of smell and interpretation; speech areas for thought before speech.
- Occipital lobes—visual areas for vision; interpretation areas for spatial relationships.
- Association areas—in all lobes, for abstract thinking, reasoning, learning, memory, and personality.
- Basal ganglia—gray matter within the cerebral hemispheres; regulate accessory movements and muscle tone.

Meninges and Cerebrospinal Fluid (CSF) (see Figs. 8–9 and 8–10)

1. Three meningeal layers made of connective tissue: outer—dura mater; middle—arachnoid membrane; inner—pia mater; all three enclose the brain and spinal cord.
2. Subarachnoid space contains CSF, the tissue fluid of the CNS.
3. CSF is formed continuously in the ventricles of the brain by choroid plexuses, from blood plasma.
4. CSF circulates from the ventricles to the central canal of the spinal cord and to the cranial and spinal subarachnoid spaces.
5. CSF is reabsorbed from the cranial subarachnoid space through arachnoid villi into the blood in the cranial venous sinuses. The rate of reabsorption equals the rate of production.
6. As tissue fluid, CSF brings nutrients to CNS neurons and removes waste products. CSF also acts as a shock absorber to cushion the CNS.

Cranial Nerves—12 pairs of nerves that emerge from the brain (see Fig. 8–11)

1. Concerned with vision, hearing and equilibrium, taste and smell, and many other functions.
2. See Table 8–4 for the functions of each pair.

The Autonomic Nervous System (ANS) (see Fig.8–12 and Table 8–5)

1. Has two divisions: sympathetic and parasympathetic; their functioning is integrated by the hypothalamus.
2. Consists of motor neurons to visceral effectors: smooth muscle, cardiac muscle, and glands.
3. An ANS pathway consists of two neurons that synapse in a ganglion:
   - Preganglionic neurons—from the CNS to the ganglia
   - Postganglionic neurons—from the ganglia to the effectors

   Most sympathetic ganglia are in two chains just outside the vertebral column; parasympathetic ganglia are very near or in the visceral effectors.
4. Neurotransmitters: acetylcholine is released by all preganglionic neurons and by parasympathetic postganglionic neurons; the inactivator is cholinesterase. Norepinephrine is released by most sympathetic postganglionic neurons; the inactivator is COMT or MAO.
5. Sympathetic division—dominates during stress situations; responses prepare the body to meet physical demands.
6. Parasympathetic division—dominates in relaxed situations to permit normal functioning.

REVIEW QUESTIONS

1. Name the divisions of the nervous system and state the parts of each. (p. 156)

2. State the function of the following parts of nerve tissue: (pp. 156, 158)
   a. Axon
   b. Dendrites
   c. Myelin sheath
   d. Neurolemma
   e. Microglia
   f. Astrocytes

3. Explain the difference between: (pp. 160–161)
   a. Sensory neurons and motor neurons
   b. Interneurons and nerve tracts

4. Describe an electrical nerve impulse in terms of charges on either side of the neuron membrane. Describe how a nerve impulse crosses a synapse. (pp. 158, 161)

5. With respect to the spinal cord: (p. 161–162)
   a. Describe its location
   b. State what gray matter and white matter are made of
   c. State the function of the dorsal root, ventral root, and dorsal root ganglion

6. State the names and number of pairs of spinal nerves. State the part of the body supplied by the phrenic nerves, radial nerves, sciatic nerves. (pp. 162, 164)

7. Define reflex, and name the five parts of a reflex arc. (p. 165)

8. Define stretch reflexes, and explain their practical importance. Define flexor reflexes, and explain their practical importance. (p. 166)

9. Name the part of the brain concerned with each of the following: (pp. 168–169)
   a. Regulates body temperature
   b. Regulates heart rate *Hypothalamus*
   c. Suppresses unimportant sensations
   d. Regulates respiration (two parts)
   e. Regulates food intake
   f. Regulates coordination of voluntary movement
   g. Regulates secretions of the anterior pituitary gland
   h. Regulates coughing and sneezing
   i. Regulates muscle tone *cerebellum*
   j. Regulates visual and auditory reflexes *Midbrain*
   k. Regulates blood pressure *medulla*

10. Name the part of the cerebrum concerned with each of the following: (pp. 170–173)
    a. Feels the cutaneous sensations
    b. Contains the auditory areas
    c. Contains the visual areas
    d. Connects the cerebral hemispheres
    e. Regulates accessory movements
    f. Contains the olfactory areas
    g. Initiates voluntary movement
    h. Contains the speech areas (for most people)

11. Name the three layers of the meninges, beginning with the outermost. (p. 174)

12. State all the locations of cerebrospinal fluid. What is CSF made from? Into what is CSF reabsorbed? State the functions of CSF. (p. 174)

13. State a function of each of the following cranial nerves: (p. 179)
    a. Glossopharyngeal
    b. Olfactory
    c. Trigeminal
    d. Facial
    e. Vagus (three functions)

14. Explain how the sympathetic division of the ANS helps the body adapt to a stress situation; give three specific examples. (pp. 178–179)

15. Explain how the parasympathetic division of the ANS promotes normal body functioning; give three specific examples. (p. 179)

FOR FURTHER THOUGHT

1. Your friend Fred was telling a story, with eloquent gestures, while making a salad. He missed the tomato with the knife, cut his hand badly, and needed quite a few stitches. A local anesthetic was used. How might a local anesthetic stop nerve impulses? (Remember that a nerve impulse is very simple.) What part of Fred's brain got him into trouble?

2. Some pesticides kill insects by interfering with cholinesterase. We have cholinesterase too, and may be adversely affected. What would be the symptoms of such pesticide poisoning?

3. We cannot live without a central nervous system. Describe all the ways the central nervous system is protected.

4. Older drivers are sometimes said to have "lost their reflexes." Is this really true? Explain.

5. Look at Question Figure 8–A below. Starting at the top of column A, read the words down as fast as you can. For column B, start at the top and name the colors as fast as you can. Did you have any trouble? Now column C: start at the top and name the colors—do not read the words—as fast as you can. Was there any difference? Explain why.

Question Figure 8–A

CHAPTER 9

Student Objectives

- Explain the general purpose of sensations.
- Name the parts of a sensory pathway, and state the function of each.
- Describe the characteristics of sensations.
- Name the cutaneous senses and explain their purpose.
- Explain referred pain and its importance.
- Explain the importance of muscle sense.
- Describe the pathways for the senses of smell and taste, and explain how these senses are interrelated.
- Name the parts of the eye and their functions.
- Describe the physiology of vision.
- Name the parts of the ear and their functions.
- Describe the physiology of hearing.
- Describe the physiology of equilibrium.
- Explain the importance of the arterial pressoreceptors and chemoreceptors.

The Senses

*Terms that appear in **bold type** in the chapter text are defined in the glossary, which begins on page 521.*

Our senses constantly provide us with information about our surroundings: We see, hear, and touch. The senses of taste and smell enable us to enjoy the flavor of our food or warn us that food has spoiled and may be dangerous to eat. Our sense of equilibrium keeps us upright. We also get information from our senses about what is happening inside the body. The pain of a headache, for example, prompts us to do something about it, such as take aspirin. In general, this is the purpose of sensations: to enable the body to respond appropriately to ever-changing situations and maintain homeostasis.

SENSORY PATHWAY

The impulses involved in sensations follow very precise pathways, which all have the following parts:

1. **Receptors**—detect changes **(stimuli)** and generate impulses. Receptors are usually very specific with respect to the kinds of changes they respond to. Those in the retina detect light rays, those in the nasal cavities detect vapors, and so on. Once a specific stimulus has affected receptors, however, they all respond the same way by generating electrical nerve impulses.
2. **Sensory neurons**—transmit impulses from receptors to the central nervous system. These sensory neurons are found in both spinal nerves and cranial nerves, but each carries impulses from only one type of receptor.
3. **Sensory tracts**—white matter in the spinal cord or brain that transmits the impulses to a specific part of the brain.
4. **Sensory area**—most are in the cerebral cortex. These areas feel and interpret the sensations. Learning to interpret sensations begins in infancy, without our awareness of it, and continues throughout life.

CHARACTERISTICS OF SENSATIONS

Certain characteristics of sensations will help you understand how the sensory areas work with information from the receptors.

1. **Projection**—the sensation seems to come from the area where the receptors were stimulated. If you touch this book, the sensation of touch seems to be in your hand but is actually being felt by your cerebral cortex. That it is indeed the brain that feels sensations is demonstrated by patients who feel **phantom pain** after amputation of a limb. After loss of a hand, for example, the person may still feel that the hand is really there. Why does this happen? The receptors in the hand are no longer present, but the severed nerve endings continue to generate impulses. These impulses arrive in the parietal lobe area for the hand, and the brain does what it has always done and creates the projection, the feeling that the hand is still there. For most amputees, phantom pain diminishes as the severed nerves heal, but the person often experiences a phantom "presence" of the missing part. This may be helpful when learning to use an artificial limb.
2. **Intensity**—some sensations are felt more distinctly and to a greater degree than are others. A weak stimulus such as dim light will affect a small number of receptors, but a stronger stimulus, such as bright sunlight, will stimulate many more receptors. When more receptors are stimulated, more impulses will arrive in the sensory area of the brain. The brain "counts" the impulses and projects a more intense sensation.
3. **Contrast**—the effect of a previous or simultaneous sensation on a current sensation, which may then be exaggerated or diminished. Again, this is a function of the brain, which constantly compares sensations. If, on a very hot day, you jump into a swimming pool, the water may feel quite cold at first. The brain compares the new sensation to the previous one, and since there is a significant difference between the two, the water will seem colder than it actually is.
4. **Adaptation**—becoming unaware of a continuing stimulus. Receptors detect changes, but if the stimulus continues it may not be much of a change, and the receptors will generate fewer impulses. The water in the swimming pool that seemed cold at first seems to "warm up" after a few minutes. The water has not changed temperature, and the receptors for cold have no changes to detect, therefore they generate fewer impulses. The sensation of cold lessens, and we interpret or feel that as increasing warmth. For another example, look at your left wrist (or perhaps the right one). Many of us wear a watch and are probably unaware of its presence on the arm most of the time. The cutaneous receptors for touch or pressure adapt very quickly to a

continuing stimulus, and if there is no change, there is nothing for the receptors to detect.

5. **After-image**—the sensation remains in the consciousness even after the stimulus has stopped. A familiar example is the bright after-image seen after watching a flashbulb go off. The very bright light strongly stimulates receptors in the retina, which generate many impulses that are perceived as an intense sensation that lasts longer than the actual stimulus.

CUTANEOUS SENSES

The dermis of the skin contains receptors for the sensations of touch, pressure, heat, cold, and pain. The receptors for pain, heat, and cold are **free nerve endings**, which also respond to any intense stimulus. Intense pressure, for example, may be felt as pain. The receptors for touch and pressure are **encapsulated nerve endings**, meaning that there is a cellular structure around the nerve ending (Fig. 9–1).

The **cutaneous senses** provide us with information about the external environment and also about the skin itself. If you have ever had chickenpox, you may remember the itching sensation of the rash. An itch is actually a mild pain sensation, which may become real pain if not scratched (how scratching relieves the itch has not yet been discovered).

The sensory areas for the skin are in the parietal lobes. You may recall from Chapter 5 that the sensitivity of an area of skin is determined by the number of receptors present. The number of receptors corresponds to the size of the sensory area in the cerebral

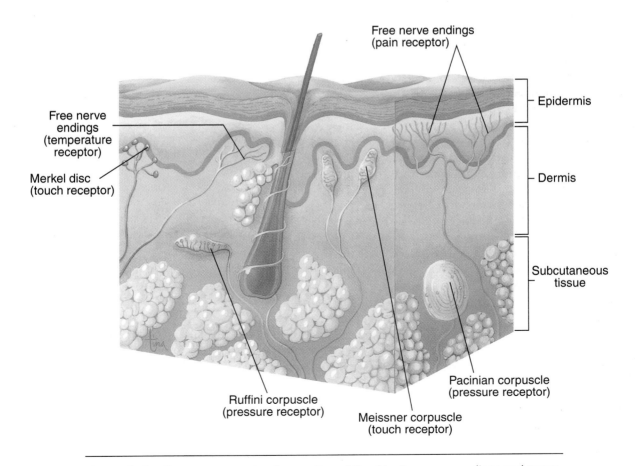

Figure 9–1   Cutaneous receptors in a section of the skin. Free nerve endings and encapsulated nerve endings are shown.

cortex. The largest parts of this sensory cortex are for the parts of the skin with the most receptors, that is, the hands and face.

As mentioned previously, sensory areas are not merely passive recipients of impulses. Consider the sensation of wetness. It is a distinct sensation, but there are no receptors for "wet" in the skin. Where does the sensation come from? Where all sensation comes from: the brain. The parietal lobes have learned to associate the simultaneous reception of temperature and pressure impulses with "wet." You can demonstrate this for yourself by putting on a plastic glove and dunking your fingers in a cup of water. Your fingers will feel wet, though they are perfectly dry inside the glove. Wetness is a learned sensation, created by the brain.

REFERRED PAIN

Free nerve endings are also found in internal organs. The smooth muscle of the small intestine, for example, has free nerve endings that are stimulated by excessive stretching or contraction; the resulting pain is called visceral pain. Sometimes pain that originates in an internal organ may be felt in a cutaneous area; this is called **referred pain**. The pain of a heart attack (myocardial infarction) may be felt in the left arm and shoulder, or the pain of gallstones may be felt in the right shoulder.

This referred pain is actually a creation of the brain. Within the spinal cord are sensory tracts that are shared by cutaneous impulses and visceral impulses. Cutaneous impulses are much more frequent, and the brain correctly projects the sensation to the skin. When the impulses have come from an organ such as the heart, however, the brain may still project the sensation to the "usual" cutaneous area. The brain projects sensation based on past experience, and cutaneous pain is far more common than visceral pain. Knowledge of referred pain, as in the examples mentioned earlier, may often be helpful in diagnosis.

MUSCLE SENSE

Muscle sense (also called kinesthetic sense) was discussed in Chapter 7 and will be reviewed only briefly here. Stretch receptors (also called proprioceptors or muscle spindles) detect stretching of muscles and generate impulses, which enable the brain to create a mental picture to know where the muscles are and how they are positioned. Conscious muscle sense is felt by the parietal lobes. Unconscious muscle sense is used by the cerebellum to coordinate voluntary movements. We do not have to see our muscles to be sure that they are performing their intended actions.

SENSE OF TASTE

The receptors for taste are found in **taste buds**, most of which are in papillae on the tongue (Fig. 9–2). These **chemoreceptors** detect chemicals in solution in the mouth. The chemicals are foods and the solvent is saliva (if the mouth is very dry, taste is very indistinct). It is believed that there are four general types of taste receptors: sweet, sour, salty, and bitter. (There is a proposed fifth, glutamate, which has been described as "savory," like grilled meat.) We experience many different tastes, however, because foods stimulate different combinations of receptors, and the sense of smell also contributes to our perception of food.

Some taste preferences have been found to be genetic. People with more than the average number of taste buds find broccoli very bitter, whereas people with fewer taste buds may like the taste.

The impulses from taste buds are transmitted by the facial and glossopharyngeal (7th and 9th cranial) nerves to the taste areas in the parietal-temporal cortex. The sense of taste is important because it makes eating enjoyable. Some medications may interfere with the sense of taste, and this sense becomes less acute as we get older. These may be contributing factors to poor nutrition in certain patients and in the elderly.

SENSE OF SMELL

The receptors for smell (**olfaction**) are **chemoreceptors** that detect vaporized chemicals that have been sniffed into the upper nasal cavities (see Fig. 9–2). Just as there are basic tastes, there are also believed to be basic scents, and research indicates that their number is a thousand or more. When stimulated by vapor molecules, **olfactory receptors** generate impulses carried by the olfactory nerves (1st cranial) through the ethmoid bone to the olfactory bulbs. The pathway for these impulses ends in the olfactory areas of the temporal lobes.

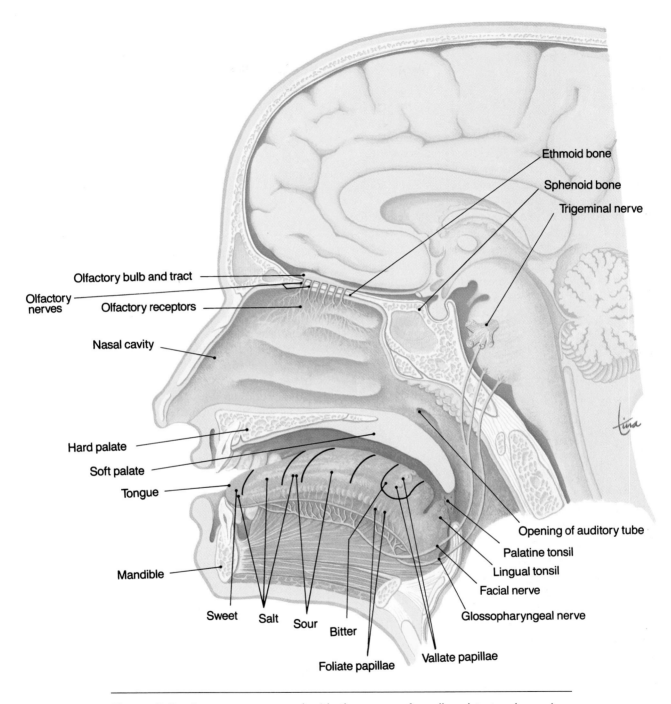

Figure 9–2   Structures concerned with the senses of smell and taste, shown in a midsagittal section of the head.

The human sense of smell is very poorly developed compared to those of other animals. Dogs, for example, have a sense of smell at least 200 times more acute than that of people. As mentioned earlier, however, much of what we call taste is actually the smell of food. If you have a cold and your nasal cavities are stuffed up, food just doesn't taste as good as it usually does. Adaptation occurs relatively quickly with odors. Pleasant scents may be sharply distinct at first but rapidly seem to dissipate or fade, and even unpleasant scents may fade with long exposure.

HUNGER AND THIRST

Hunger and thirst may be called **visceral sensations**, in that they are triggered by internal changes. Hunger is a sensation that seems to be far more complex than was first thought, but thirst seems to be somewhat simpler. The receptors for both senses are specialized cells in the hypothalamus. Receptors for hunger are believed to detect changes in blood nutrient levels, the blood levels of hormones from the stomach and small intestine, and a hormone released by adipose tissue; all of these chemical signals are collected by the hypothalamus. The receptors for thirst detect changes in the body water content, which is actually the water to salt proportion.

Naturally we do not feel these sensations in the hypothalamus: They are projected. Hunger is projected to the stomach, which contracts. Thirst is projected to the mouth and pharynx, and less saliva is produced.

If not satisfied by eating, the sensation of hunger gradually diminishes, that is, adaptation occurs. The reason is that after blood nutrient levels decrease, they become stable as fat in adipose tissue is used for energy. With little or no digestive activity in the gastrointestinal tract, secretion of hormones diminishes. With no sharp fluctuations of the chemical signals, the receptors in the hypothalamus have few changes to detect, and hunger becomes much less intense. As body fat is depleted, however, blood nutrient levels decrease again. This is a change, and hunger may be felt sharply.

In contrast, the sensation of thirst, if not satisfied by drinking, continues to worsen. There is no adaptation. As body water is lost, the amount keeps decreasing and does not stabilize. Therefore, there are constant changes for the receptors to detect, and prolonged thirst may be very painful.

THE EYE

The eye contains the receptors for vision and a refracting system that focuses light rays on the receptors in the retina. We will begin our discussion, however, with the accessory structures of the eye, then later return to the eye itself and the physiology of vision.

EYELIDS AND THE LACRIMAL APPARATUS

The eyelids contain skeletal muscle that enables the eyelids to close and cover the front of the eyeball. Eyelashes along the border of each eyelid help keep dust out of the eyes. The eyelids are lined with a thin membrane called the **conjunctiva**, which is also folded over the white of the eye. Inflammation of this membrane, called **conjunctivitis**, is often caused by allergies and makes the eyes red, itchy, and watery.

Tears are produced by the **lacrimal glands**, located at the upper, outer corner of the eyeball, within the orbit (Fig. 9–3). Small ducts take tears to the anterior of the eyeball, and blinking spreads the tears and washes the surface of the eye. Tears are mostly water, with about 1% sodium chloride, similar to other body fluids. Tears also contain **lysozyme**, an enzyme that inhibits the growth of most bacteria on the wet, warm surface of the eye. At the medial corner of the eyelids are two small openings into the superior and inferior lacrimal canals. These ducts take tears to the **lacrimal sac** (in the lacrimal bone), which leads to the **nasolacrimal duct** that empties tears into the nasal cavity. This is why crying often makes the nose run.

EYEBALL

Most of the eyeball is within and protected by the **orbit**, formed by the lacrimal, maxilla, zygomatic, frontal, sphenoid, and ethmoid bones. The six **extrinsic muscles** of the eye are attached to this bony socket and to the surface of the eyeball. There are four rectus muscles that move the eyeball up and down or side to side and two oblique muscles that rotate the eye. These are shown in Fig. 9–4. The cranial nerves that innervate these muscles are the oculomotor, trochlear, and abducens (3rd, 4th, and 6th cranial). The complex coordination of these muscles in both eyes is, fortunately, not something we have to think about, and is very important to prevent double vision.

Layers of the Eyeball

In its wall, the eyeball has three layers: the outer sclera, middle choroid layer, and inner retina (Fig. 9–5). The **sclera** is the thickest layer and is made of fibrous connective tissue that is visible as the white of the eye.

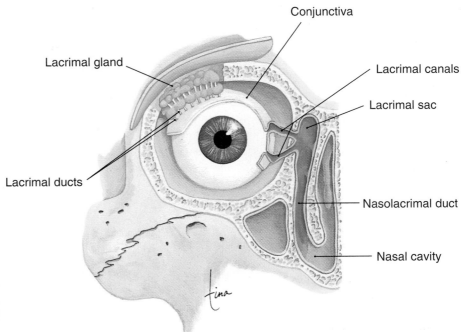

Figure 9–3 Lacrimal apparatus shown in an anterior view of the right eye.

The most anterior portion is the **cornea**, which differs from the rest of the sclera in that it is transparent and has no capillaries. The cornea is the first part of the eye that **refracts**, or bends, light rays.

The **choroid layer** contains blood vessels and a dark blue pigment (derived from melanin) that absorbs light within the eyeball and thereby prevents glare (just as does the black interior of a camera). The anterior portion of the choroid is modified into more specialized structures: the ciliary body and the iris. The **ciliary body** (muscle) is a circular muscle that surrounds the edge of the lens and is connected to the

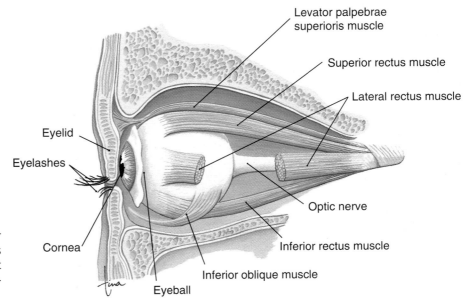

Figure 9–4 Extrinsic muscles of the eye. Lateral view of left eye (the medial rectus and superior oblique ar not shown).

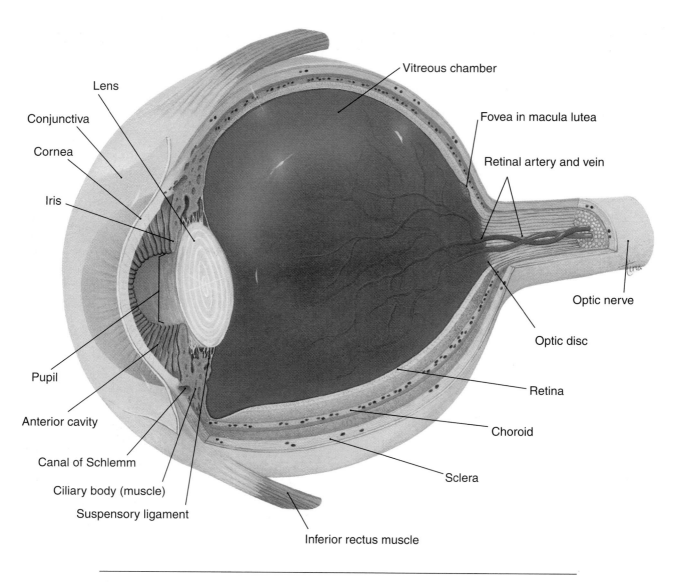

Lens

Conjunctiva

Cornea

Iris

Pupil

Anterior cavity

Canal of Schlemm

Ciliary body (muscle)

Suspensory ligament

Inferior rectus muscle

Vitreous chamber

Fovea in macula lutea

Retinal artery and vein

Optic nerve

Optic disc

Retina

Choroid

Sclera

Figure 9–5   Internal anatomy of the eyeball.

lens by **suspensory ligaments**. The **lens** is made of a transparent, elastic protein, and like the cornea, has no capillaries (see Box 9–1: Cataracts). The shape of the lens is changed by the ciliary muscle, which enables the eye to focus light from objects at varying distances from the eye.

Just in front of the lens is the circular **iris**, the colored part of the eye; its pigment is a form of melanin. What we call "eye color" is the color of the iris and is a genetic characteristic, just as skin color is. Two sets of smooth muscle fibers in the iris change

the diameter of the **pupil**, the central opening. Contraction of the radial fibers dilates the pupil; this is a sympathetic response. Contraction of the circular fibers constricts the pupil; this is a parasympathetic response (oculomotor nerves). Pupillary constriction is a reflex that protects the retina from intense light or that permits more acute near vision, as when reading.

The **retina** lines the posterior two-thirds of the eyeball and contains the visual receptors, the rods and cones (Fig. 9–6). **Rods** detect only the presence of light, whereas **cones** detect colors, which, as you may

Box 9–1   CATARACTS

The lens of the eye is normally transparent but may become opaque; this cloudiness or opacity is called a **cataract**. Cataract formation is most common among elderly people. With age, the proteins of the lens break down and lose their transparency. Long-term exposure to ultraviolet light (sunlight) also seems to be a contributing factor.

The cloudy lens does not refract light properly, and blurred vision is often an early symptom. Treatment of cataracts requires surgical removal of the lens and the use of glasses or contact lenses to replace the refractive function of the lens. The use of very precise laser surgery to destroy small cataracts may permit the lens to retain a portion of its function.

know from physics, are the different wavelengths of visible light. Cones are most abundant in the center of the retina, especially an area called the **macula lutea** directly behind the center of the lens. The **fovea**, which contains only cones, is a small depression in the macula and is the area for best color vision. Rods are proportionally more abundant toward the periphery, or edge, of the retina. Our best vision in dim light

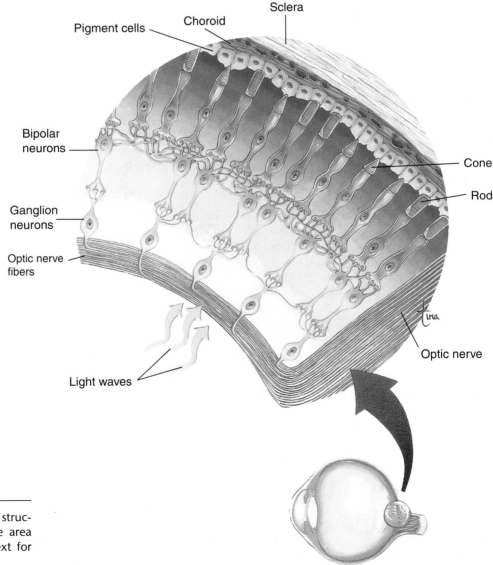

Figure 9–6 Microscopic structure of the retina in the area of the optic disc. See text for description.

Box 9–2   GLAUCOMA

The presence of aqueous humor in the anterior cavity of the eye creates a pressure called intraocular pressure. An increase in this pressure is an important risk factor for **glaucoma**, which is now defined as a group of disorders that damages the optic nerve and causes loss of vision. Other risk factors include high blood pressure and diabetes. In the most common form of glaucoma, aqueous humor is not reabsorbed properly into the canal of Schlemm. Increased pressure in the anterior cavity is transmitted to the lens, the vitreous humor, and to the retina and optic nerve. As pressure on the retina increases, halos may be seen around bright lights. Frequently, however, there are no symptoms. A person with glaucoma may not notice the shrinking visual field in one eye before vision loss is far advanced. This happens because the brain will suppress a faulty image from one eye that it cannot easily integrate with the normal image of the other eye. When both eyes are affected, the person may not become aware of the gradual loss of peripheral vision because close work such as reading does not require the edges of the visual fields.

Glaucoma may often be controlled with medications that constrict the pupil and flatten the iris, thus opening up access to the canal of Schlemm. If these or other medications are not effective, laser surgery may be used to create a larger drainage canal.

Anyone over the age of 40 should have a test for glaucoma; anyone with a family history of glaucoma should have this test annually, as should those with diabetes or high blood pressure. If diagnosed early, glaucoma is treatable, and blindness can usually be prevented.

or at night, for which we depend on the rods, is at the sides of our visual fields.

Neurons called **ganglion neurons** carry the impulses generated by the rods and cones. These neurons all converge at the **optic disc** (see Figs. 9–5 and 9–6) and pass through the wall of the eyeball as the **optic nerve**. There are no rods or cones in the optic disc, so this part of the retina is sometimes called the "blind spot." We are not aware of a blind spot in our field of vision, however, in part because the eyes are constantly moving, and in part because the brain "fills in" the blank spot to create a "complete" picture.

Cavities of the Eyeball

There are two cavities within the eye: the posterior cavity and the anterior cavity. The larger, **posterior cavity** is found between the lens and retina and contains **vitreous humor**. This semisolid substance keeps the retina in place. If the eyeball is punctured and vitreous humor is lost, the retina may fall away from the choroid; this is one possible cause of a **detached retina**.

The **anterior cavity** is found between the front of the lens and the cornea and contains **aqueous humor**, the tissue fluid of the eyeball. Aqueous humor is formed by capillaries in the ciliary body, flows anteriorly through the pupil, and is reabsorbed by the **canal of Schlemm** (small veins also called the scleral venous sinus) at the junction of the iris and cornea. Because aqueous humor is tissue fluid, you would expect it to have a nourishing function, and it does. Recall that the lens and cornea have no capillaries; they are nourished by the continuous flow of aqueous humor (see Box 9–2: Glaucoma).

PHYSIOLOGY OF VISION

In order for us to see, light rays must be focused on the retina, and the resulting nerve impulses must be transmitted to the visual areas of the cerebral cortex in the brain.

Refraction of light rays is the deflection or bending of a ray of light as it passes through one object and into another object of greater or lesser density. The refraction of light within the eye takes place in the following pathway of structures: the cornea, aqueous humor, lens, and vitreous humor. The lens is the only adjustable part of the refraction system. When looking at distant objects, the ciliary muscle is relaxed and the lens is elongated and thin. When looking at near objects, the ciliary muscle contracts to form a smaller circle, the elastic lens recoils and bulges in the middle, and has greater refractive power (see Box 9–3: Errors of Refraction).

When light rays strike the retina, they stimulate chemical reactions in the rods and cones. In rods, the chemical **rhodopsin** breaks down to form scotopsin and retinal (a derivative of vitamin A). This chemical reaction generates an electrical impulse, and rhodopsin is then resynthesized in a slower reaction. Chemical reactions in the cones, also involving retinal, are brought about by different wavelengths of light. It is believed that there are three types of cones: red-absorbing, blue-absorbing, and green-absorbing cones. Each type absorbs wavelengths over about a third of the visible light spectrum, so red cones, for example, absorb light of the red, orange, and yellow wavelengths. The chemical reactions in cones also generate electrical impulses (see Box 9–4: Night Blindness and Color Blindness).

The impulses from the rods and cones are transmitted to **ganglion neurons** (see Fig. 9–6); these converge at the optic disc and become the **optic nerve**, which passes posteriorly through the wall of the eyeball. Ganglion neurons also seem to have a photoreceptor chemical (called melanopsin) that may contribute to the daily resetting of our biological clocks.

The optic nerves from both eyes converge at the **optic chiasma** (or chiasm), just in front of the pituitary gland. Here, the medial fibers of each optic nerve cross to the other side. This crossing permits each visual area to receive impulses from both eyes, which is important for binocular vision.

The visual areas are in the **occipital lobes** of the cerebral cortex. Although each eye transmits a slightly different picture, the visual areas put them together or integrate them to make a single image. This is called **binocular vision**. The visual areas also right the image, because the image on the retina is upside down. The image on film in a camera is also upside down, but we don't even realize that because we look at the pictures right side up. The brain just as automatically ensures that we see our world right side up.

Also for near vision, the pupils constrict to block out peripheral light rays that would otherwise blur the image, and the eyes converge to keep the images on the corresponding parts of both retinas. The importance of pupil constriction can be demonstrated by looking at this page through a pinhole in a piece of paper. You will be able to read with the page much closer to your eye because the paper blocks out light from the sides.

Try looking at your finger placed on the tip of your nose. You can feel your eyes move medially ("cross") in maximum convergence. If the eyes don't converge, the result is double vision; the brain can't make the very different images into one, and settles for two. This is temporary, however, because the brain does not like seeing double, and will eventually suppress one image.

THE EAR

The ear consists of three areas: the outer ear, the middle ear, and the inner ear (Fig. 9–7). The ear contains the receptors for two senses: hearing and **equilibrium**. These receptors are all found in the inner ear.

OUTER EAR

The **outer ear** consists of the auricle and the ear canal. The **auricle**, or **pinna**, is made of cartilage covered with skin. For animals such as dogs, whose ears are movable, the auricle may act as a funnel for sound waves. For people, however, the flat and stationary auricle is not important. Hearing would not be negatively affected without it, although those of us who

---

Box 9–3   ERRORS OF REFRACTION

Normal visual acuity is referred to as 20/20, that is, the eye should and does clearly see an object 20 feet away. **Nearsightedness (myopia)** means that the eye sees near objects well but not distant ones. If an eye has 20/80 vision, this means that what the normal eye can see at 80 feet, the nearsighted eye can see only if the object is brought to 20 feet away. The nearsighted eye focuses images from distant objects in front of the retina, because the eyeball is too long or the lens too thick (see diagram on the next page). These structural characteristics of the eye are hereditary. Correction of nearsightedness requires a concave lens to spread out light rays before they strike the eye.

Farsightedness (hyperopia) means that the eye sees distant objects well. Such an eye may have an acuity of 20/10, that is, it sees at 20 feet what the normal eye can see only at 10 feet. The farsighted eye focuses light from near objects "behind" the retina, because the eyeball is too short or the lens too thin. Correction of the farsighted eye requires a convex lens to converge light rays before they strike the eye.

As we get older, most of us will become more farsighted **(presbyopia)**. As the aging lens loses its elasticity, it is not as able to recoil and thicken for near vision, and glasses for reading are often necessary.

Box 9–3   ERRORS OF REFRACTION (Continued)

Astigmatism is another error of refraction, caused by an irregular curvature of the cornea or lens that scatters light rays and blurs the image on the retina. Correction of astigmatism requires a lens ground specifically for the curvature of the individual eye.

Normal eye

Astigmatic

Nearsighted

Corrected

Farsighted

Corrected

Box Figure 9–A   Errors of refraction compared to normal eye. Corrective lenses are shown for nearsightedness and farsightedness.

Box 9–4   NIGHT BLINDNESS AND COLOR BLINDNESS

Night blindness, the inability to see well in dim light or at night is usually caused by a deficiency of vitamin A, although some night blindness may occur with aging. Vitamin A is necessary for the synthesis of rhodopsin in the rods. Without sufficient vitamin A, there is not enough rhodopsin present to respond to low levels of light.

Color blindness is a genetic disorder in which one of the three sets of cones is lacking or nonfunctional. Total color blindness, the inability to see any colors at all, is very rare. The most common form is red-green color blindness, which is the inability to distinguish between these colors. If either the red cones or green cones are missing, the person will still see most of the colors, but will not have the contrast that the missing set of cones would provide. So red and green shades will look somewhat similar, without the definite difference most of us see. (See the accompanying illustration.) This is a sex-linked trait; the recessive gene is on the X chromosome. A woman with one gene for color blindness and a gene for normal color vision on her other X chromosome will not be color blind but may pass the gene for color blindness to her children. A man with a gene for color blindness on his X chromosome has no gene at all for color vision on his Y chromosome and will be color blind.

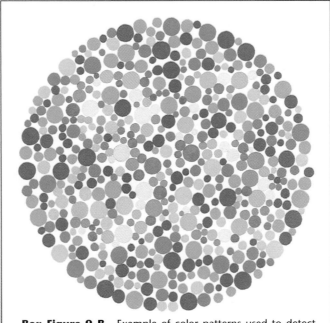

Box Figure 9–B   Example of color patterns used to detect color blindness.

wear glasses would have our vision impaired without our auricles. The **ear canal** is lined with skin that contains ceruminous glands. It may also be called the **external auditory meatus**, and is a tunnel into the temporal bone, curving slightly forward and down.

MIDDLE EAR

The **middle ear** is an air-filled cavity in the temporal bone. The **eardrum**, or **tympanic membrane**, is stretched across the end of the ear canal and vibrates when sound waves strike it. These vibrations are transmitted to the three auditory bones: the **malleus, incus**, and **stapes** (see Fig. 9–7). The stapes then transmits vibrations to the fluid-filled inner ear at the **oval window**.

The **eustachian tube** (auditory tube) extends from the middle ear to the nasopharynx and permits air to enter or leave the middle ear cavity. The air pressure in the middle ear must be the same as the exter-

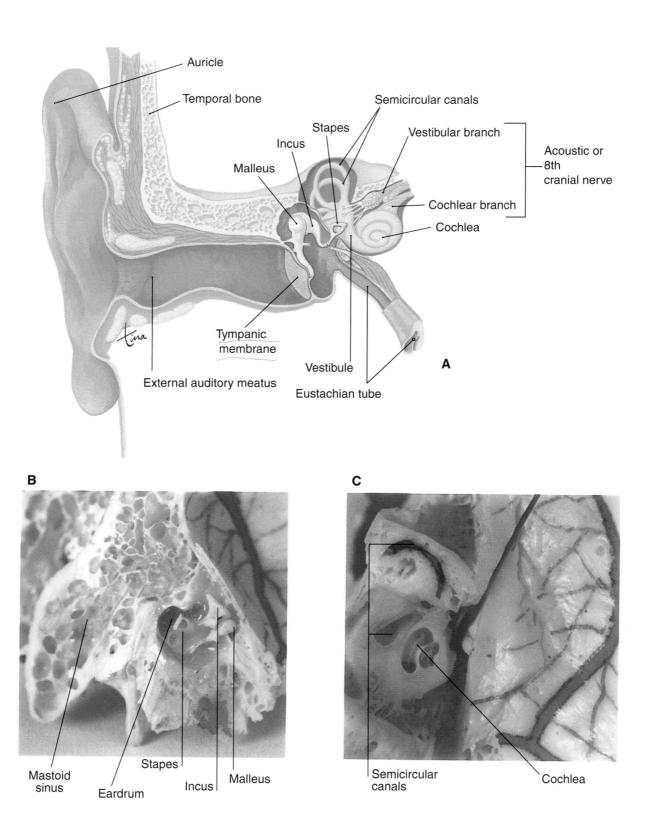

Figure 9–7 **(A)** Outer, middle, and inner ear structures as shown in a frontal section through the right temporal bone. **(B)** Section of temporal bone with the auditory bones. **(C)** Section of temporal bone showing bony labyrinth of inner ear. The colors on the bone are artificial. (Photographs by Dan Kaufman.)

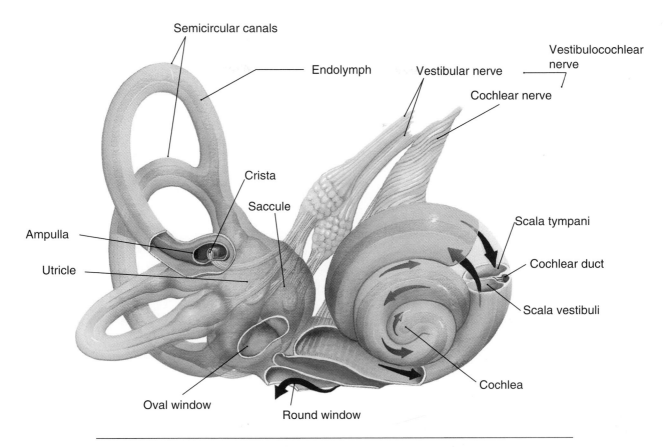

Figure 9–8 Inner ear structures. The arrows show the transmission of vibrations during hearing.

nal atmospheric pressure in order for the eardrum to vibrate properly. You may have noticed your ears "popping" when in an airplane or when driving to a higher or lower altitude. Swallowing or yawning creates the "pop" by opening the eustachian tubes and equalizing the air pressures.

The eustachian tubes of children are short and nearly horizontal and may permit bacteria to spread from the pharynx to the middle ear. This is why **otitis media** may be a complication of a strep throat.

INNER EAR

Within the temporal bone, the **inner ear** is a cavity called the **bony labyrinth** (a labyrinth is a maze—see Fig. 9–7), which is lined with membrane called the **membranous labyrinth. Perilymph** is the fluid found between bone and membrane, and **endolymph** is the fluid within the membranous structures of the inner ear. These structures are the

cochlea, concerned with hearing, and the utricle, saccule, and semicircular canals, all concerned with equilibrium (Fig. 9–8).

Cochlea

The **cochlea** is shaped like a snail shell with two-and-a-half structural turns. Internally, the cochlea is partitioned into three fluid-filled canals. The medial canal is the cochlear duct, which contains the receptors for hearing in the **organ of Corti (spiral organ)**. The receptors are called hair cells (their projections are not "hair," of course, but rather are specialized microvilli called stereocilia), which contain endings of the cochlear branch of the 8th cranial nerve. Overhanging the hair cells is the tectorial membrane (Fig. 9–9).

Very simply, the process of hearing involves the transmission of vibrations and the generation of nerve impulses. When sound waves enter the ear canal, vibrations are transmitted by the following sequence

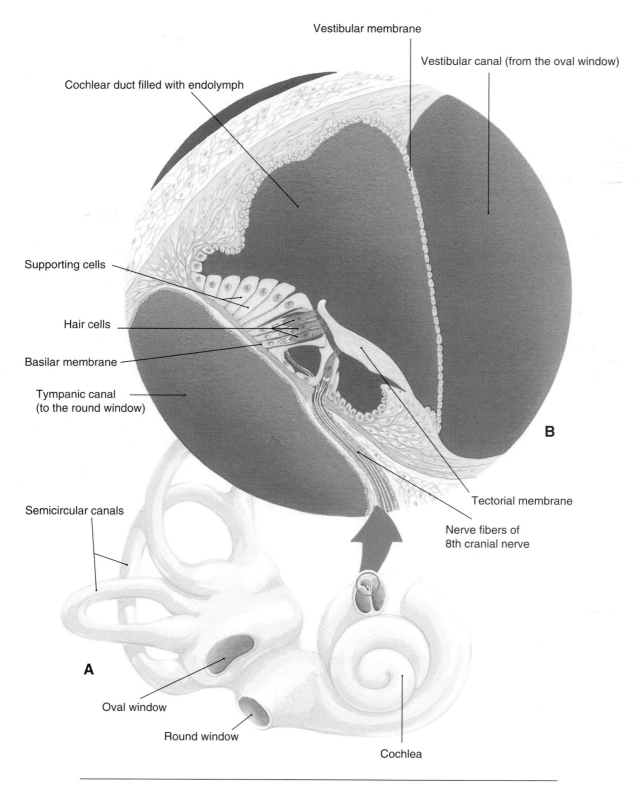

Vestibular membrane

Vestibular canal (from the oval window)

Cochlear duct filled with endolymph

Supporting cells

Hair cells

Basilar membrane

Tympanic canal
(to the round window)

B

Tectorial membrane

Nerve fibers of
8th cranial nerve

Semicircular canals

A

Oval window

Round window

Cochlea

Figure 9–9　Organ of Corti. **(A)** Inner ear structures. **(B)** Magnification of organ of Corti within the cochlea.

of structures: eardrum, malleus, incus, stapes, oval window of the inner ear, perilymph and endolymph within the cochlea, and hair cells of the organ of Corti. When the hair cells bend, they generate impulses that are carried by the 8th cranial nerve to the brain. As you may recall, the auditory areas are in the **temporal lobes** of the cerebral cortex. It is here that sounds are heard and interpreted (see Box 9–5: Deafness).

The auditory areas also enable us to determine from which direction a sound is coming. Simply stated, the auditory areas count and compare the number of impulses coming from each inner ear. For example, if more impulses arrive from the left cochlea than from the right one, the sound will be projected to the left. If the source of a sound is directly above your head, the sound may seem to come from all directions, because each auditory area is receiving approximately the same number of impulses and cannot project the sensation to one side or the other.

The final structure in the hearing pathway is the round window (Fig. 9–8). The membrane-covered **round window**, just below the oval window, is

---

Box 9–5   DEAFNESS

Deafness is the inability to hear properly; the types are classified according to the part of the hearing process that is not functioning normally.

Conduction deafness—impairment of one of the structures that transmits vibrations. Examples of this type are a punctured eardrum, arthritis of the auditory bones, or a middle ear infection in which fluid fills the middle ear cavity.

Nerve deafness—impairment of the 8th cranial nerve or the receptors for hearing in the cochlea. The 8th cranial nerve may be damaged by some antibiotics used to treat bacterial infections. Nerve deafness is a rare complication of some viral infec-

tions such as mumps or congenital rubella (German measles). Deterioration of the hair cells in the cochlea is a natural consequence of aging, and the acuity of hearing diminishes as we get older. For example, it may be more difficult for an elderly person to distiguish conversation from background noise. Chronic exposure to loud noise accelerates degeneration of the hair cells and onset of this type of deafness.

Central deafness—damage to the auditory areas in the temporal lobes. This type of deafness is rare but may be caused by a brain tumor, meningitis, or a CVA in the temporal lobe.

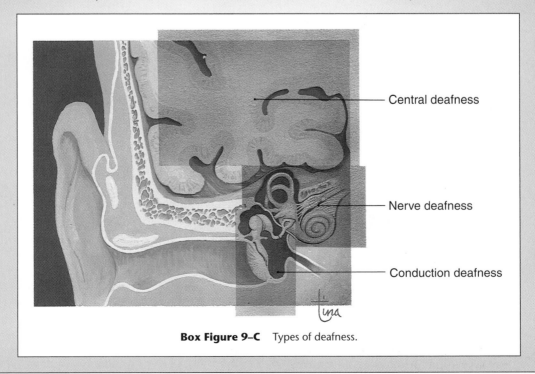

Box Figure 9–C   Types of deafness.

important to relieve pressure. When the stapes pushes in the oval window, the round window bulges out, which prevents damage to the hair cells.

Utricle and Saccule

The **utricle** and **saccule** are membranous sacs in an area called the **vestibule**, between the cochlea and semicircular canals. Within the utricle and saccule are hair cells embedded in a gelatinous membrane with tiny crystals of calcium carbonate called **otoliths**. Gravity pulls on the otoliths and bends the hair cells as the position of the head changes (see Fig. 9–10). The impulses generated by these hair cells are carried by the vestibular portion of the 8th cranial nerve to the cerebellum, midbrain, and the temporal lobes of the cerebrum.

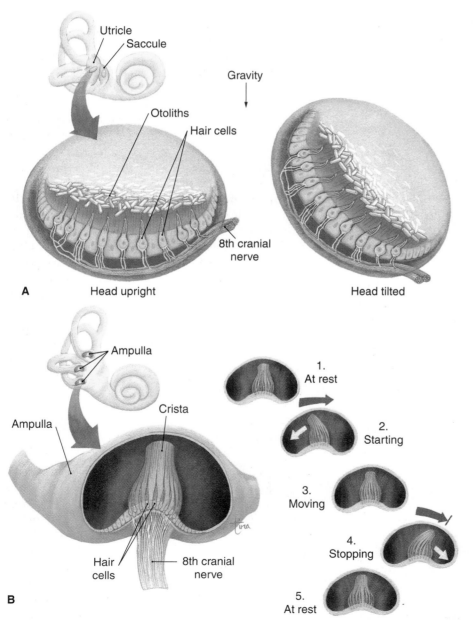

Figure 9–10 Physiology of equilibrium. **(A)** Utricle and saccule. **(B)** Semicircular canals. See text for description.

Box 9–6   MOTION SICKNESS

Motion sickness is characterized by cold sweats, hyperventilation, nausea, and vomiting when the person is exposed to repetitive motion that is unexpected or unfamiliar, or that cannot be controlled. Seasickness is a type of motion sickness, as is carsickness (why children are carsick more often than adults is not known).

Some people are simply not affected by the rolling of a ship or train; for others, the constant stimulation of the receptors for position first becomes uncomfortable, then nauseating. For those who know they are susceptible to motion sickness, medications are available for use before traveling by plane, train, or car.

The cerebellum and midbrain use this information to maintain equilibrium at a subconscious level. We can, of course, be aware of the position of the head, and it is the cerebrum that provides awareness.

Semicircular Canals

The three **semicircular canals** are fluid-filled membranous ovals oriented in three different planes. At the base of each is an enlarged portion called the ampulla (see Fig. 9–8), which contains hair cells (the crista) that are affected by movement. As the body moves forward, for example, the hair cells are bent backward at first and then straighten (see Fig. 9–10). The bending of the hair cells generates impulses carried by the vestibular branch of the 8th cranial nerve to the cerebellum, midbrain, and temporal lobes of the cerebrum. These impulses are interpreted as starting or stopping, and accelerating or decelerating, or changing direction, and this information is used to maintain equilibrium while we are moving (see Box 9–6: Motion Sickness).

In summary then, the utricle and saccule provide information about the position of the body at rest, while the semicircular canals provide information about the body in motion. Of course, there is some overlap, and the brain puts all the information together to create a single sense of body position.

ARTERIAL RECEPTORS

The aorta and carotid arteries contain receptors that detect changes in the blood. The **aortic arch**, which receives blood pumped by the left ventricle of the heart, curves over the top of the heart. The left and right **carotid arteries** are branches of the aortic arch that take blood through the neck on the way to the brain. In each of these vessels are pressoreceptors and chemoreceptors (see Fig. 12-7).

Pressoreceptors in the carotid sinuses and aortic sinus detect changes in blood pressure. **Chemoreceptors** in the carotid bodies and the aortic body detect changes in the oxygen and carbon dioxide content, and the pH, of blood. The impulses generated by these receptors do not give rise to sensations that we feel but rather are information used to make any necessary changes in respiration or circulation. We will return to this in later chapters, so one example will suffice for now.

If the blood level of oxygen decreases significantly, this change (hypoxia) is detected by carotid and aortic chemoreceptors. The sensory impulses are carried by the glossopharyngeal (9th cranial) and vagus (10th cranial) nerves to the medulla. Centers in the medulla may then increase the respiratory rate and the heart rate to obtain and circulate more oxygen. These are the respiratory and cardiac reflexes that were mentioned in Chapter 8 as functions of the glossopharyngeal and vagus nerves. The importance of these reflexes is readily apparent: to maintain normal blood levels of oxygen and carbon dioxide and to maintain normal blood pressure.

AGING AND THE SENSES

All of the senses may be diminished in old age. In the eye, cataracts may make the lens opaque. The lens also loses its elasticity and the eye becomes more farsighted, a condition called presbyopia. The risk of glaucoma increases, and elderly people should be tested for it because treatment is available that can prevent blindness. Macular degeneration, in which central vision becomes impaired, is a major cause of vision loss for people over 65. In the ear, cumulative damage to the hair cells in the organ of Corti usually becomes apparent some time after the age of 60. Hair cells that have been damaged in a lifetime of noise cannot be replaced. The deafness of old age ranges from slight to profound; very often high-pitched sounds are lost first, while hearing may still be adequate for low-pitched sounds. Both taste and smell become less acute with age, which may contribute to poor nutrition in elderly people.

SUMMARY

Changes take place all around us as well as within us. If the body could not respond appropriately to environmental and internal changes, homeostasis would soon be disrupted, resulting in injury, illness, or even death. In order to respond appropriately to changes, the brain must know what they are. Conveying this information to our brains is the function of our senses. Although we may sometimes take our senses for granted, we could not survive for very long without them.

You have just read about the great variety of internal and external changes that are detected by the sense organs. You are also familiar with the role of the nervous system in the regulation of the body's responses. In the next chapter we will discuss the other regulatory system, the endocrine system. The hormones of the endocrine glands are produced in response to changes, and their regulatory effects all contribute to homeostasis.

STUDY OUTLINE

Purpose of Sensations—to detect changes in the external or internal environment to enable the body to respond appropriately to maintain homeostasis

Sensory Pathway—pathway of impulses for a sensation
1. Receptors—detect a change (usually very specific) and generate impulses.
2. Sensory neurons—transmit impulses from receptors to the CNS.
3. Sensory tracts—white matter in the CNS.
4. Sensory area—most are in the cerebral cortex; feels and interprets the sensation.

Characteristics of Sensations
1. Projection—the sensation seems to come from the area where the receptors were stimulated, even though it is the brain that truly feels the sensation.
2. Intensity—the degree to which a sensation is felt; a strong stimulus affects more receptors, more impulses are sent to the brain and are interpreted as a more intense sensation.
3. Contrast—the effect of a previous or simultaneous sensation on a current sensation as the brain compares them.
4. Adaptation—becoming unaware of a continuing stimulus; if the stimulus remains constant, there is no change for receptors to detect.

5. After-image—the sensation remains in the consciousness after the stimulus has stopped.

Cutaneous Senses—provide information about the external environment and the skin itself
1. In the dermis are free nerve endings for pain, heat, and cold, and encapsulated nerve endings for touch and pressure (see Fig. 9–1).
2. Sensory areas are in parietal lobes.
3. Referred pain is visceral pain that is felt as cutaneous pain. Common pathways in the CNS carry both cutaneous and visceral impulses; the brain usually projects sensation to the cutaneous area.

Muscle Sense—knowing where our muscles are without looking at them
1. Stretch receptors in muscles detect stretching.
2. Sensory areas for conscious muscle sense are in parietal lobes.
3. Cerebellum uses unconscious muscle sense to coordinate voluntary movement.

Sense of Taste (see Fig. 9–2)
1. Chemoreceptors are in taste buds on the tongue; detect chemicals (foods) in solution (saliva) in the mouth.
2. Four basic tastes: sweet, sour, salty, bitter; foods stimulate combinations of receptors.

3. Pathway: Facial and glossopharyngeal nerves to taste areas in parietal-temporal lobes.

Sense of Smell (see Fig. 9–2)
1. Chemoreceptors are in upper nasal cavities; detect vaporized chemicals.
2. Pathway: olfactory nerves to olfactory bulbs to olfactory areas in the temporal lobes.
3. Smell contributes greatly to what we call taste.

Hunger and Thirst—visceral (internal) sensations
1. Receptors for hunger: in hypothalamus, detect changes in GI hormones and nutrient levels in the blood; hunger is projected to the stomach; adaptation does occur.
2. Receptors for thirst: in hypothalamus, osmoreceptors detect changes in body water (water–salt proportions); thirst is projected to the mouth and pharynx; adaptation does not occur.

The Eye (see Figs. 9–3 through 9–6)
1. Eyelids and eyelashes keep dust out of eyes; conjunctiva line the eyelids and cover white of eye.
2. Lacrimal glands produce tears which flow across eyeball to two lacrimal ducts, to lacrimal sac to nasolacrimal duct to nasal cavity. Tears wash the anterior eyeball and contain lysozyme to inhibit bacterial growth.
3. The eyeball is protected by the bony orbit (socket).
4. The six extrinsic muscles move the eyeball; innervated by the 3rd, 4th, and 6th cranial nerves.
5. Sclera—outermost layer of the eyeball, made of fibrous connective tissue; anterior portion is the transparent cornea, the first light-refracting structure.
6. Choroid layer—middle layer of eyeball; dark blue pigment absorbs light to prevent glare within the eyeball.
7. Ciliary body (muscle) and suspensory ligaments—change shape of lens, which is made of a transparent, elastic protein and which refracts light.
8. Iris—two sets of smooth muscle fibers regulate diameter of pupil, that is, how much light strikes the retina.
9. Retina—innermost layer of eyeball; contains rods and cones.

- Rods—detect light; abundant toward periphery of retina.
- Cones—detect color; abundant in center of retina. Fovea—in the center of the macula lutea; contains only cones; area of best color vision.
- Optic disc—no rods or cones; optic nerve passes through eyeball.
10. Posterior cavity contains vitreous humor (semi-solid) that keeps the retina in place.
11. Anterior cavity contains aqueous humor that nourishes the lens and cornea; made by capillaries of the ciliary body, flows through pupil, is reabsorbed to blood at the canal of Schlemm.

Physiology of Vision
1. Refraction (bending and focusing) pathway of light: cornea, aqueous humor, lens, vitreous humor.
2. Lens is adjustable: ciliary muscle relaxes for distant vision, and lens is thin. Ciliary muscle contracts for near vision, and elastic lens thickens and has greater refractive power.
3. Light strikes retina and stimulates chemical reactions in the rods and cones.
4. In rods: rhodopsin breaks down to scotopsin and retinal (from vitamin A), and an electrical impulse is generated. In cones: specific wavelengths of light are absorbed (red, blue, green); chemical reactions generate nerve impulses.
5. Ganglion neurons from the rods and cones form the optic nerve, which passes through the eyeball at the optic disc.
6. Optic chiasma—site of the crossover of medial fibers of both optic nerves, permitting binocular vision.
7. Visual areas in occipital lobes—each area receives impulses from both eyes; both areas create one image from the two slightly different images of each eye; both areas right the upside-down retinal image.

The Ear (see Figs. 9–7 through 9–10)
1. Outer ear—auricle or pinna has no real function for people; ear canal curves forward and down into temporal bone.
2. Middle ear—eardrum at end of ear canal vibrates when sound waves strike it. Auditory bones: malleus, incus, stapes; transmit vibrations to inner ear at oval window.
- Eustachian tube—extends from middle ear to nasopharynx; allows air in and out of middle ear

to permit eardrum to vibrate; air pressure in middle ear should equal atmospheric pressure.

3. Inner ear—bony labyrinth in temporal bone, lined with membranous labyrinth. Perilymph is fluid between bone and membrane; endolymph is fluid within membrane. Membranous structures are the cochlea, utricle and saccule, and semicircular canals.

4. Cochlea—snail-shell shaped; three internal canals; cochlear duct contains receptors for hearing: hair cells in the organ of Corti; these cells contain endings of the cochlear branch of the 8th cranial nerve.

5. Physiology of hearing—sound waves stimulate vibration of eardrum, malleus, incus, stapes, oval window of inner ear, perilymph and endolymph of cochlea, and hair cells of organ of Corti. When hair cells bend, impulses are generated and carried by the 8th cranial nerve to the auditory areas in the temporal lobes. Round window prevents pressure damage to the hair cells.

6. Utricle and saccule—membranous sacs in the vestibule; each contains hair cells that are affected by gravity. When position of the head changes, otoliths bend the hair cells, which generate impulses along the vestibular branch of the 8th cranial nerve to the cerebellum, midbrain, and cerebrum. Impulses are interpreted as position of the head at rest.

7. Semicircular canals—three membranous ovals in three planes; enlarged base is the ampulla, which contains hair cells (crista) that are affected by movement. As body moves, hair cells bend in opposite direction, generate impulses along vestibular branch of 8th cranial nerve to cerebellum, midbrain, and cerebrum. Impulses are interpreted as movement of the body, changing speed, stopping or starting.

Arterial Receptors—in large arteries; detect changes in blood

1. Aortic arch—curves over top of heart. Aortic sinus contains pressoreceptors; aortic body contains chemoreceptors; sensory nerve is vagus (10th cranial).

2. Right and left carotid arteries in the neck; carotid sinus contains pressoreceptors; carotid body contains chemoreceptors; sensory nerve is the glossopharyngeal (9th cranial).

3. Pressoreceptors detect changes in blood pressure; chemoreceptors detect changes in pH or oxygen and CO_2 levels in the blood. This information is used by the vital centers in the medulla to change respiration or circulation to maintain normal blood oxygen and CO_2 and normal blood pressure.

REVIEW QUESTIONS

1. State the two general functions of receptors. Explain the purpose of sensory neurons and sensory tracts. (p. 188)

2. Name the receptors for the cutaneous senses, and explain the importance of this information. (p. 189)

3. Name the receptors for muscle sense and the parts of the brain concerned with muscle sense. (p. 190)

4. State what the chemoreceptors for taste and smell detect. Name the cranial nerve(s) for each of these senses and the lobe of the cerebrum where each is felt. (p. 190)

5. Name the part of the eye with each of the following functions: (pp. 192–196)
   a. Change the shape of the lens

   b. Contains the rods and cones
   c. Forms the white of the eye
   d. Form the optic nerve
   e. Keep dust out of eye
   f. Changes the size of the pupil
   g. Produce tears
   h. Absorbs light within the eyeball to prevent glare

6. With respect to vision: (p. 196–197)
   a. Name the structures and substances that refract light rays (in order).
   b. State what cones detect and what rods detect. What happens within these receptors when light strikes them?
   c. Name the cranial nerve for vision and the lobe of the cerebrum that contains the visual area.

7. With respect to the ear: (pp. 199–205)
   a. Name the parts of the ear that transmit the vibrations of sound waves (in order).
   b. State the location of the receptors for hearing.
   c. State the location of the receptors that respond to gravity.
   d. State the location of the receptors that respond to motion.
   e. State the two functions of the 8th cranial nerve.
   f. Name the lobe of the cerebrum concerned with hearing.
   g. Name the two parts of the brain concerned with maintaining balance and equilibrium.

8. Name the following (p. 205):
   a. The locations of arterial chemoreceptors, and state what they detect
   b. The locations of arterial pressoreceptors, and state what they detect
   c. The cranial nerves involved in respiratory and cardiac reflexes, and state the part of the brain that regulates these vital functions

9. Explain each of the following: adaptation, afterimage, projection, contrast. (pp. 188–189)

FOR FURTHER THOUGHT

1. Why are the inner ear labyrinths filled with fluid rather than air? One reason is directly concerned with hearing, the other with survival.

2. Michael's summer job in his town was collecting garbage. At first he thought the garbage and the truck smelled awful, but by lunchtime he decided that he didn't mind it at all. Explain what happened.

3. When we are out in very cold weather, why don't our eyes freeze shut? Try to think of two reasons.

4. You probably have at one time hit your "funny bone," which is really the ulnar nerve where it crosses the elbow. Such a whack is very painful, and not just in the elbow but all the way down the forearm to the ring and little fingers of the hand. This is referred pain. Explain why it happens, and name the characteristic of sensations that it illustrates.

5. Albinism is a genetic characteristic in which melanin is not produced; it may occur in just about any type of animal. As you probably know, an albino person will have white skin and hair. Describe the consequences for the person's eyes.

6. We sometimes hear that blind people have a better sense of hearing than do sighted people. Do you think this is really true? Explain. Name two other senses a blind person may especially depend upon. Explain.

7. Look at Question Figure 9–A below. In part A, which rectangle seems wider, the upper one or the lower one? Measure them, and explain your answer. Part B shows a Necker cube. Look at the cube and let your eyes relax. What seems to happen? Why do you think this happens? Part C has some lines and some shaded blocks. But what do we see? Explain.

Question Figure 9–A

CHAPTER 10

Box 10–1	DISORDERS OF GROWTH HORMONE
Box 10–2	DISORDERS OF THYROXINE
Box 10–3	DIABETES MELLITUS
Box 10–4	DISORDERS OF THE ADRENAL CORTEX

Student Objectives

- Name the endocrine glands and the hormones secreted by each.
- Explain how a negative feedback mechanism works.
- Explain how the hypothalamus is involved in the secretion of hormones from the posterior pituitary gland and anterior pituitary gland.
- State the functions of oxytocin and antidiuretic hormone, and explain the stimulus for secretion of each.
- State the functions of the hormones of the anterior pituitary gland, and state the stimulus for secretion of each.
- State the functions of thyroxine and T_3, and describe the stimulus for their secretion.

The Endocrine System

*Terms that appear in **bold type** in the chapter text are defined in the glossary, which begins on page 521.*

We have already seen how the nervous system regulates body functions by means of nerve impulses and integration of information by the spinal cord and brain. The other regulating system of the body is the **endocrine system**, which consists of endocrine glands that secrete chemicals called **hormones**. These glands, and the names of the hormones they secrete, are shown in Fig. 10–1.

Endocrine glands are ductless, that is, they do not have ducts to take their secretions to specific sites. Instead, hormones are secreted directly into capillaries and circulate in the blood throughout the body. Each hormone then exerts very specific effects on certain organs, called **target organs** or **target tissues**. Some hormones, such as insulin and thyroxine, have many target organs. Other hormones, such as calcitonin and some pituitary gland hormones, have only one or a few target organs.

In general, the endocrine system and its hormones help regulate growth, the use of foods to produce energy, resistance to stress, the pH of body fluids and fluid balance, and reproduction. In this chapter we will discuss the specific functions of the hormones and how each contributes to homeostasis.

CHEMISTRY OF HORMONES

With respect to their chemical structure, hormones may be classified into three groups: amines, proteins, and steroids.

1. **Amines**—these simple hormones are structural variations of the amino acid tyrosine. This group includes thyroxine from the thyroid gland and epinephrine and norepinephrine from the adrenal medulla.
2. **Proteins**—these hormones are chains of amino acids. Insulin from the pancreas, growth hormone from the anterior pituitary gland, and calcitonin from the thyroid gland are all proteins. Short chains of amino acids may be called **peptides**. Antidiuretic hormone and oxytocin, synthesized by the hypothalamus, are peptide hormones.
3. **Steroids**—cholesterol is the precursor for the steroid hormones, which include cortisol and aldosterone from the adrenal cortex, estrogen and progesterone from the ovaries, and testosterone from the testes.

REGULATION OF HORMONE SECRETION

Hormones are secreted by endocrine glands when there is a need for them, that is, for their effects on their target organs. The cells of endocrine glands respond to changes in the blood, or perhaps to other hormones in the blood. These stimuli are the information they use to increase or decrease secretion of their own hormones. When a hormone brings about its effects, the stimulus is reversed, and secretion of the hormone decreases until the stimulus reoccurs. A specific example will be helpful here; let us use insulin.

Insulin is secreted by the pancreas when the blood glucose level is high, that is, hyperglycemia is the stimulus for secretion of insulin. Once circulating in the blood, insulin enables cells to remove glucose from the blood to use for energy production and enables the liver to store glucose as glycogen. As a result of these actions of insulin, the blood glucose level decreases, reversing the stimulus for secretion of insulin. Insulin secretion then decreases until the blood glucose level increases again.

This is an example of a **negative feedback mechanism**, in which information about the effects of the hormone is "fed back" to the gland, which then decreases its secretion of the hormone. This is why the mechanism is called "negative": The effects of the hormone reverse the stimulus and decrease the secretion of the hormone. The secretion of many other hormones is regulated in a similar way.

The hormones of the anterior pituitary gland are secreted in response to **releasing hormones** (also called releasing factors) secreted by the hypothalamus. You may recall this from Chapter 8. Growth hormone, for example, is secreted in response to growth hormone releasing hormone (GHRH) from the hypothalamus. As growth hormone exerts its effects, the secretion of GHRH decreases, which in turn decreases the secretion of growth hormone. This is another type of negative feedback mechanism.

For each of the hormones to be discussed in this chapter, the stimulus for its secretion will also be mentioned. Some hormones function as an **antagonistic pair** to regulate a particular aspect of blood chemistry; these mechanisms will also be covered.

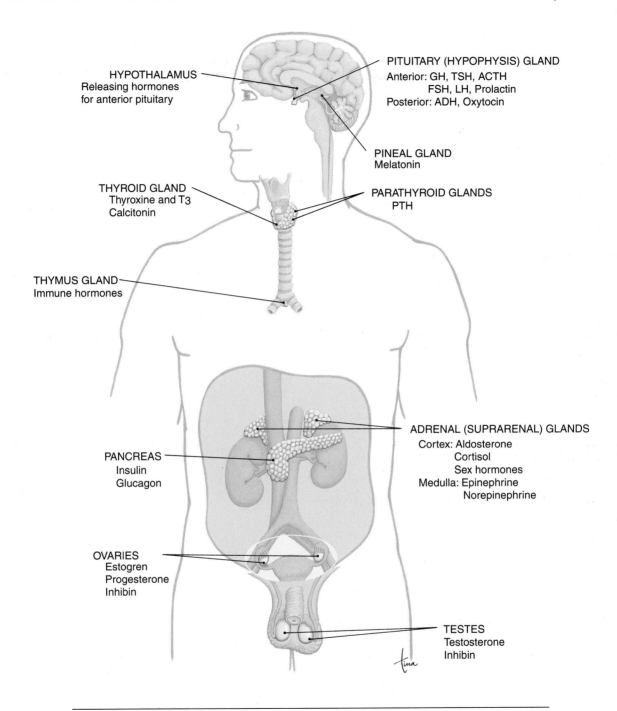

HYPOTHALAMUS
Releasing hormones
for anterior pituitary

PITUITARY (HYPOPHYSIS) GLAND
Anterior: GH, TSH, ACTH
FSH, LH, Prolactin
Posterior: ADH, Oxytocin

PINEAL GLAND
Melatonin

THYROID GLAND
Thyroxine and T3
Calcitonin

PARATHYROID GLANDS
PTH

THYMUS GLAND
Immune hormones

ADRENAL (SUPRARENAL) GLANDS
Cortex: Aldosterone
Cortisol
Sex hormones
Medulla: Epinephrine
Norepinephrine

PANCREAS
Insulin
Glucagon

OVARIES
Estogren
Progesterone
Inhibin

TESTES
Testosterone
Inhibin

Figure 10–1 The endocrine system. Locations of many endocrine glands. Both male and female gonads (testes and ovaries) are shown.

THE PITUITARY GLAND

The **pituitary gland** (or **hypophysis**) hangs by a short stalk (infundibulum) from the hypothalamus and is enclosed by the sella turcica of the sphenoid bone. Despite its small size, the pituitary gland regulates many body functions. Its two major portions are the posterior pituitary gland **(neurohypophysis)**, which is an extension of the nerve tissue of the hypothalamus, and the anterior pituitary gland **(adenohypophysis)**, which is separate glandular tissue.

POSTERIOR PITUITARY GLAND

The two hormones of the **posterior pituitary gland** are actually produced by the hypothalamus and simply stored in the posterior pituitary until needed. Their release is stimulated by nerve impulses from the hypothalamus (Fig. 10–2).

Antidiuretic Hormone

Antidiuretic hormone (ADH) increases the reabsorption of water by kidney tubules, which decreases the amount of urine formed. The water is reabsorbed into the blood, so as urinary output is decreased, blood volume is increased, which helps maintain normal blood pressure.

The stimulus for secretion of ADH is decreased water content of the body. If too much water is lost in sweating or diarrhea, for example, **osmoreceptors** in the hypothalamus detect the increased "saltiness" of body fluids. The hypothalamus then transmits impulses to the posterior pituitary to increase the secretion of ADH and decrease the loss of more water in urine.

Any type of dehydration stimulates the secretion of ADH to conserve body water. In the case of severe hemorrhage, ADH is released in large amounts and will also cause vasoconstriction, which will contribute to the maintenance of normal blood pressure.

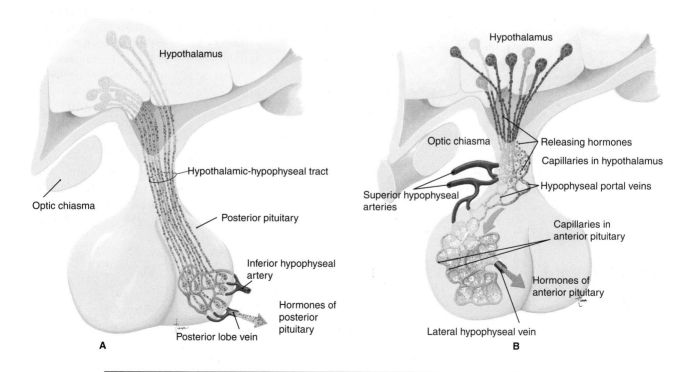

Figure 10–2 Structural relationships of hypothalamus and pituitary gland. **(A)** Posterior pituitary stores hormones produced in the hypothalamus. **(B)** Releasing hormones of the hypothalamus circulate directly to the anterior pituitary and influence its secretions. Notice the two networks of capillaries.

Ingestion of alcohol inhibits the secretion of ADH and increases urinary output. If alcohol intake is excessive and fluid is not replaced, a person will feel thirsty and dizzy the next morning. The thirst is due to the loss of body water, and the dizziness is the result of low blood pressure.

Oxytocin

Oxytocin stimulates contraction of the uterus at the end of pregnancy and stimulates release of milk from the mammary glands.

As labor begins, the cervix of the uterus is stretched, which generates sensory impulses to the hypothalamus, which in turn stimulates the posterior pituitary to release oxytocin. Oxytocin then causes strong contractions of the smooth muscle (myometrium) of the uterus to bring about delivery of the baby and the placenta. The secretion of oxytocin is one of the few positive feedback mechanisms within the body, and the external brake or shutoff of the feedback cycle is delivery of the baby.

It has been discovered that the placenta itself secretes oxytocin at the end of gestation and in an amount far higher than that from the posterior pituitary gland. Research is continuing to determine the exact mechanism and precise role of the placenta in labor.

When a baby is breast-fed, the sucking of the baby stimulates sensory impulses from the mother's nipple to the hypothalamus. Nerve impulses from the hypothalamus to the posterior pituitary cause the release of oxytocin, which stimulates contraction of the smooth muscle cells around the mammary ducts. This release of milk is sometimes called the "milk let-down" reflex. The hormones of the posterior pituitary are summarized in Table 10–1.

ANTERIOR PITUITARY GLAND

The hormones of the **anterior pituitary gland** regulate many body functions. They are in turn regulated by **releasing hormones** from the hypothalamus. These releasing hormones are secreted into capillaries in the hypothalamus and pass through the **hypophyseal portal** veins to another capillary network in the anterior pituitary gland. Here, the releasing hormones are absorbed and stimulate secretion of the anterior pituitary hormones. This small but specialized pathway of circulation is shown in Fig. 10–2. This pathway permits the releasing hormones to rapidly stimulate the anterior pituitary, without having to pass through general circulation.

Growth Hormone

Growth hormone (GH) may also be called **somatotropin**, and does indeed stimulate growth (see Fig. 10–3). GH increases the transport of amino acids into cells, and increases the rate of protein synthesis. Amino acids cannot be stored in the body, so when they are available, they must be used in protein synthesis. Excess amino acids are changed to carbohydrates or fat, for energy storage. Growth hormone ensures that amino acids will be used for whatever protein synthesis is necessary, before the amino acids can be changed to carbohydrates. Growth hormone also stimulates cell division in those tissues capable of mitosis. These functions contribute to the growth of the body during childhood, especially growth of bones and muscles.

You may now be wondering if GH is secreted in adults, and the answer is yes. The use of amino acids for the synthesis of proteins is still necessary, even if the body is not growing in height. GH also stimulates the release of fat from adipose tissue and the use of

Table 10–1	HORMONES OF THE POSTERIOR PITUITARY GLAND	
Hormone	**Function(s)**	**Regulation of Secretion**
Oxytocin	• Promotes contraction of myometrium of uterus (labor) • Promotes release of milk from mammary glands	Nerve impulses from hypothalamus, the result of stretching of cervix or stimulation of nipple. Secretion from placenta at end of gestation—stimulus unknown
Antidiuretic hormone (ADH)	• Increases water reabsorption by the kidney tubules (water returns to the blood)	Decreased water content in the body (alcohol inhibits secretion)

Figure 10–3   Functions of growth hormone.

fats for energy production. This is important any time we go for extended periods without eating, no matter what our ages.

The secretion of GH is regulated by two releasing hormones from the hypothalamus. Growth hormone releasing hormone (GHRH), which increases the secretion of GH, is produced during hypoglycemia and during exercise. Another stimulus for GHRH is a high blood level of amino acids; the GH then secreted will ensure the conversion of these amino acids into protein. **Somatostatin** may also be called growth hormone inhibiting hormone (GHIH), and as its name tells us, it decreases the secretion of GH. Somatostatin is produced during states of hyperglycemia. Disorders of GH secretion are discussed in Box 10–1.

Thyroid-Stimulating Hormone

Thyroid-stimulating hormone (TSH) may also be called thyrotropin, and its target organ is the thyroid gland. TSH stimulates the normal growth of the thyroid and the secretion of thyroxine (T_4) and triiodothyronine (T_3). The functions of these thyroid hormones will be covered later in this chapter.

The secretion of TSH is stimulated by thyrotropin releasing hormone (TRH) from the hypothalamus. When metabolic rate (energy production) decreases, TRH is produced.

Adrenocorticotropic Hormone

Adrenocorticotropic hormone (ACTH) stimulates the secretion of cortisol and other hormones by the

Box 10–1   DISORDERS OF GROWTH HORMONE

A deficiency or excess of growth hormone (GH) during childhood will have marked effects on the growth of a child. Hyposecretion of GH results in **pituitary dwarfism**, in which the person may attain a final height of only 3 to 4 feet but will have normal body proportions. GH can now be produced using genetic engineering and may be used to stimulate growth in children with this disorder. GH will not increase growth of children with the genetic potential for short stature. Reports that GH will reverse the effects of aging are simply not true.

Hypersecretion of GH results in **giantism**, in which the long bones grow excessively and the person may attain a height of 8 feet. Most very tall people, such as basketball players, do *not* have this condition; they are tall as a result of their genetic makeup and good nutrition.

In an adult, hypersecretion of GH is caused by a pituitary tumor, and results in **acromegaly**. The long bones cannot grow because the epiphyseal discs are closed, but the growth of other bones is stimulated. The jaw and other facial bones become disproportionally large, as do the bones of the hands and feet. The skin becomes thicker, and the tongue also grows and may protrude. Other consequences include compression of nerves by abnormally growing bones and growth of the articular cartilages, which then erode and bring on arthritis. Treatment of acromegaly requires surgical removal of the tumor or its destruction by radiation.

adrenal cortex. Secretion of ACTH is increased by corticotropin releasing hormone (CRH) from the hypothalamus. CRH is produced in any type of physiological stress situation such as injury, disease, exercise, or hypoglycemia (being hungry is stressful).

Prolactin

Prolactin, as its name suggests, is responsible for lactation. More precisely, prolactin initiates and maintains milk production by the mammary glands. The regulation of secretion of prolactin is complex, involving both prolactin releasing hormone (PRH) and prolactin inhibiting hormone (PIH) from the hypothalamus. The mammary glands must first be acted upon by other hormones such as estrogen and progesterone, which are secreted in large amounts by the placenta during pregnancy. Then, after delivery of the baby, prolactin secretion increases and milk is produced. If the mother continues to breast-feed, prolactin levels remain high.

Follicle-Stimulating Hormone

Follicle-stimulating hormone (FSH) is one of the gonadotropic hormones, that is, it has its effects on the gonads: the ovaries or testes. FSH is named for one of its functions in women. Within the ovaries are ovarian follicles that contain potential ova (egg cells). FSH stimulates the growth of ovarian follicles, that is, it initiates egg development in cycles of approximately 28 days. FSH also stimulates secretion of estrogen by the follicle cells. In men, FSH initiates sperm production within the testes.

The secretion of FSH is stimulated by the hypothalamus, which produces **gonadotropin releasing hormone (GnRH)**. FSH secretion is decreased by inhibin, a hormone produced by the ovaries or testes.

Luteinizing Hormone

Luteinizing hormone (LH) is another gonadotropic hormone. In women, LH is responsible for ovulation, the release of a mature ovum from an ovarian follicle. LH then stimulates that follicle to develop into the corpus luteum, which secretes progesterone, also under the influence of LH. In men, LH stimulates the interstitial cells of the testes to secrete testosterone. (LH is also called ICSH, interstitial cell stimulating hormone.)

Secretion of LH is also regulated by GnRH from the hypothalamus. We will return to FSH and LH, as well as to the sex hormones, in Chapter 20.

All of the target organs of the pituitary gland are shown in Fig. 10–4. The hormones of the anterior pituitary are summarized in Table 10–2.

THYROID GLAND

The **thyroid gland** is located on the front and sides of the trachea just below the larynx. Its two lobes are connected by a middle piece called the isthmus. The

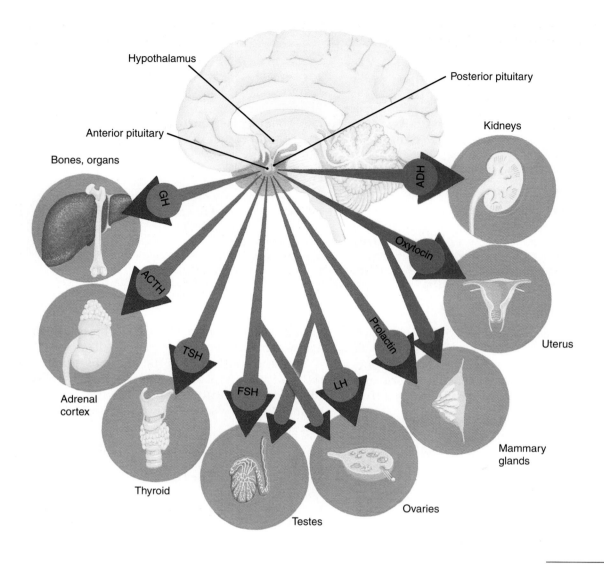

Hypothalamus

Posterior pituitary

Anterior pituitary

Kidneys

Bones, organs

ADH

GH

Oxytocin

ACTH

TSH

Prolactin

FSH

LH

Uterus

Adrenal
cortex

Mammary
glands

Thyroid

Testes

Ovaries

Anterior pituitary hormones

Posterior pituitary hormones

Figure 10–4 Hormones of the pituitary gland and their target organs.

structural units of the thyroid gland are thyroid folli-cles, which produce **thyroxine (T_4)** and **triiodothy-ronine (T_3)**. Iodine is necessary for the synthesis of these hormones; thyroxine contains four atoms of iodine, and T_3 contains three atoms of iodine.

The third hormone produced by the thyroid gland is **calcitonin**, which is secreted by parafollicular cells. Its function is very different from those of thyroxine and T_3, which you may recall from Chapter 6.

THYROXINE AND T_3

Thyroxine (T_4) and T_3 have the same functions: regu-lation of energy production and protein synthesis, which contribute to growth of the body and to normal body functioning throughout life (see Fig. 10–5). Thyroxine and T_3 increase cell respiration of all food types (carbohydrates, fats, and excess amino acids) and thereby increase energy and heat production.

Table 10–2	HORMONES OF THE ANTERIOR PITUITARY GLAND	

Hormone	Function(s)	Regulation of Secretion
Growth hormone (GH)	• Increases rate of mitosis • Increases amino acid transport into cells • Increases rate of protein synthesis • Increases use of fats for energy	• GHRH (hypothalamus) stimulates secretion • GHIH—somatostatin (hypothalamus) inhibits secretion
Thyroid-stimulating hormone (TSH)	• Increases secretion of thyroxine and T_3 by thyroid gland	• TRH (hypothalamus)
Adrenocorticotropic hormone (ACTH)	• Increases secretion of cortisol by the adrenal cortex	• CRH (hypothalamus)
Prolactin	• Stimulates milk production by the mammary glands	• PRH (hypothalamus) stimulates secretion • PIH (hypothalamus) inhibits secretion
Follicle-stimulating hormone (FSH)	*In women:* • Initiates growth of ova in ovarian follicles • Increases secretion of estrogen by follicle cells *In men:* • Initiates sperm production in the testes	• GnRH (hypothalamus) stimulates secretion • Inhibin (ovaries or testes) inhibits secretion
Luteinizing hormone (LH) (ICSH)	*In women:* • Causes ovulation • Causes the ruptured ovarian follicle to become the corpus luteum • Increases secretion of progesterone by the corpus luteum *In men:* • Increases secretion of testosterone by the interstitial cells of the testes	• GnRH (hypothalamus)

They also increase the rate of protein synthesis within cells. Normal production of thyroxine and T_3 is essential for physical growth, normal mental development, and maturation of the reproductive system. These hormones are the most important day-to-day regulators of metabolic rate; their activity is reflected in the functioning of the brain, muscles, heart, and virtually all other organs. Although thyroxine and T_3 are not vital hormones, in that they are not crucial to survival, their absence greatly diminishes physical and mental growth and abilities (see Box 10–2: Disorders of Thyroxine).

Secretion of thyroxine and T_3 is stimulated by **thyroid-stimulating hormone (TSH)** from the anterior pituitary gland. When metabolic rate (energy production) decreases, this change is detected by the hypothalamus, which secretes thyrotropin releasing hormone (TRH). TRH stimulates the anterior pituitary to secrete TSH, which stimulates the thyroid to release thyroxine and T_3, which raise the metabolic rate by increasing energy production. This negative feedback mechanism then shuts off TRH from the hypothalamus until the metabolic rate decreases again.

CALCITONIN

Calcitonin decreases the reabsorption of calcium and phosphate from the bones to the blood, thereby lowering blood levels of these minerals. This function of calcitonin helps maintain normal blood levels of calcium and phosphate and also helps maintain a stable, strong bone matrix. It is believed that calcitonin exerts its most important effects during childhood, when bones are growing. A form of calcitonin obtained from salmon is used to help treat osteoporosis.

The stimulus for secretion of calcitonin is **hypercalcemia**, that is, a high blood calcium level. When blood calcium is high, calcitonin ensures that no more will be removed from bones until there is a real need

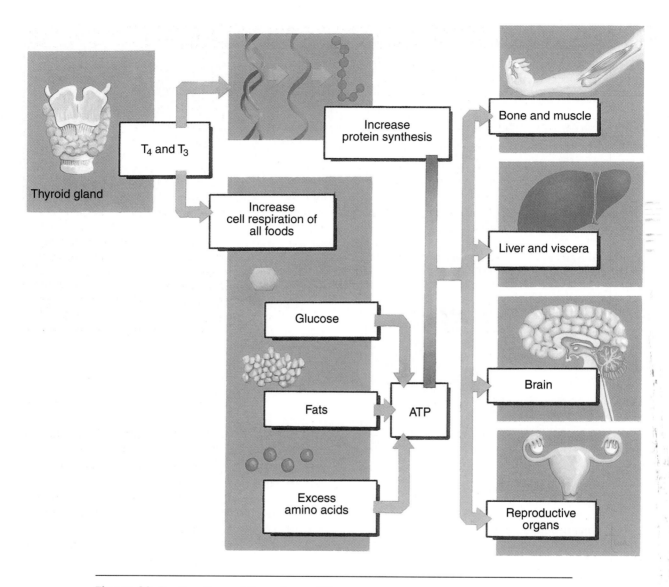

Figure 10–5   Functions of thyroxine and T_3.

for more calcium in the blood (Fig. 10–6). The hormones of the thyroid gland are summarized in Table 10–3.

PARATHYROID GLANDS

There are four **parathyroid glands**: two on the back of each lobe of the thyroid gland (see Fig. 10–7). The hormone they produce is called parathyroid hormone.

PARATHYROID HORMONE

Parathyroid hormone (PTH) is an antagonist to calcitonin and is important for the maintenance of normal blood levels of calcium and phosphate. The target organs of PTH are the bones, small intestine, and kidneys.

PTH increases the reabsorption of calcium and phosphate from bones to the blood, thereby raising their blood levels. Absorption of calcium and phosphate from food in the small intestine, which also

Box 10–2   DISORDERS OF THYROXINE

Iodine is an essential component of thyroxine (and T_3), and a dietary deficiency of iodine causes **goiter**. In an attempt to produce more thyroxine, the thyroid cells become enlarged, and the thyroid gland becomes apparent on the front of the neck. The use of iodized salt has made goiter a rare condition.

Hyposecretion of thyroxine in a newborn has devastating effects on the growth of the child. Without thyroxine, physical growth is diminished, as is mental development. This condition is called **cretinism**, characterized by severe physical and mental retardation. If the thyroxine deficiency is detected shortly after birth, the child may be treated with thyroid hormones to promote normal development.

Hyposecretion of thyroxine in an adult is called **myxedema**. Without thyroxine, the metabolic rate (energy production) decreases, resulting in lethargy, muscular weakness, slow heart rate, a feeling of cold, weight gain, and a characteristic puffiness of the face. The administration of thyroid hormones will return the metabolic rate to normal.

Graves' disease is a hypersecretion of thyroxine that is believed to be an immune disorder. The autoantibodies seem to bind to TSH receptors on the thyroid cells and stimulate secretion of excess thyroxine. The symptoms are those that would be expected when the metabolic rate is abnormally elevated: weight loss accompanied by increased appetite, increased sweating, fast heart rate, feeling of warmth, and fatigue. Also present may be goiter and exophthalmos, which is protrusion of the eyes. Treatment is aimed at decreasing the secretion of thyroxine by the thyroid, and medications or radioactive iodine may be used to accomplish this.

---

requires vitamin D, is increased by PTH. This too raises the blood levels of these minerals. In the kidneys, PTH stimulates the activation of vitamin D and increases the reabsorption of calcium and the excretion of phosphate (more than is obtained from bones). Therefore, the overall effect of PTH is to raise the blood calcium level and lower the blood phosphate level. The functions of PTH are summarized in Table 10–4).

Secretion of PTH is stimulated by **hypocalcemia**, a low blood calcium level, and inhibited by hypercalcemia. The antagonistic effects of PTH and calcitonin are shown in Fig. 10–6. Together, these hormones maintain blood calcium within a normal range. Calcium in the blood is essential for the process of blood clotting and for normal activity of neurons and muscle cells.

As you might expect, a sustained hypersecretion of PTH, such as is caused by a parathyroid tumor, would remove calcium from bones and weaken them. It has been found, however, that an intermittent, brief excess of PTH, such as can occur by injection, will stimulate the formation of more bone matrix, rather than matrix reabsorption. This may seem very strange, the opposite of what we would expect, but it shows how much we have yet to learn about the body. PTH is being investigated as a possible way to help prevent osteoporosis.

PANCREAS

The **pancreas** is located in the upper left quadrant of the abdominal cavity, extending from the curve of the duodenum to the spleen. Although the pancreas is both an exocrine (digestive) gland as well as an endocrine gland, only its endocrine function will be discussed here. The hormone-producing cells of the pancreas are called **islets of Langerhans** (pancreatic islets; see Fig. 16-7); they contain **alpha cells** that produce glucagon and **beta cells** that produce insulin.

GLUCAGON

Glucagon stimulates the liver to change glycogen to glucose (this process is called **glycogenolysis**, which literally means "glycogen breakdown") and to increase the use of fats and excess amino acids for energy production. The process of **gluconeogenesis** (literally, "making new glucose") is the conversion of excess amino acids into simple carbohydrates that may enter the reactions of cell respiration. The overall effect of glucagon, therefore, is to raise the blood glucose level and to make all types of food available for energy production.

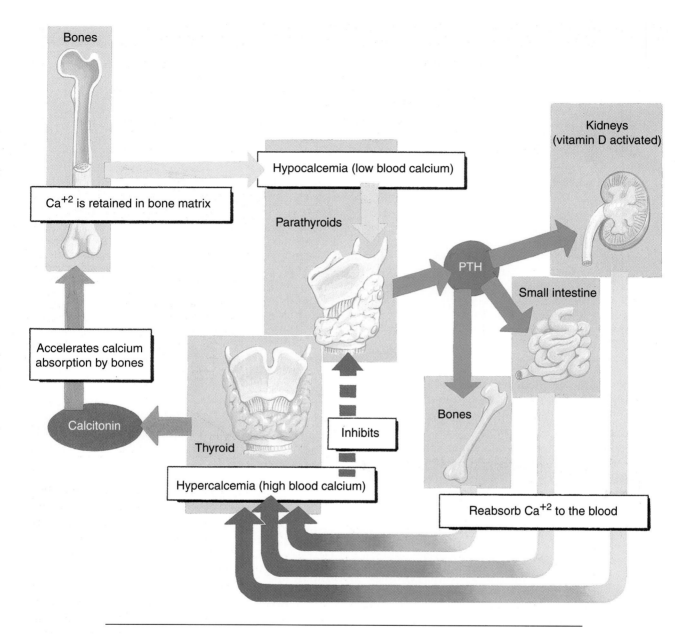

Bones

Hypocalcemia (low blood calcium)

Ca^{+2} is retained in bone matrix

Parathyroids

Kidneys (vitamin D activated)

PTH

Small intestine

Accelerates calcium absorption by bones

Calcitonin

Thyroid

Inhibits

Bones

Hypercalcemia (high blood calcium)

Reabsorb Ca^{+2} to the blood

Figure 10–6   Calcitonin and parathyroid hormone (PTH) and their functions related to the maintenance of the blood calcium level.

The secretion of glucagon is stimulated by **hypoglycemia**, a low blood glucose level. Such a state may occur between meals or during physiological stress situations such as exercise (Fig. 10–8).

INSULIN

Insulin increases the transport of glucose from the blood into cells by increasing the permeability of cell membranes to glucose. (Brain, liver, and kidney cells, however, are not dependent on insulin for glucose intake.) Once inside cells, glucose is used in cell respiration to produce energy. The liver and skeletal muscles also change glucose to glycogen (**glycogenesis**, which literally means "glycogen production") to be stored for later use. Insulin also enables cells to take in fatty acids and amino acids to use in the synthesis of lipids and proteins (*not* energy production).

Table 10–3	HORMONES OF THE THYROID GLAND	
Hormone	**Function(s)**	**Regulation of Secretion**
Thyroxine (T_4) and triiodothyronine (T_3)	• Increase energy production from all food types • Increase rate of protein synthesis	TSH (anterior pituitary)
Calcitonin	• Decreases the reabsorption of calcium and phosphate from bones to blood	Hypercalcemia

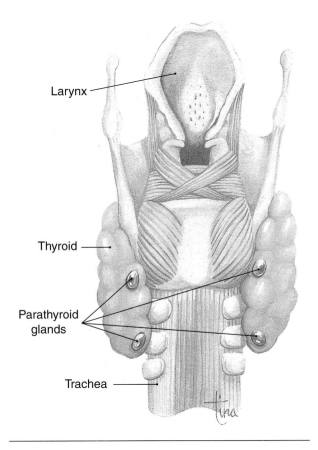

Figure 10–7 Parathyroid glands in posterior view, on lobes of the thyroid gland.

Table 10–4	HORMONE OF THE PARATHYROID GLANDS	
Hormone	**Functions**	**Regulation of Secretion**
Parathyroid hormone (PTH)	• Increases the reabsorption of calcium and phosphate from bone to blood • Increases absorption of calcium and phosphate by the small intestine • Increases the reabsorption of calcium and the excretion of phosphate by the kidneys; activates vitamin D	Hypocalcemia stimulates secretion. Hypercalcemia inhibits secretion.

With respect to blood glucose, insulin decreases its level by promoting the use of glucose for energy production. The antagonistic functions of insulin and glucagon are shown in Fig. 10–8.

Insulin is a vital hormone; we cannot survive for very long without it. A deficiency of insulin or in its functioning is called **diabetes mellitus**, which is discussed in Box 10–3: Diabetes Mellitus.

Secretion of insulin is stimulated by **hyperglycemia**, a high blood glucose level. This state occurs after eating, especially of meals high in carbohydrates. As glucose is absorbed from the small intestine into the blood, insulin is secreted to enable cells to use the glucose for immediate energy. At the same time, any excess glucose will be stored in the liver and muscles as glycogen.

You will also notice in Fig. 16-7 the cells called delta cells. These produce the hormone somatostatin, which is identical to growth hormone inhibiting hormone from the hypothalamus. Pancreatic somatostatin acts locally to inhibit the secretion of insulin and glucagon, and it seems to slow the absorption of the end products of digestion in the small intestine. The hormones of the pancreas are summarized in Table 10–5.

ADRENAL GLANDS

The two **adrenal glands** are located one on top of each kidney, which gives them their other name of **suprarenal glands**. Each adrenal gland consists of

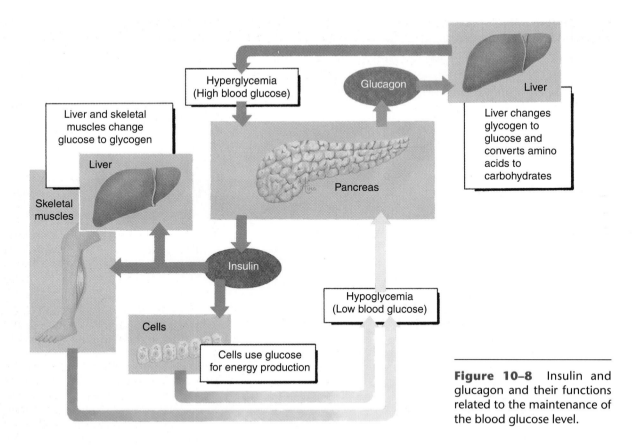

Figure 10–8 Insulin and glucagon and their functions related to the maintenance of the blood glucose level.

two parts: an inner adrenal medulla and an outer adrenal cortex. The hormones produced by each part have very different functions.

ADRENAL MEDULLA

The cells of the **adrenal medulla** secrete epinephrine and norepinephrine, which collectively are called **catecholamines**, and are **sympathomimetic**. The secretion of both hormones is stimulated by sympathetic impulses from the hypothalamus, and their functions duplicate and prolong those of the sympathetic division of the autonomic nervous system (*mimetic* means "to mimic").

Epinephrine and Norepinephrine

Epinephrine (adrenalin) and norepinephrine (noradrenalin) are both secreted in stress situations and help prepare the body for "fight or flight." **Norepinephrine** is secreted in small amounts, and its most

significant function is to cause vasoconstriction in the skin, viscera, and skeletal muscles (that is, throughout the body), which raises blood pressure.

Epinephrine, secreted in larger amounts, increases heart rate and force of contraction and stimulates vasoconstriction in skin and viscera and vasodilation in skeletal muscles. It also dilates the bronchioles, decreases peristalsis, stimulates the liver to change glycogen to glucose, increases the use of fats for energy, and increases the rate of cell respiration. Many of these effects do indeed seem to be an echo of sympathetic responses, don't they? Responding to stress is so important that the body is redundant (it repeats itself) and has both a nervous mechanism and a hormonal mechanism. Epinephrine is actually more effective than sympathetic stimulation, however, because the hormone increases energy production and cardiac output to a greater extent. The hormones of the adrenal medulla are summarized in Table 10–6, and their functions are shown in Fig. 10–9.

Box 10–3   DIABETES MELLITUS

There are two types of **diabetes mellitus**: Type 1 is called insulin-dependent diabetes and its onset is usually in childhood (juvenile onset). Type 2 is called non–insulin-dependent diabetes, and its onset is usually later in life (maturity onset).

Type 1 diabetes is characterized by destruction of the beta cells of the islets of Langerhans and a complete lack of insulin (see below). Destruction of the beta cells is believed to be an autoimmune response, perhaps triggered by a virus; onset of diabetes is usually abrupt. This form of diabetes occurs most often in children, and there may be a genetic predisposition for it (certain HLA types are found more frequently in juvenile-onset diabetics than in other children—see Box 11–5: White Blood Cell Types: HLA). Insulin by injection is essential to control this form of diabetes. Recently, however, an immunosuppressant medication (usually used to prevent rejection of transplanted organs) has been found to slow or stop the progression of type 1 diabetes if given as the disease is developing. By blocking the autoimmune response, this drug seems to permit the survival of some beta cells, which will continue to produce insulin.

In **type 2** diabetes, insulin is produced but cannot exert its effects on cells because of a deficiency of insulin receptors on cell membranes (see below). Onset of type 2 diabetes is usually gradual, and risk factors include a family history of diabetes and being over-weight. Control may not require insulin, but rather medications that enable insulin to react with the remaining cell membrane receptors. Some newer medications seem to stimulate the same reactions that insulin does. For those with a family history of diabetes, a low-fat diet and regular exercise greatly reduce the risk of development of the disease.

The commitment to exercise must be lifelong but is well worth the effort, because diabetes is a very destructive disease.

Without insulin (or its effects) blood glucose level remains high, and glucose is lost in urine. Since more water is lost as well, symptoms include greater urinary output (polyuria) and thirst (polydipsia).

The long-term effects of hyperglycemia produce distinctive vascular changes. The capillary walls thicken, and exchange of gases and nutrients diminishes. The most damaging effects are seen in the skin (especially of the feet), the retina, and the kidneys. Poorly controlled diabetes may lead to dry gangrene, blindness, and severe kidney damage. In non–insulin-dependent diabetics, atherosclerosis is quite common. It is now possible for diabetics to prevent much of this tissue damage by precise monitoring of blood glucose level and more frequent administration of insulin. The new insulin pumps are able to more closely mimic the natural secretion of insulin.

A very serious potential problem for the insulin-dependent diabetic is **ketoacidosis**. When glucose cannot be used for energy, the body turns to fats and proteins, which are converted by the liver to ketones. Ketones are organic acids (acetone, acetoacetic acid) that can be used in cell respiration, but cells are not able to utilize them rapidly so ketones accumulate in the blood. Since ketones are acids, they lower the pH of the blood as they accumulate. The kidneys excrete excess ketones, but in doing so excrete more water as well, which leads to dehydration and worsens the acidosis. Without administration of insulin to permit the use of glucose for energy, and IV fluids to restore blood volume to normal, ketoacidosis will progress to coma and death.

A Normal   **B** Type 1   **C** Type 2

Box Figure 10–A   **(A)** Cell membrane in normal state, with insulin receptors and insulin to regulate glucose intake. **(B)** Cell membrane in type 1 diabetes: Insulin not present, glucose remains outside cell. **(C)** Cell membrane in type 2 diabetes: without insulin receptors, glucose remains outside cell.

Table 10–5 | HORMONES OF THE PANCREAS

Hormone	Functions	Regulation of Secretion
Glucagon (alpha cells)	• Increases conversion of glycogen to glucose in the liver • Increases the use of excess amino acids and of fats for energy	Hypoglycemia
Insulin (beta cells)	• Increases glucose transport into cells and the use of glucose for energy production • Increases the conversion of excess glucose to glycogen in the liver and muscles • Increases amino acid and fatty acid transport into cells, and their use in synthesis reactions	Hyperglycemia
Somatostatin (delta cells)	• Decreases secretion of insulin and glucagon • Slows absorption of nutrients	Rising levels of insulin and glucagon

ADRENAL CORTEX

The **adrenal cortex** secretes three types of steroid hormones: mineralocorticoids, glucocorticoids, and sex hormones. The sex hormones, "female" estrogens and "male" androgens (similar to testosterone), are produced in very small amounts, and their importance is not known with certainty. They may contribute to rapid body growth during early puberty. They may also be important to supply estrogen to women after menopause, and to men throughout life (see section on Estrogen, later in this chapter).

The functions of the other adrenal cortical hormones are well known, however, and these are considered vital hormones.

Aldosterone

Aldosterone is the most abundant of the **mineralocorticoids**, and we will use it as a representative of this group of hormones. The target organs of aldosterone are the kidneys, but there are important secondary effects as well. Aldosterone increases the reabsorption of sodium and the excretion of potassium by the kidney tubules. Sodium ions (Na^+) are returned to the blood, and potassium ions (K^+) are excreted in urine.

As Na^+ ions are reabsorbed, hydrogen ions (H^+) may be excreted in exchange. This is one mechanism to prevent the accumulation of excess H^+ ions that would cause acidosis of body fluids. Also, as Na^+ ions are reabsorbed, negative ions such as chloride (Cl^-) and bicarbonate (HCO_3^-) follow the Na^+ ions back to the blood, and water follows by osmosis. This indirect effect of aldosterone, the reabsorption of water by the kidneys, is very important to maintain normal blood volume and blood pressure. In summary, then, aldosterone maintains normal blood levels of sodium and potassium, and contributes to the maintenance of normal blood pH, blood volume, and blood pressure.

A number of factors stimulate the secretion of aldosterone. These are a deficiency of sodium, loss of blood or dehydration that lowers blood pressure, or an elevated blood level of potassium. Low blood

Table 10–6 | HORMONES OF THE ADRENAL MEDULLA

Hormone	Function(s)	Regulation of Secretion
Norepinephrine	• Causes vasoconstriction in skin, viscera, and skeletal muscles	
Epinephrine	• Increases heart rate and force of contraction • Dilates bronchioles • Decreases peristalsis • Increases conversion of glycogen to glucose in the liver • Causes vasodilation in skeletal muscles • Causes vasoconstriction in skin and viscera • Increases use of fats for energy • Increases the rate of cell respiration	Sympathetic impulses from the hypothalamus in stress situations

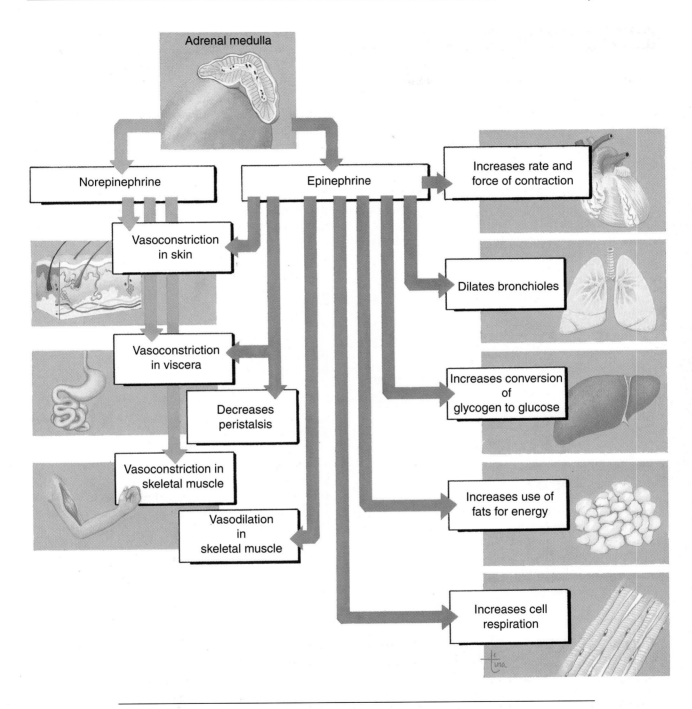

Figure 10–9   Functions of epinephrine and norepinephrine.

pressure or blood volume activates the **renin-angiotensin mechanism** of the kidneys. This mechanism is discussed in Chapters 13 and 18, so we will say for now that the process culminates in the formation of a chemical called **angiotensin II**. Angiotensin II causes vasoconstriction and stimulates the secretion of aldosterone by the adrenal cortex. Aldosterone then increases sodium and water retention by the kidneys to help restore blood volume and blood pressure to normal.

Cortisol

We will use **cortisol** as a representative of the group of hormones called **glucocorticoids**, since it is responsible for most of the actions of this group (see Fig. 10–10). Cortisol increases the use of fats and excess amino acids (gluconeogenesis) for energy, and decreases the use of glucose. This is called the *glucose-sparing effect,* and it is important because it conserves glucose for use by the brain. Cortisol is secreted in any type of physiological stress situation: disease, physical injury, hemorrhage, fear or anger, exercise, and hunger. Although most body cells easily use fatty acids and excess amino acids in cell respiration, brain cells do not and must have glucose. By enabling other cells to use the alternative energy sources, cortisol ensures that whatever glucose is present will be available to the brain.

Cortisol also has an **anti-inflammatory effect**. During inflammation, **histamine** from damaged tissues makes capillaries more permeable, and the lysosomes of damaged cells release their enzymes, which help break down damaged tissue but may also cause destruction of nearby healthy tissue. Cortisol blocks the effects of histamine and stabilizes lysosomal membranes, preventing excessive tissue destruction. Inflammation is a beneficial process up to a point, and is an essential first step if tissue repair is to take

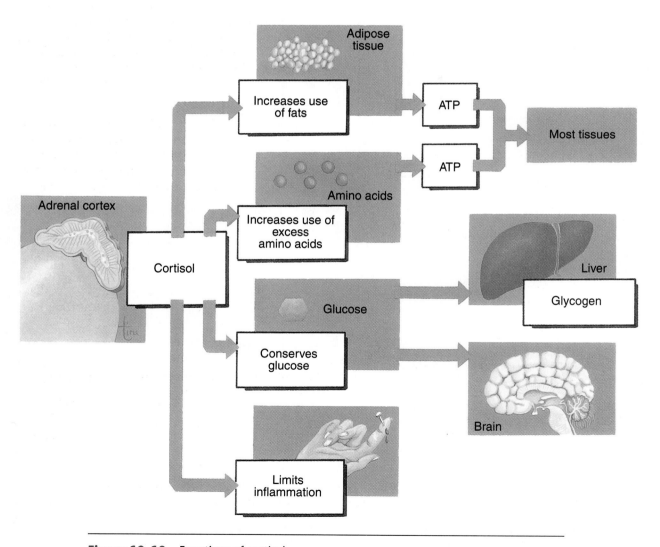

Figure 10–10 Functions of cortisol.

Box 10–4   DISORDERS OF THE ADRENAL CORTEX

Addison's disease is the result of hyposecretion of the adrenal cortical hormones. Most cases are idiopathic, that is, of unknown cause; atrophy of the adrenal cortex decreases both cortisol and aldosterone secretion.

Deficiency of cortisol is characterized by hypoglycemia, decreased gluconeogenesis, and depletion of glycogen in the liver. Consequences are muscle weakness and the inability to resist physiological stress. Aldosterone deficiency leads to retention of potassium and excretion of sodium and water in urine. The result is severe dehydration, low blood volume, and low blood pressure. Without treatment, circulatory shock and death will follow. Treatment involves administration of hydrocortisone; in high doses this will also compensate for the aldosterone deficiency.

Cushing's syndrome is the result of hypersecretion of the adrenal cortex, primarily cortisol.

The cause may be a pituitary tumor that increases ACTH secretion or a tumor of the adrenal cortex itself.

Excessive cortisol promotes fat deposition in the trunk of the body, while the extremities remain thin. The skin becomes thin and fragile, and healing after injury is slow. The bones also become fragile because osteoporosis is accelerated. Also characteristic of this syndrome is the rounded appearance of the face. Treatment is aimed at removal of the cause of the hypersecretion, whether it be a pituitary or adrenal tumor.

Cushing's syndrome may also be seen in people who receive corticosteroids for medical reasons. Transplant recipients or people with rheumatoid arthritis of severe asthma who must take corticosteroids may exhibit any of the above symptoms. In such cases, the disadvantages of this medication must be weighed against the benefits provided.

place. It may, however, become a vicious cycle of damage, inflammation, more damage, more inflammation, and so on. Normal cortisol secretion seems to limit the inflammation process to what is useful for tissue repair, and to prevent excessive tissue destruction. Too much cortisol, however, decreases the immune response, leaving the body susceptible to infection and significantly slowing the healing of damaged tissue (see Box 10–4: Disorders of the Adrenal Cortex).

The direct stimulus for cortisol secretion is **ACTH** from the anterior pituitary gland, which in turn is stimulated by corticotropin releasing hormone (CRH) from the hypothalamus. CRH is produced in the physiological stress situations mentioned above. Although we often think of epinephrine as a hormone important in stress, cortisol is also important. The hormones of the adrenal cortex are summarized in Table 10–7.

OVARIES

The **ovaries** are located in the pelvic cavity, one on each side of the uterus. The hormones produced by

Table 10–7   HORMONES OF THE ADRENAL CORTEX

Hormone	Functions	Regulation of Secretion
Aldosterone	• Increases reabsorption of Na$^+$ ions by the kidneys to the blood • Increases excretion of K$^+$ ions by the kidneys in urine	• Low blood Na$^+$ level • Low blood volume or blood pressure • High blood K$^+$ level
Cortisol	• Increases use of fats and excess amino acids for energy • Decreases use of glucose for energy (except for the brain) • Increases conversion of glucose to glycogen in the liver • Anti-inflammatory effect: stabilizes lysosomes and blocks the effects of histamine	• ACTH (anterior pituitary) during physiological stress

the ovaries are the steroids estrogen and progesterone, and the protein inhibin. Although their functions are an integral part of Chapters 20 and 21, we will briefly discuss some of them here.

ESTROGEN

Estrogen is secreted by the follicle cells of the ovary; secretion is stimulated by **FSH** from the anterior pituitary gland. Estrogen promotes the maturation of the ovum in the ovarian follicle and stimulates the growth of blood vessels in the endometrium (lining) of the uterus in preparation for a possible fertilized egg.

The **secondary sex characteristics** in women also develop in response to estrogen. These include growth of the duct system of the mammary glands, growth of the uterus, and the deposition of fat subcutaneously in the hips and thighs. The closure of the epiphyseal discs in long bones is brought about by estrogen, and growth in height stops. Estrogen is also believed to lower blood levels of cholesterol and triglycerides. For women before the age of menopause this is beneficial in that it decreases the risk of atherosclerosis and coronary artery disease.

Research suggests that estrogen no longer be considered only a "female" hormone. Estrogen seems to have effects on many organs, including the brain, the heart, and blood vessels. In the brain, testosterone from the testes or the adrenal cortex can be converted to estrogen, which may be important for memory, especially for older people. Estrogen seems to have non-reproductive functions in both men and women, though we cannot yet be as specific as we can be with the reproductive functions in women, mentioned previously.

PROGESTERONE

When a mature ovarian follicle releases an ovum, the follicle becomes the **corpus luteum** and begins to secrete **progesterone** in addition to estrogen. This is stimulated by **LH** from the anterior pituitary gland.

Progesterone promotes the storage of glycogen and the further growth of blood vessels in the endometrium, which thus becomes a potential placenta. The secretory cells of the mammary glands also develop under the influence of progesterone.

Both progesterone and estrogen are secreted by the placenta during pregnancy; these functions are covered in Chapter 21.

INHIBIN

The corpus luteum secretes another hormone, called **inhibin**. Inhibin helps decrease the secretion of FSH by the anterior pituitary gland, and GnRH by the hypothalamus.

TESTES

The **testes** are located in the scrotum, a sac of skin between the upper thighs. Two hormones, testosterone and inhibin, are secreted by the testes.

TESTOSTERONE

Testosterone is a steroid hormone secreted by the interstitial cells of the testes; the stimulus for secretion is LH from the anterior pituitary gland.

Testosterone promotes maturation of sperm in the seminiferous tubules of the testes; this process begins at puberty and continues throughout life. At puberty, testosterone stimulates development of the male **secondary sex characteristics**. These include growth of all the reproductive organs, growth of facial and body hair, growth of the larynx and deepening of the voice, and growth (protein synthesis) of the skeletal muscles. Testosterone also brings about closure of the epiphyses of the long bones.

INHIBIN

The hormone **inhibin** is secreted by the sustentacular cells of the testes; the stimulus for secretion is increased testosterone. The function of inhibin is to decrease the secretion of FSH by the anterior pituitary gland. The interaction of inhibin, testosterone, and the anterior pituitary hormones maintains spermatogenesis at a constant rate.

OTHER HORMONES

Melatonin is a hormone produced by the **pineal gland**, which is located at the back of the third ventricle of the brain. The secretion of melatonin is greatest during darkness and decreases when light enters the eye and the retina signals the hypothalamus. A recent discovery is that the retina also produces melatonin, which seems to indicate that the eyes and pineal gland work with the biological clock of the hypothalamus. In other mammals, melatonin helps regulate seasonal reproductive cycles. For people, melatonin definitely stimulates the onset of sleep and increases its duration. Other claims, such as that melatonin strengthens the immune system or prevents cellular damage and aging, are simply without evidence as yet.

There are other organs that produce hormones that have only one or a few target organs. For example, the stomach and duodenum produce hormones that regulate aspects of digestion. The thymus gland produces hormones necessary for the normal functioning of the immune system, and the kidneys produce a hormone that stimulates red blood cell production. All of these will be discussed in later chapters.

PROSTAGLANDINS

Prostaglandins (PG) are made by virtually all cells from the phospholipids of their cell membranes. They differ from other hormones in that they do not circulate in the blood to target organs, but rather exert their effects locally, where they are produced.

There are many types of prostaglandins, designated by the letters A–I, as in PGA, PGB, and so on. The functions of prostaglandins are also many, and we will list only a few of them here. Prostaglandins are known to be involved in inflammation, pain mechanisms, blood clotting, vasoconstriction and vasodilation, contraction of the uterus, reproduction, secretion of digestive glands, and nutrient metabolism. Current research is directed at determining the normal functioning of prostaglandins in the hope that many of them may eventually be used clinically.

One familiar example may illustrate the widespread activity of prostaglandins. For minor pain such as a headache, many people take aspirin. Aspirin inhibits the synthesis of prostaglandins involved in pain mechanisms, and usually relieves the pain. Some people, however, such as those with rheumatoid arthritis, may take large amounts of aspirin to diminish pain and inflammation. These people may bruise easily because blood clotting has been impaired. This too is an effect of aspirin, which blocks the synthesis of prostaglandins necessary for blood clotting.

MECHANISMS OF HORMONE ACTION

Exactly how hormones exert their effects on their target organs involves a number of complex processes, which will be presented simply here.

A hormone must first bond to a **receptor** for it on or in the target cell. Cells respond to certain hormones and not to others because of the presence of specific receptors, which are proteins. These receptor proteins may be part of the cell membrane or within the cytoplasm or nucleus of the target cells. A hormone will affect only those cells that have its specific receptors. Liver cells, for example, have cell membrane receptors for insulin, glucagon, growth hormone, and epinephrine; bone cells have receptors for growth hormone, PTH, and calcitonin. Cells of the ovaries and testes do not have receptors for PTH and calcitonin, but do have receptors for FSH and LH, which bone cells and liver cells do not have. Once a hormone has bonded to a receptor on or in its target cell, other reactions will take place.

THE TWO-MESSENGER THEORY—PROTEIN HORMONES

The Two-Messenger Theory of hormone action involves "messengers" that make something happen, that is, stimulate specific reactions. **Protein hormones** usually bond to receptors of the cell membrane, and the hormone is called the first messenger. The hormone–receptor bonding activates the enzyme adenyl cyclase on the inner surface of the cell membrane. Adenyl cyclase synthesizes a substance called cyclic adenosine monophosphate **(cyclic AMP)** from ATP, and cyclic AMP is the second messenger.

Cyclic AMP activates specific enzymes within the cell, which bring about the cell's characteristic response to the hormone. These responses include a change in the permeability of the cell membrane to a specific substance, an increase in protein synthesis, activation of other enzymes, or the secretion of a cellular product.

In summary, a cell's response to a hormone is determined by the enzymes within the cell, that is, the reactions of which the cell is capable. These reactions are brought about by the first messenger, the hormone, which stimulates the formation of the second messenger, cyclic AMP. Cyclic AMP then acti-

Figure 10–11 Mechanisms of hormone action. **(A)** Two-Messenger model of the action of protein hormones. **(B)** Action of steroid hormones. See text for description.

vates the cell's enzymes to elicit a response to the hormone (Fig. 10–11).

ACTION OF STEROID HORMONES

Steroid hormones are soluble in the lipids of the cell membrane, and diffuse easily into a target cell. Once inside the cell, the steroid hormone combines with a protein receptor in the cytoplasm, and this steroid-protein complex enters the nucleus of the cell. Within the nucleus, the steroid-protein complex activates specific genes, which begin the process of **protein synthesis**. The enzymes produced bring about the cell's characteristic response to the hormone (see Fig. 10–11).

AGING AND THE ENDOCRINE SYSTEM

Most of the endocrine glands decrease their secretions with age, but normal aging usually does not lead to serious hormone deficiencies. There are decreases in adrenal cortical hormones, for example, but the levels are usually sufficient to maintain homeostasis of water, electrolytes, and nutrients. The decreased secretion of growth hormone leads to a decrease in muscle mass and an increase in fat storage. A lower basal metabolic rate is common in elderly people as the thyroid slows its secretion of thyroxine. Unless specific pathologies develop, however, the endocrine system usually continues to function adequately in old age.

SUMMARY

The hormones of endocrine glands are involved in virtually all aspects of normal body functioning. The growth and repair of tissues, the utilization of food to produce energy, responses to stress, the maintenance of the proper levels and pH of body fluids, and the continuance of the human species all depend on hormones. Some of these topics will be discussed in later chapters. As you might expect, you will be reading about the functions of many of these hormones again, and reviewing their important contributions to the maintenance of homeostasis.

STUDY OUTLINE

Endocrine glands are ductless glands that secrete hormones into the blood. Hormones exert their effects on target organs or tissues.

Chemistry of Hormones

1. Amines—structural variations of the amino acid tyrosine; thyroxine, epinephrine.
2. Proteins—chains of amino acids; peptides are short chains. Insulin, GH, glucagon are proteins; ADH and oxytocin are peptides.
3. Steroids—made from cholesterol; cortisol, aldosterone, estrogen, testosterone.

Regulation of Hormone Secretion

1. Hormones are secreted when there is a need for their effects. Each hormone has a specific stimulus for secretion.
2. The secretion of most hormones is regulated by negative feedback mechanisms: as the hormone exerts its effects, the stimulus for secretion is reversed, and secretion of the hormone decreases.

Pituitary Gland (Hypophysis)—hangs from hypothalamus by the infundibulum; enclosed by sella turcica of sphenoid bone (see Fig. 10–1)

Posterior Pituitary (Neurohypophysis)—stores hormones produced by the hypothalamus (Figs. 10–2 and 10–4 and Table 10–1).

- ADH—increases water reabsorption by the kidneys. Result: decreases urinary output and increases blood volume. Stimulus: nerve impulses from hypothalamus when body water decreases.
- Oxytocin—stimulates contraction of myometrium of uterus during labor and release of milk from mammary glands. Stimulus: nerve impulses from hypothalamus as cervix is stretched or as infant sucks on nipple.

Anterior Pituitary (Adenohypophysis)—secretions are regulated by releasing hormones from the hypothalamus (Figs. 10–2 and 10–4 and Table 10–2).

- GH—increases amino acid transport into cells and increases protein synthesis; increases rate of mitosis; increases use of fats for energy (Fig. 10–3). Stimulus: GHRH from the hypothalamus.
- TSH—increases secretion of thyroxine and T_3 by the thyroid. Stimulus: TRH from the hypothalamus.
- ACTH—increases secretion of cortisol by the adrenal cortex. Stimulus: CRH from the hypothalamus.

- Prolactin—initiates and maintains milk production by the mammary glands. Stimulus: PRH from the hypothalamus.
- FSH—*In women:* initiates development of ova in ovarian follicles and secretion of estrogen by follicle cells.
  In men: initiates sperm development in the testes. Stimulus: GnRH from the hypothalamus.
- LH—*In women:* stimulates ovulation, transforms mature follicle into corpus luteum and stimulates secretion of progesterone.
  In men: stimulates secretion of testosterone by the testes. Stimulus: GnRH from the hypothalamus.

Thyroid Gland—on front and sides of trachea below the larynx (see Fig. 10–1 and Table 10–3)

- Thyroxine (T_4) and T_3—(Fig. 10–5) produced by thyroid follicles. Increase use of all food types for energy and increase protein synthesis. Necessary for normal physical, mental, and sexual development. Stimulus: TSH from the anterior pituitary.
- Calcitonin—produced by parafollicular cells. Decreases reabsorption of calcium from bones and lowers blood calcium level. Stimulus: hypercalcemia.

Parathyroid Glands—four; two on posterior of each lobe of thyroid (see Figs. 10–6 and 10–7 and Table 10–4)

- PTH—increases reabsorption of calcium and phosphate from bones to the blood; increases absorption of calcium and phosphate by the small intestine; increases reabsorption of calcium and excretion of phosphate by the kidneys, and activates vitamin D. Result: raises blood calcium and lowers blood phosphate levels. Stimulus: hypocalcemia. Inhibitor: hypercalcemia.

Pancreas—extends from curve of duodenum to the spleen. Islets of Langerhans consist of alpha cells and beta cells (see Figs. 10–1 and 10–8 and Table 10–5)

- Glucagon—secreted by alpha cells. Stimulates liver to change glycogen to glucose; increases use of fats and amino acids for energy. Result: raises blood glucose level. Stimulus: hypoglycemia.

- Insulin—secreted by beta cells. Increases use of glucose by cells to produce energy; stimulates liver and muscles to change glucose to glycogen; increases cellular intake of fatty acids and amino acids to use for synthesis of lipids and proteins. Result: lowers blood glucose level. Stimulus: hyperglycemia.

Adrenal Glands—one on top of each kidney; each has an inner adrenal medulla and an outer adrenal cortex (see Fig. 10–1)

Adrenal Medulla—produces catecholamines in stress situations (Table 10–6 and Fig. 10–9).

- Norepinephrine—stimulates vasoconstriction and raises blood pressure.
- Epinephrine—increases heart rate and force, causes vasoconstriction in skin and viscera and vasodilation in skeletal muscles; dilates bronchioles; slows peristalsis; causes liver to change glycogen to glucose; increases use of fats for energy; increases rate of cell respiration. Stimulus: sympathetic impulses from the hypothalamus.

Adrenal Cortex—produces mineralocorticoids, glucocorticoids, and very small amounts of sex hormones (function not known with certainty) (Table 10–7).

- Aldosterone—increases reabsorption of sodium and excretion of potassium by the kidneys. Results: hydrogen ions are excreted in exchange for sodium; chloride and bicarbonate ions and water follow sodium back to the blood; maintains normal blood pH, blood volume, and blood pressure. Stimulus: decreased blood sodium or elevated blood potassium; decreased blood volume or blood pressure (activates the renin-angiotensin mechanism of the kidneys).
- Cortisol—(Fig. 10–10) increases use of fats and amino acids for energy; decreases use of glucose to conserve glucose for the brain; anti-inflammatory effect: blocks effects of histamine and stabilizes lysosomes to prevent excessive tissue damage. Stimulus: ACTH from hypothalamus during physiological stress.

Ovaries—in pelvic cavity on either side of uterus (see Fig. 10–1)

- Estrogen—produced by follicle cells. Promotes maturation of ovum; stimulates growth of blood vessels in endometrium; stimulates development of secondary sex characteristics: growth of duct system of mammary glands, growth of uterus, fat deposition. Promotes closure of epiphyses of long bones; lowers blood levels of cholesterol and triglycerides. Stimulus: FSH from anterior pituitary.
- Progesterone—produced by the corpus luteum. Promotes storage of glycogen and further growth of blood vessels in the endometrium; promotes growth of secretory cells of mammary glands. Stimulus: LH from anterior pituitary.
- Inhibin—inhibits secretion of FSH.

Testes—in scrotum between the upper thighs (see Fig. 10–1)

- Testosterone—produced by interstitial cells. Promotes maturation of sperm in testes; stimulates development of secondary sex characteristics: growth of reproductive organs, facial and body hair, larynx, skeletal muscles; promotes closure of epiphyses of long bones. Stimulus: LH from anterior pituitary.
- Inhibin—produced by sustentacular cells. Inhibits secretion of FSH to maintain a constant rate of sperm production. Stimulus: increased testosterone.

Other Hormones

- Melatonin—secreted by the pineal gland during darkness; brings on sleep.
- Prostaglandins—synthesized by cells from the phospholipids of their cell membranes; exert their effects locally. Are involved in inflammation and pain, reproduction, nutrient metabolism, changes in blood vessels, blood clotting.

Mechanisms of Hormone Action (see Fig. 10–11)

- A hormone affects cells that have receptors for it. Receptors are proteins that may be part of the cell membrane, or within the cytoplasm or nucleus of the target cell.
- The Two-Messenger Theory: a protein hormone (1st messenger) bonds to a membrane receptor; stimulates formation of cyclic AMP (2nd messenger), which activates the cell's enzymes to bring about the cell's characteristic response to the hormone.
- Steroid hormones diffuse easily through cell membranes and bond to cytoplasmic receptors. Steroid-protein complex enters the nucleus and activates certain genes which initiate protein synthesis.

REVIEW QUESTIONS

1. Use the following to describe a negative feedback mechanism: TSH, TRH, decreased metabolic rate, thyroxine, and T_3. (pp. 216, 219)

2. Name the two hormones stored in the posterior pituitary gland. Where are these hormones produced? State the functions of each of these hormones. (pp. 214–215)

3. Name the two hormones of the anterior pituitary gland that affect the ovaries or testes, and state their functions. (p. 217)

4. Describe the antagonistic effects of PTH and calcitonin on bones and on blood calcium level. State the other functions of PTH. (p. 222)

5. Describe the antagonistic effects of insulin and glucagon on the liver and on blood glucose level. (p. 224)

6. Describe how cortisol affects the use of foods for energy. Explain the anti-inflammatory effects of cortisol. (p. 228)

7. State the effect of aldosterone on the kidneys. Describe the results of this effect on the composition of the blood. (p. 226)

8. When are epinephrine and norepinephrine secreted? Describe the effects of these hormones. (pp. 224, 227)

9. Name the hormones necessary for development of egg cells in the ovaries. Name the hormones necessary for development of sperm in the testes. (pp. 217, 230)

10. State what prostaglandins are made from. State three functions of prostaglandins. (p. 231)

11. Name the hormones that promote the growth of the endometrium of the uterus in preparation for a fertilized egg, and state precisely where each hormone is produced. (p. 230)

12. State the functions of thyroxine and T_3. For what aspects of growth are these hormones necessary? (pp. 218–220)

13. Explain the functions of GH as they are related to normal growth. (pp. 215–216)

14. State the direct stimulus for secretion of each of these hormones: (pp. 214, 216, 219, 221–223, 226, 229, 230)
    a. Thyroxine
    b. Insulin
    c. Cortisol
    d. PTH
    e. Aldosterone
    f. Calcitonin
    g. GH
    h. Glucagon
    i. Progesterone
    j. ADH

FOR FURTHER THOUGHT

1. During a soccer game, 12-year-old Alicia got in a tangle with another player, fell hard on her hand, and fractured her radius. She is going to be fine, though she will be wearing a cast for a few weeks. What hormones were secreted immediately after the injury? What functions do they have? What hormones will contribute to the healing of the fracture, and how?

2. Darren is 15 years old, tall for his age, but he wants to build more muscle. He decides that he will eat only protein foods, because, he says, "Muscle is protein, so protein will make protein, and the more protein, the more muscle." In part he is correct, and in part incorrect. Explain, and name the hormones involved in protein metabolism; state how for each.

3. Many people love pasta, others love potatoes. Name the hormones involved in carbohydrate metabolism, and, for each, explain its specific function.

4. Unfortunately, many fast-food meals are well over 50% fat. Name the hormones involved in fat metabolism, and, for each, explain its specific function.

5. You have read about the liver several times in this chapter, and often seen its picture as a target organ. Many functions of the liver are stimulated by hormones. Name as many hormones as you can think of with effects on the liver, and state the function of each.

CHAPTER 11

Student Objectives

- Describe the composition and explain the functions of blood plasma.
- Name the hemopoietic tissues and the kinds of blood cells each produces.
- State the function of red blood cells, including the protein and the mineral involved.
- Name the nutrients necessary for red blood cell production, and state the function of each.
- Explain how hypoxia may change the rate of red blood cell production.
- Describe what happens to red blood cells that have reached the end of their life span; what happens to the hemoglobin?
- Explain the ABO and Rh blood types.
- Name the five kinds of white blood cells and describe the function of each.
- State what platelets are, and explain how they are involved in hemostasis.
- Describe the three stages of chemical blood clotting.
- Explain how abnormal clotting is prevented in the vascular system.
- State the normal values in a complete blood count (CBC).

Blood

New Terminology

ABO group (A-B-O GROOP)
Albumin (al-**BYOO**-min)
Bilirubin (**BILL**-ee-roo-bin)
Chemical clotting (**KEM**-i-kuhl **KLAH**-ting)
Embolism (**EM**-boh-lizm)
Erythrocyte (e-**RITH**-roh-sight)
Hemoglobin (**HEE**-muh-GLOW-bin)
Hemostasis (HEE-moh-**STAY**-sis)
Heparin (**HEP**-ar-in)
Immunity (im-**YOO**-ni-tee)
Leukocyte (**LOO**-koh-sight)
Macrophage (**MAK**-roh-fahj)
Normoblast (**NOR**-moh-blast)
Reticulocyte (re-**TIK**-yoo-loh-sight)
Rh factor (R-H **FAK**-ter)
Thrombocyte (**THROM**-boh-sight)
Thrombus (**THROM**-bus)

Related Clinical Terminology

Anemia (uh-**NEE**-mee-yah)
Differential count (**DIFF**-er-EN-shul KOWNT)
Erythroblastosis fetalis (e-RITH-roh-blass-**TOH**-sis
 fee-**TAL**-is)
Hematocrit (hee-**MAT**-oh-krit)
Hemophilia (HEE-moh-**FILL**-ee-ah)
Jaundice (**JAWN**-diss)
Leukemia (loo-**KEE**-mee-ah)
Leukocytosis (LOO-koh-sigh-**TOH**-sis)
RhoGAM (**ROH**-gam)
Tissue-typing (**TISH**-yoo-TIGH-ping)
Typing and cross-matching (**TIGH**-ping and
 KROSS-match-ing)

*Terms that appear in **bold type** in the chapter text are defined in the glossary, which begins on page 521.*

One of the simplest and most familiar life-saving medical procedures is a blood transfusion. As you know, however, the blood of one individual is not always compatible with that of another person. The ABO blood types were discovered in the early 1900s by Karl Landsteiner, an Austrian-American. He also contributed to the discovery of the Rh factor in 1940. In the early 1940s, Charles Drew, an African-American, developed techniques for processing and storing blood plasma, which could then be used in transfusions for people with any blood type. When we donate blood today, our blood may be given to a recipient as whole blood, or it may be separated into its component parts, and recipients will then receive only those parts they need, such as red cells, plasma, Factor VIII, or platelets. Each of these parts has a specific function, and all of the functions of blood are essential to our survival.

The general functions of blood are transportation, regulation, and protection. Materials transported by the blood include nutrients, waste products, gases, and hormones. The blood helps regulate fluid–electrolyte balance, acid–base balance, and the body temperature. Protection against pathogens is provided by white blood cells, and the blood clotting mechanism prevents excessive loss of blood after injuries. Each of these functions is covered in more detail in this chapter.

CHARACTERISTICS OF BLOOD

Blood has distinctive physical characteristics:

Amount—a person has 4 to 6 liters of blood, depending on his or her size. Of the total blood volume in the human body, 38% to 48% is composed of the various blood cells, also called *formed elements*. The remaining 52% to 62% of the blood volume is plasma, the liquid portion of blood (Fig. 11–1).

Color—you're probably saying to yourself, "of course, it's red!" Mention is made of this obvious fact, however, because the color does vary. Arterial blood is bright red because it contains high levels of oxygen. Venous blood has given up much of its oxygen in tissues, and has a darker, dull red color. This may be important in the assessment of the source of bleeding. If blood is bright red it is prob-

ably from a severed artery, and dark red blood is probably venous blood.

pH—the normal pH range of blood is 7.35 to 7.45, which is slightly alkaline. Venous blood normally has a lower pH than does arterial blood because of the presence of more carbon dioxide.

Viscosity—this means thickness or resistance to flow. Blood is about three to five times thicker than water. Viscosity is increased by the presence of blood cells and the plasma proteins, and this thickness contributes to normal blood pressure.

PLASMA

Plasma is the liquid part of blood and is approximately 91% water. The solvent ability of water enables the plasma to transport many types of substances. Nutrients absorbed in the digestive tract are circulated to all body tissues, and waste products of the tissues circulate through the kidneys and are excreted in urine. Hormones produced by endocrine glands are carried in the plasma to their target organs, and antibodies are also transported in plasma. Most of the carbon dioxide produced by cells is carried in the plasma in the form of bicarbonate ions (HCO_3^-). When the blood reaches the lungs, the CO_2 is re-formed, diffuses into the alveoli, and is exhaled.

Also in the plasma are the **plasma proteins**. The clotting factors **prothrombin, fibrinogen**, and others are synthesized by the liver and circulate until activated to form a clot in a ruptured or damaged blood vessel. **Albumin** is the most abundant plasma protein. It too is synthesized by the liver. Albumin contributes to the colloid osmotic pressure of blood, which pulls tissue fluid into capillaries. This is important to maintain normal blood volume and blood pressure. Other plasma proteins are called **globulins**. Alpha and beta globulins are synthesized by the liver and act as carriers for molecules such as fats. The gamma globulins are antibodies produced by lymphocytes. Antibodies initiate the destruction of pathogens and provide us with immunity.

Plasma also carries body heat. Blood is warmed by flowing through active organs such as the liver and muscles. This heat is distributed to cooler parts of the body as blood continues to circulate.

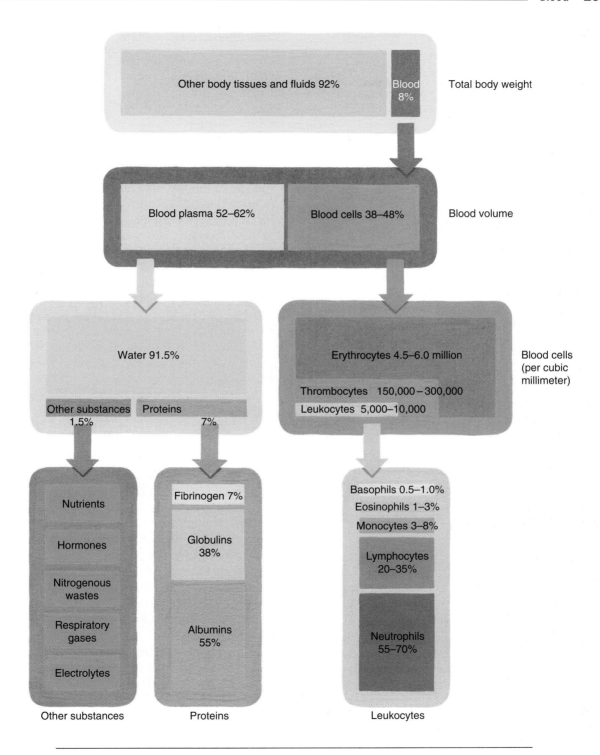

Figure 11–1   Components of blood and the relationship of blood to other body tissues.

BLOOD CELLS

There are three kinds of blood cells: red blood cells, white blood cells, and platelets. Blood cells are produced in **hemopoietic tissues**, of which there are two: **red bone marrow**, found in flat and irregular bones, and **lymphatic tissue**, found in the spleen, lymph nodes, and thymus gland.

RED BLOOD CELLS

Also called **erythrocytes**, red blood cells (RBCs) are biconcave discs, which means their centers are thinner than their edges. You may recall from Chapter 3 that red blood cells are the only human cells without nuclei. Their nuclei disintegrate as the red blood cells mature and are not needed for normal functioning.

A normal RBC count ranges from 4.5 to 6.0 million cells per mm^3 of blood (the volume of a cubic millimeter is approximately that of a very small droplet). RBC counts for men are often toward the high end of this range; those for women are often toward the low end. Another way to measure the amount of RBCs is the **hematocrit**. This test involves drawing blood into a thin glass tube called a capillary tube, and centrifuging the tube to force all the cells to one end. The percentages of cells and plasma can then be determined. Because RBCs are by far the most abundant of the blood cells, a normal hematocrit range is just like that of the total blood cells: 38% to 48%. Both RBC count and hematocrit (Hct) are part of a complete blood count (CBC).

Function

Red blood cells contain the protein **hemoglobin** (Hb), which gives them the ability to carry oxygen. Each red blood cell contains approximately 300 million hemoglobin molecules, each of which can bond to four oxygen molecules. In the pulmonary capillaries, RBCs pick up oxygen and oxyhemoglobin is formed. In the systemic capillaries, hemoglobin gives up much of its oxygen and becomes reduced hemoglobin. A determination of hemoglobin level is also part of a CBC; the normal range is 12 to 18 grams per 100 ml of blood. Essential to the formation of hemoglobin is the mineral iron; there are four atoms of iron in each molecule of hemoglobin. It is the iron that actually bonds to the oxygen and also makes RBCs red.

Production and Maturation

Red blood cells are formed in red bone marrow (RBM) in flat and irregular bones. Within the red bone marrow are precursor cells called **stem cells**. Recall from Chapter 3 that stem cells are unspecialized cells that may develop, or differentiate, in several ways. The stem cells of the red bone marrow may also be called hemocytoblasts (hemo = blood, cyto = cell, blast = producing), and they constantly undergo mitosis to produce all the kinds of blood cells, most of which are RBCs (Figs. 11–2 and 11–3). The rate of production is very rapid (estimated at several million new RBCs per second) and a major regulating factor is oxygen. If the body is in a state of **hypoxia**, or lack of oxygen, the kidneys produce a hormone called **erythropoietin**, which stimulates the red bone marrow to increase the rate of RBC production (that is, the rate of stem cell mitosis). This will occur following hemorrhage, or if a person stays for a time at a higher altitude. As a result of the action of erythropoietin, more RBCs will be available to carry oxygen and correct the hypoxic state.

The stem cells that will become RBCs go through a number of developmental stages, only the last two of which we will mention (see Fig. 11–2). The **normoblast** is the last stage with a nucleus, which then disintegrates. The **reticulocyte** has fragments of the endoplasmic reticulum, which are visible when blood smears are stained for microscopic evaluation. These immature cells are usually found in the red bone marrow, although a small number of reticulocytes in the peripheral circulation is considered normal. Large numbers of reticulocytes or normoblasts in the circulating blood mean that the number of mature RBCs is not sufficient to carry the oxygen needed by the body. Such situations include hemorrhage, or when mature RBCs have been destroyed, as in Rh disease of the newborn, and malaria.

The maturation of red blood cells requires many nutrients. Protein and iron are necessary for the synthesis of hemoglobin and become part of hemoglobin molecules. Copper is part of some enzymes involved in hemoglobin synthesis. The vitamins folic acid and B$_{12}$ are required for DNA synthesis in the stem cells of the red bone marrow. As these cells undergo mitosis they must continually produce new sets of chromosomes. Vitamin B$_{12}$ is also called the **extrinsic factor** because its source is external, our food. Parietal cells of the stomach lining produce the

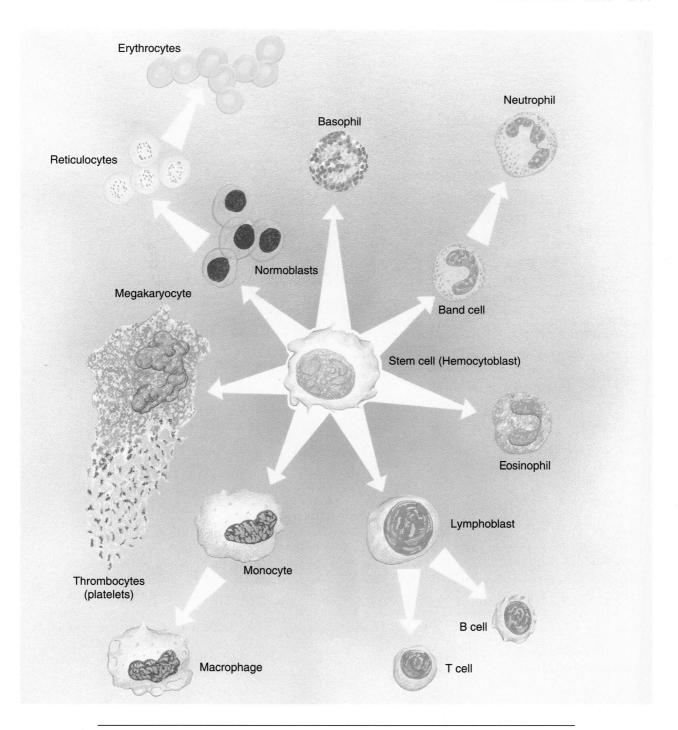

Figure 11–2   Production of blood cells. Stem cells are found in red bone marrow and in lymphatic tissue, and are the precursor cells for all the types of blood cells.

Figure 11–3 Blood cells. **(A)** Red blood cells, platelets, and a basophil. **(B)** Lymphocyte (left) and neutrophil (right). **(C)** Eosinophil. **(D)** Monocytes. **(E)** Megakaryocyte with platelets. (A–E ×600) **(F)** Normal bone marrow (× 200). (From Harmening, DM: Clinical Hematology and Fundamentals of Hemostasis, ed. 3. FA Davis, Philadelphia, 1997, pp 14, 17, 19, 26, 48, with permission.)

intrinsic factor, a chemical that combines with the vitamin B_{12} in food to prevent its digestion and promote its absorption in the small intestine. A deficiency of either vitamin B_{12} or the intrinsic factor results in **pernicious anemia** (see Box 11–1: Anemia).

Life Span

Red blood cells live for approximately 120 days. As they reach this age they become fragile and are removed from circulation by cells of the **tissue macrophage system** (formerly called the reticuloendothelial or RE system). The organs that contain macrophages (literally, "big eaters") are the liver, spleen, and red bone marrow. Look at Fig. 11–4 as you read the following. The old RBCs are phagocytized and digested by macrophages, and the iron they

contained is put into the blood to be returned to the red bone marrow to be used for the synthesis of new hemoglobin. If not needed immediately for this purpose, excess iron is stored in the liver. The iron of RBCs is actually recycled over and over again. The globin or protein portion of the hemoglobin molecule is also recycled. It is digested to its amino acids, which may then be used for the synthesis of new proteins.

Another part of the hemoglobin molecule is the heme portion, which cannot be recycled and is a waste product. The heme is converted to **bilirubin** by macrophages. The liver removes bilirubin from circulation and excretes it into bile; bilirubin is called a bile pigment. Bile is secreted by the liver into the duodenum and passes through the small intestine and colon, so bilirubin is eliminated in feces, and gives feces their characteristic brown color. In the colon

Box 11–1   ANEMIA

Anemia is a deficiency of red blood cells, or insufficient hemoglobin within the red blood cells. There are many different types of anemia.

Iron-deficiency anemia is caused by a lack of dietary iron, and there is not enough of this mineral to form sufficient hemoglobin. A person with this type of anemia may have a normal RBC count and a normal hematocrit, but the hemoglobin level will be below normal.

A deficiency of vitamin B_{12}, which is found only in animal foods, leads to **pernicious anemia**, in which the RBCs are large, misshapen, and fragile. Another cause of this form of anemia is lack of the intrinsic factor due to autoimmune destruction of the parietal cells of the stomach lining.

Sickle-cell anemia has already been discussed in Chapter 3. It is a genetic disorder of hemoglobin, which causes RBCs to sickle, clog capillaries, and rupture.

Aplastic anemia is suppression of the red bone marrow, with decreased production of RBCs, the granular WBCs, and platelets. This is a very serious disorder which may be caused by exposure to radiation, certain chemicals such as benzene, or some medications. There are several antibiotics that must be used with caution since they may have this potentially fatal side effect.

Hemolytic anemia is any disorder that causes rupture of RBCs before the end of their normal life span. Sickle cell anemia and Rh disease of the newborn are examples. Another example is malaria, in which a protozoan parasite reproduces in RBCs and destroys them. Hemolytic anemias are often characterized by jaundice because of the increased production of bilirubin.

Box Figure 11–A   Anemia. **(A)** Iron-deficiency anemia; notice the pale, oval RBCs ($\times$400). **(B)** Pernicious anemia, with large, misshapen RBCs ($\times$400). **(C)** Sickle-cell anemia ($\times$ 400). **(D)** Aplastic anemia, bone marrow ($\times$200). (**A**, **B**, and **C** from Listen, Look, and Learn, Vol 3; coagulation, Hematology. The American Society of Clinical Pathologists Press, Chicago, 1973, with permission. **D** from Harmening, DM: Clinical Hematology and Fundamentals of Hemostasis, ed 3. FA Davis, Philadelphia, 1997, p 49, with permission.)

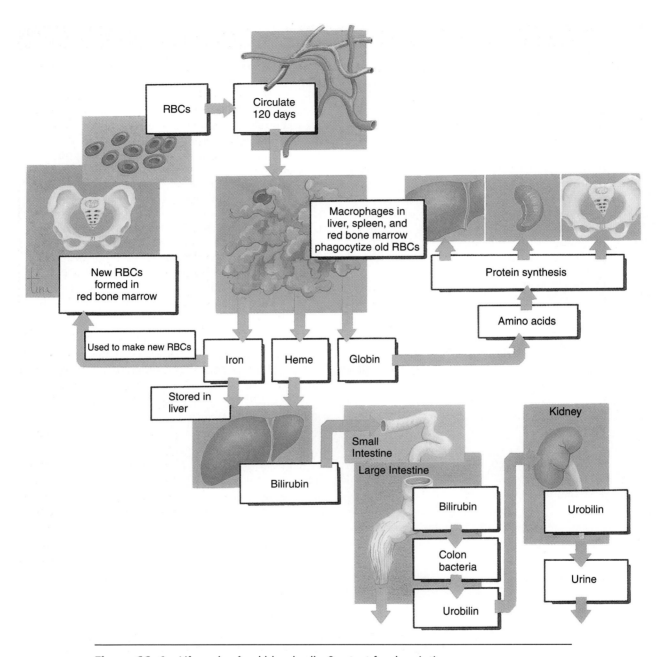

Figure 11–4 Life cycle of red blood cells. See text for description.

some bilirubin is changed to urobilinogen by the colon bacteria. Some urobilinogen may be absorbed into the blood, but it is changed to urobilin and excreted by the kidneys in urine. If bilirubin is not excreted properly, perhaps because of liver disease such as hepatitis, it remains in the blood. This may cause **jaundice**, a condition in which the whites of the eyes appear yellow. This yellow color may also be seen in the skin of light-skinned people (see Box 11–2: Jaundice).

Box 11–2   JAUNDICE

Jaundice is not a disease, but rather a sign caused by excessive accumulation of bilirubin in the blood. Because one of the liver's many functions is the excretion of bilirubin, jaundice may be a sign of liver disease such as hepatitis or cirrhosis. This may be called **hepatic jaundice,** because the problem is with the liver.

Other types of jaundice are prehepatic jaundice and posthepatic jaundice: The name of each tells us where the problem is. Recall that bilirubin is the waste product formed from the heme portion of the hemoglobin of old RBCs. **Prehepatic jaundice** means that the problem is "before" the liver, that is, hemolysis of RBCs is taking place at a more rapid rate. Rapid hemolysis is characteristic of sickle-cell anemia, malaria, and Rh disease of the newborn;

these are hemolytic anemias. As excessive numbers of RBCs are destroyed, bilirubin is formed at a faster rate than the liver can excrete it. The bilirubin that the liver cannot excrete remains in the blood and causes jaundice. Another name for this type is **hemolytic jaundice.**

Posthepatic jaundice means that the problem is "after" the liver. The liver excretes bilirubin into bile, which is stored in the gallbladder and then moves to the small intestine. If the bile ducts are obstructed, perhaps by gall stones or inflammation of the gallbladder, bile cannot pass to the small intestine and backs up in the liver. Bilirubin may then be reabsorbed back into the blood and cause jaundice. Another name for this type is **obstructive jaundice.**

Blood Types

Our blood types are genetic; that is, we inherit genes from our parents that determine our own types. There are many red blood cell factors or types; we will discuss the two most important ones: the **ABO group** and the **Rh factor**.

The **ABO group** contains four blood types: A, B, AB, and O. The letters A and B represent antigens (protein-oligosaccharides) on the red blood cell membrane. A person with type A blood has the A antigen on the RBCs, and someone with type B blood has the B antigen. Type AB means that both A and B antigens are present, and type O means that neither the A nor the B antigen is present.

Circulating in the plasma of each person are natural antibodies for those antigens *not* present on the

RBCs. Therefore, a type A person has anti-B antibodies in the plasma; a type B person has anti-A antibodies; a type AB person has neither anti-A nor anti-B antibodies, and a type O person has both anti-A and anti-B antibodies (see Table 11–1 and Fig. 11–5).

These natural antibodies are of great importance for transfusions. If possible, a person should receive blood of his or her own type; only if this type is not available should another type be given. For example, let us say that a type A person needs a transfusion to replace blood lost in hemorrhage. If this person were to receive type B blood, what would happen? The type A recipient has anti-B antibodies that would bind to the type B antigens of the RBCs of the donated blood. The type B RBCs would first clump **(agglutination)** then rupture **(hemolysis)**, thus defeating the purpose of the transfusion. An even more serious consequence

Table 11–1   ABO BLOOD TYPES

Type	Antigens Present on RBCs	Antibodies Present in Plasma	Percentage in U.S. Population* White	Black	Asian
A	A	anti-B	40	27	31
B	B	anti-A	11	20	26
AB	both A and B	neither anti-A nor anti-B	4	4	8
O	neither A nor B	both anti-A and anti-B	45	49	35

* Average.

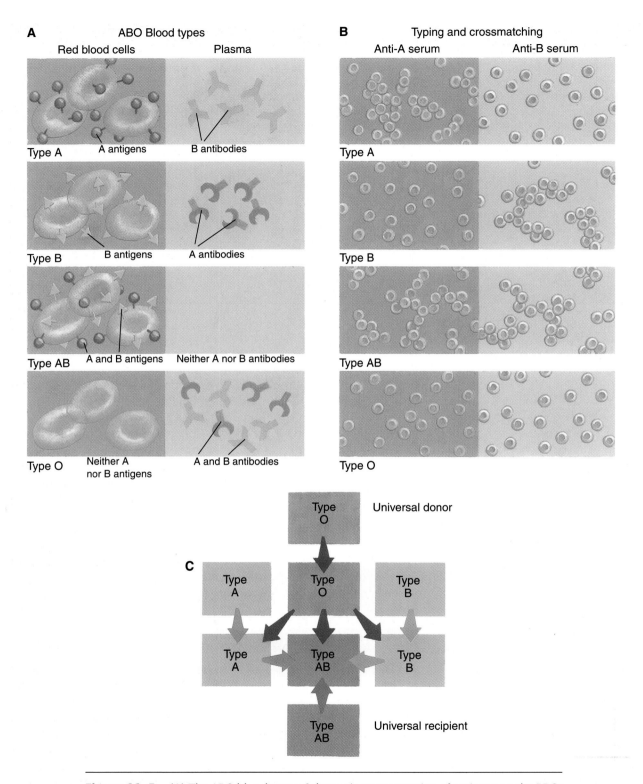

Figure 11–5   (A) The ABO blood types. Schematic representation of antigens on the RBCs and antibodies in the plasma. (B) Typing and cross-matching. The A or B antiserum causes agglutination of RBCs with the matching antigen. (C) Acceptable transfusions are diagrammed and presuppose compatible Rh factors.

Box 11–3   Rh DISEASE OF THE NEWBORN

Rh disease of the newborn may also be called **erythroblastosis fetalis** and is the result of an Rh incompatibility between mother and fetus. During a normal pregnancy, maternal blood and fetal blood do not mix in the placenta. However, during delivery of the placenta (the "afterbirth" that follows the birth of the baby), some fetal blood may enter maternal circulation.

If the woman is Rh negative and her baby is Rh positive, this exposes the woman to Rh-positive RBCs. In response, her immune system will now produce anti-Rh antibodies following this first delivery. In a subsequent pregnancy, these maternal antibodies will cross the placenta and enter fetal circulation. If this next fetus is also Rh positive, the maternal antibodies will cause destruction (hemolysis) of the fetal RBCs. In severe cases this may result in the death of the fetus. In less severe cases, the baby

will be born anemic and jaundiced from the loss of RBCs. Such an infant may require a gradual exchange transfusion to remove the blood with the maternal antibodies and replace it with Rh-negative blood. The baby will continue to produce its own Rh-positive RBCs, which will not be destroyed once the maternal antibodies have been removed.

Much better than treatment, however, is prevention. If an Rh-negative woman delivers an Rh-positive baby, she should be given **RhoGAM** within 72 hours after delivery. RhoGAM is an anti-Rh antibody that will destroy any fetal RBCs that have entered the mother's circulation *before* her immune system can respond and produce antibodies. The RhoGAM antibodies themselves break down within a few months. The woman's next pregnancy will be like the first, as if she had never been exposed to Rh-positive RBCs.

is that the hemoglobin of the ruptured RBCs, now called free hemoglobin, may clog the capillaries of the kidneys and lead to renal damage or renal failure. You can see why **typing** and **cross-matching** of donor and recipient blood in the hospital laboratory is so important before any transfusion is given (see Fig. 11–5). This procedure helps ensure that donated blood will not bring about a hemolytic transfusion reaction in the recipient.

You may have heard of the concept that type O is the "universal donor." Usually, type O negative blood may be given to people with any other blood type. This is so because type O RBCs have neither the A nor the B antigens and will not react with whatever antibodies the recipient may have. The term *negative* refers to the Rh factor, which we will now consider.

The **Rh factor** is another antigen (often called D) that may be present on RBCs. People whose RBCs have the Rh antigen are Rh positive; those without the antigen are Rh negative. Rh-negative people do not have natural antibodies to the Rh antigen, and for them this antigen is foreign. If an Rh-negative person receives Rh-positive blood by mistake, antibodies will be formed just as they would be to bacteria or viruses. A first mistaken transfusion often does not cause problems, because antibody production is slow upon the first exposure to Rh-positive RBCs. A second transfusion, however, when anti-Rh antibodies are already present, will bring about a transfusion reaction, with

hemolysis and possible kidney damage (see also Box 11–3: Rh Disease of the Newborn).

WHITE BLOOD CELLS

White blood cells (WBCs) are also called **leukocytes**. There are five kinds of WBCs; all are larger than RBCs and have nuclei when mature. The nucleus may be in one piece or appear as several lobes. Special staining for microscopic examination gives each kind of WBC a distinctive appearance (see Figs. 11–2 and 11–3).

A normal WBC count (part of a CBC) is 5,000 to 10,000 per mm³. Notice that this number is quite small compared to a normal RBC count. Many of our WBCs are not within blood vessels but are carrying out their functions in tissue fluid.

Classification and Sites of Production

The five kinds of white blood cells may be classified in two groups: granular and agranular. The granular leukocytes are produced in the red bone marrow; these are the **neutrophils, eosinophils**, and **basophils**, which have distinctly colored granules when stained. The agranular leukocytes are **lymphocytes** and **monocytes**, which are produced in the lymphatic tissue of the spleen, lymph nodes, and thymus, as well as in the red bone marrow. A **differential WBC count** (part of a CBC) is the percentage of each kind of leukocyte. Normal ranges are listed

Table 11–2	COMPLETE BLOOD COUNT
Measurement	**Normal Range***
Red blood cells	• 4.5–6.0 million/mm^3
Hemoglobin	• 12–18 grams/100 ml
Hematocrit	• 38%–48%
Reticulocytes	• 0%–1.5%
White blood cells (total)	• 5000–10,000/mm^3
Neutrophils	• 55%–70%
Eosinophils	• 1%–3%
Basophils	• 0.5%–1%
Lymphocytes	• 20%–35%
Monocytes	• 3%–8%
Platelets	• 150,000–300,000/mm^3

* The values on hospital lab slips may vary somewhat but will be very similar to the normal ranges given here.

in Table 11–2, along with other normal values of a CBC.

Functions

White blood cells all contribute to the same general function, which is to protect the body from infectious disease and to provide **immunity** to certain diseases. Each kind of leukocyte makes a contribution to this very important aspect of homeostasis.

Neutrophils and monocytes are capable of the **phagocytosis** of pathogens. Neutrophils are the more abundant phagocytes, but the monocytes are the more efficient phagocytes, because they differentiate into **macrophages**, which also phagocytize dead or damaged tissue at the site of any injury, helping to make tissue repair possible.

Eosinophils are believed to detoxify foreign proteins. This is especially important in allergic reactions and parasitic infections such as trichinosis (a worm parasite). Basophils contain granules of heparin and histamine. **Heparin** is an anticoagulant that helps prevent abnormal clotting within blood vessels. **Histamine**, you may recall, is released as part of the inflammation process, and it makes capillaries more permeable, allowing tissue fluid, proteins, and white blood cells to accumulate in the damaged area.

There are two major kinds of lymphocytes: T cells and B cells. For now we will say that **T cells** (or T lymphocytes) recognize foreign antigens, may directly destroy some foreign antigens, and stop the immune response when the antigen has been destroyed. **B cells** (or B lymphocytes) become plasma cells that produce antibodies to foreign antigens. These functions of T cells and B cells, as well as a third kind of lymphocyte called a natural killer cell, are discussed in the context of the mechanisms of immunity in Chapter 14.

As mentioned earlier, leukocytes function in tissue fluid as well as in the blood. Many WBCs are capable of self-locomotion (ameboid movement) and are able to squeeze between the cells of capillary walls and out into tissue spaces. Macrophages provide a good example of the dual locations of leukocytes. Some macrophages are "fixed," that is, stationary in organs such as the liver, spleen, and red bone marrow (part of the tissue macrophage or RE system—the same macrophages that phagocytize old RBCs) and in the lymph nodes. They phagocytize pathogens that circulate in blood or lymph through these organs. Other "wandering" macrophages move about in tissue fluid, especially in the areolar connective tissue of mucous membranes and below the skin. Pathogens that gain entry into the body through natural openings or through breaks in the skin are usually destroyed by the macrophages and other leukocytes in connective tissue before they can cause serious disease.

A high WBC count, called **leukocytosis**, is often an indication of infection. **Leukopenia** is a low WBC count, which may be present in the early stages of diseases such as tuberculosis. Exposure to radiation or to chemicals such as benzene may destroy WBCs and lower the total count. Such a person is then very susceptible to infection. **Leukemia**, or malignancy of leukocyte-forming tissues, is discussed in Box 11–4: Leukemia.

The white blood cell types (analogous to RBC types such as the ABO group) are called **human leukocyte antigens (HLAs)** and are discussed in Box 11–5: White Blood Cell Types: HLA.

PLATELETS

The more formal name for platelets is **thrombocytes**, which are not whole cells but rather fragments or pieces of cells. A normal platelet count (part of a CBC) is 150,000 to 300,000/mm^3 (the high end of the range may be extended to 500,000). **Thrombocytopenia** is the term for a low platelet count.

Box 11–4   LEUKEMIA

Leukemia is the term for malignancy of the blood-forming tissues, the red bone marrow or lymphatic tissue. There are many types of leukemia, which are classified as acute or chronic, by the types of abnormal cells produced, and by either childhood or adult onset.

In general, leukemia is characterized by an overproduction of immature white blood cells. These immature cells cannot perform their normal functions, and the person becomes very susceptible to infection. As a greater proportion of the body's nutrients are used by malignant cells, the production of other blood cells decreases. Severe anemia is a consequence of decreased red blood cell production, and the tendency to hemorrhage is the result of decreased platelets.

Chemotherapy may bring about cure or remission for some forms of leukemia, but other forms remain resistant to treatment and may be fatal within a few months of diagnosis. In such cases, the cause of death is often pneumonia or some other serious infection, because the abnormal white blood cells cannot prevent the growth of pathogens within the body.

Box Figure 11–B   Leukemia. Notice the many darkly staining WBCs (×300). (From Sacher, RA, and McPherson, RA: Widmann's Clinical Interpretation of Laboratory Tests, ed 11. FA Davis, Philadelphia, 2000, with permission.)

Site of Production

Some of the stem cells in the red bone marrow differentiate into large cells called **megakaryocytes** (see Figs. 11–2 and 11–3), which break up into small pieces that enter circulation. These circulating pieces are platelets, which may survive for 5 to 9 days, if not utilized before that.

Function

Platelets are necessary for **hemostasis**, which means prevention of blood loss. There are three mechanisms, and platelets are involved in each. Two of these mechanisms are shown in Fig. 11–6.

1. **Vascular spasm**—when a large vessel such as an artery or vein is severed, the smooth muscle in its wall contracts in response to the damage (called the myogenic response). Platelets in the area of the rupture release serotonin, which also brings about vasoconstriction. The diameter of the vessel is thereby made smaller, and the smaller opening may then be blocked by a blood clot. If the vessel did not constrict first, the clot that forms would quickly be washed out by the force of the blood pressure.

2. **Platelet plugs**—when capillaries rupture, the damage is too slight to initiate the formation of a blood clot. The rough surface, however, causes platelets to become sticky and stick to the edges of the break and to each other. The platelets form a mechanical barrier or wall to close off the break in the capillary. Capillary ruptures are quite frequent, and platelet plugs, although small, are all that is needed to seal them.

Box 11–5   WHITE BLOOD CELL TYPES: HLA

Human leukocyte antigens (HLA) are antigens on WBCs that are representative of the antigens present on all the cells of an individual. These are our "self" antigens that identify cells that belong in the body.

Recall that in the ABO blood group of RBCs, there are only two antigens, A and B, and four possible types: A, B, AB, and O. HLA antigens are also given letter names. HLA-A, -B, and -C are called class I proteins, with from 100 to more than 400 possibilities for the specific protein each can be. The several class II proteins are given various D designations, and again, there are many possibilities for each. Each person has two genes for each HLA type, because these types are inherited, just as RBC types are inherited. Members of the same family may have some of the same HLA types, and identical twins have exactly the same HLA types.

The purpose of the HLA types is to provide a "self" comparison for the immune system to use when pathogens enter the body. The T lymphocytes compare the "self" antigens on macrophages to the antigens on bacteria and viruses. Because these antigens do not match ours, they are recognized as foreign; this is the first step in the destruction of a pathogen.

The surgical transplantation of organs has also focused on the HLA. The most serious problem for the recipient of a transplanted heart or kidney is rejection of the organ and its destruction by the immune system. You may be familiar with the term **tissue-typing.** This involves determining the HLA types of a donated organ to see if one or several will match the HLA types of the potential recipient. If even one HLA type matches, the chance of rejection is significantly lessened. Although all transplant recipients (except corneal) must receive immunosuppressive medications to prevent rejection, such medications make them more susceptible to infection. The closer the HLA match of the donated organ, the lower the dosage of such medications, and the less chance of serious infections. (The chance of finding a perfect HLA match in the general population is estimated at 1 in 20,000.)

There is yet another aspect of the importance of HLA: People with certain HLA types seem to be more likely to develop certain non-infectious diseases. For example, insulin-dependent diabetes mellitus is often found in people with HLA DR3 or DR4, and a form of arthritis of the spine called ankylosing spondylitis is often found in those with HLA B27. These are *not* genes for these diseases, but may be predisposing factors. What may happen is this: A virus enters the body and stimulates the immune system to produce antibodies. The virus is destroyed, but one of the person's own antigens is so similar to the viral antigen that the immune system continues its activity and begins to destroy this similar part of the body. Another possibility is that a virus damages a self-antigen to the extent that it is now so different that it will be perceived as foreign. These are two theories of how autoimmune diseases are triggered, which is the focus of much research in the field of immunology.

Would platelet plugs be effective for breaks in larger vessels? No, they are too small, and though they do form, they are washed away (until a clot begins to form that can contain them). Would vascular spasm be effective for capillaries? Again, the answer is no, because capillaries have no smooth muscle and cannot constrict at all.

3. **Chemical clotting**—The stimulus for clotting is a rough surface within a vessel, or a break in the vessel, which also creates a rough surface. The more damage there is, the faster clotting begins, usually within 15 to 120 seconds.

The clotting mechanism is a series of reactions involving chemicals that normally circulate in the blood and others that are released when a vessel is damaged.

The chemicals involved in clotting include platelet factors, chemicals released by damaged tissues, calcium ions, and the plasma proteins prothrombin, fibrinogen, Factor 8, and others synthesized by the liver. (These clotting factors are also designated by Roman numerals; Factor 8 would be Factor VIII.) Vitamin K is necessary for the liver to synthesize prothrombin and several other clotting factors (Factors 7, 9, and 10). Most of our vitamin K is produced by the bacteria that live in the colon; the vitamin is absorbed as the colon absorbs water, and may be stored in the liver.

Chemical clotting is usually described in three stages, which are listed in Table 11–3 and illustrated in Fig. 11–7. As you follow the pathway, notice that the product of stage 1 is prothrombin activator, which may also be called prothrombinase. Each name tells

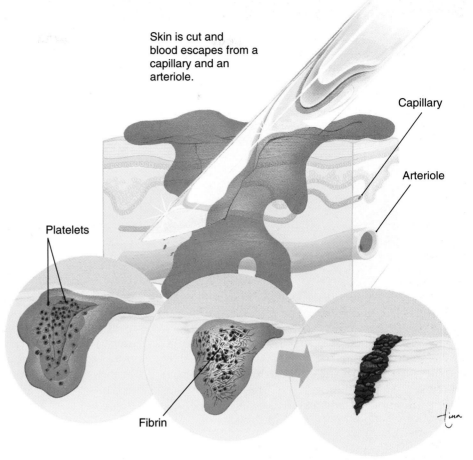

Figure 11–6 Hemostasis. Platelet plug formation in a capillary and chemical clotting and clot retraction in an arteriole.

Skin is cut and blood escapes from a capillary and an arteriole.

Capillary

Arteriole

Platelets

Fibrin

In the capillary, platelets stick to the ruptured wall and form a platelet plug.

In the arteriole, chemical clotting forms a fibrin clot.

Clot retraction pulls the edges of the break together.

us something. The first name suggests that this chemical activates prothrombin, and that is true. The second name ends in "ase," which indicates that this is an enzyme. The traditional names for enzymes use the substrate of the enzyme as the first part of the name, and add "ase." So this chemical must be an enzyme whose substrate is prothrombin, and that is also true. The stages of clotting may be called a cascade, where one leads to the next, as inevitable as water flowing downhill. Prothrombin activator, the product of stage 1, brings about the stage 2 reaction. The product of stage 2, thrombin, brings about the stage 3 reaction (see Box 11–6: Hemophilia).

The clot itself is made of **fibrin**, the product of stage 3. Fibrin is a thread-like protein. Many strands of fibrin form a mesh that traps RBCs and platelets, and creates a wall across the break in the vessel.

Once the clot has formed and bleeding has stopped, **clot retraction** and **fibrinolysis** occur. Clot retraction requires platelets, ATP, and Factor 13 and involves folding of the fibrin threads to pull the edges of the rupture in the vessel wall closer together. This will make the area to be repaired smaller. As repair begins, the clot is dissolved, a process called fibrinolysis. It is important that the clot be dissolved, because it is a rough surface, and if inside a vessel would stimulate more and unnecessary clotting, which might eventually obstruct blood flow.

Prevention of Abnormal Clotting

Clotting should take place to stop bleeding, but too much clotting would obstruct vessels and interfere with normal circulation of blood. Clots do not usually

Table 11–3	CHEMICAL CLOTTING	
Clotting Stage	**Factors Needed**	**Reaction**
Stage 1	• Platelet factors • Chemicals from damaged tissue (tissue thromboplastin) • Factors 5,7,8,9,10,11,12 • Calcium ions	Platelet factors + tissue thromboplastin + other clotting factors + calcium ions form prothrombin activator
Stage 2	• Prothrombin activator from stage 1 • Prothrombin • Calcium ions	Prothrombin activator converts prothrombin to thrombin
Stage 3	• Thrombin from stage 2 • Fibrinogen • Calcium ions • Factor 13 (fibrin stabilizing factor)	Thrombin converts fibrinogen to fibrin

form in intact vessels because the simple squamous epithelial lining is very smooth and repels the platelets and clotting factors. If the lining becomes roughened, as happens with the lipid deposits of atherosclerosis, a clot will form.

Heparin, produced by basophils, is a natural anticoagulant that inhibits the clotting process. The liver produces a globulin called **antithrombin**, which combines with and inactivates excess thrombin. Excess thrombin would exert a positive feedback effect on the clotting cascade, and result in the splitting of more prothrombin to thrombin, more clotting, more thrombin formed, and so on. Antithrombin helps to prevent this, as does fibrin, which absorbs excess thrombin. All of these factors are the external brake for this positive feedback mechanism. Together they usually limit the fibrin formed to what is needed to create a useful clot but not an obstructive one.

Thrombosis refers to clotting in an intact vessel; the clot itself is called a **thrombus**. Coronary thrombosis, for example, is abnormal clotting in a coronary artery, which will decrease the blood (oxygen) supply to part of the heart muscle. An **embolism** is a clot or other tissue transported from elsewhere that lodges in and obstructs a vessel (see Box 11–7: Dissolving Clots).

SUMMARY

All of the functions of blood described in this chapter contribute to the homeostasis of the body as a whole.

Box 11–6	HEMOPHILIA

There are several forms of **hemophilia;** all are genetic and are characterized by the inability of the blood to clot properly. Hemophilia A is the most common form and involves a deficiency of clotting Factor 8. The gene for hemophilia A is located on the X chromosome, so this is a **sex-linked trait,** with the same pattern of inheritance as red-green color blindness and Duchenne's muscular dystrophy.

Without Factor 8, the first stage of chemical clotting cannot be completed, and prothrombin activator is not formed. Without treatment, a hemophiliac experiences prolonged bleeding after even minor injuries and extensive internal bleeding, especially in joints subjected to the stresses of weight bearing. In recent years, treatment (but not cure) has become possible with Factor 8 obtained from blood donors. The Factor 8 is extracted from the plasma of donated blood and administered in concentrated form to hemophiliacs, enabling them to live normal lives.

In what is perhaps the most tragic irony of medical progress, many hemophiliacs were inadvertently infected with HIV, the virus that causes AIDS. Prior to 1985, there was no test to detect HIV in donated blood, and the virus was passed to hemophiliacs in the very blood product that was meant to control their disease and prolong their lives. Today, all donated blood and blood products are tested for HIV, and the risk of AIDS transmission to hemophiliacs, or anyone receiving donated blood, is now very small.

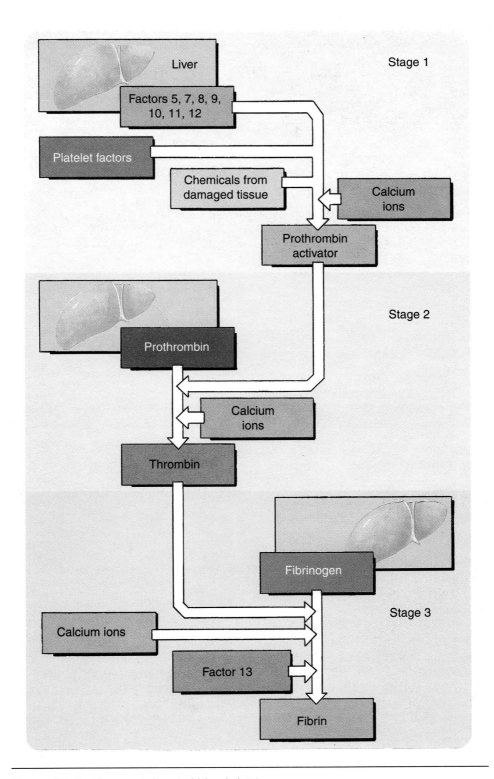

Figure 11–7   Stages of chemical blood clotting.

Box 11–7   DISSOLVING CLOTS

Abnormal clots may cause serious problems in coronary arteries, pulmonary arteries, cerebral vessels, and even veins in the legs. However, if clots can be dissolved before they cause death of tissue, normal circulation and tissue functioning may be restored.

One of the first substances used to dissolve clots in coronary arteries was **streptokinase,** which is actually a bacterial toxin produced by some members of the genus *Streptococcus*. Streptokinase does indeed dissolve clots, but its use creates the possibility of clot destruction throughout the body, with hemorrhage a potential consequence.

A natural clot-dissolving enzyme has been produced by genetic engineering; this is tissue plas-minogen activator, or t–PA. When a blood clot forms, a plasma protein called plasminogen is incorporated into the clot. Plasminogen is converted to plasmin by a substance present in the blood vessel lining and lysosomes, and by thrombin. Plasmin then begins to dissolve the fibrin of which the clot is made. The synthetic t–PA functions in a similar way: It converts the plasminogen in an abnormal clot to plasmin, which dissolves the clot and permits blood to flow through the vessel. In a case of coronary thrombo-sis, if t–PA can be administered within a few hours, the clot may be dissolved and permanent heart damage prevented. The enzyme t–PA is also used to prevent permanent brain damage after strokes (CVAs) caused by blood clots.

However, these functions could not be carried out if the blood did not circulate properly. The circulation of blood throughout the blood vessels is dependent upon the proper functioning of the heart, the pump of the circulatory system.

STUDY OUTLINE

The general functions of blood are transportation, regulation, and protection.

Characteristics of Blood

1. Amount—4 to 6 liters; 38% to 48% is cells; 52% to 62% is plasma (Fig. 11–1).
2. Color—arterial blood has a high oxygen content and is bright red; venous blood has less oxygen and is dark red.
3. pH—7.35 to 7.45; venous blood has more CO_2 and a lower pH than arterial blood.
4. Viscosity—thickness or resistance to flow; due to the presence of cells and plasma proteins; contributes to normal blood pressure.

Plasma—the liquid portion of blood

1. 91% water.
2. Plasma transports nutrients, wastes, hormones, antibodies, CO_2 as HCO_3^-.
3. Plasma proteins: clotting factors are synthesized by the liver; albumin is synthesized by the liver and provides colloid osmotic pressure that pulls tissue fluid into capillaries to maintain normal blood volume and blood pressure; alpha and beta globulins are synthesized by the liver and are carriers for fats and other substances in the blood; gamma globulins are antibodies produced by lymphocytes.

Blood Cells

1. Formed elements are RBCs, WBCs, and platelets (Figs. 11–2 and 11–3).
2. The hemopoietic tissues are red bone marrow (RBM) and lymphatic tissue of the spleen, lymph nodes, and thymus.

Red Blood Cells—erythrocytes (see Table 11–2 for normal values)

1. Biconcave discs; no nuclei when mature.
2. RBCs carry O_2 bonded to the iron in hemoglobin.
3. RBCs are formed in the RBM from hemocytoblasts (stem cells, the precursor cells).
4. Hypoxia stimulates the kidneys to produce the hormone erythropoietin, which increases the rate of RBC production in the RBM.

5. Immature RBCs: normoblasts (have nuclei) and reticulocytes (large numbers in peripheral circulation indicate a need for more RBCs to carry oxygen).
6. Vitamin B_{12} is the extrinsic factor, needed for DNA synthesis (mitosis) in stem cells in the RBM. Intrinsic factor is produced by the parietal cells of the stomach lining; it combines with B_{12} to prevent its digestion and promote its absorption.
7. RBCs live for 120 days and are then phagocytized by macrophages in the liver, spleen, and RBM. The iron is returned to the RBM or stored in the liver. The heme of the hemoglobin is converted to bilirubin, which the liver excretes into bile to be eliminated in feces. Colon bacteria change bilirubin to urobilinogen. Any urobilinogen absorbed is converted to urobilin and excreted by the kidneys in urine (Fig. 11–4). Jaundice is the accumulation of bilirubin in the blood, perhaps due to liver disease.
8. ABO blood types are hereditary. The type indicates the antigen(s) on the RBCs (see Table 11–1 and Fig. 11–5); antibodies in plasma are for those antigens not present on the RBCs and are important for transfusions.
9. The Rh type is also hereditary. Rh positive means that the D antigen is present on the RBCs; Rh negative means that the D antigen is not present on the RBCs. Rh-negative people do not have natural antibodies but will produce them if given Rh-positive blood.

White Blood Cells—leukocytes (see Table 11–2 for normal values)
1. Larger than RBCs; have nuclei when mature (Figs. 11–2 and 11–3).
2. Granular WBCs are the neutrophils, eosinophils, and basophils and are produced in the RBM.
3. Agranular WBCs are the lymphocytes and monocytes and are produced in lymphatic tissue, as well as in RBM.
4. Neutrophils and monocytes phagocytize pathogens; monocytes become macrophages, which also phagocytize dead tissue.
5. Eosinophils detoxify foreign proteins during allergic reactions and parasitic infections.
6. Basophils contain the anticoagulant heparin and histamine, which contributes to inflammation.
7. Lymphocytes: T cells and B cells. T cells recognize foreign antigens and stop the immune response once the antigen has been destroyed. B cells become plasma cells, which produce antibodies to foreign antigens.
8. WBCs carry out their functions in tissue fluid as well as in the blood.

Platelets—thrombocytes (see Table 11–2 for normal values)
1. Platelets are formed in the RBM and are fragments of megakaryocytes.
2. Platelets are involved in all mechanisms of hemostasis (prevention of blood loss) (Fig. 11–6).
3. Vascular spasm—large vessels constrict when damaged, the myogenic response. Platelets release serotonin, which also causes vasoconstriction. The break in the vessel is made smaller and may be closed with a blood clot.
4. Platelet plugs—rupture of a capillary creates a rough surface to which platelets stick and form a barrier over the break.
5. Chemical clotting involves platelet factors, chemicals from damaged tissue, prothrombin, fibrinogen and other clotting factors synthesized by the liver, and calcium ions. See Table 11–3 and Fig. 11–7 for the three stages of chemical clotting. The clot is formed of fibrin threads that form a mesh over the break in the vessel.
6. Clot retraction is the folding of the fibrin threads to pull the cut edges of the vessel closer together. Fibrinolysis is the dissolving of the clot once it has served its purpose.
7. Abnormal clotting (thrombosis) is prevented by the very smooth simple squamous epithelium (endothelium), which lines blood vessels; heparin, which inhibits the clotting process; and antithrombin (synthesized by the liver), which inactivates excess thrombin.

REVIEW QUESTIONS

1. Name four different kinds of substances transported in blood plasma. (p. 238)

2. Name the precursor cell of all blood cells. Name the two types of hemopoietic tissue, their locations, and the types of blood cells produced by each. (pp. 240, 247, 249)

3. State the normal values (CBC) for RBCs, WBCs, platelets, hemoglobin, and hematocrit. (p. 248)

4. State the function of RBCs; include the protein and mineral needed. (p. 240)

5. Explain why iron, protein, folic acid, vitamin B_{12}, and the intrinsic factor are needed for RBC production. (pp. 240, 242)

6. Explain how bilirubin is formed and excreted. (pp. 242, 244)

7. Explain what will happen if a person with type O positive blood receives a transfusion of type A negative blood. (p. 245)

8. Name the WBC with each of the following functions: (p. 248)
   a. Become macrophages and phagocytize dead tissue
   b. Produce antibodies
   c. Detoxify foreign proteins
   d. Phagocytize pathogens
   e. Contain the anticoagulant heparin
   f. Recognize antigens as foreign
   g. Secrete histamine during inflammation

9. Explain how and why platelet plugs form in ruptured capillaries. (p. 249)

10. Explain how vascular spasm prevents excessive blood loss when a large vessel is severed. (p. 249)

11. With respect to chemical blood clotting: (p. 253)
    a. Name the mineral necessary.
    b. Name the organ that produces many of the clotting factors.
    c. Name the vitamin necessary for prothrombin synthesis.
    d. State what the clot itself is made of.

12. Explain what is meant by clot retraction and fibrinolysis. (p. 251)

13. State two ways abnormal clotting is prevented in the vascular system. (p. 252)

14. Explain what is meant by blood viscosity, the factors that contribute, and why viscosity is important. (p. 238)

15. State the normal pH range of blood. What gas has an effect on blood pH? (p. 238)

16. Define anemia, leukocytosis, and thrombocytopenia. (pp. 243, 248)

FOR FURTHER THOUGHT

1. The liver has many functions that are directly related to the composition and functions of blood. Think of as many as you can.

2. Constructing a brick wall requires bricks *and* bricklayers. List all the nutrients that are needed for RBC production, and indicate which are bricks and which are bricklayers.

3. Anthony moved from New Jersey to a mountain cabin in Colorado, 8,000 feet above sea level. When he first arrived, his hematocrit was 44 %. After six months in his new home, what would you expect his hematocrit to be? Explain your answer, and what brought about the change.

4. The lab results for a particular patient show these CBC values:
   RBCs—4.2 million/mm^3
   Hct—40%
   Hb—13 g/100 ml
   WBCs—8,500/mm^3
   platelets—60,000/mm^3

   Is this patient healthy, or would you expect any symptoms of a disorder? Explain your answer.

5. Using the model in Question 4, make a list of possible CBC values for a patient with iron-deficiency anemia. Then make a list of possible CBC values for a person with aplastic anemia.

6. An artificial blood may soon be available; many are being tested. What specific function of blood will it definitely have? Are there any advantages to an artificial blood compared with blood from a human donor?

7. Disseminated intravascular coagulation (DIC) is a serious condition that may follow certain kinds of infections or traumas. First, explain what the name means. This is best done one word at a time. In DIC, clotting becomes a vicious cycle, and the blood is depleted of clotting factors. What do you think will be the consequence for the affected person?

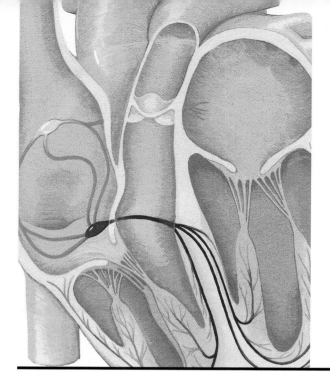

CHAPTER 12

Student Objectives

- Describe the location of the heart, the pericardial membranes, and the endocardium.
- Name the chambers of the heart and the vessels that enter or leave each.
- Name the valves of the heart, and explain their functions.
- Describe coronary circulation, and explain its purpose.
- Describe the cardiac cycle.
- Explain how heart sounds are created.
- Name the parts of the cardiac conduction pathway, and explain why it is the SA node that initiates each beat.
- Explain stroke volume, cardiac output, and Starling's Law of the Heart.
- Explain how the nervous system regulates heart rate and force of contraction.

The Heart

New Terminology

Aorta (ay-**OR**-tah)

Atrium (**AY**-tree-um)

Cardiac cycle (**KAR**-dee-yak **SIGH**-kuhl)

Cardiac output (**KAR**-dee-yak **OUT**-put)

Coronary arteries (**KOR**-uh-na-ree **AR**-tuh-rees)

Diastole (dye-**AS**-tuh-lee)

Endocardium (EN-doh-**KAR**-dee-um)

Epicardium (EP-ee-**KAR**-dee-um)

Mediastinum (ME-dee-ah-**STYE**-num)

Mitral valve (**MYE**-truhl VALV)

Myocardium (MY-oh-**KAR**-dee-um)

Sinoatrial (SA) node (**SIGH**-noh-AY-tree-al NOHD)

Stroke volume (STROHK **VAHL**-yoom)

Systole (**SIS**-tuh-lee)

Tricuspid valve (try-**KUSS**-pid VALV)

Venous return (**VEE**-nus ree-**TURN**)

Ventricle (**VEN**-tri-kuhl)

Related Clinical Terminology

Arrhythmia (uh-**RITH**-me-yah)

Ectopic focus (ek-**TOP**-ik **FOH**-kus)

Electrocardiogram (ECG) (ee-LEK-troh-**KAR**-dee-oh-GRAM)

Fibrillation (fi-bri-**LAY**-shun)

Heart murmur (HART **MUR**-mur)

Ischemic (iss-**KEY**-mik)

Myocardial infarction (MY-oh-**KAR**-dee-yuhl in-**FARK**-shun)

Pulse (**PULS**)

Stenosis (ste-**NOH**-sis)

*Terms that appear in **bold type** in the chapter text are defined in the glossary, which begins on page 521.*

In the embryo, the heart begins to beat at 4 weeks of age, even before its nerve supply has been established. If a person lives to be 80 years old, his or her heart continues to beat an average of 100,000 times a day, every day for each of those 80 years. Imagine trying to squeeze a tennis ball 70 times a minute. After a few minutes, your arm muscles would begin to tire. Then imagine increasing your squeezing rate to 120 times a minute. Most of us could not keep that up very long, but that is what the heart does during exercise. A healthy heart can increase its rate and force of contraction to meet the body's need for more oxygen, then return to its resting rate and keep on beating as if nothing very extraordinary had happened. In fact, it isn't extraordinary at all; this is the job the heart is meant to do.

The primary function of the heart is to pump blood through the arteries, capillaries, and veins. As you learned in the last chapter, blood transports oxygen and nutrients and has other important functions as well. The heart is the pump that keeps blood circulating properly.

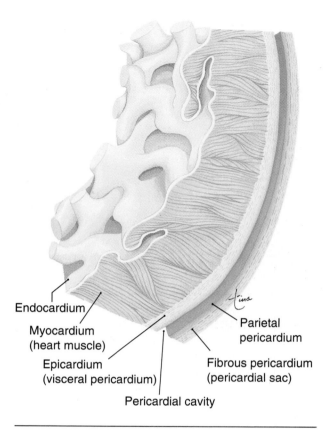

Endocardium

Myocardium (heart muscle)

Epicardium (visceral pericardium)

Pericardial cavity

Parietal pericardium

Fibrous pericardium (pericardial sac)

Figure 12–1 Layers of the wall of the heart and the pericardial membranes. The endocardium is the lining of the chambers of the heart. The fibrous pericardium is the outermost layer.

LOCATION AND PERICARDIAL MEMBRANES

The heart is located in the thoracic cavity between the lungs. This area is called the **mediastinum**. The cone-shaped heart has its tip (apex) just above the diaphragm to the left of the midline. This is why we may think of the heart as being on the left side, because the strongest beat can be heard or felt here.

The heart is enclosed in the **pericardial membranes**, of which there are three (Fig. 12–1). The outermost is the **fibrous pericardium**, a loose-fitting sac of fibrous connective tissue that extends inferiorly over the diaphragm and superiorly over the bases of the large vessels that enter and leave the heart. Lining the fibrous pericardium is the **parietal pericardium**, a serous membrane. On the surface of the heart muscle is the **visceral pericardium**, also called the **epicardium**, another serous membrane. Between the parietal and visceral pericardial membranes is **serous fluid**, which prevents friction as the heart beats.

CHAMBERS—VESSELS AND VALVES

The walls of the four chambers of the heart are made of cardiac muscle called the **myocardium**. The chambers are lined with **endocardium**, simple squamous epithelium that also covers the valves of the heart and continues into the vessels as their lining. The important physical characteristic of the endocardium is not its thinness, but rather its smoothness. This very smooth tissue prevents abnormal blood clotting, because clotting would be initiated by contact of blood with a rough surface.

The upper chambers of the heart are the right and left **atria** (singular: **atrium**), which have relatively thin walls and are separated by a common wall of myocardium called the **interatrial septum**. The lower chambers are the right and left **ventricles**, which have thicker walls and are separated by the **interventricular septum** (Fig. 12–2). As you will see, the atria receive blood, either from the body or the lungs, and the ventricles pump blood to either the lungs or the body.

RIGHT ATRIUM

Two large veins return blood from the body to the right atrium (see Fig. 12–2). The **superior vena cava** carries blood from the upper body, and the **inferior vena cava** carries blood from the lower body. From the right atrium, blood will flow through the right **atrioventricular (AV) valve**, or **tricuspid valve**, into the right ventricle.

The tricuspid valve is made of three flaps (or cusps) of endocardium reinforced with connective tissue. The general purpose of all valves in the circulatory system is to prevent backflow of blood. The specific purpose of the tricuspid valve is to prevent backflow of blood from the right ventricle to the right atrium when the right ventricle contracts. As the ventricle contracts, blood is forced behind the three valve flaps, forcing them upward and together to close the valve.

LEFT ATRIUM

The left atrium receives blood from the lungs, by way of four **pulmonary veins**. This blood will then flow into the left ventricle through the left atrioventricular (AV) valve, also called the **mitral valve** or **bicuspid** (two flaps) valve. The mitral valve prevents backflow of blood from the left ventricle to the left atrium when the left ventricle contracts.

Another function of the atria is the production of a hormone involved in blood pressure maintenance. When the walls of the atria are stretched, for instance, by increased blood volume or blood pressure, the cells produce **atrial natriuretic hormone**, abbreviated ANH, and also called atrial natriuretic peptide, or ANP. (The ventricles of the heart produce a similar hormone, but we will use ANH as the representative cardiac hormone.) ANH decreases the reabsorption of sodium ions by the kidneys, so that more sodium ions are excreted in urine, which in turn increases the elimination of water. The loss of water lowers blood volume and blood pressure. You may have noticed that ANH is an antagonist to the hormone aldosterone, which raises blood pressure.

RIGHT VENTRICLE

When the right ventricle contracts, the tricuspid valve closes, and the blood is pumped to the lungs through the pulmonary artery (or trunk). At the junction of this large artery and the right ventricle is the **pulmonary semilunar valve**. Its three flaps are forced open when the right ventricle contracts and pumps blood into the pulmonary artery. When the right ventricle relaxes, blood tends to come back, but this fills the valve flaps and closes the pulmonary semilunar valve to prevent backflow of blood into the right ventricle.

Projecting into the lower part of the right ventricle are columns of myocardium called **papillary muscles** (see Fig. 12–2). Strands of fibrous connective tissue, the **chordae tendineae**, extend from the papillary muscles to the flaps of the tricuspid valve. When the right ventricle contracts, the papillary muscles also contract and pull on the chordae tendineae to prevent inversion of the tricuspid valve. If you have ever had your umbrella blown inside out by a strong wind, you can see what would happen if the flaps of the tricuspid valve were not anchored by the chordae tendineae and papillary muscles.

LEFT VENTRICLE

The walls of the left ventricle are thicker than those of the right ventricle, which enables the left ventricle to contract more forcefully. The left ventricle pumps blood to the body through the **aorta**, the largest artery of the body. At the junction of the aorta and the left ventricle is the **aortic semilunar valve** (see Fig. 12–2). This valve is opened by the force of contraction of the left ventricle, which also closes the mitral valve. The aortic semilunar valve closes when the left ventricle relaxes, to prevent backflow of blood from the aorta to the left ventricle. When the mitral (left AV) valve closes, it prevents backflow of blood to the left atrium; the flaps of the mitral valve are also anchored by chordae tendineae and papillary muscles. All of the valves are shown in Fig. 12–3, which also depicts the skeleton of the heart. This is fibrous connective tissue that anchors the outer edges of the valve flaps. It also prevents the contraction of the atria from reaching the ventricles, except by way of the normal conduction pathway.

As you can see from this description of the chambers and their vessels, the heart is really a double, or two-sided, pump. The right side of the heart receives

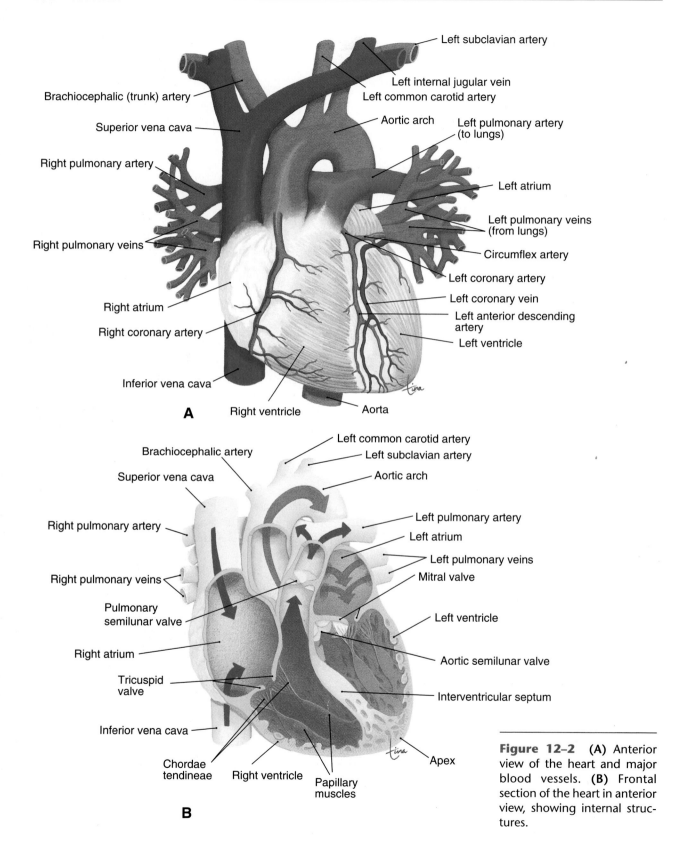

Left subclavian artery

Left internal jugular vein
Left common carotid artery

Brachiocephalic (trunk) artery

Superior vena cava

Aortic arch

Left pulmonary artery
(to lungs)

Right pulmonary artery

Left atrium

Left pulmonary veins
(from lungs)

Right pulmonary veins

Circumflex artery

Left coronary artery

Right atrium

Left coronary vein

Right coronary artery

Left anterior descending
artery

Left ventricle

Inferior vena cava

A   Right ventricle   Aorta

Brachiocephalic artery

Left common carotid artery
Left subclavian artery

Superior vena cava

Aortic arch

Right pulmonary artery

Left pulmonary artery
Left atrium

Left pulmonary veins
Mitral valve

Right pulmonary veins

Pulmonary
semilunar valve

Left ventricle

Right atrium

Aortic semilunar valve

Tricuspid
valve

Interventricular septum

Inferior vena cava

Chordae
tendineae   Right ventricle   Papillary
muscles

Apex

B

Figure 12–2 **(A)** Anterior view of the heart and major blood vessels. **(B)** Frontal section of the heart in anterior view, showing internal structures.

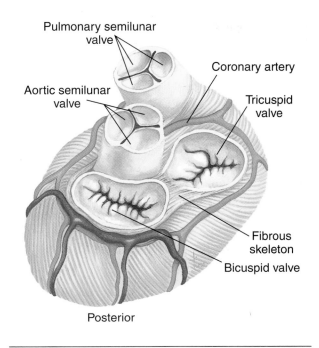

Pulmonary semilunar valve

Aortic semilunar valve

Coronary artery

Tricuspid valve

Fibrous skeleton

Bicuspid valve

Posterior

Figure 12–3   Heart valves in superior view. The atria have been removed. The fibrous skeleton of the heart is fibrous connective tissue that anchors the valve flaps and prevents enlargement of the valve openings.

deoxygenated blood from the body and pumps it to the lungs to pick up oxygen and release carbon dioxide. The left side of the heart receives oxygenated blood from the lungs and pumps it to the body. Both pumps work simultaneously; that is, both atria contract together, followed by the contraction of both ventricles.

CORONARY VESSELS

The right and left **coronary arteries** are the first branches of the ascending aorta, just beyond the aortic semilunar valve (Fig. 12–4). The two arteries branch into smaller arteries and arterioles, then to capillaries. The coronary capillaries merge to form coronary veins, which empty blood into a large coronary sinus that returns blood to the right atrium.

The purpose of the coronary vessels is to supply blood to the myocardium itself, because oxygen is essential for normal myocardial contraction. If a coronary artery becomes obstructed, by a blood clot for example, part of the myocardium becomes **ischemic**, that is, deprived of its blood supply. Prolonged ischemia will create an **infarct**, an area of

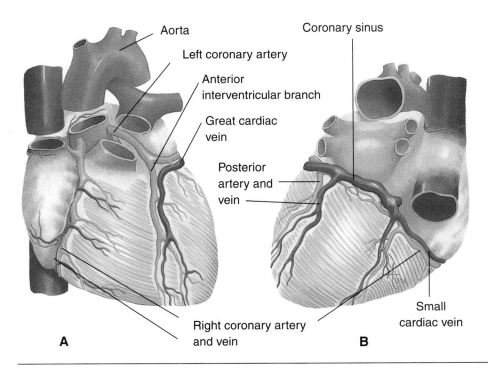

Aorta

Left coronary artery

Anterior interventricular branch

Great cardiac vein

Posterior artery and vein

Coronary sinus

Small cardiac vein

Right coronary artery and vein

A

B

Figure 12–4   (A) Coronary vessels in anterior view. The pulmonary artery has been cut to show the left coronary artery emerging from the ascending aorta. (B) Coronary vessels in posterior view. The coronary sinus empties blood into the right atrium.

necrotic (dead) tissue. This is a myocardial infarction, commonly called a heart attack (see also Box 12–1: Risk Factors for Heart Disease).

CARDIAC CYCLE AND HEART SOUNDS

The **cardiac cycle** is the sequence of events in one heartbeat. In its simplest form, the cardiac cycle is the simultaneous contraction of the two atria, followed a fraction of a second later by the simultaneous contraction of the two ventricles. **Systole** is another term for contraction. The term for relaxation is **diastole**. You are probably familiar with these terms as they apply to blood pressure readings. If we apply them to the cardiac cycle, we can say that atrial systole is followed by ventricular systole. There is, however, a significant difference between the movement of blood from the atria to the ventricles and the movement of blood from the ventricles to the arteries. The events of the cardiac cycle are shown in Fig. 12–5. In this traditional representation, the cardiac cycle is depicted in a circle, because one heartbeat follows another, and the beginning event is atrial systole (at 12 o'clock). The size of the segment or arc of the circle indicates how long it takes. Find the segment for atrial systole and the one for ventricular systole, and notice how much larger (meaning: longer) ventricular systole is. Do you think this might mean that ventricular contraction is more important than atrial contraction? It does, as you will see. Refer to Fig. 12–5 as you read the following. We will begin at the bottom (6 o'clock) where the atria are in the midst of diastole and the ventricles have just completed their systole. The entire heart is relaxed and the atria are filling with blood.

Blood is constantly flowing from the veins into both atria. As more blood accumulates, its pressure forces open the right and left AV valves. Two thirds of the atrial blood flows passively into the ventricles (which brings us to 12 o'clock); the atria then contract to pump the remaining blood into the ventricles.

Following their contraction, the atria relax and the ventricles begin to contract. Ventricular contraction forces blood against the flaps of the right and left AV valves and closes them; the force of blood also opens the aortic and left semilunar valves. As the ventricles continue to contract, they pump blood into the arteries. Notice that blood that enters the arteries must all be pumped. The ventricles then relax, and at the same time blood continues to flow into the atria, and the cycle will begin again.

The important distinction here is that most blood flows passively from atria to ventricles, but *all* blood to the arteries is actively pumped by the ventricles. For this reason, the proper functioning of the ventricles is much more crucial to survival than is atrial functioning.

You may be asking: all this in one heartbeat? The answer is yes. The cardiac cycle is this precise sequence of events that keeps blood moving from the veins, through the heart, and into the arteries.

The cardiac cycle also creates the **heart sounds:** each heartbeat produces two sounds, often called lub-dup, that can be heard with a stethoscope. The first sound, the loudest and longest, is caused by ventricular systole closing the AV valves. The second sound is caused by the closure of the aortic and pulmonary semilunar valves. If any of the valves do not close properly, an extra sound called a **heart murmur** may be heard (see Box 12–2: Heart Murmur).

CARDIAC CONDUCTION PATHWAY

The cardiac cycle is a sequence of mechanical events that is regulated by the electrical activity of the myocardium. Cardiac muscle cells have the ability to contract spontaneously, that is, nerve impulses are not required to cause contraction. The heart generates its own beat, and the electrical impulses follow a very specific route throughout the myocardium. You may find it helpful to refer to Fig. 12–6 as you read the following.

The natural pacemaker of the heart is the **sinoatrial (SA) node**, a specialized group of cardiac muscle cells located in the wall of the right atrium. The SA node is considered specialized because it has the most rapid rate of contraction, that is, it depolarizes more rapidly than any other part of the myocardium. As you may recall, depolarization is the rapid entry of Na^+ ions and the reversal of charges on either side of the cell membrane. The cells of the SA node are more permeable to Na^+ ions than are other cardiac muscle cells. Therefore, they depolarize more rapidly, then contract and initiate each heartbeat.

From the SA node, impulses for contraction travel to the **atrioventricular (AV) node**, located in the lower interatrial septum. The transmission of impulses

Box 12–1   RISK FACTORS FOR HEART DISEASE

Coronary artery disease results in decreased blood flow to the myocardium. If blood flow is diminished but not completely obstructed, the person may experience angina, which is chest pain caused by lack of oxygen to part of the heart muscle. If blood flow is completely blocked, however, the result is a myocardial infarction (necrosis of cardiac muscle).

The most common cause of coronary artery disease is **atherosclerosis**. Plaques of cholesterol from in the walls of a coronary artery; this narrows the lumen (cavity) and creates a rough surface where a clot (thrombus) may form (see Box Figure 12–A). Predisposing factors for atherosclerosis include cigarette smoking, diabetes mellitus, and high blood pressure. Any one of these may cause damage to the lining of coronary arteries, which is the first step in the abnormal deposition of cholesterol. A diet high in cholesterol and saturated fats and high blood levels of these lipids will increase the rate of cholesterol deposition.

A possible risk factor is a high blood level of homocysteine. Homocysteine is a metabolic product of the essential amino acid methionine, and may be converted back to methionine or further changed and excreted by the kidneys. Research indicates that homocysteine contributes to inflammation of the walls of arteries. A diet low in meat and high in the vitamins B_6, B_{12}, and folic acid helps lower the blood homocysteine level.

Another predisposing factor is a family history of coronary artery disease. There is no "gene for heart attacks," but we do have genes for the enzymes involved in cholesterol metabolism. Many of these are liver enzymes that regulate the transport of cholesterol in the blood in the form of lipoproteins and regulate the liver's excretion of excess cholesterol in bile. Some people, therefore, have a greater tendency than others to have higher blood levels of cholesterol and certain lipoproteins. In women before menopause, estrogen is believed to exert a protective effect by lowering blood lipid levels. This is why heart attacks in the 30- to 50-year-old age range are more frequent in men than in women.

What can an individual do to minimize the risk of coronary artery disease? There is no way to change a hereditary predisposition, but other sensible steps can be taken. First, don't smoke. Second, maintain a diet low in cholesterol and saturated fats. Third, maintain normal body weight through exercise and a diet with a variety of fruits and vegetables. Fourth, have regular blood pressure checks and, if hypertension develops, follow the recommendations of a physician to maintain normal blood pressure.

When coronary artery disease may be life-threatening, coronary artery **bypass surgery** may be performed. In this procedure, a synthetic vessel or a vein (such as the saphenous vein of the leg) is grafted around the obstructed coronary vessel to restore blood flow to the myocardium. This is not a cure, for atherosclerosis may occur in a grafted vein or at other sites in the coronary arteries. The person who has such surgery should follow the guidelines described previously.

Normal artery   Atherosclerotic artery

A   B

Box Figure 12–A   **(A)** Cross-section of normal coronary artery. **(B)** Coronary artery with atherosclerosis narrowing the lumen.

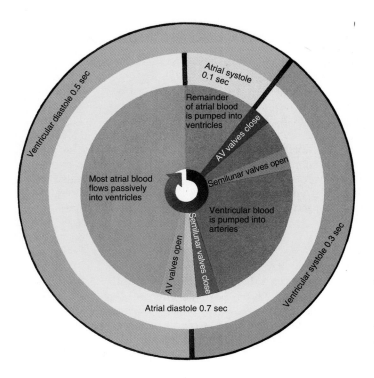

Ventricular diastole 0.5 sec

Atrial systole
0.1 sec

Remainder
of atrial blood
is pumped into
ventricles

AV valves close

Semilunar valves open

Most atrial blood
flows passively
into ventricles

Ventricular blood
is pumped into
arteries

Semilunar valves close

AV valves open

Atrial diastole 0.7 sec

Ventricular systole 0.3 sec

Figure 12–5 The cardiac cycle depicted in one heartbeat (pulse: 75). The outer circle represents the ventricles, the middle circle the atria, and the inner circle the movement of blood and its effect on the heart valves. See text for description.

from the SA node to the AV node and to the rest of the atrial myocardium brings about atrial systole.

Within the upper interventricular septum is the **bundle of His** (AV bundle), which receives impulses from the AV node and transmits them to the right and left **bundle branches**. From the bundle branches, impulses travel along **Purkinje fibers** to the rest of the ventricular myocardium and bring about

ventricular systole. The electrical activity of the atria and ventricles is depicted by an electrocardiogram (ECG); this is discussed in Box 12–3: Electrocardiogram.

If the SA node does not function properly, the AV node will initiate the heartbeat, but at a slower rate (50 to 60 beats per minute). The bundle of His is also capable of generating the beat of the ventricles, but

Box 12–2 HEART MURMUR

A heart murmur is an abnormal or extra heart sound caused by a malfunctioning heart valve. The function of heart valves is to prevent backflow of blood, and when a valve does not close properly, blood will regurgitate (go backward), creating turbulence that may be heard with a stethoscope.

Rheumatic heart disease is a now uncommon complication of a streptococcal infection. In rheumatic fever, the heart valves are damaged by an abnormal response by the immune system. Erosion of the valves makes them "leaky" and inefficient, and a murmur of backflowing blood will be heard. Mitral valve regurgitation, for example, will be heard as a systolic murmur, because this valve is meant to close and prevent backflow during ventricular systole.

Some valve defects involve a narrowing **(stenosis)** and are congenital, that is, the child is born with an abnormally narrow valve. In aortic stenosis, for example, blood cannot easily pass from the left ventricle to the aorta. The ventricle must then work harder to pump blood through the narrow valve to the arteries, and the turbulence created is also heard as a systolic murmur.

Children sometimes have heart murmurs that are called "functional" because no structural cause can be found. These murmurs usually disappear with no adverse effects on the child.

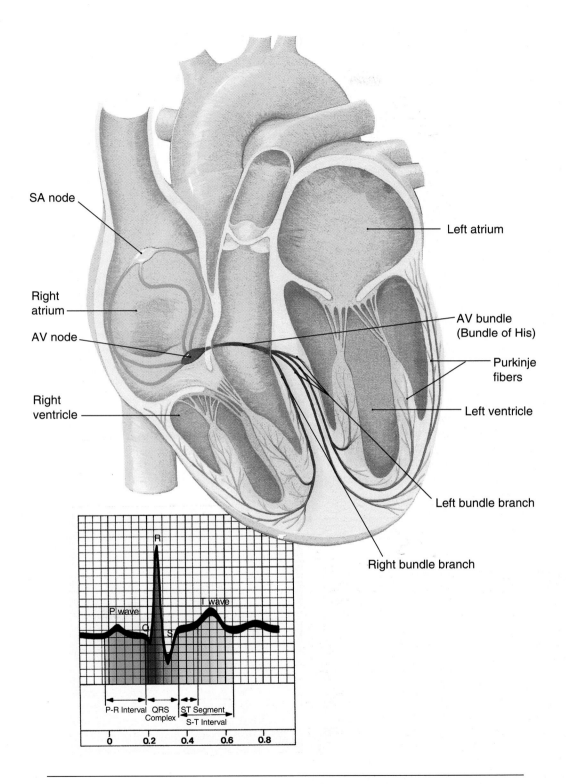

Figure 12–6 Conduction pathway of the heart. Anterior view of the interior of the heart. The electrocardiogram tracing is of one normal heartbeat. See text and Box 12–3 for description.

Box 12–3   ELECTROCARDIOGRAM

A heartbeat is a series of electrical events, and the electrical changes generated by the myocardium can be recorded by placing electrodes on the body surface. Such a recording is called an **electrocardiogram (ECG)** (see Fig. 12–6).

A typical ECG consists of three distinguishable waves or deflections: the P wave, the QRS complex, and the T wave. Each represents a specific electrical event; all are shown in Fig. 12–6 in a normal ECG tracing.

The P wave represents depolarization of the atria, that is, the transmission of electrical impulses from the SA node throughout the atrial myocardium.

The QRS complex represents depolarization of the ventricles as the electrical impulses spread throughout the ventricular myocardium. The T wave represents repolarization of the ventricles (atrial repolarization does not appear as a separate wave because it is masked by the QRS complex).

Detailed interpretation of abnormal ECGs is beyond the scope of this book, but in general, the length of each wave and the time intervals between waves are noted. An ECG may be helpful in the diagnosis of coronary atherosclerosis, which deprives the myocardium of oxygen, or of rheumatic fever or other valve disorders that result in enlargement of a chamber of the heart and prolong a specific wave of an ECG. For example, the enlargement of the left ventricle that is often a consequence of hypertension may be indicated by an abnormal QRS complex.

---

at a much slower rate (15 to 40 beats per minute). This may occur in certain kinds of heart disease in which transmission of impulses from the atria to the ventricles is blocked.

Arrhythmias are irregular heartbeats; their effects range from harmless to life-threatening. Nearly everyone experiences heart **palpitations** (becoming aware of an irregular beat) from time to time. These are usually not serious and may be the result of too much caffeine, nicotine, or alcohol. Much more serious is ventricular **fibrillation**, a very rapid and uncoordinated ventricular beat that is totally ineffective for pumping blood (see Box 12–4: Arrhythmias).

HEART RATE

A healthy adult has a resting heart rate **(pulse)** of 60 to 80 beats per minute, which is the rate of depolarization of the SA node. A rate less than 60 (except for

---

Box 12–4   ARRHYTHMIAS

Arrhythmias (also called dysrhythmias) are irregular heartbeats caused by damage to part of the conduction pathway, or by an **ectopic focus**, which is a beat generated in part of the myocardium other than the SA node.

Flutter is a very rapid but fairly regular heartbeat. In atrial flutter, the atria may contract up to 300 times per minute. Because atrial pumping is not crucial, however, blood flow to the ventricles may be maintained for a time, and flutter may not be immediately life-threatening. Ventricular flutter is usually only a brief transition between ventricular tachycardia and fibrillation.

Fibrillation is very rapid and uncoordinated contractions. Ventricular fibrillation is a medical emergency that must be rapidly corrected to prevent death. Normal contraction of the ventricles is necessary to pump blood into the arteries, but fibrillating ventricles are not pumping, and cardiac output decreases sharply.

Ventricular fibrillation may follow a non-fatal heart attack (myocardial infarction). Damaged cardiac muscle cells may not be able to maintain a normal state of polarization, and they depolarize spontaneously and rapidly. From this ectopic focus, impulses spread to other parts of the ventricular myocardium in a rapid and haphazard pattern, and the ventricles quiver rather than contract as a unit.

It is often possible to correct ventricular fibrillation with the use of an electrical defibrillator. This instrument delivers an electric shock to the heart, which causes the entire myocardium to depolarize and contract, then relax. If the first part of the heart to recover is the SA node (which usually has the most rapid rate of contraction), a normal heartbeat may be restored.

athletes) is called **bradycardia**; a prolonged or consistent rate greater than 100 beats per minute is called **tachycardia**.

A child's normal heart rate may be as high as 100 beats per minute, that of an infant as high as 120, and that of a near-term fetus as high as 140 beats per minute. These higher rates are not related to age, but rather to size: the smaller the individual, the higher the metabolic rate and the faster the heart rate. Parallels may be found among animals of different sizes; the heart rate of a mouse is about 200 beats per minute and that of an elephant about 30 beats per minute.

Let us return to the adult heart rate and consider the person who is in excellent physical condition. As you may know, well-conditioned athletes have low resting pulse rates. Those of basketball players are often around 50 beats per minute, and the pulse of a marathon runner often ranges from 35 to 40 beats per minute. To understand why this is so, remember that the heart is a muscle. When our skeletal muscles are exercised, they become stronger and more efficient. The same is true for the heart; consistent exercise makes it a more efficient pump, as you will see in the next discussion.

CARDIAC OUTPUT

Cardiac output is the amount of blood pumped by a ventricle in 1 minute. A certain level of cardiac output is needed at all times to transport oxygen to tissues and to remove waste products. During exercise, cardiac output must increase to meet the body's need for more oxygen. We will return to exercise after first considering resting cardiac output.

In order to calculate cardiac output, we must know the pulse rate and how much blood is pumped per beat. **Stroke volume** is the term for the amount of blood pumped by a ventricle per beat; an average resting stroke volume is 60 to 80 ml per beat. A simple formula then enables us to determine cardiac output:

Cardiac output = stroke volume × pulse (heart rate)

Let us put into this formula an average resting stroke volume, 70 ml, and an average resting pulse, 70 beats per minute (bpm):

Cardiac output = 70 ml × 70 bpm

Cardiac output = 4900 ml per minute
(approximately 5 liters)

Naturally, cardiac output varies with the size of the person, but the average resting cardiac output is 5 to 6 liters per minute.

If we now reconsider the athlete, you will be able to see precisely why the athlete has a low resting pulse. In our formula, we will use an average resting cardiac output (5 liters) and an athlete's pulse rate (50):

Cardiac output = stroke volume × pulse

5000 ml = stroke volume × 50 bpm

5000/50 = stroke volume

100 ml = stroke volume

Notice that the athlete's resting stroke volume is significantly higher than the average. The athlete's more efficient heart pumps more blood with each beat and so can maintain a normal resting cardiac output with fewer beats.

Now let us see how the heart responds to exercise. Heart rate (pulse) increases during exercise, and so does stroke volume. The increase in stroke volume is the result of **Starling's Law of the Heart**, which states that the more the cardiac muscle fibers are stretched, the more forcefully they contract. During exercise, more blood returns to the heart; this is called **venous return**. Increased venous return stretches the myocardium of the ventricles, which contract more forcefully and pump more blood, thereby increasing stroke volume. Therefore, during exercise, our formula might be the following:

Cardiac output = stoke volume × pulse

Cardiac output = 100 ml × 100 bpm

Cardiac output = 10,000 ml (10 liters)

This exercise cardiac output is twice the resting cardiac output we first calculated, which should not be considered unusual. The cardiac output of a healthy young person may increase up to four times the resting level during strenuous exercise. The marathon runner's cardiac output may increase six times or more compared to the resting level; this is the result of the marathoner's extremely efficient heart.

Also related to cardiac output, and another measure of the health of the heart, is the **ejection fraction**. This is the percent of the blood in a ventricle that is pumped during systole. A ventricle doesn't empty completely when it contracts, but should pump out 60% to 70% of the blood within it. A lower percentage would indicate that the ventricle is weakening.

REGULATION OF HEART RATE

Although the heart generates and maintains its own beat, the rate of contraction can be changed to adapt to different situations. The nervous system can and does bring about necessary changes in heart rate as well as in force of contraction.

The **medulla** of the brain contains the two cardiac centers, the **accelerator center** and the **inhibitory center**. These centers send impulses to the heart along autonomic nerves. Recall from Chapter 8 that the autonomic nervous system has two divisions: sympathetic and parasympathetic. Sympathetic impulses from the accelerator center along sympathetic nerves increase heart rate and force of contraction. Parasympathetic impulses from the inhibitory center along the vagus nerves decrease the heart rate.

Our next question might be: What information is received by the medulla to initiate changes? Because the heart pumps blood, it is essential to maintain normal blood pressure. Blood contains oxygen, which all tissues must receive continuously. Therefore, changes in blood pressure and oxygen level of the blood are stimuli for changes in heart rate.

You may also recall from Chapter 9 that pressoreceptors and chemoreceptors are located in the carotid arteries and aortic arch. **Pressoreceptors** in the carotid sinuses and aortic sinus detect changes in blood pressure. **Chemoreceptors** in the carotid bodies and aortic body detect changes in the oxygen content of the blood. The sensory nerves for the carotid receptors are the glossopharyngeal (9th cranial) nerves; the sensory nerves for the aortic arch receptors are the vagus (10th cranial) nerves. If we now put all of these facts together in a specific example, you will see that the regulation of heart rate is a reflex. Figure 12–7 depicts all of the structures mentioned above.

A person who stands up suddenly from a lying position may feel light-headed or dizzy for a few moments, because blood pressure to the brain has decreased abruptly. The drop in blood pressure is detected by pressoreceptors in the carotid sinuses—notice that they are "on the way" to the brain, a very strategic location. The drop in blood pressure causes fewer impulses to be generated by the pressoreceptors. These impulses travel along the glossopharyngeal nerves to the medulla, and the decrease in the frequency of impulses stimulates the accelerator center. The accelerator center generates impulses that are carried by sympathetic nerves to the SA node, AV node, and the ventricular myocardium. As heart rate and force increase, blood pressure to the brain is raised to normal, and the sensation of light-headedness passes. When blood pressure to the brain is restored to normal, the heart receives more parasympathetic impulses from the inhibitory center along the vagus nerves to the SA node and AV node. These parasympathetic impulses slow the heart rate to a normal resting pace.

The heart will also be the effector in a reflex stimulated by a decrease in the oxygen content of the blood. The aortic receptors are strategically located so as to detect such an important change as soon as blood leaves the heart. The reflex arc in this situation would be (1) aortic chemoreceptors, (2) vagus nerves (sensory), (3) accelerator center in the medulla, (4) sympathetic nerves, and (5) the heart muscle, which will increase its rate and force of contraction to circulate more oxygen to correct the hypoxia.

Recall also from Chapter 10 that the hormone epinephrine is secreted by the adrenal medulla in stressful situations. One of the many functions of epinephrine is to increase heart rate and force of contraction. This will help supply more blood to tissues in need of more oxygen.

AGING AND THE HEART

The heart muscle becomes less efficient with age, and there is a decrease in both maximum cardiac output and heart rate, although resting levels may be more than adequate. The health of the myocardium depends on its blood supply, and with age there is greater likelihood that atherosclerosis will narrow the coronary arteries. Atherosclerosis is the deposition of cholesterol on and in the walls of the arteries, which decreases blood flow and forms rough surfaces that may cause intravascular clot formation.

High blood pressure (hypertension) causes the left ventricle to work harder; it may enlarge and outgrow its blood supply, thus becoming weaker. A weak ventricle is not an efficient pump, and such weakness may progress to congestive heart failure; such a progression may be slow, or may be rapid. The heart valves may become thickened by fibrosis, leading to heart murmurs and less efficient pumping. Arrhythmias are also more common with age, as the cells of the conduction pathway become less efficient.

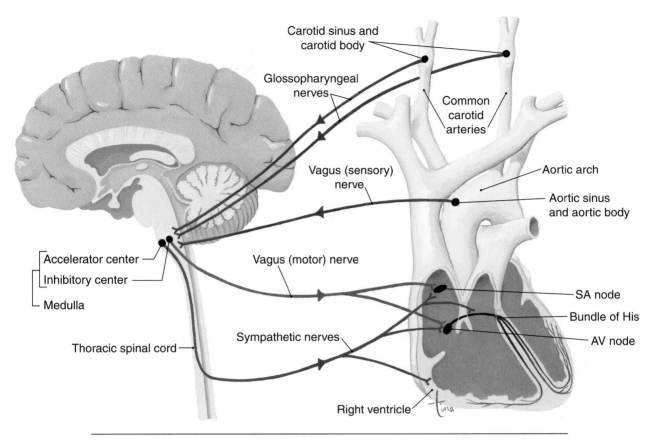

Figure 12–7 Nervous regulation of the heart. The brain and spinal cord are shown on the left. The heart and major blood vessels are shown on the right.

SUMMARY

As you can see, the nervous system regulates the functioning of the heart based on what the heart is supposed to do. The pumping of the heart maintains normal blood pressure and proper oxygenation of tissues, and the nervous system ensures that the heart will be able to meet these demands in different situations. Blood pressure and the blood vessels are the subjects of the next chapter.

STUDY OUTLINE

The heart pumps blood, which creates blood pressure, and circulates oxygen, nutrients, and other substances. The heart is located in the mediastinum, the area between the lungs in the thoracic cavity.

Pericardial Membranes—three layers that enclose the heart (see Fig. 12–1)

1. The outer, fibrous pericardium, made of fibrous connective tissue, is a loose-fitting sac that surrounds the heart and extends over the diaphragm and the bases of the great vessels.
2. The parietal pericardium is a serous membrane that lines the fibrous pericardium.
3. The visceral pericardium, or epicardium, is a serous membrane on the surface of the myocardium.

4. Serous fluid between the parietal and visceral pericardial membranes prevents friction as the heart beats.

Chambers of the Heart (see Fig. 12–2)

1. Cardiac muscle tissue, the myocardium, forms the walls of the four chambers of the heart.
2. Endocardium lines the chambers and covers the valves of the heart; is simple squamous epithelium that is very smooth and prevents abnormal clotting.
3. The right and left atria are the upper chambers, separated by the interatrial septum. The atria receive blood from veins.
4. The right and left ventricles are the lower chambers, separated by the interventricular septum. The ventricles pump blood into arteries.

Right Atrium

1. Receives blood from the upper body by way of the superior vena cava and receives blood from the lower body by way of the inferior vena cava.
2. The tricuspid (right AV) valve prevents backflow of blood from the right ventricle to the right atrium when the right ventricle contracts.

Left Atrium

1. Receives blood from the lungs by way of four pulmonary veins.
2. The mitral (left AV or bicuspid) valve prevents backflow of blood from the left ventricle to the left atrium when the left ventricle contracts.
3. The walls of the atria produce atrial natriuretic hormone when stretched by increased blood volume or BP. ANH increases the loss of Na^+ ions and water in urine, which decreases blood volume and BP to normal.

Right Ventricle—has relatively thin walls

1. Pumps blood to the lungs through the pulmonary artery.
2. The pulmonary semilunar valve prevents backflow of blood from the pulmonary artery to the right ventricle when the right ventricle relaxes.
3. Papillary muscles and chordae tendineae prevent inversion of the right AV valve when the right ventricle contracts.

Left Ventricle—has thicker walls than does the right ventricle

1. Pumps blood to the body through the aorta.

2. The aortic semilunar valve prevents backflow of blood from the aorta to the left ventricle when the left ventricle relaxes.
3. Papillary muscles and chordae tendineae prevent inversion of the left AV valve when the left ventricle contracts.
4. The heart is a double pump: The right heart receives deoxygenated blood from the body and pumps it to the lungs; the left heart receives oxygenated blood from the lungs and pumps it to the body. Both sides of the heart work simultaneously.

Coronary Vessels (see Fig. 12–4)

1. Pathway: ascending aorta to right and left coronary arteries, to smaller arteries, to capillaries, to coronary veins, to the coronary sinus, to the right atrium.
2. Coronary circulation supplies oxygenated blood to the myocardium.
3. Obstruction of a coronary artery causes a myocardial infarction: death of an area of myocardium due to lack of oxygen.

Cardiac Cycle—the sequence of events in one heartbeat (see Fig. 12–5)

1. The atria continually receive blood from the veins; as pressure within the atria increases, the AV valves are opened.
2. Two-thirds of the atrial blood flows passively into the ventricles; atrial contraction pumps the remaining blood into the ventricles; the atria then relax.
3. The ventricles contract, which closes the AV valves and opens the aortic and pulmonary semilunar valves.
4. Ventricular contraction pumps all blood into the arteries. The ventricles then relax. Meanwhile, blood is filling the atria, and the cycle begins again.
5. Systole means contraction; diastole means relaxation. In the cardiac cycle, atrial systole is followed by ventricular systole. When the ventricles are in systole, the atria are in diastole.
6. The mechanical events of the cardiac cycle keep blood moving from the veins through the heart and into the arteries.

Heart Sounds—two sounds per heartbeat: lub-dup

1. The first sound is created by closure of the AV valves during ventricular systole.

2. The second sound is created by closure of the aortic and pulmonary semilunar valves.
3. Improper closing of a valve results in a heart murmur.

Cardiac Conduction Pathway—the pathway of impulses during the cardiac cycle (see Fig. 12–6)

1. The SA node in the wall of the right atrium initiates each heartbeat; the cells of the SA node are more permeable to Na^+ ions and depolarize more rapidly than any other part of the myocardium.
2. The AV node is in the lower interatrial septum. Depolarization of the SA node spreads to the AV node and to the atrial myocardium and brings about atrial systole.
3. The bundle of His is in the upper interventricular septum; the first part of the ventricles to depolarize.
4. The right and left bundle branches in the interventricular septum transmit impulses to the Purkinje fibers in the ventricular myocardium, which complete ventricular systole.
5. An electrocardiogram (ECG) depicts the electrical activity of the heart (see Fig. 12–6).
6. If part of the conduction pathway does not function properly, the next part will initiate contraction, but at a slower rate.
7. Arrhythmias are irregular heartbeats; their effects range from harmless to life-threatening.

Heart Rate

1. Healthy adult: 60 to 80 beats per minute (heart rate equals pulse); children and infants have faster pulses because of their smaller size and higher metabolic rate.
2. A person in excellent physical condition has a slow resting pulse because the heart is a more efficient pump and pumps more blood per beat.

Cardiac Output

1. Cardiac output is the amount of blood pumped by a ventricle in 1 minute.

2. Stroke volume is the amount of blood pumped by a ventricle in one beat; average is 60 to 80 ml.
3. Cardiac output equals stroke volume × pulse; average resting cardiac output is 5 to 6 liters.
4. Starling's Law of the Heart—the more that cardiac muscle fibers are stretched, the more forcefully they contract.
5. During exercise, stroke volume increases as venous return increases and stretches the myocardium of the ventricles (Starling's Law).
6. During exercise, the increase in stroke volume and the increase in pulse result in an increase in cardiac output: two to four times the resting level.
7. The ejection fraction is the percent of its total blood that a ventricle pumps; average is 60% to 70%.

Regulation of Heart Rate (see Fig. 12–7)

1. The heart generates its own beat, but the nervous system brings about changes to adapt to different situations.
2. The medulla contains the cardiac centers: the accelerator center and the inhibitory center.
3. Sympathetic impulses to the heart increase rate and force of contraction; parasympathetic impulses (vagus nerves) to the heart decrease heart rate.
4. Pressoreceptors in the carotid and aortic sinuses detect changes in blood pressure.
5. Chemoreceptors in the carotid and aortic bodies detect changes in the oxygen content of the blood.
6. The glossopharyngeal nerves are sensory for the carotid receptors. The vagus nerves are sensory for the aortic receptors.
7. If blood pressure to the brain decreases, pressoreceptors in the carotid sinuses detect this decrease and send fewer sensory impulses along the glossopharyngeal nerves to the medulla. The accelerator center dominates and sends motor impulses along sympathetic nerves to increase heart rate and force to restore blood pressure to normal.
8. A similar reflex is activated by hypoxia.
9. Epinephrine from the adrenal medulla increases heart rate and force of contraction during stressful situations.

REVIEW QUESTIONS

1. Describe the location of the heart with respect to the lungs and to the diaphragm. (p. 260)

2. Name the three pericardial membranes. Where is serous fluid found and what is its function? (p. 260)

3. Describe the location and explain the function of endocardium. (p. 260)

4. Name the veins that enter the right atrium; name those that enter the left atrium. For each, where does the blood come from? (p. 261)

5. Name the artery that leaves the right ventricle; name the artery that leaves the left ventricle. For each, where is the blood going? (p. 261)

6. Explain the purpose of the right and left AV valves and the purpose of the aortic and pulmonary semilunar valves. (p. 261)

7. Describe the coronary system of vessels and explain the purpose of coronary circulation. (p. 263)

8. Define systole, diastole, and cardiac cycle. (p. 264)

9. Explain how movement of blood from atria to ventricles differs from movement of blood from ventricles to arteries. (p. 264)

10. Explain why the heart is considered a double pump. Trace the path of blood from the right atrium back to the right atrium, naming the chambers of the heart and their vessels through which the blood passes. (pp. 261, 263)

11. Name the parts, in order, of the cardiac conduction pathway. Explain why it is the SA node that generates each heartbeat. State a normal range of heart rate for a healthy adult. (pp. 264, 266)

12. Calculate cardiac output if stroke volume is 75 ml and pulse is 75 bpm. Using the cardiac output you just calculated as a resting normal, what is the stroke volume of a marathoner whose resting pulse is 40 bpm? (p. 269)

13. Name the two cardiac centers and state their location. Sympathetic impulses to the heart have what effect? Parasympathetic impulses to the heart have what effect? Name the parasympathetic nerves to the heart. (p. 270)

14. State the locations of arterial pressoreceptors and chemoreceptors; what they detect, and their sensory nerves. (p. 270)

15. Describe the reflex arc to increase heart rate and force when blood pressure to the brain decreases. (p. 270)

FOR FURTHER THOUGHT

1. Endocarditis may be caused by bacteria or fungi that erode, or wear away, the heart valves, or in some cases make the valves bumpy (these bumps are called *vegetations*—think cauliflower). Explain the possible consequences of this.

2. Bob, a college freshman, is telling his new friends that he has been running seriously for 6 years, and can run a marathon in a little over 3 hours. His friends aren't sure they should believe him, but don't want to spend 3 hours waiting while Bob runs 26 miles. Bob says that he can prove he is telling the truth in 1 minute. Can he? Explain why or why not.

3. A neighbor, Mrs. G., age 62, tells you that she "doesn't feel right" and is suddenly tired for no apparent reason. She denies having chest pain, though she admits to a "full" feeling she calls indigestion. You suspect that she may be having a heart attack. What question can you ask to help you be more sure? Explain the physiological basis for your question.

4. Several types of artificial hearts are being developed and tested. What are the three essential characteristics a truly useful artificial heart must have? One is obvious, the others, perhaps not as much so.

CHAPTER 13

The Vascular System

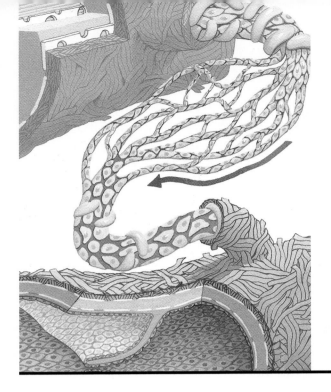

CHAPTER 13

Student Objectives

- Describe the structure of arteries and veins, and relate their structure to function.
- Explain the purpose of arterial and venous anastomoses.
- Describe the structure of capillaries, and explain the exchange processes that take place in capillaries.
- Describe the pathway and purpose of pulmonary circulation.
- Name the branches of the aorta and their distributions.
- Name the major systemic veins, and the parts of the body they drain of blood.
- Describe the pathway and purpose of hepatic portal circulation.
- Describe the modifications of fetal circulation, and explain the purpose of each.
- Explain the importance of slow blood flow in capillaries.
- Define blood pressure, and state the normal ranges for systemic and pulmonary blood pressure.
- Explain the factors that maintain systemic blood pressure.
- Explain how the heart and kidneys are involved in the regulation of blood pressure.
- Explain how the medulla and the autonomic nervous system regulate the diameter of blood vessels.

The Vascular System

New Terminology

Anastomosis (a-NAS-ti-**MOH**-sis)
Arteriole (ar-**TIR**-ee-ohl)
Circle of Willis (**SIR**-kuhl of **WILL**-iss)
Ductus arteriosus (**DUK**-tus ar-TIR-ee-**OH**-sis)
Endothelium (EN-doh-**THEEL**-ee-um)
Foramen ovale (for-**RAY**-men oh-**VAHL**-ee)
Hepatic portal (hep-**PAT**-ik **POOR**-tuhl)
Peripheral resistance (puh-**RIFF**-uh-ruhl
   ree-**ZIS**-tense)
Placenta (pluh-**SEN**-tah)
Precapillary sphincter (pre-**KAP**-i-lar-ee **SFINK**-ter)
Sinusoid (**SIGH**-nuh-soyd)
Umbilical arteries (uhm-**BILL**-i-kull **AR**-tuh-rees)
Umbilical vein (uhm-**BILL**-i-kull VAIN)
Venule (**VEN**-yool)

Related Clinical Terminology

Anaphylactic (AN-uh-fi-**LAK**-tik)
Aneurysm (**AN**-yur-izm)
Arteriosclerosis (ar-TIR-ee-oh-skle-**ROH**-sis)
Hypertension (HIGH-per-**TEN**-shun)
Hypovolemic (HIGH-poh-voh-**LEEM**-ik)
Phlebitis (fle-**BY**-tis)
Pulse deficit (PULS **DEF**-i-sit)
Septic shock (**SEP**-tik SHAHK)
Varicose veins (**VAR**-i-kohs VAINS).

*Terms that appear in **bold type** in the chapter text are defined in the glossary, which begins on page 521.*

The role of blood vessels in the circulation of blood has been known since 1628, when William Harvey, an English anatomist, demonstrated that blood in veins always flowed toward the heart. Before that time, it was believed that blood was static or stationary, some of it within the vessels but the rest sort of in puddles throughout the body. Harvey showed that blood indeed does move, and only in the blood vessels. In the centuries that followed, the active (rather than merely passive) roles of the vascular system were discovered, and all contribute to homeostasis.

The vascular system consists of the arteries, capillaries, and veins through which the heart pumps blood throughout the body. As you will see, the major "business" of the vascular system, which is the exchange of materials between the blood and tissues, takes place in the capillaries. The arteries and veins, however, are just as important, transporting blood between the capillaries and the heart.

Another important topic of this chapter will be blood pressure (BP), which is the force the blood exerts against the walls of the vessels. Normal blood pressure is essential for circulation and for some of the material exchanges that take place in capillaries.

ARTERIES

Arteries carry blood from the heart to capillaries; smaller arteries are called **arterioles**. If we look at an artery in cross-section, we find three layers (or tunics) of tissues, each with different functions (Fig. 13–1).

The innermost layer, the **tunica intima**, is simple squamous epithelium called **endothelium**. This lining is the same type of tissue that forms the endocardium, the lining of the chambers of the heart. As you might guess, its function is also the same: Its extreme smoothness prevents abnormal blood clotting. The **tunica media**, or middle layer, is made of smooth muscle and elastic connective tissue. Both of these tissues are involved in the maintenance of normal blood pressure, especially diastolic blood pressure when the heart is relaxed. Fibrous connective tissue forms the outer layer, the **tunica externa**. This tissue is very strong, which is important to prevent the rupture or bursting of the larger arteries that carry blood under high pressure (see Box 13–1: Disorders of Arteries).

The outer and middle layers of large arteries are quite thick. In the arterioles, only individual smooth muscle cells encircle the tunica intima. The smooth muscle layer enables arteries to constrict or dilate. This is regulated by the medulla and autonomic nervous system and will be discussed in a later section on blood pressure.

VEINS

Veins carry blood from capillaries back to the heart; the smaller veins are called **venules**. The same three tissue layers are present in veins as in the walls of arteries, but there are some differences when compared to the arterial layers. The inner layer of veins is smooth endothelium, but at intervals this lining is folded to form **valves** (see Fig. 13–1). Valves prevent backflow of blood and are most numerous in veins of the legs, where blood must often return to the heart against the force of gravity.

The middle layer of veins is a thin layer of smooth muscle. It is thin because veins do not regulate blood pressure and blood flow into capillaries as arteries do. Veins can constrict extensively, however, and this function becomes very important in certain situations such as severe hemorrhage. The outer layer of veins is also thin; not as much fibrous connective tissue is necessary because blood pressure in veins is very low.

ANASTOMOSES

An **anastomosis** is a connection, or joining, of vessels, that is, artery to artery or vein to vein. The general purpose of these connections is to provide alternate pathways for the flow of blood if one vessel becomes obstructed.

An arterial anastomosis helps ensure that blood will get to the capillaries of an organ to deliver oxygen and nutrients, and to remove waste products. There are arterial anastomoses, for example, between some of the coronary arteries that supply blood to the myocardium.

A venous anastomosis helps ensure that blood will be able to return to the heart in order to be pumped again. Venous anastomoses are most numerous among the veins of the legs, where the possibility of obstruction increases as a person gets older (see Box 13–2: Disorders of Veins).

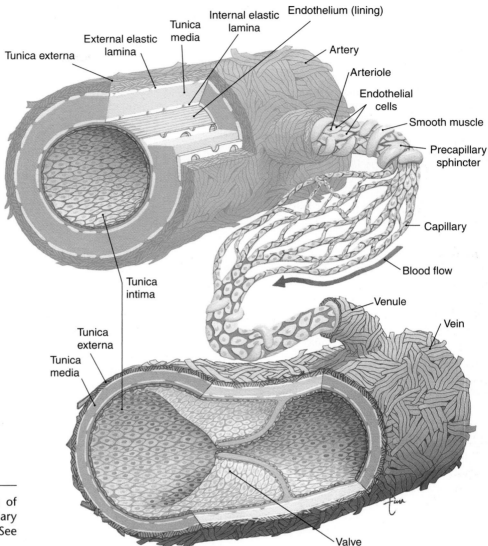

Figure 13–1 Structure of an artery, arteriole, capillary network, venule, and vein. See text for description.

CAPILLARIES

Capillaries carry blood from arterioles to venules. Their walls are only one cell in thickness; capillaries are actually the extension of just the simple squamous lining of arteries and veins (see Fig. 13–1). Some tissues do not have capillaries; these are the epidermis, cartilage, and the lens and cornea of the eye.

Most tissues, however, have extensive capillary networks. Blood flow into these networks is regulated by smooth muscle cells called **precapillary sphincters**, found at the beginning of each network (see Fig.

13–1). Precapillary sphincters are not regulated by the nervous system but rather constrict or dilate depending on the needs of the tissues. Because there is not enough blood in the body to fill all of the capillaries at once, precapillary sphincters are usually slightly constricted. In an active tissue that requires more oxygen, such as exercising muscle, the precapillary sphincters dilate to increase blood flow. These automatic responses ensure that blood, the volume of which is constant, will circulate where it is needed most.

Some organs have another type of capillary called **sinusoids**, which are larger and more permeable than

Box 13–1   DISORDERS OF ARTERIES

Arteriosclerosis—although commonly called "hardening of the arteries," arteriosclerosis really means that the arteries lose their elasticity, and their walls become weakened. Arteries carry blood under high pressure, so deterioration of their walls is part of the aging process.

Aneurysm—a weak portion of an arterial wall may bulge out, forming a sac or bubble called an aneurysm. Arteriosclerosis is a possible cause, but some aneurysms are congenital. An aneurysm may be present for many years without any symptoms and may only be discovered during diagnostic

procedures for some other purpose.

The most common sites for aneurysm formation are the cerebral arteries and the aorta. Rupture of a cerebral aneurysm is a possible cause of a cerebrovascular accident (CVA). Rupture of an aortic aneurysm is life-threatening and requires immediate corrective surgery. The damaged portion of the artery is removed and replaced with a graft. Such surgery may also be performed when an aneurysm is found before it ruptures.

Atherosclerosis—this condition has been mentioned previously; see Chapter 12.

Box 13–2   DISORDERS OF VEINS

Phlebitis—inflammation of a vein. This condition is most common in the veins of the legs because they are subjected to great pressure as the blood is returned to the heart against the force of gravity. Often no specific cause can be determined, but advancing age, obesity, and blood disorders may be predisposing factors.

If a superficial vein is affected, the area may be tender or painful, but blood flow is usually maintained because there are so many anastomoses among these veins. Deep vein phlebitis is potentially more serious, with the possibility of clot formation (thrombo-phlebitis) and subsequent dislodging of the clot to form an embolism.

Varicose veins—swollen and distended veins that occur most often in the superficial veins of the legs. This condition may develop in people who must sit or stand in one place for long periods of time. Without contraction of the leg muscles, blood tends

to pool in the leg veins, stretching their walls. If the veins become overly stretched, the valves within them no longer close properly. These incompetent valves no longer prevent backflow of blood, leading to further pooling and even further stretching of the walls of the veins. Varicose veins may cause discomfort and cramping in the legs, or become even more painful. Severe varicosities may be removed surgically.

This condition may also develop during pregnancy, when the enlarged uterus presses against the iliac veins and slows blood flow into the inferior vena cava. Varicose veins of the anal canal are called **hemorrhoids**, which may also be a result of pregnancy or of chronic constipation and straining to defecate. Hemorrhoids that cause discomfort or pain may also be removed surgically. The developments in laser surgery have made this a simpler procedure than it was in the past.

are other capillaries. The permeability of sinusoids permits large substances such as proteins and blood cells to enter or leave the blood. Sinusoids are found in hemopoietic tissues such as the red bone marrow and spleen and in organs such as the liver and pituitary gland, which produce and secrete proteins into the blood.

EXCHANGES IN CAPILLARIES

Capillaries are the sites of exchanges of materials between the blood and the tissue fluid surrounding

cells. Some of these substances move from the blood to tissue fluid, and others move from tissue fluid to the blood. The processes by which these substances are exchanged are illustrated in Fig. 13–2.

Gases move by **diffusion**, that is, from their area of greater concentration to their area of lesser concentration. Oxygen, therefore, diffuses from the blood in systemic capillaries to the tissue fluid, and carbon dioxide diffuses from tissue fluid to the blood to be brought to the lungs and exhaled.

Let us now look at the blood pressure as blood enters capillaries from the arterioles. Blood pressure

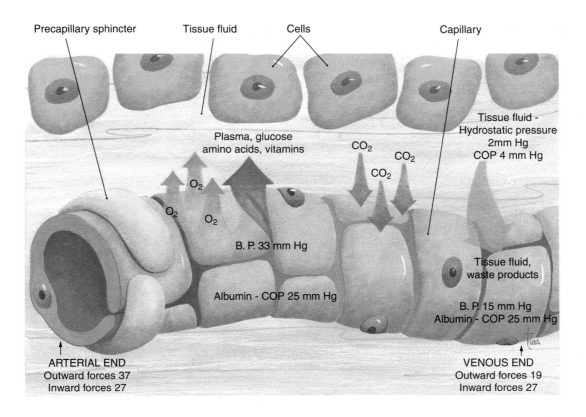

Precapillary sphincter   Tissue fluid   Cells   Capillary

Tissue fluid - Hydrostatic pressure 2mm Hg COP 4 mm Hg

Plasma, glucose amino acids, vitamins

CO_2 CO_2 CO_2

O_2 O_2 O_2

B. P. 33 mm Hg

Tissue fluid, waste products

Albumin - COP 25 mm Hg

B. P. 15 mm Hg
Albumin - COP 25 mm Hg

ARTERIAL END
Outward forces 37
Inward forces 27

VENOUS END
Outward forces 19
Inward forces 27

Figure 13–2 Exchanges between blood in a systemic capillary and the surrounding tissue fluid. Arrows depict the direction of movement. Filtration takes place at the arterial end of the capillary. Osmosis takes place at the venous end. Gases are exchanged by diffusion.

here is about 30 to 35 mmHg, and the pressure of the surrounding tissue fluid is much lower, about 2 mmHg. Because the capillary blood pressure is higher, the process of **filtration** occurs, which forces plasma and dissolved nutrients out of the capillaries and into tissue fluid. This is how nutrients such as glucose, amino acids, and vitamins are brought to cells.

Blood pressure decreases as blood reaches the venous end of capillaries, but notice that proteins such as albumin have remained in the blood. Albumin contributes to the **colloid osmotic pressure** of blood; this is an "attracting" pressure, a "pulling" rather than a "pushing" pressure. At the venous end of capillaries, the presence of albumin in the blood pulls tissue fluid into the capillaries, which also brings into the blood the waste products produced by cells. The tissue fluid that returns to the blood also helps maintain normal blood volume and blood pressure.

The amount of tissue fluid formed is slightly greater than the amount returned to the capillaries. If this were to continue, blood volume would be gradually depleted. The excess tissue fluid, however, enters lymph capillaries. Now called lymph, it will be returned to the blood to be recycled again as plasma, thus maintaining blood volume. This is discussed further in Chapter 14.

PATHWAYS OF CIRCULATION

The two major pathways of circulation are pulmonary and systemic. Pulmonary circulation begins at the right ventricle, and systemic circulation begins at the left ventricle. Hepatic portal circulation is a special segment of systemic circulation that will be covered separately. Fetal circulation involves pathways that are present only before birth and will also be discussed separately.

PULMONARY CIRCULATION

The right ventricle pumps blood into the pulmonary artery (or trunk), which divides into the right and left pulmonary arteries, one going to each lung. Within the lungs each artery branches extensively into smaller arteries and arterioles, then to capillaries. The pulmonary capillaries surround the alveoli of the lungs; it is here that exchanges of oxygen and carbon dioxide take place. The capillaries unite to form venules, which merge into veins, and finally into the two pulmonary veins from each lung that return blood to the left atrium. This oxygenated blood will then travel through the systemic circulation. (Notice that the pulmonary veins contain oxygenated blood; these are the only veins that carry blood with a high oxygen content. The blood in systemic veins has a low oxygen content; it is systemic arteries that carry oxygenated blood.)

SYSTEMIC CIRCULATION

The left ventricle pumps blood into the aorta, the largest artery of the body. We will return to the aorta and its branches in a moment, but first we will summarize the rest of systemic circulation. The branches of the aorta take blood into arterioles and capillary networks throughout the body. Capillaries merge to form venules and veins. The veins from the lower body take blood to the inferior vena cava; veins from the upper body take blood to the superior vena cava. These two caval veins return blood to the right atrium. The major arteries and veins are shown in Figs. 13–3 to 13–5, and their functions are listed in Tables 13–1 and 13–2.

The aorta is a continuous vessel, but for the sake of precise description it is divided into sections that are named anatomically: ascending aorta, aortic arch, thoracic aorta, and abdominal aorta. The ascending aorta is the first inch that emerges from the top of the left ventricle. The arch of the aorta curves posteriorly over the heart and turns downward. The thoracic aorta continues down through the chest cavity and through the diaphragm. Below the level of the diaphragm, the abdominal aorta continues to the level of the 4th lumbar vertebra, where it divides into the two common iliac arteries. Along its course,

the aorta has many branches through which blood travels to specific organs and parts of the body.

The ascending aorta has only two branches: the right and left coronary arteries, which supply blood to the myocardium. This pathway of circulation was described previously in Chapter 12.

The aortic arch has three branches that supply blood to the head and arms: the brachiocephalic artery, left common carotid artery, and left subclavian artery. The brachiocephalic (literally, "arm-head") artery is very short and divides into the right common carotid artery and right subclavian artery. The right and left common carotid arteries extend into the neck, where each divides into an internal carotid artery and external carotid artery, which supply the head. The right and left subclavian arteries are in the shoulders behind the clavicles and continue into the arms. The branches of the carotid and subclavian arteries are diagrammed in Figs. 13–3 and 13–5. As you look at these diagrams, keep in mind that the name of the vessel often tells us where it is. The facial artery, for example, is found in the face.

Some of these vessels contribute to an important arterial anastomosis, the **circle of Willis** (or cerebral arterial circle), which is a "circle" of arteries around the pituitary gland (Fig. 13–6). The circle of Willis is formed by the right and left internal carotid arteries and the basilar artery, which is the union of the right and left vertebral arteries (branches of the subclavian arteries). The brain must have a constant flow of blood to supply oxygen and remove waste products, and there are four vessels that bring blood to the circle of Willis. From this anastomosis, several paired arteries (the cerebral arteries) extend into the brain itself.

The thoracic aorta and its branches supply the chest wall and the organs within the thoracic cavity. These vessels are listed in Table 13–1.

The abdominal aorta gives rise to arteries that supply the abdominal wall and organs and to the common iliac arteries, which continue into the legs. These vessels are also listed in Table 13–1 (see Box 13–3: Pulse Sites).

The systemic veins drain blood from organs or parts of the body and often parallel their corresponding arteries. The most important veins are diagrammed in Fig. 13–4 and listed in Table 13–2.

HEPATIC PORTAL CIRCULATION

Hepatic portal circulation is a subdivision of systemic circulation in which blood from the abdominal diges-

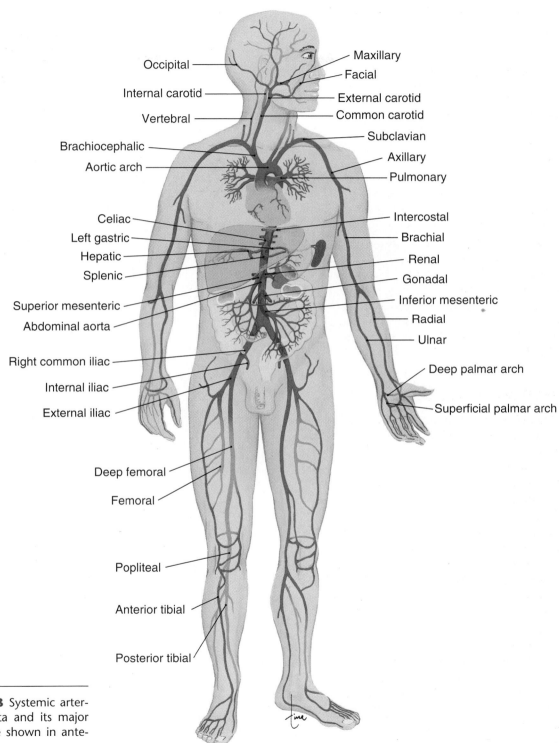

Occipital

Maxillary

Facial

Internal carotid

External carotid

Common carotid

Vertebral

Subclavian

Brachiocephalic

Axillary

Aortic arch

Pulmonary

Celiac

Intercostal

Left gastric

Brachial

Hepatic

Renal

Splenic

Gonadal

Superior mesenteric

Inferior mesenteric

Abdominal aorta

Radial

Ulnar

Right common iliac

Deep palmar arch

Internal iliac

External iliac

Superficial palmar arch

Deep femoral

Femoral

Popliteal

Anterior tibial

Posterior tibial

Figure 13–3 Systemic arteries. The aorta and its major branches are shown in anterior view.

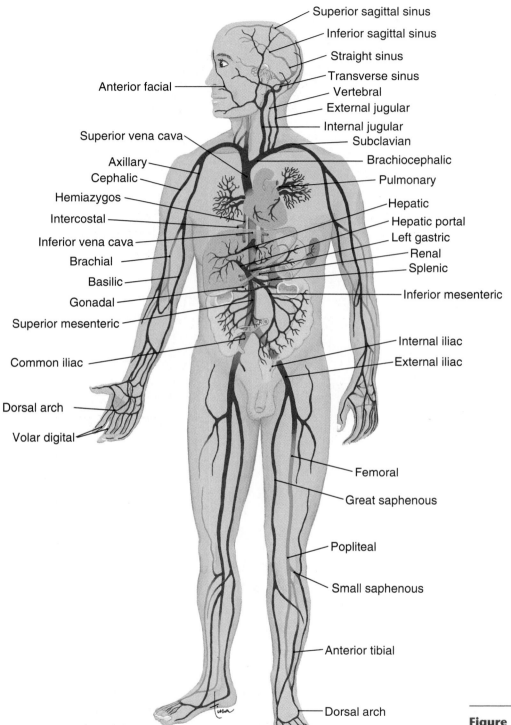

Superior sagittal sinus
Inferior sagittal sinus
Straight sinus
Transverse sinus
Vertebral
External jugular
Internal jugular
Subclavian
Brachiocephalic
Pulmonary
Hepatic
Hepatic portal
Left gastric
Renal
Splenic
Inferior mesenteric
Internal iliac
External iliac

Anterior facial
Superior vena cava
Axillary
Cephalic
Hemiazygos
Intercostal
Inferior vena cava
Brachial
Basilic
Gonadal
Superior mesenteric
Common iliac
Dorsal arch
Volar digital

Femoral
Great saphenous
Popliteal
Small saphenous
Anterior tibial
Dorsal arch

Figure 13–4 Systemic veins shown in anterior view.

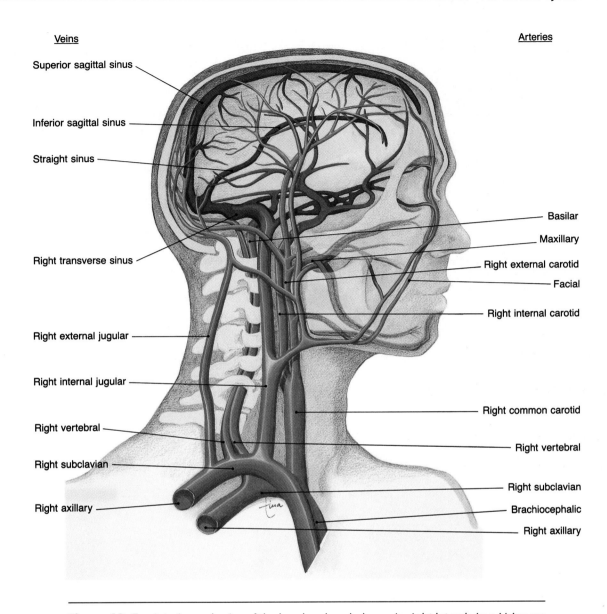

Veins

Superior sagittal sinus

Inferior sagittal sinus

Straight sinus

Right transverse sinus

Right external jugular

Right internal jugular

Right vertebral

Right subclavian

Right axillary

Arteries

Basilar

Maxillary

Right external carotid

Facial

Right internal carotid

Right common carotid

Right vertebral

Right subclavian

Brachiocephalic

Right axillary

Figure 13–5 Arteries and veins of the head and neck shown in right lateral view. Veins are labeled on the left. Arteries are labeled on the right.

tive organs and spleen circulates through the liver before returning to the heart.

Blood from the capillaries of the stomach, small intestine, colon, pancreas, and spleen flows into two large veins, the superior mesenteric vein and the splenic vein, which unite to form the portal vein (Fig. 13–7). The portal vein takes blood into the liver, where

it branches extensively and empties blood into the sinusoids, the capillaries of the liver (see also Fig. 16-6). From the sinusoids, blood flows into hepatic veins, to the inferior vena cava and back to the right atrium. Notice that in this pathway there are two sets of capillaries, and keep in mind that it is in capillaries that exchanges take place. Let us use some specific exam-

Table 13–1 | MAJOR SYSTEMIC ARTERIES

A. Branches of the Ascending Aorta and Aortic Arch

Artery	Branch of	Region supplied
Coronary a.	Ascending aorta	• Myocardium
Brachiocephalic a.	Aortic arch	• Right arm and head
Right common carotid a.	Brachiocephalic a.	• Right side of head
Right subclavian a.	Brachiocephalic a.	• Right shoulder and arm
Left common carotid a.	Aortic arch	• Left side of head
Left subclavian a.	Aortic arch	• Left shoulder and arm
External carotid a.	Common carotid a.	• Superficial head
Superficial temporal a.	External carotid a.	• Scalp
Internal carotid a.	Common carotid a.	• Brain (circle of Willis)
Ophthalamic a.	Internal carotid a.	• Eye
Vertebral a.	Subclavian a.	• Cervical vertebrae and circle of Willis
Axillary a.	Subclavian a.	• Armpit
Brachial a.	Axillary a.	• Upper arm
Radial a.	Brachial a.	• Forearm
Ulnar a.	Brachial a.	• Forearm
Volar arch	Radial and ulnar a.	• Hand

B. Branches of the Thoracic Aorta

Artery	Region Supplied
Intercostal a. (9 pairs)	• Skin, muscles, bones of trunk
Superior phrenic a.	• Diaphragm
Pericardial a.	• Pericardium
Esophageal a.	• Esophagus
Bronchial a.	• Bronchioles and connective tissue of the lungs

C. Branches of the Abdominal Aorta

Artery	Region Supplied
Inferior phrenic a.	• Diaphragm
Lumbar a.	• Lumbar area of back
Middle sacral a.	• Sacrum, coccyx, buttocks
Celiac a.	• (see branches)
Hepatic a.	• Liver
Left gastric a.	• Stomach
Splenic a.	• Spleen, pancreas
Superior mesenteric a.	• Small intestine, part of colon
Suprarenal a.	• Adrenal glands
Renal a.	• Kidneys
Inferior mesenteric a.	• Most of colon and rectum
Testicular or ovarian a.	• Testes or ovaries

Table 13–1	MAJOR SYSTEMIC ARTERIES (Continued)

C. Branches of the Abdominal Aorta (Continued)

Artery	Branch of
Common iliac a.	• The two large vessels that receive blood from the abdominal aorta; each branches as follows:
Internal iliac a.	• Bladder, rectum, reproductive organs
External iliac a.	• Lower pelvis to leg
Femoral a.	• Thigh
Popliteal a.	• Back of knee
Anterior tibial a.	• Front of lower leg
Dorsalis pedis	• Top of ankle and foot
Plantar arches	• Foot
Posterior tibial a.	• Back of lower leg
Peroneal a.	• Medial lower leg
Plantar arches	• Foot

ples to show the purpose and importance of portal circulation.

Glucose from carbohydrate digestion is absorbed into the capillaries of the small intestine; after a big meal this may greatly increase the blood glucose level. If this blood were to go directly back to the heart and then circulate through the kidneys, some of the glucose might be lost in urine. However, blood from the small intestine passes first through the liver sinusoids, and the liver cells remove the excess glucose and store it as glycogen. The blood that returns to the heart will then have a blood glucose level in the normal range.

Another example: Alcohol is absorbed into the capillaries of the stomach. If it were to circulate directly throughout the body, the alcohol would rapidly impair the functioning of the brain. Portal circulation, however, takes blood from the stomach to the liver, the organ that can detoxify the alcohol and prevent its detrimental effects on the brain. Of course, if alcohol consumption continues, the blood alcohol level rises faster than the liver's capacity to detoxify, and the well-known signs of alcohol intoxication appear.

As you can see, this portal circulation pathway enables the liver to modify the blood from the digestive organs and spleen. Some nutrients may be stored or changed, bilirubin from the spleen is excreted into bile, and potential poisons are detoxified before the blood returns to the heart and the rest of the body.

FETAL CIRCULATION

The fetus depends upon the mother for oxygen and nutrients and for the removal of carbon dioxide and other waste products. The site of exchange between fetus and mother is the **placenta**, which contains fetal and maternal blood vessels that are very close to one another (see Figs. 13–8 and 21-5). The blood of the fetus does not mix with the blood of the mother; substances are exchanged by diffusion and active transport mechanisms.

The fetus is connected to the placenta by the umbilical cord, which contains two umbilical arteries and one umbilical vein (see Fig. 13–8). The **umbilical arteries** are branches of the fetal internal iliac arteries; they carry blood from the fetus to the placenta. In the placenta, carbon dioxide and waste products in the fetal blood enter maternal circulation, and oxygen and nutrients from the mother's blood enter fetal circulation.

The **umbilical vein** carries this oxygenated blood from the placenta to the fetus. Within the body of the fetus, the umbilical vein branches: One branch takes some blood to the fetal liver, but most of the blood passes through the **ductus venosus** to the inferior vena cava, to the right atrium. After birth, when the umbilical cord is cut, the remnants of these fetal vessels constrict and become nonfunctional.

The other modifications of fetal circulation concern the fetal heart and large arteries (also shown

Table 13–2 | MAJOR SYSTEMIC VEINS

Vein	Vein Joined	Region Drained
Head and Neck		
Cranial venous sinuses	Internal jugular v.	• Brain, including reabsorbed CSF
Internal jugular v.	Brachiocephalic v.	• Face and neck
External jugular v.	Subclavian v.	• Superficial face and neck
Subclavian v.	Brachiocephalic v.	• Shoulder
Brachiocephalic v.	Superior vena cava	• Upper body
Superior vena cava	Right atrium	• Upper body
Arm and Shoulder		
Radial v.	Brachial v.	• Forearm and hand
Ulnar v.	Brachial v.	• Forearm and hand
Cephalic v.	Axillary v.	• Superficial arm and forearm
Basilic v.	Axillary v.	• Superficial upper arm
Brachial v.	Axillary v.	• Upper arm
Axillary v.	Subclavian v.	• Armpit
Subclavian v.	Brachiocephalic v.	• Shoulder
Trunk		
Brachiocephalic v.	Superior vena cava	• Upper body
Azygos v.	Superior vena cava	• Deep structures of chest and abdomen; links inferior vena cava to superior vena cava
Hepatic v.	Inferior vena cava	• Liver
Renal v.	Inferior vena cava	• Kidney
Testicular or ovarian v.	Inferior vena cava and left renal v.	• Testes or ovaries
Internal iliac v.	Common iliac v.	• Rectum, bladder, reproductive organs
External iliac v.	Common iliac v.	• Leg and abdominal wall
Common iliac v.	Inferior vena cava	• Leg and lower abdomen
Leg		
Anterior and posterior tibial v.	Popliteal v.	• Lower leg and foot
Popliteal v.	Femoral v.	• Knee
Small saphenous v.	Popliteal v.	• Superficial leg and foot
Great saphenous v.	Femoral v.	• Superficial foot, leg, and thigh
Femoral v.	External iliac v.	• Thigh
External iliac v.	Common iliac v.	• Leg and abdominal wall
Common iliac v.	Inferior vena cava	• Leg and lower abdomen
Inferior vena cava	Right atrium	• Lower body

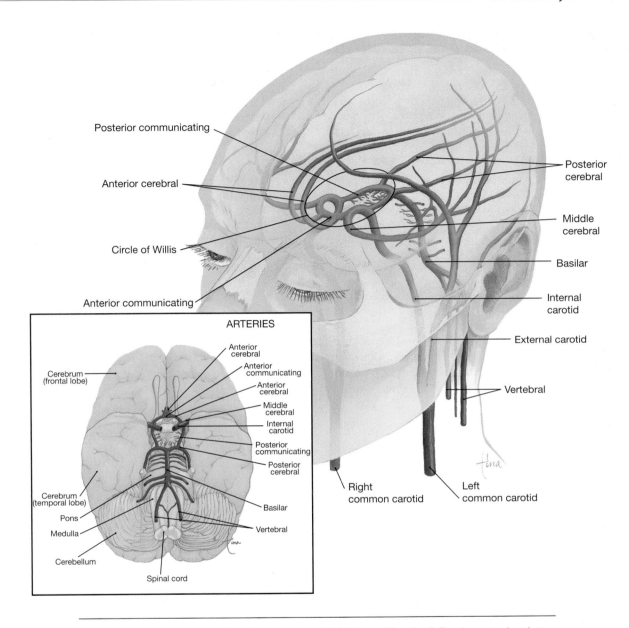

Figure 13–6   Circle of Willis. This anastomosis is formed by the following arteries: internal carotid, anterior communicating, posterior communicating, and basilar. The cerebral arteries extend from the circle of Willis into the brain. The box shows these vessels in an inferior view of the brain.

in Fig. 13–8). Because the fetal lungs are deflated and do not provide for gas exchange, blood is shunted away from the lungs and to the body. The **foramen ovale** is an opening in the interatrial septum that permits some blood to flow from the right atrium to the left atrium, not, as usual, to the right ventricle. The

blood that does enter the right ventricle is pumped into the pulmonary artery. The **ductus arteriosus** is a short vessel that diverts most of the blood in the pulmonary artery to the aorta, to the body. Both the foramen ovale and the ductus arteriosus permit blood to bypass the fetal lungs.

Box 13–3   PULSE SITES

A pulse is the heartbeat that is felt at an arterial site. What is felt is not actually the force exerted by the blood, but the force of ventricular contraction transmitted through the walls of the arteries. This is why pulses are not felt in veins; they are too far from the heart for the force to be detectable.

The most commonly used pulse sites are:

Radial—the radial artery on the thumb side of the wrist.

Carotid—the carotid artery lateral to the larynx in the neck.

Temporal—the temporal artery just in front of the ear.

Femoral—the femoral artery at the top of the thigh.

Popliteal—the popliteal artery at the back of the knee.

Dorsalis pedis—the dorsalis pedis artery on the top of the foot (commonly called the pedal pulse).

Pulse rate is, of course, the heart rate. However, if the heart is beating weakly, a radial pulse may be lower than an **apical pulse** (listening to the heart itself with a stethoscope). This is called a **pulse deficit** and indicates heart disease of some kind.

When taking a pulse, the careful observer also notes the rhythm and force of the pulse. Abnormal rhythms may reflect cardiac arrhythmias, and the force of the pulse (strong or weak) is helpful in assessing the general condition of the heart and arteries.

Just after birth, the baby breathes and expands its lungs, which pulls more blood into the pulmonary circulation. More blood then returns to the left atrium, and a flap on the left side of the foramen ovale is closed. The ductus arteriosus constricts, probably in response to the higher oxygen content of the blood, and pulmonary circulation becomes fully functional within a few days.

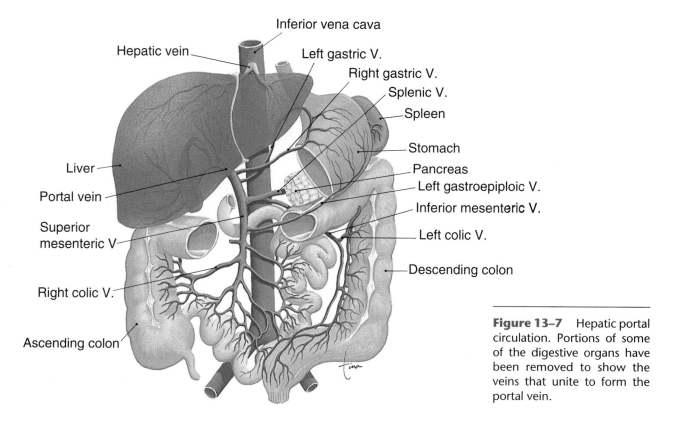

Figure 13–7 Hepatic portal circulation. Portions of some of the digestive organs have been removed to show the veins that unite to form the portal vein.

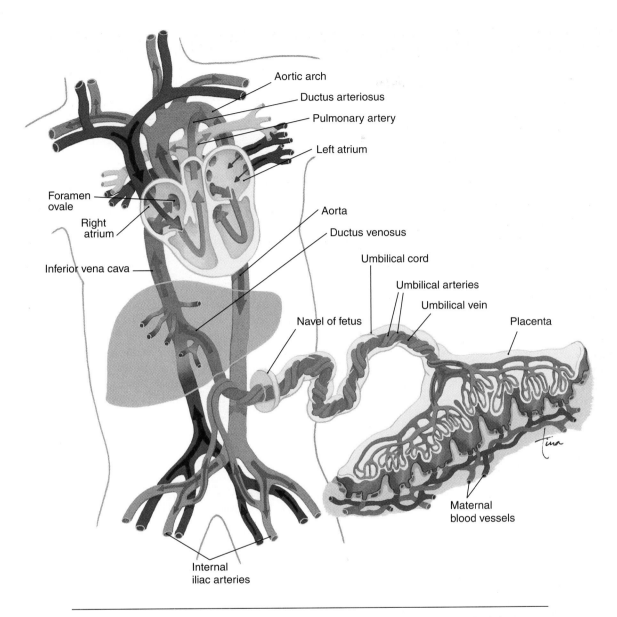

Figure 13–8   Fetal circulation. Fetal heart and blood vessels are shown on the left. Arrows depict the direction of blood flow. The placenta and umbilical blood vessels are shown on the right.

VELOCITY OF BLOOD FLOW

The velocity, or speed, with which blood flows differs in the various parts of the vascular system. Velocity is inversely related (meaning as one value goes up, the other goes down) to the cross-sectional area of the particular segment of the vascular system. Refer to Figure 13–9 as you read the following. The aorta receives all the blood from the left ventricle, its cross-sectional area is small, about 3 cm² (1 sq. inch), and the blood moves very rapidly, at least 30 cm per second (about 12 inches). Each time the aorta or any artery branches, the total cross-sectional area becomes larger, and the speed of blood flow decreases. Think of a river that begins in a narrow bed and is flowing rapidly. If the river bed widens, the water spreads out to fill it and flows more slowly. If the river were to narrow again, the water would flow faster. This is just what happens in the vascular system.

The capillaries in total have the greatest cross-sectional area, and blood velocity there is slowest, less than 0.1 cm per second. When capillaries unite to form venules, and then veins, the cross-sectional area decreases and blood flow speeds up.

Recall that it is in capillary networks that exchanges of nutrients, wastes, and gases take place between the blood and tissue fluid. The slow rate of blood flow in capillaries permits sufficient time for these essential exchanges. Think of a train slowing down (not actually stopping) at stations to allow people to jump on and off, then speeding up again to get to the next station. The capillaries are the "stations" of the vascular system.

The more rapid blood velocity in other vessels makes circulation time quite short. This is the time it takes for blood to go from the right ventricle to the lungs, back to the heart to be pumped by the left ventricle to the body, and return to the heart again. Circulation time is about 1 minute or less, and ensures an adequate exchange of gases.

BLOOD PRESSURE

Blood pressure is the force the blood exerts against the walls of the blood vessels. Filtration in capillaries depends upon blood pressure; filtration brings nutrients to tissues, and as you will see in Chapter 18, is the first step in the formation of urine. Blood pressure is one of the "vital signs" often measured, and indeed a normal blood pressure is essential to life.

The pumping of the ventricles creates blood pressure, which is measured in mmHg (millimeters of mercury). When a systemic blood pressure reading is taken, two numbers are obtained: systolic and diastolic, as in 110/70 mmHg. **Systolic** pressure is always the higher of the two and represents the blood pressure when the left ventricle is contracting. The lower number is the **diastolic** pressure, when the left ventricle is relaxed and does not exert force. Diastolic pressure is maintained by the arteries and arterioles and is discussed in a later section.

Systemic blood pressure is highest in the aorta, which receives all of the blood pumped by the left ventricle. As blood travels farther away from the heart,

blood pressure decreases (see Fig. 13–9). The brachial artery is most often used to take a blood pressure reading; here a normal systolic range is 90 to 130 mmHg, and a normal diastolic range is 60 to 85 mmHg. In the arterioles, blood pressure decreases further, and systolic and diastolic pressures merge into one pressure. At the arterial end of capillary networks, blood pressure is about 30 to 35 mmHg, decreasing to 12 to 15 mmHg at the venous end of capillaries. This is high enough to permit filtration but low enough to prevent rupture of the capillaries. As blood flows through veins, the pressure decreases further, and in the caval veins, blood pressure approaches zero as blood enters the right atrium.

A systemic blood pressure consistently higher than the normal range is called **hypertension** (see also Box 13–4: Hypertension). A lower than normal blood pressure is called **hypotension**. The regulation of systemic blood pressure is discussed in a later section.

Pulmonary blood pressure is created by the right ventricle, which has relatively thin walls and thus exerts about one-sixth the force of the left ventricle. The result is that pulmonary arterial pressure is always low: 20 to 25/8 to 10 mmHg, and in pulmonary capillaries is lower still. This is important to *prevent* filtration in pulmonary capillaries, to prevent tissue fluid from accumulating in the alveoli of the lungs.

MAINTENANCE OF SYSTEMIC BLOOD PRESSURE

Because blood pressure is so important, many physiological factors and processes interact to keep blood pressure within normal limits:

1. **Venous return**—the amount of blood that returns to the heart by way of the veins. Venous return is important because the heart can pump only the blood it receives. If venous return decreases, the cardiac muscle fibers will not be stretched, the force of ventricular systole will decrease (Starling's Law), and blood pressure will decrease. This is what might happen following a severe hemorrhage.

   When the body is horizontal, venous return can be maintained fairly easily, but when the body is vertical, gravity must be overcome to return blood from the lower body to the heart. Three mechanisms help promote venous return: constriction of veins, the skeletal muscle pump, and the respiratory pump.

Figure 13–9 Characteristics of the vascular system. **(A)** Schematic of the branching of vessels. **(B)** Cross-sectional area in square centimeters. **(C)** Blood velocity in centimeters per second. **(D)** Systemic blood pressure changes. Notice that systolic and diastolic pressures become one pressure in the capillaries.

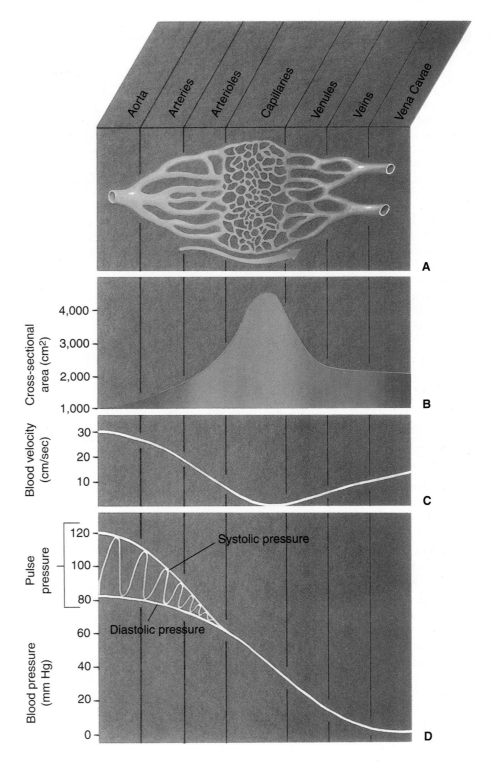

Box 13–4   HYPERTENSION

Hypertension is high blood pressure, that is, a resting systemic pressure consistently above 130/85. The term "essential hypertension" means that no specific cause can be determined; most cases are in this category. For some people, however, an overproduction of renin by the kidneys is the cause of their hypertension. Excess renin increases the production of angiotensin II, which raises blood pressure. Although hypertension often produces no symptoms, the long-term consequences may be very serious. Chronic hypertension has its greatest effects on the arteries and on the heart.

Although the walls of arteries are strong, hypertension weakens them and contributes to arteriosclerosis. Such weakened arteries may rupture or develop aneurysms, which may in turn lead to a CVA or kidney damage.

Hypertension affects the heart because the left ventricle must now pump blood against the higher arterial pressure. The left ventricle works harder and, like any other muscle, enlarges as more work is demanded; this is called **left ventricular hypertrophy.** This abnormal growth of the myocardium, however, is not accompanied by a corresponding growth in coronary capillaries, and the blood supply of the left ventricle may not be adequate for all situations. Exercise, for example, puts further demands on the heart, and the person may experience angina due to a lack of oxygen or a myocardial infarction if there is a severe oxygen deficiency.

Although several different kinds of medications are used to treat hypertension, people with moderate hypertension may limit their dependence on medications by following certain guidelines.

1. *Don't smoke,* because nicotine stimulates vasoconstriction, which raises BP. Smoking also damages arteries, contributing to arteriosclerosis.
2. *Lose weight* if overweight. A weight loss of as little as 10 pounds can lower BP. A diet high in fruits and vegetables may, for some people, contribute to lower BP.
3. *Cut salt intake* in half. Although salt consumption may not be the *cause* of hypertension, reducing salt intake may help lower blood pressure by decreasing blood volume.
4. *Exercise* on a regular basis. A moderate amount of aerobic exercise (such as a halfhour walk every day) is beneficial for the entire cardiovascular system and may also contribute to weight loss.

Veins contain smooth muscle, which enables them to constrict and force blood toward the heart; the valves prevent backflow of blood. The second mechanism is the **skeletal muscle pump,** which is especially effective for the deep veins of the legs. These veins are surrounded by skeletal muscles that contract and relax during normal activities such as walking. Contractions of the leg muscles squeeze the veins to force blood toward the heart. The third mechanism is the **respiratory pump,** which affects veins that pass through the chest cavity. The pressure changes of inhalation and exhalation alternately expand and compress the veins, and blood is returned to the heart.

2. **Heart rate and force**—in general, if heart rate and force increase, blood pressure increases; this is what happens during exercise. However, if the heart is beating extremely rapidly, the ventricles may not fill completely between beats, and cardiac output and blood pressure will decrease.
3. **Peripheral resistance**—this term refers to the resistance the vessels offer to the flow of blood.

The arteries and veins are usually slightly constricted, which maintains normal diastolic blood pressure. It may be helpful to think of the vessels as the "container" for the blood. If a person's body has 5 liters of blood, the "container" must be smaller in order for the blood to exert a pressure against its walls. This is what normal vasoconstriction does: It makes the container (the vessels) smaller than the volume of blood so that the blood will exert pressure even when the left ventricle is relaxed.

If more vasoconstriction occurs, blood pressure will increase (the container has become even smaller). This is what happens in a stress situation, when greater vasoconstriction is brought about by sympathetic impulses. If vasodilation occurs, blood pressure will decrease (the container is larger). After eating a large meal, for example, there is extensive vasodilation in the digestive tract to supply more oxygenated blood for digestive activities. To keep blood pressure within the normal range, vasoconstriction must, and does, occur elsewhere in the body. This is why strenuous exercise should be avoided right after eating; there is not enough blood to completely supply oxygen to exercising muscles and an active digestive tract at the same time.

4. **Elasticity of the large arteries**—when the left ventricle contracts, the blood that enters the large arteries stretches their walls. The arterial walls are elastic and absorb some of the force. When the left ventricle relaxes, the arterial walls recoil or snap back, which helps keep diastolic pressure within the normal range. Normal elasticity, therefore, lowers systolic pressure, raises diastolic pressure, and maintains a normal pulse pressure. (Pulse pressure is the difference between systolic and diastolic pressure. The usual ratio of systolic to diastolic to pulse pressure is approximately 3:2:1. For example, with a blood pressure of 120/80, the pulse pressure is 40, and the ratio is 120:80:40, or 3:2:1.)

5. **Viscosity of the blood**—normal blood viscosity depends upon the presence of red blood cells and plasma proteins, especially albumin. Having too many red blood cells is rare but does occur in the disorder called polycythemia vera and in people who are heavy smokers. This will increase blood viscosity and blood pressure.

   A decreased number of red blood cells, as is seen with severe anemia, or decreased albumin, as may occur in liver disease or kidney disease, will decrease blood viscosity and blood pressure. In these situations, other mechanisms such as vasoconstriction will maintain blood pressure as close to normal as is possible.

6. **Loss of blood**—a small loss of blood, as when donating a pint of blood, will cause a temporary drop in blood pressure followed by rapid compensation in the form of more rapid heart rate and greater vasoconstriction. After a severe hemorrhage, however, these compensating mechanisms may not be sufficient to maintain normal blood pressure and blood flow to the brain. Although a person may survive loss of 50% of the body's total blood, the possibility of brain damage increases as more blood is lost and not rapidly replaced.

7. **Hormones**—several hormones have effects on blood pressure. You may recall them from Chapters 10 and 12, but let us summarize them here. The adrenal medulla secretes norepinephrine and epinephrine in stress situations. Norepinephrine stimulates vasoconstriction, which raises blood pressure. Epinephrine also causes vasoconstriction, and increases heart rate and force of contraction, both of which increase blood pressure.

Antidiuretic hormone (ADH) is secreted by the posterior pituitary gland when the water content of the body decreases. ADH increases the reabsorption of water by the kidneys to prevent further loss of water in urine and a further decrease in blood pressure.

Aldosterone, a hormone from the adrenal cortex, has a similar effect on blood volume. When blood pressure decreases, secretion of aldosterone stimulates the reabsorption of Na^+ ions by the kidneys. Water follows sodium back to the blood, which maintains blood volume to prevent a further drop in blood pressure.

Atrial natriuretic hormone (ANH), secreted by the atria of the heart, functions in opposition to aldosterone. ANH increases the excretion of Na^+ ions and water by the kidneys, which decreases blood volume and lowers blood pressure.

DISTRIBUTION OF BLOOD FLOW

An individual's blood volume remains relatively constant within the normal range appropriate to the size of the person. Active tissues, however, require more blood, that is, more oxygen, than do less active tissues. As active tissues and organs receive a greater proportion of the total blood flow, less active organs must receive less, or blood pressure will decrease markedly.

As mentioned previously, precapillary sphincters dilate in active tissues and constrict in less active ones. The arterioles also constrict to reduce blood flow to less active organs. This ensures that metabolically active organs will receive enough oxygen to function properly, and that blood pressure for the body as a whole will be maintained within normal limits.

An example will be helpful here; let us use the body at rest and the body during exercise. Consult Figure 13–10 as you read the following. Resting cardiac output is approximately 5,000 ml per minute. Exercise cardiac output is three times that, about 15,000 ml per minute. Keep in mind that the volume of blood is the same in both cases, but that during exercise the blood is being circulated more rapidly.

Compare the amounts of blood flowing to various organs and tissues, during exercise and at rest. During exercise, the heart receives about three times as much blood as it does when the body is at rest. The very active skeletal muscles receive about ten times as much blood. The skin, as an organ of heat loss,

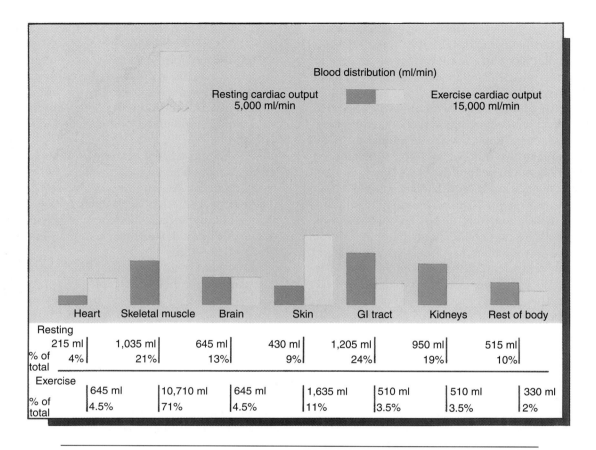

Figure 13–10   Blood flow through various organs when the body is at rest and during exercise. For each organ, the percentage of the total blood flow is given.

receives about four times as much blood. Other organs, however, can function adequately with less blood. Blood flow is reduced to the digestive tract, to the kidneys, and to other parts of the body such as bones.

When the exercise ceases, cardiac output will gradually return to the resting level, as will blood flow to the various organs. These changes in the distribution of blood ensure sufficient oxygen for active tissues and an appropriate blood pressure for the body as a whole.

REGULATION OF BLOOD PRESSURE

The mechanisms that regulate systemic blood pressure may be divided into two types: intrinsic mechanisms and nervous mechanisms. The nervous mechanisms involve the nervous system, and the intrinsic mechanisms do not require nerve impulses.

INTRINSIC MECHANISMS

The term *intrinsic* means "within." Intrinsic mechanisms work because of the internal characteristics of certain organs. The first such organ is the heart. When venous return increases, cardiac muscle fibers are stretched, and the ventricles pump more forcefully (Starling's Law). Thus, cardiac output and blood pressure increase. This is what happens during exercise, when a higher blood pressure is needed. When exercise ends and venous return decreases, the heart pumps less forcefully, which helps return blood pressure to a normal resting level.

The second intrinsic mechanism involves the kidneys. When blood flow through the kidneys decreases, the process of filtration decreases and less urine is formed. This decrease in urinary output preserves blood volume so that it does not decrease further. Following severe hemorrhage or any other type of dehydration, this is very important to maintain blood pressure.

The kidneys are also involved in the **renin-angiotensin mechanism**. When blood pressure decreases, the kidneys secrete the enzyme **renin**, which initiates a series of reactions that result in the formation of **angiotensin II**. These reactions are described in Table 13–3 and depicted in Fig. 13–11. Angiotensin II causes vasoconstriction and stimulates secretion of aldosterone by the adrenal cortex, both of which will increase blood pressure.

NERVOUS MECHANISMS

The medulla and the autonomic nervous system are directly involved in the regulation of blood pressure.

Table 13–3	THE RENIN-ANGIOTENSIN MECHANISM

1. Decreased blood pressure stimulates the kidneys to secrete renin.
2. Renin splits the plasma protein angiotensinogen (synthesized by the liver) to angiotensin I.
3. Angiotensin I is converted to angiotensin II by an enzyme (called converting enzyme) found primarily in lung tissue.
4. Angiotensin II:
   • causes vasoconstriction
   • stimulates the adrenal cortex to secrete aldosterone

The first of these nervous mechanisms concerns the heart; this was described previously, so we will not review it here but refer you to Chapter 12 and Fig. 12–7, as well as Fig. 13–12.

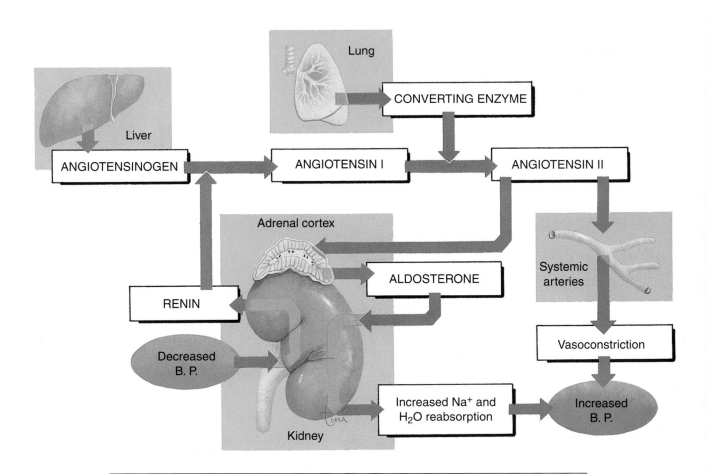

Figure 13–11   The renin-angiotensin mechanism. Begin at "Decreased B.P." and see Table 13–3 for numbered steps.

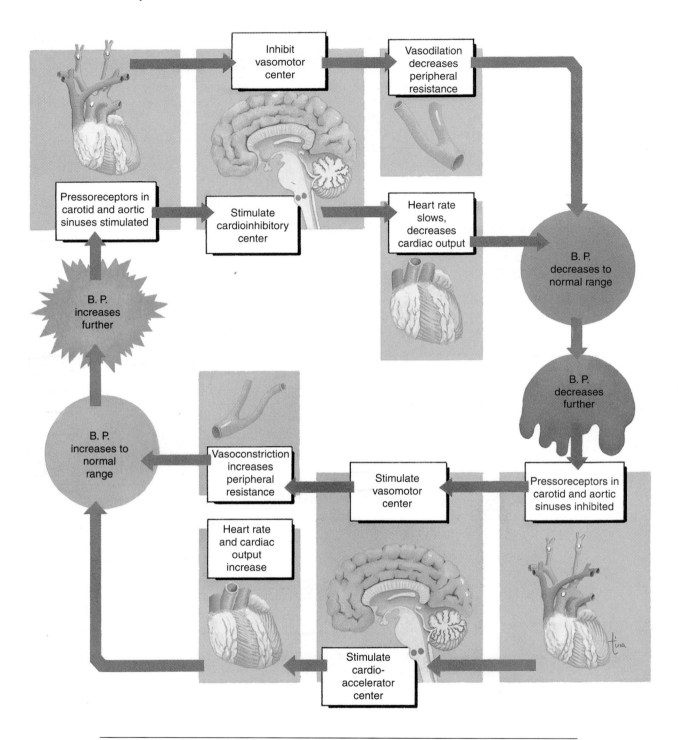

Figure 13–12 Nervous mechanisms that regulate blood pressure. See text for description.

The second nervous mechanism involves peripheral resistance, that is, the degree of constriction of the arteries and arterioles and, to a lesser extent, the veins (see Fig. 13–12). The medulla contains the **vasomotor center**, which consists of a vasoconstrictor area and a vasodilator area. The vasodilator area may depress the vasoconstrictor area to bring about vasodilation, which will decrease blood pressure. The vasoconstrictor area may bring about more vasoconstriction by way of the sympathetic division of the autonomic nervous system.

Sympathetic vasoconstrictor fibers innervate the smooth muscle of all arteries and veins, and several impulses per second along these fibers maintain normal vasoconstriction. More impulses per second bring about greater vasoconstriction, and fewer impulses per second cause vasodilation. The medulla receives the information to make such changes from the pressoreceptors in the carotid sinuses and the aortic sinus. The inability to maintain normal blood pressure is one aspect of circulatory shock (see Box 13–5: Circulatory Shock).

AGING AND THE VASCULAR SYSTEM

It is believed that the aging of blood vessels, especially arteries, begins in childhood, although the effects are not apparent for decades. The cholesterol deposits of atherosclerosis are to be expected with

---

Box 13–5   CIRCULATORY SHOCK

Circulatory shock is any condition in which cardiac output decreases to the extent that tissues are deprived of oxygen and waste products accumulate.

Causes of Shock

Cardiogenic shock occurs most often after a severe myocardial infarction but may also be the result of ventricular fibrillation. In either case, the heart is no longer an efficient pump, and cardiac output decreases.

Hypovolemic shock is the result of decreased blood volume, often due to severe hemorrhage. Other possible causes are extreme sweating (heat stroke) or extreme loss of water through the kidneys (diuresis) or intestines (diarrhea). In these situations, the heart simply does not have enough blood to pump, and cardiac output decreases. Anaphylactic shock, also in this category, is a massive allergic reaction in which great amounts of histamine increase capillary permeability and vasodilation throughout the body. Much plasma is then lost to tissue spaces, which decreases blood volume, blood pressure, and cardiac output.

Septic shock is the result of septicemia, the presence of bacteria in the blood. The bacteria and damaged tissues release inflammatory chemicals that cause vasodilation and extensive loss of plasma into tissue spaces.

Stages of Shock

Compensated shock—the responses by the body maintain cardiac output. Following a small hemorrhage, for example, the heart rate increases, the blood vessels constrict, and the kidneys decrease urinary output to conserve water. These responses help preserve blood volume and maintain blood pressure, cardiac output, and blood flow to tissues.

Progressive shock—the state of shock leads to more shock. Following a severe hemorrhage, cardiac output decreases, and the myocardium itself is deprived of blood. The heart weakens, which further decreases cardiac output. Arteries that are deprived of their blood supply cannot remain constricted. As the arteries dilate, venous return decreases, which in turn decreases cardiac output. Progressive shock is a series of such vicious cycles, and medical intervention is required to restore cardiac output to normal.

Irreversible shock—no amount of medical assistance can restore cardiac output to normal. The usual cause of death is that the heart has been damaged too much to recover. A severe myocardial infarction, massive hemorrhage, or septicemia may all be fatal despite medical treatment.

advancing age, with the most serious consequences in the coronary arteries. A certain degree of arteriosclerosis is to be expected, and average resting blood pressure may increase, which further damages arterial walls. Consequences include stroke and left-sided heart failure.

The veins also deteriorate with age; their thin walls weaken and stretch, making their valves incompetent. This is most likely to occur in the veins of the legs; their walls are subject to great pressure as blood is returned to the heart against the force of gravity. Varicose veins and phlebitis are more likely to occur among elderly people.

SUMMARY

Although the vascular system does form passageways for the blood, you can readily see that the blood vessels are not simply pipes through which the blood flows. The vessels are not passive tubes, but rather active contributors to homeostasis. The arteries and veins help maintain blood pressure, and the capillaries provide sites for the exchanges of materials between the blood and the tissues. Some very important sites of exchange are discussed in the following chapters: the lungs, the digestive tract, and the kidneys.

STUDY OUTLINE

The vascular system consists of the arteries, capillaries, and veins through which blood travels.

Arteries (and arterioles) (see Fig. 13–1)
1. Carry blood from the heart to capillaries; three layers in their walls.
2. Inner layer (tunica intima): simple squamous epithelial tissue (endothelium), very smooth to prevent abnormal blood clotting.
3. Middle layer (tunica media): smooth muscle and elastic connective tissue; contributes to maintenance of diastolic blood pressure (BP).
4. Outer layer (tunica externa): fibrous connective tissue to prevent rupture.
5. Constriction or dilation is regulated by the autonomic nervous system.

Veins (and venules) (see Fig. 13–1)
1. Carry blood from capillaries to the heart; three layers in walls.
2. Inner layer: endothelium folded into valves to prevent the backflow of blood.
3. Middle layer: thin smooth muscle, because veins are not as important in the maintenance of BP.
4. Outer layer: thin fibrous connective tissue because veins do not carry blood under high pressure.

Anastomoses—connections between vessels of the same type
1. Provide alternate pathways for blood flow if one vessel is blocked.

2. Arterial anastomoses provide for blood flow to the capillaries of an organ (e.g., circle of Willis to the brain).
3. Venous anastomoses provide for return of blood to the heart and are most numerous in veins of the legs.

Capillaries (see Fig. 13–1 and Fig. 13–2)
1. Carry blood from arterioles to venules.
2. Walls are one cell thick (simple squamous epithelial tissue) to permit exchanges between blood and tissue fluid.
3. Oxygen and carbon dioxide are exchanged by diffusion.
4. BP in capillaries brings nutrients to tissues and forms tissue fluid in the process of filtration.
5. Albumin in the blood provides colloid osmotic pressure, which pulls waste products and tissue fluid into capillaries. The return of tissue fluid maintains blood volume and BP.
6. Precapillary sphincters regulate blood flow into capillary networks based on tissue needs; in active tissues they dilate; in less active tissues they constrict.
7. Sinusoids are very permeable capillaries found in the liver, spleen, pituitary gland, and red bone marrow to permit proteins and blood cells to enter or leave the blood.

Pathways of Circulation
1. Pulmonary: Right ventricle → pulmonary artery → pulmonary capillaries (exchange of gases) → pulmonary veins → left atrium.

2. Systemic: left ventricle → aorta → capillaries in body tissues → superior and inferior caval veins → right atrium (see Table 13–1 and Fig. 13–3 for systemic arteries and Table 13–2 and Fig. 13–4 for systemic veins).

3. Hepatic portal circulation: blood from the digestive organs and spleen flows through the portal vein to the liver before returning to the heart. Purpose: the liver stores some nutrients or regulates their blood levels and detoxifies potential poisons before blood enters the rest of peripheral circulation (see Fig. 13–7).

Fetal Circulation—the fetus depends on the mother for oxygen and nutrients and for the removal of waste products (see Fig. 13–8)

1. The placenta is the site of exchange between fetal blood and maternal blood.
2. Umbilical arteries (two) carry blood from the fetus to the placenta, where CO_2 and waste products enter maternal circulation.
3. The umbilical vein carries blood with O_2 and nutrients from the placenta to the fetus.
4. The umbilical vein branches: some blood flows through the fetal liver; most blood flows through the ductus venosus to the fetal inferior vena cava.
5. The foramen ovale permits blood to flow from the right atrium to the left atrium to bypass the fetal lungs.
6. The ductus arteriosus permits blood to flow from the pulmonary artery to the aorta to bypass the fetal lungs.
7. These fetal structures become nonfunctional after birth, when the umbilical cord is cut and breathing takes place.

Velocity of Blood Flow (see Fig. 13–9)

1. Velocity is inversely related to the cross-sectional area of a segment of the vascular system.
2. The total capillaries have the greatest cross-sectional area and slowest blood flow.
3. Slow flow is important to permit sufficient time for exchange of gases, nutrients, and wastes.

Blood Pressure (BP)—the force exerted by the blood against the walls of the blood vessels

1. BP is measured in mmHg: systolic/diastolic. Systolic pressure occurs during ventricular contrac-

tion; diastolic pressure occurs during ventricular relaxation (see Fig. 13–9).
2. Normal range of systemic arterial BP: 90 to 130/60 to 85 mmHg.
3. BP in capillaries is 30 to 35 mmHg at the arterial end and 12 to 15 mmHg at the venous end—high enough to permit filtration but low enough to prevent rupture of the capillaries.
4. BP decreases in the veins and approaches zero in the caval veins.
5. Pulmonary BP is always low (the right ventricle pumps with less force): 20 to 25/8 to 10 mmHg. This low BP prevents filtration and accumulation of tissue fluid in the alveoli.

Maintenance of Systemic BP

1. Venous return—the amount of blood that returns to the heart. If venous return decreases, the heart contracts less forcefully (Starling's Law) and BP decreases. The mechanisms that maintain venous return when the body is vertical are:
   - constriction of veins with the valves preventing backflow of blood
   - skeletal muscle pump—contraction of skeletal muscles, especially in the legs, squeezes the deep veins
   - respiratory pump—the pressure changes of inhalation and exhalation expand and compress the veins in the chest cavity
2. Heart rate and force—if heart rate and force increase, BP increases.
3. Peripheral resistance—the resistance of the arteries and arterioles to the flow of blood. These vessels are usually slightly constricted to maintain normal diastolic BP. Greater vasoconstriction will increase BP; vasodilation will decrease BP. In the body, vasodilation in one area requires vasoconstriction in another area to maintain normal BP.
4. Elasticity of the large arteries—ventricular systole stretches the walls of large arteries, which recoil during ventricular diastole. Normal elasticity lowers systolic BP, raises diastolic BP, and maintains normal pulse pressure.
5. Viscosity of blood—depends on RBCs and plasma proteins, especially albumin. Severe anemia tends to decrease BP. Deficiency of albumin as in liver or kidney disease tends to decrease BP. In these cases, compensation such as greater vasoconstriction will keep BP close to normal.

6. Loss of blood—a small loss will be rapidly compensated for by faster heart rate and greater vasoconstriction. After severe hemorrhage, these mechanisms may not be sufficient to maintain normal BP.

7. Hormones—(a) Norepinephrine stimulates vasoconstriction, which raises BP; (b) epinephrine increases cardiac output and raises BP; (c) ADH increases water reabsorption by the kidneys, which increases blood volume and BP; (d) aldosterone increases reabsorption of Na$^+$ ions by the kidneys; water follows Na$^+$ and increases blood volume and BP; (e) ANH increases excretion of Na$^+$ ions and water by the kidneys, which decreases blood volume and BP.

Distribution of Blood Flow

1. Metabolically active tissues require more oxygen, and receive a greater proportion of the blood volume as it circulates (see Fig. 13–10).

2. Blood flow is increased by the dilation of arterioles and precapillary sphincters.

3. In less active tissues, arterioles and precapillary sphincters constrict.

4. Organs receive sufficient oxygen, and BP for the body is maintained within the normal range.

Regulation of Blood Pressure—intrinsic mechanisms and nervous mechanisms

Intrinsic Mechanisms

1. The heart—responds to increased venous return by pumping more forcefully (Starling's Law), which increases cardiac output and BP.

2. The kidneys—decreased blood flow decreases filtration, which decreases urinary output to preserve blood volume. Decreased BP stimulates the kidneys to secrete renin, which initiates the renin-angiotensin mechanism (Table 13–3 and Fig. 13–11) that results in the formation of angiotensin II, which causes vasoconstriction and stimulates secretion of aldosterone.

Nervous Mechanisms (see Fig. 13–12)

1. Heart rate and force—see also Chapter 12.

2. Peripheral resistance—the medulla contains the vasomotor center, which consists of a vasoconstrictor area and a vasodilator area. The vasodilator area brings about vasodilation by suppressing the vasoconstrictor area. The vasoconstrictor area maintains normal vasoconstriction by generating several impulses per second along sympathetic vasoconstrictor fibers to all arteries and veins. More impulses per second increase vasoconstriction and raise BP; fewer impulses per second bring about vasodilation and a drop in BP.

REVIEW QUESTIONS

1. Describe the structure of the three layers in the walls of arteries, and state the function of each layer. Describe the structural differences in these layers in veins, and explain the reason for each difference. (p. 278)

2. Describe the structure and purpose of anastomoses, and give a specific example. (p. 278)

3. Describe the structure of capillaries. State the process by which each of the following is exchanged between capillaries and tissue fluid: nutrients, oxygen, waste products, and carbon dioxide. (pp. 279–281)

4. State the part of the body supplied by each of the following arteries: (pp. 286–287)
   a. Bronchial
   b. Femoral
   c. Hepatic
   d. Brachial
   e. Inferior mesenteric
   f. Internal carotid
   g. Subclavian
   h. Intercostal

5. Describe the pathway of blood flow in hepatic portal circulation. Use a specific example to explain the purpose of portal circulation. (pp. 285, 287)

6. Begin at the right ventricle and describe the pathway of pulmonary circulation. Explain the purpose of this pathway. (p. 282)

7. Name the fetal structure with each of the following functions: (pp. 287, 289)

a. Permits blood to flow from the right atrium to the left atrium

b. Carries blood from the placenta to the fetus

c. Permits blood to flow from the pulmonary artery to the aorta

d. Carry blood from the fetus to the placenta

e. Carries blood from the umbilical vein to the inferior vena cava

8. Describe the three mechanisms that promote venous return when the body is vertical. (pp. 292, 294)

9. Explain how the normal elasticity of the large arteries affects both systolic and diastolic blood pressure. (p. 295)

10. Explain how Starling's Law of the Heart is involved in the maintenance of blood pressure. (p. 292)

11. Name two hormones involved in the maintenance of blood pressure, and state the function of each. (p. 295)

12. Describe two different ways the kidneys respond to decreased blood flow and blood pressure. (pp. 296–297)

13. State two compensations that will maintain blood pressure after a small loss of blood. (p. 295)

14. State the location of the vasomotor center and name its two parts. Name the division of the autonomic nervous system that carries impulses to blood vessels. Which blood vessels? Which tissue in these vessels? Explain why normal vasoconstriction is important. Explain how greater vasoconstriction is brought about. Explain how vasodilation is brought about. How will each of these changes affect blood pressure? (pp. 298–299)

FOR FURTHER THOUGHT

1. Some old textbooks used the term *descending aorta*. Explain what is meant by that, and why it is not a very good term. Explain why an aneurysm of the aorta is quite likely to rupture sooner or later.

2. Renee, a nurse, is first on the scene of a car accident. The driver has been thrown from the car, and even from 15 feet away, Renee knows that a large artery in the man's leg has been severed. How does she know this? What two things does she see? Renee stops the bleeding, but the ambulance has not arrived. She wants to assess the man's condition after he has lost so much blood. She cannot take a blood pressure, but what other vital sign can be helpful? Explain. If Renee could take a blood pressure reading, what might it be? Might it be within the normal range? Explain.

3. A friend tells you that her grandmother has a tendency to develop blood clots in the veins of her legs. Your friend fears that her grandmother will have a stroke as a result. How would you explain that a stroke is not likely? Because you are a good friend, you want to explain the serious result that may occur. How would you do that?

4. Some people with hypertension take prescribed diuretics. Some call these "water pills." Is this an accurate name? How can a diuretic help lower blood pressure? What disadvantage does the use of diuretics have?

5. Sinusoids are found in the liver and pituitary gland. For each of these organs, name 4 specific large molecules that enter the blood by way of sinusoids.

CHAPTER 14

Student Objectives

- Describe the functions of the lymphatic system.
- Describe how lymph is formed.
- Describe the system of lymph vessels, and explain how lymph is returned to the blood.
- State the locations and functions of the lymph nodes and nodules.
- State the location and functions of the spleen.
- Explain the role of the thymus in immunity.
- Explain what is meant by immunity.
- Describe humoral immunity and cell-mediated immunity.
- Describe the responses to a first and second exposure to a pathogen.
- Explain the difference between genetic immunity and acquired immunity.
- Explain the difference between passive acquired immunity and active acquired immunity.
- Explain how vaccines work.

The Lymphatic System and Immunity

New Terminology

Acquired immunity (uh-**KWHY**-erd)
Active immunity (**AK**-tiv)
Antibody (**AN**-ti-BAH-dee)
Antigen (**AN**-ti-jen)
B cells (B SELLS)
Cell-mediated immunity (SELL **ME**-dee-ay-ted)
Genetic immunity (je-**NET**-ik)
Humoral immunity (**HYOO**-mohr-uhl)
Lymph (LIMF)
Lymph nodes (LIMF NOHDS)
Lymph nodules (LIMF **NAHD**-yools)
Opsonization (OP-sah-ni-**ZAY**-shun)
Passive immunity (**PASS**-iv)
Plasma cell (**PLAZ**-mah SELL)
Spleen (**SPLEEN**)
T cells (T SELLS)
Thymus (**THIGH**-mus)
Tonsils (**TAHN**-sills)

Related Clinical Terminology

AIDS (AYDS)
Allergy (**AL**-er-jee)
Antibody titer (**AN**-ti-BAH-dee **TIGH**-ter)
Attenuated (uh-**TEN**-yoo-AY-ted)
Complement fixation test (**KOM**-ple-ment fik-**SAY**-shun)
Fluorescent antibody test (floor-**ESS**-ent)
Hodgkin's disease (**HODJ**-kinz)
Interferon (in-ter-**FEER**-on)
Tonsillectomy (TAHN-si-**LEK**-toh-mee)
Toxoid (**TOK**-soyd)
Vaccine (vak-**SEEN**)

*Terms that appear in **bold type** in the chapter text are defined in the glossary, which begins on page 521.*

A child falls and scrapes her knee. Is this likely to be a life-threatening injury? Probably not, even though the breaks in the skin have permitted the entry of thousands or even millions of bacteria. Those bacteria, however, will be quickly destroyed by the cells and organs of the lymphatic system.

Although the lymphatic system may be considered part of the circulatory system, we will consider it separately because its functions are so different from those of the heart and blood vessels. Keep in mind, however, that all of these functions are interdependent. The lymphatic system is responsible for returning tissue fluid to the blood and for protecting the body against foreign material. The parts of the lymphatic system are the lymph, the system of lymph vessels, lymph nodes and nodules, the spleen, and the thymus gland.

LYMPH

Lymph is the name for tissue fluid that enters lymph capillaries. As you may recall from Chapter 13, filtration in capillaries creates tissue fluid, most of which returns almost immediately to the blood in the capillaries by osmosis. Some tissue fluid, however, remains in interstitial spaces and must be returned to the blood by way of the lymphatic vessels. Without this return, blood volume and blood pressure would very soon decrease. The relationship of the lymphatic vessels to the cardiovascular system is depicted in Fig. 14–1.

LYMPH VESSELS

The system of lymph vessels begins as dead-end **lymph capillaries** found in most tissue spaces (Fig. 14–2). Lymph capillaries are very permeable and collect tissue fluid and proteins. **Lacteals** are specialized lymph capillaries in the villi of the small intestine; they absorb the fat-soluble end products of digestion, such as fatty acids and vitamin A.

Lymph capillaries unite to form larger lymph vessels, whose structure is very much like that of veins. There is no pump for lymph (as the heart is the pump for blood), but the lymph is kept moving within lymph vessels by the same mechanisms that promote venous return. The smooth muscle layer of the larger lymph vessels constricts, and the one-way valves (just

like those of veins) prevent backflow of lymph. Lymph vessels in the extremities, especially the legs, are compressed by the skeletal muscles that surround them; this is the **skeletal muscle pump**. The **respiratory pump** alternately expands and compresses the lymph vessels in the chest cavity and keeps the lymph moving.

Where is the lymph going? Back to the blood to become plasma again. Refer to Fig. 14–3 as you read the following. The lymph vessels from the lower body unite in front of the lumbar vertebrae to form a vessel called the **cisterna chyli**, which continues upward in front of the backbone as the **thoracic duct**. Lymph vessels from the upper left quadrant of the body join the thoracic duct, which empties lymph into the left subclavian vein. Lymph vessels from the upper right quadrant of the body unite to form the right lymphatic duct, which empties lymph into the right subclavian vein. Flaps in both subclavian veins permit the entry of lymph but prevent blood from flowing into the lymph vessels.

LYMPH NODES AND NODULES

Lymph nodes and **nodules** are masses of lymphatic tissue. Recall that lymphatic tissue is one of the hemopoietic tissues and that one of its functions is to produce lymphocytes and monocytes. Nodes and nodules differ with respect to size and location. Nodes are usually larger, 10 to 20 mm in length; nodules range from a fraction of a millimeter to several millimeters in length.

Lymph nodes are found in groups along the pathways of lymph vessels, and lymph flows through these nodes on its way to the subclavian veins. Lymph enters a node through several afferent lymph vessels and leaves through one or two efferent vessels (Fig. 14–4). As lymph passes through a lymph node, bacteria and other foreign materials are phagocytized by fixed (stationary) **macrophages**. Fixed **plasma cells** (from lymphocytes) produce antibodies to any pathogens in the lymph; these antibodies, as well as lymphocytes and monocytes, will eventually reach the blood.

There are many groups of lymph nodes along all the lymph vessels throughout the body, but three paired groups deserve mention because of their strategic locations. These are the **cervical, axillary,** and **inguinal** lymph nodes (see Fig. 14–3). Notice that these are at the junctions of the head and extremities

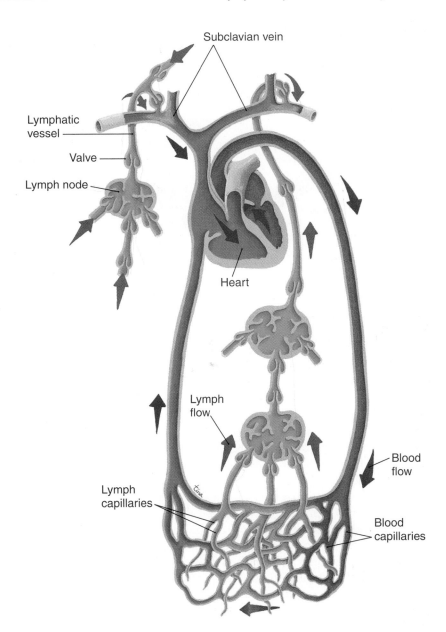

Subclavian vein

Lymphatic
vessel

Valve

Lymph node

Heart

Lymph
flow

Blood
flow

Lymph
capillaries

Blood
capillaries

Figure 14–1   Relationship of lymphatic vessels to the cardiovascular system. Lymph capillaries collect tissue fluid, which is returned to the blood. The arrows indicate the direction of flow of the blood and lymph.

with the trunk of the body. Breaks in the skin, with entry of pathogens, are much more likely to occur in the arms or legs or head rather than in the trunk. If these pathogens get to the lymph, they will be destroyed by the lymph nodes before they get to the trunk, before the lymph is returned to the blood in the subclavian veins.

You may be familiar with the expression "swollen glands," as when a child has a strep throat (an inflammation of the pharynx caused by *Streptococcus* bacte-

ria). These "glands" are the cervical lymph nodes that have enlarged as their macrophages attempt to destroy the bacteria in the lymph from the pharynx (see Box 14–1: Hodgkin's Disease).

Lymph nodules are small masses of lymphatic tissue found just beneath the epithelium of all **mucous membranes**. The body systems lined with mucous membranes are those that have openings to the environment: the respiratory, digestive, urinary, and reproductive tracts. You can probably see that

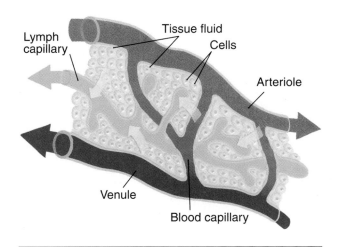

Figure 14–2   Dead-end lymph capillaries found in tissue spaces. Arrows indicate the movement of plasma, lymph, and tissue fluid.

these are also strategic locations for lymph nodules, because any natural body opening is a possible portal of entry for pathogens. For example, if bacteria in inhaled air get through the epithelium of the trachea, lymph nodules with their macrophages are in position to destroy these bacteria before they get to the blood.

Some of the lymph nodules have specific names. Those of the small intestine are called **Peyer's patches**, and those of the pharynx are called **tonsils**. The palatine tonsils are on the lateral walls of the pharynx, the adenoid (pharyngeal tonsil) is on the posterior wall, and the lingual tonsils are on the base of the tongue. The tonsils, therefore, form a ring of lymphatic tissue around the pharynx, which is a common pathway for food and air and for the pathogens they contain. A **tonsillectomy** is the surgical removal of the palatine tonsils and the adenoid and may be performed if the tonsils are chronically inflamed and swollen, as may happen in children. As mentioned earlier, the body has redundant structures to help ensure survival if one structure is lost or seriously impaired. Thus, there are many other lymph nodules in the pharynx to take over the function of the surgically removed tonsils.

SPLEEN

The **spleen** is located in the upper left quadrant of the abdominal cavity, just below the diaphragm,

behind the stomach. The lower rib cage protects the spleen from physical trauma (see Fig. 14–3).

In the fetus, the spleen produces red blood cells, a function assumed by the red bone marrow after birth.

The functions of the spleen after birth are:

1. Produces lymphocytes and monocytes, which enter the blood.
2. Contains fixed plasma cells that produce antibodies to foreign antigens.
3. Contains fixed macrophages (RE cells) that phagocytize pathogens or other foreign material in the blood. The macrophages of the spleen also phagocytize old red blood cells and form bilirubin. By way of portal circulation, the bilirubin is sent to the liver for excretion in bile.

The spleen is not considered a vital organ, because other organs compensate for its functions if the spleen must be removed. The liver and red bone marrow will remove old red blood cells from circulation, and the many lymph nodes and nodules will produce lymphocytes and monocytes and phagocytize pathogens (as will the liver). Despite this redundancy, a person without a spleen is somewhat more susceptible to certain bacterial infections such as pneumonia and meningitis.

THYMUS

The **thymus** is located inferior to the thyroid gland. In the fetus and infant, the thymus is large and extends under the sternum (Fig. 14–5). With increasing age, the thymus shrinks, and relatively little thymus tissue is found in adults.

The lymphocytes produced by the thymus are called T lymphocytes or **T cells**; their functions are discussed in the next section. Thymic hormones are necessary for what may be called "immunological competence." To be competent means to be able to do something well. The thymic hormones enable the T cells to participate in the recognition of foreign antigens and to provide immunity. This capability of T cells is established early in life and then is perpetuated by the lymphocytes themselves. The newborn's immune system is not yet fully mature, and infants are more susceptible to certain infections than are older children and adults. Usually by the age of 2 years, the immune system matures and becomes fully functional. This is why some vaccines, such as the

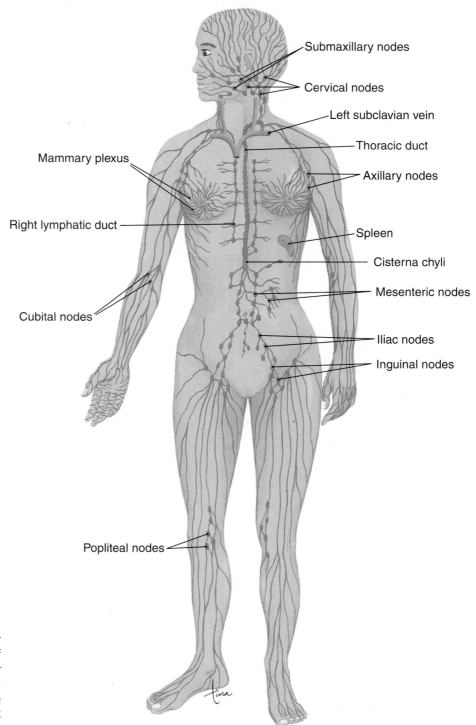

Submaxillary nodes

Cervical nodes

Left subclavian vein

Thoracic duct

Mammary plexus

Axillary nodes

Right lymphatic duct

Spleen

Cisterna chyli

Mesenteric nodes

Cubital nodes

Iliac nodes

Inguinal nodes

Popliteal nodes

Figure 14–3 System of lymph vessels and the major groups of lymph nodes. Lymph is returned to the blood in the right and left subclavian veins.

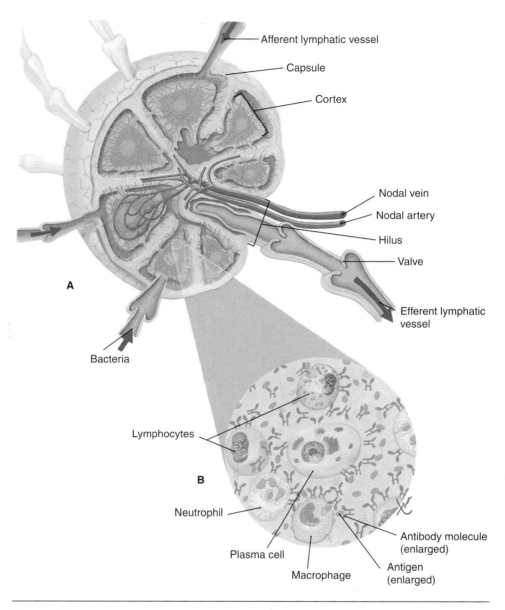

Afferent lymphatic vessel

Capsule

Cortex

Nodal vein

Nodal artery

Hilus

Valve

Efferent lymphatic vessel

A

Bacteria

Lymphocytes

B

Neutrophil

Plasma cell

Macrophage

Antibody molecule (enlarged)

Antigen (enlarged)

Figure 14–4   Lymph node. **(A)** Section through a lymph node, showing the flow of lymph. **(B)** Microscopic detail of bacteria being destroyed within the lymph node.

Box 14–1   HODGKIN'S DISEASE

Hodgkin's disease is a malignant disorder of the lymph nodes; the cause is not known. The first symptom is usually a swollen but painless lymph node, often in the cervical region. The individual is prompted to seek medical attention by other symptoms: chronic fever, fatigue, and weight loss. The diagnosis involves biopsy of the lymph node and the finding of characteristic cells.

Treatment of Hodgkin's disease requires chemotherapy, radiation, or both. With early diagnosis and proper treatment, this malignancy is very often curable.

Trachea

Clavicle

First rib

Thymus gland

Figure 14–5   Location of the thymus in a young child.

measles vaccine, are not recommended for infants younger than 15 to 18 months of age. Their immune systems are not mature enough to respond strongly to the vaccine, and the protection provided by the vaccine may be incomplete.

IMMUNITY

Immunity may be defined as the ability to destroy pathogens or other foreign material and to prevent further cases of certain infectious diseases. This ability is of vital importance because the body is exposed to pathogens from the moment of birth.

Malignant cells, which may be formed within the body as a result of mutations of normal cells, are also recognized as foreign and are usually destroyed before they can establish themselves and cause cancer. Unfortunately, organ transplants are also foreign tissue, and the immune system may reject (destroy) a transplanted kidney or heart. Sometimes the immune system mistakenly reacts to part of the body itself and causes an autoimmune disease; several of these were mentioned in previous chapters. Most often, however, the immune mechanisms function to protect the body from the microorganisms around us and within us.

LYMPHOCYTES

There are three types of lymphocytes: natural killer cells, T lymphocytes, and B lymphocytes. Each has different functions.

Natural killer cells (NK cells) circulate in the blood but are also found in the red bone marrow, spleen, and lymph nodes. They are a small portion (about 10%) of the total lymphocytes, but are able to destroy many kinds of pathogens and tumor cells. NK cells make direct contact with foreign cells, and kill them by rupturing their cell membranes or inflicting some other kind of chemical damage. Foreign cells are recognized as such because they lack the normal antigens found on an individual's cells.

The majority of lymphocytes are the T lymphocytes and B lymphocytes, or, more simply, **T cells** and **B cells**. In the embryo, T cells are produced in the bone marrow and thymus. They must pass through the thymus, where the thymic hormones bring about their maturation. The T cells then migrate to the spleen, lymph nodes, and lymph nodules, where they are found after birth.

Produced in the embryo bone marrow, B cells then migrate directly to the spleen and lymph nodes and nodules. When activated during an immune response, some B cells will become plasma cells that produce antibodies to a specific foreign antigen.

The mechanisms of immunity that involve T cells and B cells are specific, meaning that one foreign antigen is the target each time a mechanism is activated. A macrophage has receptor sites for foreign chemicals such as those of bacterial cell walls or flagella, and may phagocytize just about any foreign material it comes across (as will the Langerhans or dendritic cells of the skin). T cells and B cells, however, become very specific, as you will see.

ANTIGENS AND ANTIBODIES

Antigens are chemical markers that identify cells. Human cells have their own antigens that identify all the cells in an individual as "self" (recall the HLA types mentioned in Chapter 11). When antigens are foreign, or "non-self," they may be recognized as such and destroyed. Bacteria, viruses, fungi, protozoa, malignant cells, and organ transplants are all foreign antigens that activate immune responses.

Antibodies, also called **immune globulins** or **gamma globulins**, are proteins produced by plasma cells in response to foreign antigens. Antibodies do

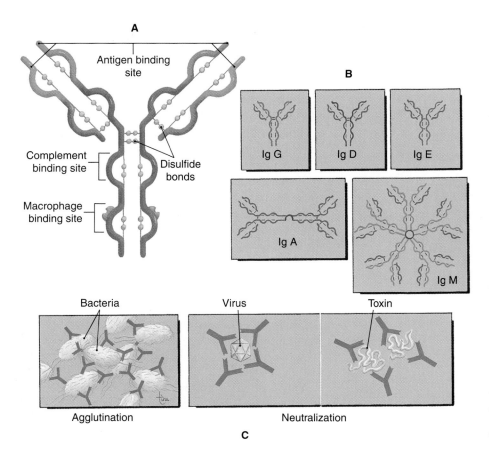

Figure 14–6 Antibodies. **(A)** Structure of one IgG molecule. Notice how the many disulfide bonds maintain the shape of the molecule. **(B)** Structure of the five classes of antibodies. **(C)** Antibody activity: Agglutination of bacteria and neutralization of viruses or toxins.

not themselves destroy foreign antigens, but rather become attached to such antigens to "label" them for destruction. Each antibody produced is specific for only one antigen. Since there are so many different pathogens, you might think that the immune system would have to be capable of producing many different antibodies, and in fact this is so. It is estimated that millions of different antigen-specific antibodies can be produced, should there be a need for them.

The structure of antibodies is shown in Fig. 14–6, and the five classes of antibodies are described in Table 14–1.

MECHANISMS OF IMMUNITY

The first step in the destruction of a pathogen or foreign cell is the recognition of its antigens as foreign. Both T cells and B cells are capable of this, but the immune mechanisms are activated especially well when this recognition is accomplished by macrophages and a specialized group of T lymphocytes called **helper T cells**. The foreign antigen is first phagocytized by a macrophage, and parts of it are "presented" on the macrophage's cell membrane. Also on the macrophage membrane are "self" antigens that are representative of the antigens found on all of the cells of the individual. Therefore, the helper T cell that encounters this macrophage is presented not only with the foreign antigen but also with "self" antigens for comparison. The helper T cell now becomes sensitized to and specific for the foreign antigen, the one that does not belong in the body (see Box 14–2: AIDS).

The recognition of an antigen as foreign initiates one or both of the mechanisms of immunity. These are **cell-mediated immunity**, in which T cells and macrophages participate, and **humoral immunity** (or antibody-mediated), which involves T cells, B cells, and macrophages.

Cell-Mediated Immunity

This mechanism of immunity does not result in the production of antibodies, but it is effective against

Table 14–1 CLASSES OF ANTIBODIES

Name	Location	Functions
IgG	Blood	• Crosses the placenta to provide passive immunity for newborns
	Extracellular fluid	• Provides long-term immunity following recovery or a vaccine
IgA	External secretions (tears, saliva, etc.)	• Present in breast milk to provide passive immunity for breast-fed infants • Found in secretions of all mucous membranes
IgM	Blood	• Produced first by the maturing immune system of infants • Produced first during an infection (IgG production follows) • Part of the ABO blood group
IgD	B lymphocytes	• Receptors on B lymphocytes
IgE	Mast cells or basophils	• Important in allergic reactions (mast cells release histamine)

intracellular pathogens (such as viruses), fungi, malignant cells, and grafts of foreign tissue. As mentioned above, the first step is the recognition of the foreign antigen by macrophages and helper T cells, which become activated and specific (you may find it helpful to refer to Fig. 14–7 as you read the following).

These activated T cells, which are antigen specific, divide many times, forming **memory T cells** and **cytotoxic (killer) T cells**. The memory T cells will remember the specific foreign antigen and become active if it enters the body again. Cytotoxic T cells are able to chemically destroy foreign antigens by disrupting cell membranes. This is how cytotoxic T cells destroy cells infected with viruses, and prevent the viruses from reproducing. These T cells also produce cytokines, which are chemicals that attract macrophages to the area and activate them to phagocytize the foreign antigen.

Other activated T cells become **suppressor T cells**, which will stop the immune response once the foreign antigen has been destroyed. The memory T cells, however, will quickly initiate the cell-mediated immune response should there be a future exposure to the antigen.

Humoral Immunity

This mechanism of immunity does involve the production of antibodies and is diagrammed in Fig. 14–8. Again, the first step is the recognition of the foreign antigen, this time by B cells as well as by macrophages and helper T cells. The sensitized helper T cell presents the foreign antigen to B cells, which provides a strong stimulus for the activation of B cells specific for this antigen. The activated B cells begin to divide many times, and two types of cells are formed. Some of the new B cells produced are **memory B cells**, which will remember the specific antigen. Other B cells become **plasma cells** that produce antibodies specific for this one foreign antigen.

The antibodies then bond to the antigen, forming an antigen–antibody complex. This complex results in **opsonization**, which means that the antigen is now "labeled" for phagocytosis by macrophages or neutrophils. The antigen–antibody complex also stimulates the process of complement fixation (see Box 14–3: Diagnostic Tests).

Complement is a group of about 20 plasma proteins that circulate in the blood until activated, or fixed, by an antigen–antibody complex. Complement fixation may be complete or partial. If the foreign antigen is cellular, the complement proteins bond to the antigen–antibody complex, then to one another, forming an enzymatic ring that punches a hole in the cell to bring about the death of the cell. This is complete (or entire) complement fixation and is what happens to bacterial cells (it is also the cause of hemolysis in a transfusion reaction).

If the foreign antigen is not a cell, a virus for example, partial complement fixation takes place, in which some of the complement proteins bond to the anti-

Box 14–2 AIDS

In 1981, young homosexual men in New York and California were diagnosed with Kaposi's sarcoma and *Pneumocystis carinii* pneumonia. At that time, Kaposi's sarcoma was known as a rare, slowly growing malignancy in elderly men. Pneumocystis pneumonia was almost unheard of; *P. carinii* is a pathogen that does not cause disease in healthy people. That in itself was a clue. These young men were not healthy; their immune systems were not functioning normally. As the number of patients increased rapidly, the disease was given a name (acquired immune deficiency syndrome—AIDS) and the pathogen was found. Human immunodeficiency virus (HIV) is a retrovirus that infects helper T cells, macrophages, and other human cells. Once infected, the human cells contain HIV genes for the rest of their lives. Without sufficient helper T cells, the immune system is seriously impaired. Foreign antigens are not recognized, B cells are not activated, and killer T cells are not stimulated to proliferate.

The person with AIDS is susceptible to opportunistic infections, that is, those infections caused by fungi and protozoa that would not affect average healthy adults. Some of these infections may be treated with medications and even temporarily cured, but the immune system cannot prevent the next infection, or the next. As of this writing, AIDS is considered an incurable disease, although with proper medical treatment, some people with AIDS may live for many years.

Where did this virus come from? The latest research suggests that HIV evolved from a harmless chimpanzee virus, in Africa sometime during the 1930s. Spread of the virus was very slow at first, and only when air travel became commonplace did the virus spread worldwide.

The incubation period of AIDS is highly variable, ranging from a few months to several years. An infected person may unknowingly spread HIV to others before any symptoms appear. It should be emphasized that AIDS, although communicable, is not a contagious disease. It is not spread by casual contact as is measles or the common cold. Transmission of AIDS occurs through sexual contact, contact with infected blood, or by placental transmission of the virus from mother to fetus.

In the United States, most of the cases of AIDS during the 1980s were in homosexual men and IV drug users who shared infected syringes contaminated with their blood. By the 1990s, however, it was clear that AIDS was becoming more of a heterosexually transmitted disease, with rapidly increasing case rates among women and teenagers. In much of the rest of the world, especially Africa and Asia, the transmission of AIDS has always been primarily by heterosexual contact, with equal numbers of women and men infected.

How can the spread of HIV be stopped? At present we still have no antiviral medications that will eradicate this virus, although certain combinations of drugs effectively suppress the virus in some people. For these people, AIDS may become a chronic but not fatal disease. Unfortunately, the medications do not work for everyone, and they are very expensive, beyond the means of most of the world's AIDS patients.

Development of an AIDS vaccine is likely by 2010, perhaps sooner, and dozens of vaccines are undergoing clinical trials. A vaccine stimulates antibody production to a specific pathogen, but everyone who has died of AIDS had antibodies to HIV, and those antibodies were not protective. Why not? HIV is a mutating virus; it constantly changes itself, making previously produced antibodies ineffective. An AIDS vaccine may not be entirely effective, may not have the 80–90% protection rate we have come to expect from vaccines.

If we cannot cure AIDS and we cannot yet prevent it by vaccination, what recourse is left? Education. Everyone should know how AIDS is spread. The obvious reason is to be able to avoid the high-risk behaviors that make acquiring HIV more likely. Yet another reason, however, is that everyone should know that they need not fear casual contact with people with AIDS. Health-care personnel have a special responsibility, not only to educate themselves, but to provide education about AIDS for their patients and the families of their patients.

gen–antibody complex. This is a chemotactic factor. Chemotaxis means "chemical movement" and is actually another label that attracts macrophages to engulf and destroy the foreign antigen.

When the foreign antigen has been destroyed, suppressor T cells that have been sensitized to it stop the immune response. This is important to limit antibody production to just what is necessary to eliminate

Figure 14–7 Cell-mediated immunity. See text for description.

ANTIBODY RESPONSES

The first exposure to a foreign antigen does stimulate antibody production, but antibodies are produced slowly and in small amounts (see Fig. 14–9). Let us take as a specific example: the measles virus. On a person's first exposure to this virus, antibody production is usually too slow to prevent the disease itself, and the person will have clinical measles. Most people

the pathogen without triggering an autoimmune response.

who get measles recover, and upon recovery have antibodies and memory cells that are specific for the measles virus.

On a second exposure to this virus, the memory cells initiate rapid production of large amounts of antibodies, enough to prevent a second case of measles. This is the reason why we develop immunity to certain diseases, and this is also the basis for the protection given by **vaccines** (see Box 14–4: Vaccines).

As mentioned previously, antibodies label pathogens or other foreign antigens for phagocytosis or complement fixation. More specifically, antibodies

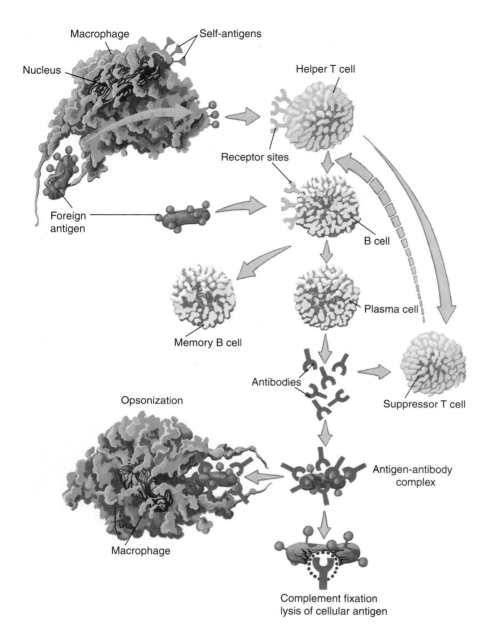

Macrophage
Self-antigens
Nucleus
Helper T cell
Receptor sites
Foreign antigen
B cell
Memory B cell
Plasma cell
Antibodies
Suppressor T cell
Opsonization
Antigen-antibody complex
Macrophage
Complement fixation lysis of cellular antigen

Figure 14–8 Humoral or antibody-mediated immunity. See text for description of events.

cause agglutination or neutralization of pathogens before their eventual destruction. **Agglutination** means "clumping," and this is what happens when antibodies bind to bacterial cells. The bacteria that are clumped together by attached antibodies are more easily phagocytized by macrophages (see Fig. 14–6).

The activity of viruses may be neutralized by antibodies. A virus must get inside a living cell in order to reproduce itself. However, a virus with antibodies attached to it is unable to enter a cell, cannot reproduce, and will soon be phagocytized. (Another aspect of antiviral defense is a chemical called **interferon**, which is discussed in Box 14–5.) Bacterial toxins may also be neutralized by attached antibodies. The antibodies change the shape of the toxin, prevent it from exerting its harmful effects, and promote its phagocytosis by macrophages.

Allergies are also the result of antibody activity (see Box 14–6).

Box 14–3   DIAGNOSTIC TESTS

Several important laboratory tests involve antibodies and may be very useful to confirm a diagnosis.

Complement Fixation Test—determines the presence of a particular antibody in the patient's blood, but does not indicate when the infection occurred.

Antibody Titer—determines the level or amount of a specific antibody in the patient's blood. If another titer is done 1 to several weeks later, an increase in the antibody level shows the infection to be current.

Fluorescent Antibody Test—uses antibodies tagged with fluorescent dyes, which are added to a clinical specimen such as blood, sputum, or a biopsy of tissue. If the suspected pathogen is present, the fluorescent antibodies will bond to it and the antigen-antibody complex will "glow" when examined with a fluorescent microscope.

Tests such as these are used in conjunction with patient history and symptoms to arrive at a diagnosis.

TYPES OF IMMUNITY

There are two major categories of immunity: genetic immunity, which is conferred by our DNA, and acquired immunity, which we must develop or acquire by natural or artificial means.

Genetic immunity does not involve antibodies or the immune system; it is the result of our genetic makeup. What it means is that some pathogens cause disease in certain host species but not in others. Dogs and cats, for example, have genetic immunity to the measles virus, which is a pathogen only for people. Plant viruses affect only plants, not people; we have genetic immunity to them. This is not because we have antibodies against these plant viruses, but rather that our genetic makeup makes

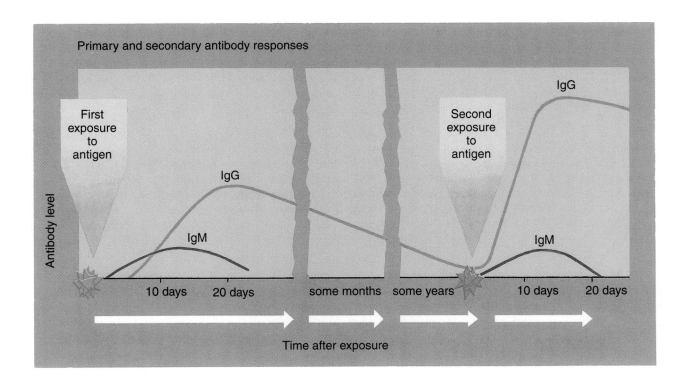

Figure 14–9   Antibody responses to first and subsequent exposures to a pathogen. See text for description.

Box 14–4   VACCINES

The purpose of vaccines is to prevent disease. A vaccine contains an antigen that the immune system will respond to, just as it would to the actual pathogen. The types of vaccine antigens are a killed or weakened **(attenuated)** pathogen, part of a pathogen such as a bacterial capsule, or an inactivated bacterial toxin called a **toxoid**.

Because the vaccine itself does not cause disease (with very rare exceptions), the fact that antibody production to it is slow is not detrimental to the person. The vaccine takes the place of the first exposure to the pathogen and stimulates production of antibodies and memory cells. On exposure to the pathogen itself, the memory cells initiate rapid production of large amounts of antibody, enough to prevent disease.

We now have vaccines for many diseases. The tetanus and diphtheria vaccines contain toxoids, the inactivated toxins of these bacteria. Vaccines for pneumococcal pneumonia and meningitis contain bacterial capsules. These vaccines cannot cause disease because the capsules are non-toxic and non-living; there is nothing that can reproduce. Influenza and rabies vaccines contain killed viruses. Measles and the oral polio vaccines contain attenuated (weakened) viruses.

Although attenuated pathogens are usually strongly antigenic and stimulate a protective immune response, there is a very small chance that the pathogen may regain its virulence and cause the disease. For example, a few cases each year of polio are caused by the oral polio vaccine itself. Although the risk is small (1 in 500,000), parents should be aware that a killed virus vaccine is available, which they may request for their children.

Box 14–5   INTERFERON

Interferon is produced by cells infected with viruses and by T cells. Viruses must be inside a living cell to reproduce, and although interferon cannot prevent the entry of viruses into cells, it does block their reproduction. When viral reproduction is blocked, the viruses cannot infect new cells and cause disease. Interferon is probably a factor in the self-limiting nature of many viral diseases.

There are several types of human interferon (alpha, beta, gamma), which were first produced in amounts sufficient for clinical research in the 1970s. At that time there was hope that interferon would be an effective anti-cancer therapy, but results against the most common forms of cancer were disappointing. Alpha interferon is effective, however, in the treatment of a rare type of leukemia called hairy-cell leukemia and has also been approved for use in cases of genital warts and Kaposi's sarcoma. Most recently, interferon has proved useful in the treatment of hepatitis B and C and multiple sclerosis, although it is not equally effective for all patients.

The research on the interferons is a good example of the way science works. Discovery, research, dead-ends, more research, other possibilities, and so on. Our knowledge is gained piece by piece and often requires many years of careful study. In the future, the interferons will probably become more useful therapeutic tools, but there is much to be learned first.

it impossible for such pathogens to reproduce in our cells and tissues. Because this is a genetic characteristic programmed in DNA, genetic immunity always lasts a lifetime.

Acquired immunity does involve antibodies. **Passive immunity** means that the antibodies are from another source, whereas **active immunity** means that the individual produces his or her own antibodies.

One type of naturally acquired passive immunity is the placental transmission of antibodies (IgG) from maternal blood to fetal circulation. The baby will then be born temporarily immune to the diseases the mother is immune to. Such passive immunity may be prolonged by breast-feeding, because breast milk also contains maternal antibodies (IgA).

Artificially acquired passive immunity is obtained by the injection of immune globulins (gamma globu-

Box 14–6   ALLERGIES

An **allergy** is a hypersensitivity to a particular foreign antigen, called an **allergen**. Allergens include plant pollens, foods, chemicals in cosmetics, antibiotics such as penicillin, dust, and mold spores. Such allergens are not themselves harmful. Most people, for example, can inhale pollen, eat peanuts, or take penicillin with no ill effects.

Hypersensitivity means that the immune system overresponds to the allergen, and produces tissue damage by doing so. Allergic responses are characterized by the production of IgE antibodies, which bond to mast cells. Mast cells are specialized cells that differentiate from basophils, and are numerous in the connective tissue of the skin and mucous membranes. One of several chemicals in mast cells is histamine, which is released by the bonding of IgE antibodies or when tissue damage occurs.

Histamine contributes to the process of inflammation by increasing the permeability of capillaries and venules. When tissue is damaged this promotes greater tissue fluid formation and brings more WBCs to the damaged area.

In an allergic reaction, the effects of histamine and other inflammatory chemicals create symptoms such as watery eyes and runny nose (hay fever) or the more serious wheezing and difficult breathing that characterize asthma. People with seasonal hay fever may take antihistamines to counteract these effects (see Chapter 15 for a description of asthma).

Anaphylactic shock is an extreme allergic response that may be elicited by exposure to penicillin or insect venoms. On the first exposure the person becomes highly sensitized to the foreign antigen. On the second exposure, histamine is released from mast cells throughout the body and causes a drastic decrease in blood volume. The resulting drop in blood pressure may be fatal in only a few minutes. People who know they are allergic to bee stings, for example, may obtain a self-contained syringe of epinephrine to carry with them. Epinephrine can delay the progression of anaphylactic shock long enough for the person to seek medical attention.

lins or preformed antibodies) after presumed exposure to a particular pathogen. Such immune globulins are available for German measles, hepatitis A and B, tetanus and botulism (anti-toxins), and rabies. These are *not* vaccines; they do not stimulate immune mechanisms, but rather provide immediate antibody protection. Passive immunity is always temporary, lasting a few weeks to a few months, because antibodies from another source eventually break down.

Active immunity is the production of one's own antibodies and may be stimulated by natural or artificial means. Naturally acquired active immunity means that a person has recovered from a disease and now has antibodies and memory cells specific for that pathogen. Artificially acquired active immunity is the result of a vaccine that has stimulated production of antibodies and memory cells (see Box 14–7: Vaccines That Have Changed Our Lives). No general statement can be made about the duration of active immunity. Recovering from plague, for example, confers lifelong immunity, but the plague vaccine does not. Duration of active immunity, therefore, varies with the particular disease or vaccine.

The types of immunity are summarized in Table 14–2.

AGING AND THE LYMPHATIC SYSTEM

The aging of the lymphatic system is apparent in the decreased efficiency of immune responses. Elderly people are more susceptible to infections such as influenza and to what are called secondary infections, such as pneumonia following a case of the flu. Vaccines for both of these are available, and elderly people should be encouraged to get them. Elderly people should also be sure to get a tetanus-diphtheria booster every 10 years.

Autoimmune disorders are also more common among older people; the immune system mistakenly perceives a body tissue as foreign and initiates its destruction. Rheumatoid arthritis and myasthenia gravis are examples of autoimmune diseases. The incidence of cancer is also higher. Malignant cells that

Box 14–7   VACCINES THAT HAVE CHANGED OUR LIVES

In 1797, Edward Jenner (in England) published his results on the use of the cowpox virus called vaccinia as the first vaccine for smallpox, a closely related virus. (He was unaware of the actual pathogens, because viruses had not yet been discovered, but he had noticed that milkmaids who got cowpox rarely got smallpox.) In 1980, the World Health Organization declared that smallpox had been eradicated throughout the world. A disease that had killed or disfigured millions of people throughout recorded history is now considered part of history (except for the possible use of the virus as a biological weapon).

In the 19th century in the northern United States, thousands of children died of diphtheria every winter. Today there are fewer than 10 cases of diphtheria each year in the entire country. In the early 1950s, 50,000 cases of paralytic polio were reported in the United States each year. Today, wild-type polio virus is not found in North America.

Smallpox, diphtheria, and polio are no longer the terrible diseases they once were, and this is because of the development and widespread use of vaccines. When people are protected by a vaccine, they are no longer possible reservoirs or sources of the pathogen for others, and the spread of disease may be greatly limited.

Other diseases that have been controlled by the use of vaccines are whooping cough, tetanus, mumps, influenza, measles, and German measles. The vaccine for hepatitis B has significantly decreased the number of cases of this disease among healthcare workers, and the CDC recommends the vaccine for all children. People who have been exposed to rabies, which is virtually always fatal, can be protected by a new and safe vaccine.

Without such vaccines our lives would be very different. Infant mortality or death in childhood would be much more frequent, and all of us would have to be much more aware of infectious diseases. In many parts of the world this is still true; many of the developing countries in Africa and Asia still cannot afford extensive vaccination programs for their children. Many of the diseases mentioned above, which we may rarely think of, are still a very significant part of the lives of millions of people.

Table 14–2   TYPES OF IMMUNITY

Type	Description
Genetic	• Does not involve antibodies; is programmed in DNA • Some pathogens affect certain host species but not others
Acquired	• Does involve antibodies
Passive	• Antibodies from another source
NATURAL	• Placental transmission of antibodies from mother to fetus • Transmission of antibodies in breast milk
ARTIFICIAL	• Injection of preformed antibodies (gamma globulins or immune globulins) after presumed exposure
Active	• Production of one's own antibodies
NATURAL	• Recovery from a disease, with production of antibodies and memory cells
ARTIFICIAL	• A vaccine stimulates production of antibodies and memory cells

once might have been quickly destroyed remain alive and proliferate.

SUMMARY

The preceding discussions of immunity will give you a small idea of the complexity of the body's defense system. However, there is still much more to be learned, especially about the effects of the nervous system and endocrine system on immunity. For example, it is known that people under great stress have immune systems that may not function as they did when stress was absent.

At present, much research is being done in this field. The goal is not to eliminate all disease, for that would not be possible. Rather, the aim is to enable people to live healthier lives by preventing certain diseases.

STUDY OUTLINE

Functions of the Lymphatic System
1. To return tissue fluid to the blood to maintain blood volume (see Fig. 14–1).
2. To protect the body against pathogens and other foreign material.

Parts of the Lymphatic System
1. Lymph
2. Lymph vessels
3. Lymph nodes and nodules
4. Spleen
5. Thymus

Lymph—the tissue fluid that enters lymph capillaries
1. Similar to plasma, but more WBCs are present.
2. Must be returned to the blood to maintain blood volume and blood pressure.

Lymph Vessels
1. Dead-end lymph capillaries are found in most tissue spaces; collect tissue fluid and proteins (see Fig. 14–2).
2. The structure of larger lymph vessels is like that of veins; valves prevent the backflow of lymph.
3. Lymph is kept moving in lymph vessels by:
   - constriction of the lymph vessels
   - the skeletal muscle pump
   - the respiratory pump
4. Lymph from the lower body and upper left quadrant enters the thoracic duct and is returned to the blood in the left subclavian vein (see Fig. 14–3).
5. Lymph from the upper right quadrant enters the right lymphatic duct and is returned to the blood in the right subclavian vein.

Lymph Nodes—masses of lymphatic tissue; produce lymphocytes and monocytes
1. Found in groups along the pathways of lymph vessels.
2. As lymph flows through the nodes:
   - lymphocytes and monocytes enter the lymph
   - foreign materials are phagocytized by fixed macrophages
   - fixed plasma cells produce antibodies to foreign antigens (see Fig. 14–4)
3. The major paired groups of lymph nodes are the cervical, axillary, and inguinal groups. These are at the junctions of the head and extremities with the trunk; remove pathogens from the lymph from the extremities before the lymph is returned to the blood.

Lymph Nodules—small masses of lymphatic tissue; produce lymphocytes and monocytes
1. Found beneath the epithelium of all mucous membranes, that is, the tracts that have natural openings to the environment.
2. Destroy pathogens that penetrate the epithelium of the respiratory, digestive, urinary, or reproductive tracts.
3. Tonsils are the lymph nodules of the pharynx; Peyer's patches are those of the small intestine.

Spleen—located in the upper left abdominal quadrant behind the stomach
1. The fetal spleen produces RBCs.
2. Functions after birth:
   - production of lymphocytes and monocytes
   - fixed plasma cells produce antibodies
   - fixed macrophages (RE cells) phagocytize pathogens and old RBCs; bilirubin is formed and sent to the liver for excretion in bile

Thymus—in the fetus and infant the thymus is large and inferior to the thyroid gland; with age the thymus shrinks (see Fig. 14–5)
1. Produces T lymphocytes (T cells).
2. Produces thymic hormones that make T cells immunologically competent, that is, able to recognize foreign antigens and provide immunity.

Immunity
1. The ability to destroy foreign antigens and prevent future cases of certain infectious diseases.
2. Foreign antigens include bacteria, viruses, fungi, protozoa, and malignant cells.

Lymphocytes
1. Natural killer cells (NK cells)—destroy foreign or malignant cells by rupturing their cell membranes.
2. T lymphocytes (T cells)—in the embryo are produced in the thymus and RBM; they require the hormones of the thymus for maturation; migrate to the spleen, lymph nodes, and nodules.

3. B lymphocytes (B cells)—in the embryo are produced in the RBM; migrate to the spleen, lymph nodes, and nodules.

Antigens

1. Chemical markers that identify cells.
2. Human cells have "self" antigens—the HLA types.
3. Foreign antigens stimulate antibody production or other immune responses.

Antibodies—immune globulins or gamma globulins (see Table 14–1 and Fig. 14–6)

1. Proteins produced by plasma cells in response to foreign antigens.
2. Each antibody is specific for only one foreign antigen.
3. Bond to the foreign antigen to label it for phagocytosis (opsonization).

Mechanisms of Immunity

1. The antigen must first be recognized as foreign; this is accomplished by B cells or by helper T cells that compare the foreign antigen to "self" antigens present on macrophages.
2. Helper T cells strongly initiate one or both of the immune mechanisms: cell-mediated immunity and humoral immunity.

Cell-Mediated Immunity (see Fig. 14–7)

1. Does not involve antibodies; is effective against intracellular pathogens, malignant cells, and grafts of foreign tissue.
2. Helper T cells recognize the foreign antigen, become antigen specific, and begin to divide to form different groups of T cells.
3. Memory T cells will remember the specific foreign antigen.
4. Cytotoxic (killer) T cells chemically destroy foreign cells and produce cytokines to attract macrophages.
5. Suppressor T cells stop the immune response once the foreign antigen has been destroyed.

Humoral (Antibody-Mediated) Immunity (see Fig. 14–8)

1. Does involve antibody production; is effective against pathogens and foreign cells.
2. B cells and helper T cells recognize the foreign antigen; the B cells are antigen-specific and begin to divide.
3. Memory B cells will remember the specific foreign antigen.
4. Other B cells become plasma cells that produce antigen-specific antibodies.
5. An antigen–antibody complex is formed, which attracts macrophages (opsonization).
6. Complement fixation is stimulated by antigen–antibody complexes. The complement proteins bind to the antigen–antibody complex and lyse cellular antigens or enhance the phagocytosis of noncellular antigens.
7. Suppressor T cells stop the immune response when the foreign antigen has been destroyed.

Antibody Responses and Functions (see Fig. 14–9)

1. On the first exposure to a foreign antigen, antibodies are produced slowly and in small amounts, and the person may develop clinical disease.
2. On the second exposure, the memory cells initiate rapid production of large amounts of antibodies, and a second case of the disease may be prevented. This is the basis for the protection given by vaccines, which take the place of the first exposure.
3. Antibodies cause agglutination (clumping) of bacterial cells; clumped cells are easier for macrophages to phagocytize (see Fig. 14–6).
4. Antibodies neutralize viruses by bonding to them and preventing their entry into cells.
5. Antibodies neutralize bacterial toxins by bonding to them and changing their shape.

Types of Immunity (see Table 14–2)

REVIEW QUESTIONS

1. Explain the relationships among plasma, tissue fluid, and lymph, in terms of movement of water throughout the body. (p. 306)

2. Describe the system of lymph vessels. Explain how lymph is kept moving in these vessels. Into which veins is lymph emptied? (p. 306)

3. State the locations of the major groups of lymph nodes, and explain their functions. (pp. 306–307)

4. State the locations of lymph nodules, and explain their functions. (pp. 307–308)

5. Describe the location of the spleen and explain its functions. If the spleen is removed, what organs will compensate for its functions? (p. 308)

6. Explain the function of the thymus, and state when (age) this function is important. (p. 308)

7. Name the different kinds of foreign antigens to which the immune system responds. (p. 311)

8. State the functions of natural killer cells, helper T cells, cytotoxic T cells, memory T cells, and suppressor T cells. (pp. 311, 313)

9. Plasma cells differentiate from which type of lymphocyte? State the function of plasma cells. What other type of cell comes from B lymphocytes? (p. 313)

10. Explain how a foreign antigen is recognized as foreign. Which mechanism of immunity involves antibody production? Explain what opsonization means. (pp. 312–313)

11. What is the stimulus for complement fixation? How does this process destroy cellular antigens and non-cellular antigens? (pp. 313–314)

12. Explain the antibody reactions of agglutination and neutralization. (p. 316)

13. Explain how a vaccine provides protective immunity in terms of first and second exposures to a pathogen. (p. 315)

14. Explain the difference between the following: (pp. 317–319)
    a. Genetic immunity and acquired immunity
    b. Passive acquired immunity and active acquired immunity
    c. Natural and artificial passive acquired immunity
    d. Natural and artificial active acquired immunity

FOR FURTHER THOUGHT

1. Bubonic plague, also called black plague, is a serious disease caused by a bacterium and spread by fleas from rats or rodents to people. It got its "black" name from "buboes," dark swellings found in the groin or armpit of people with plague. Explain what buboes are, and why they were usually found in the groin and armpit.

2. In Rh disease of the newborn, maternal antibodies enter fetal circulation and destroy the red blood cells of the fetus. A mother with type O blood has anti-A and anti-B antibodies, but may have a dozen type A children without any problem at all. Explain why. (Look at Table 14–1 and Fig. 14–6.)

3. Most vaccines are given by injection. The oral polio vaccine (OPV) is not, rather it is given by mouth. Remembering that the purpose of a vaccine is to expose the individual to the pathogen, what does this tell you about the polio viruses (there are three) and their usual site of infection?

4. Everyone should have a tetanus booster shot every 10 years. That is what we often call a "tetanus shot." Someone who sustains a soil-contaminated injury should also receive a tetanus booster (if none in the past 10 years). But someone who has symptoms of tetanus should get TIG, tetanus immune globulin. Explain the difference, and why TIG is so important.

5. People with AIDS are susceptible to many other diseases. Which of these would be least likely: pneumonia, rheumatoid arthritis, yeast infection of the mouth, protozoan infection of the intestines? Explain your answer.

6. Think back to previous organ systems. Describe all the defenses against pathogens you can remember. Begin with the skin.

CHAPTER 15

Chapter Outline

Student Objectives

- State the general function of the respiratory system.
- Describe the structure and functions of the nasal cavities and pharynx.
- Describe the structure of the larynx and explain the speaking mechanism.
- Describe the structure and functions of the trachea and bronchial tree.
- State the locations of the pleural membranes, and explain the functions of serous fluid.
- Describe the structure of the alveoli and pulmonary capillaries, and explain the importance of surfactant.
- Name and describe the important air pressures involved in breathing.
- Describe normal inhalation and exhalation and forced exhalation.
- Explain the diffusion of gases in external respiration and internal respiration.
- Describe how oxygen and carbon dioxide are transported in the blood.
- Name the pulmonary volumes and define each.
- Explain the nervous and chemical mechanisms that regulate respiration.
- Explain how respiration affects the pH of body fluids.

The Respiratory System

New Terminology

Alveoli (al-**VEE**-oh-lye)
Bronchial tree (**BRONG**-kee-uhl TREE)
Epiglottis (ep-i-**GLAH**-tis)
Glottis (**GLAH**-tis)
Intrapleural pressure (IN-trah-**PLOOR**-uhl
   PRES–shur)
Intrapulmonic pressure (IN-trah-pull-**MAHN**-ik
   PRES-shur)
Larynx (**LA**-rinks)
Partial pressure (**PAR**-shul **PRES**-shur)
Phrenic nerves (**FREN**-ik NURVZ)
Pulmonary surfactant (**PULL**-muh-ner-ee
   sir–**FAK**–tent)
Residual air (ree-**ZID**-yoo-al AYRE)
Respiratory acidosis (RES-pi-rah-**TOR**-ee
   ass–i–**DOH**-sis)
Respiratory alkalosis (RES-pi-rah-**TOR**-ee
   al–kah–**LOH**-sis)
Soft palate (SAWFT **PAL**-uht)
Tidal volume (**TIGH**-duhl **VAHL**-yoom)
Ventilation (VEN-ti-**LAY**-shun)
Vital capacity (**VY**-tuhl kuh-**PASS**-i-tee)

Related Clinical Terminology

Cyanosis (SIGH-uh-**NOH**-sis)
Dyspnea (**DISP**-nee-ah)
Emphysema (EM-fi-**SEE**-mah)
Heimlich maneuver (**HIGHM**-lik ma-**NEW**-ver)
Hyaline membrane disease (**HIGH**-e-lin **MEM**–brain
   dis-**EEZ**)
Pneumonia (new-**MOH**-nee-ah)
Pneumothorax (NEW-moh-**THAW**-raks)
Pulmonary edema (**PULL**-muh-ner-ee uh–**DEE**–muh).

*Terms that appear in **bold type** in the chapter text are defined in the glossary, which begins on page 521.*

Sometimes a person will describe a habit as being "as natural as breathing." Indeed, what could be more natural? We rarely think about breathing, and it isn't something we look forward to, as we might look forward to a good dinner. We just breathe, usually at the rate of 12 to 20 times per minute, and faster when necessary (such as during exercise). You may have heard of trained singers "learning how to breathe," but they are really learning how to make their breathing more efficient.

Most of the **respiratory system** is concerned with what we think of as breathing: moving air into and out of the lungs. The lungs are the site of the exchanges of oxygen and carbon dioxide between the air and the blood. Both of these exchanges are important. All of our cells must obtain oxygen to carry out cell respiration to produce ATP. Just as crucial is the elimination of the CO_2 produced as a waste product of cell respiration, and, as you already know, the proper functioning of the circulatory system is essential for the transport of these gases in the blood.

DIVISIONS OF THE RESPIRATORY SYSTEM

The respiratory system may be divided into the upper respiratory tract and the lower respiratory tract. The **upper respiratory tract** consists of the parts outside the chest cavity: the air passages of the nose, nasal cavities, pharynx, larynx, and upper trachea. The **lower respiratory tract** consists of the parts found within the chest cavity: the lower trachea and the lungs themselves, which include the bronchial tubes and alveoli. Also part of the respiratory system are the pleural membranes and the respiratory muscles that form the chest cavity: the diaphragm and intercostal muscles.

Have you recognized some familiar organs and structures thus far? There will be more, because this chapter includes material from Chapters 1 through 9, 11, and 12. Even though we are discussing the body system by system, the respiratory system is an excellent example of the interdependent functioning of all the body systems.

NOSE AND NASAL CAVITIES

Air enters and leaves the respiratory system through the **nose**, which is made of bone and cartilage covered with skin. Just inside the nostrils are hairs, which help block the entry of dust.

The two **nasal cavities** are within the skull, separated by the **nasal septum**, which is a bony plate made of the ethmoid bone and vomer. The **nasal mucosa** (lining) is ciliated epithelium, with goblet cells that produce mucus. The surface area of the nasal mucosa is increased by the **conchae**, shelf-like bones on the lateral wall of each nasal cavity (Figs. 15–1 and 6-6). As air passes through the nasal cavities it is warmed and humidified, so that air that reaches the lungs is warm and moist. Bacteria and particles of air pollution are trapped on the mucus; the cilia continuously sweep the mucus toward the pharynx. Most of this mucus is eventually swallowed, and any bacteria present will be destroyed by the hydrochloric acid in the gastric juice.

In the upper nasal cavities are the **olfactory receptors**, which detect vaporized chemicals that have been inhaled. The olfactory nerves pass through the ethmoid bone to the brain.

You may also recall the **paranasal sinuses**, air cavities in the maxillae, frontal, sphenoid, and ethmoid bones (see Figs. 15–1 and 6-9). These sinuses are lined with ciliated epithelium, and the mucus produced drains into the nasal cavities. The functions of the paranasal sinuses are to lighten the skull and provide resonance for the voice.

PHARYNX

The **pharynx** is a muscular tube posterior to the nasal and oral cavities and anterior to the cervical vertebrae. For descriptive purposes, the pharynx may be divided into three parts: the nasopharynx, oropharynx, and laryngopharynx (see Fig. 15–1).

The uppermost portion is the **nasopharynx**, which is behind the nasal cavities. The **soft palate** is elevated during swallowing to block the nasopharynx and prevent food or saliva from going up rather than down. The uvula is the part of the soft palate you can see at the back of the throat. On the posterior wall of the nasopharynx is the adenoid or pharyngeal tonsil, a lymph nodule that contains macrophages. Opening into the nasopharynx are the two eustachian tubes, which extend to the middle ear cavities. The purpose of the eustachian tubes is to permit air to enter or leave the middle ears, allowing the eardrums to vibrate properly.

The nasopharynx is a passageway for air only, but the remainder of the pharynx serves as both an air and

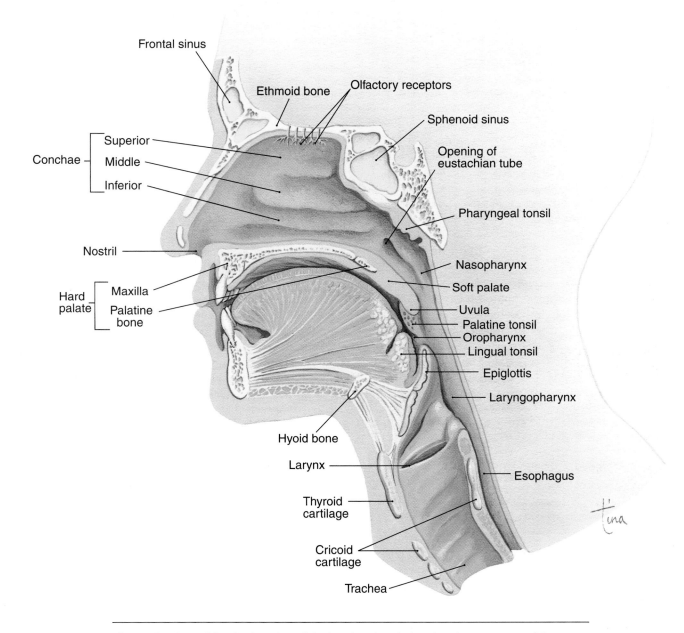

Figure 15–1   Midsagittal section of the head and neck showing the structures of the upper respiratory tract.

food passageway, although not for both at the same time. The **oropharynx** is behind the mouth; its mucosa is stratified squamous epithelium, continuous with that of the oral cavity. On its lateral walls are the palatine tonsils, also lymph nodules. Together with the adenoid and the lingual tonsils on the base of the

tongue, they form a ring of lymphatic tissue around the pharynx to destroy pathogens that penetrate the mucosa.

The **laryngopharynx** is the most inferior portion of the pharynx. It opens anteriorly into the larynx and posteriorly into the esophagus. Contraction of the muscular wall of the oropharynx and laryngopharynx is part of the swallowing reflex.

LARYNX

The **larynx** is often called the voice box, a name that indicates one of its functions, which is speaking. The other function of the larynx is to be an air passageway between the pharynx and the trachea. Air passages must be kept open at all times, and so the larynx is made of nine pieces of cartilage connected by ligaments. Cartilage is a firm yet flexible tissue that prevents collapse of the larynx. In comparison, the esophagus is a collapsed tube except when food is passing through it.

The largest cartilage of the larynx is the **thyroid cartilage** (Fig. 15–2), which you can feel on the anterior surface of your neck. The **epiglottis** is the uppermost cartilage. During swallowing, the larynx is elevated, and the epiglottis closes over the top to prevent the entry of food into the larynx.

The mucosa of the larynx is ciliated epithelium, except for the vocal cords (stratified squamous epithelium). The cilia of the mucosa sweep upward to remove mucus and trapped dust and microorganisms.

The **vocal cords** (or vocal folds) are on either side of the **glottis**, the opening between them. During

breathing, the vocal cords are held at the sides of the glottis, so that air passes freely into and out of the trachea (Fig. 15–3). During speaking, the intrinsic muscles of the larynx pull the vocal cords across the glottis, and exhaled air vibrates the vocal cords to produce sounds that can be turned into speech. It is also physically possible to speak while inhaling, but this is not what we are used to. The cranial nerves that are motor nerves to the larynx for speaking are the vagus and accessory nerves. You may also recall that for most people, the speech areas are in the left cerebral hemisphere.

TRACHEA AND BRONCHIAL TREE

The **trachea** is about 4 to 5 inches (10 to 13 cm) long and extends from the larynx to the primary bronchi. The wall of the trachea contains 16 to 20 C-shaped pieces of cartilage, which keep the trachea open. The gaps in these incomplete cartilage rings are posterior, to permit the expansion of the esophagus when food is swallowed. The mucosa of the trachea is ciliated epithelium with goblet cells. As in the larynx, the cilia sweep upward toward the pharynx.

The right and left **primary bronchi** (Fig. 15–4) are the branches of the trachea that enter the lungs. Within the lungs, each primary bronchus branches into secondary bronchi leading to the lobes of each lung (three right, two left). The further branching of the bronchial tubes is often called the **bronchial tree**. Imagine the trachea as the trunk of an upside-down tree with extensive branches that become smaller and smaller; these smaller branches are the **bronchioles**. No cartilage is present in the walls of the bronchioles; this becomes clinically important in asthma (see Box 15–1: Asthma). The smallest bronchioles terminate in clusters of alveoli, the air sacs of the lungs.

LUNGS AND PLEURAL MEMBRANES

The **lungs** are located on either side of the heart in the chest cavity and are encircled and protected by the rib cage. The base of each lung rests on the diaphragm below; the apex (superior tip) is at the level of the clavicle. On the medial surface of each lung is an indentation called the **hilus**, where the primary bronchus and the pulmonary artery and veins enter the lung.

The pleural membranes are the serous membranes of the thoracic cavity. The **parietal pleura** lines the chest wall, and the **visceral pleura** is on the surface

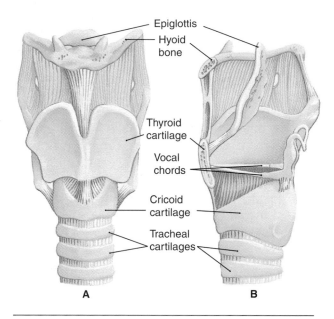

Epiglottis
Hyoid bone
Thyroid cartilage
Vocal chords
Cricoid cartilage
Tracheal cartilages

A   B

Figure 15–2 Larynx. **(A)** Anterior view. **(B)** Midsagittal section through the larynx, viewed from the left side.

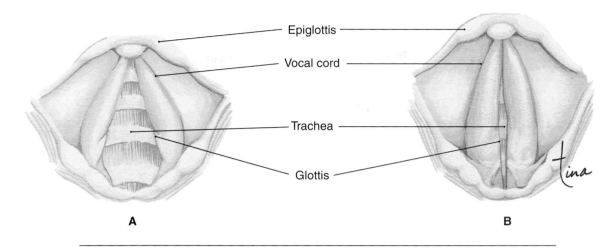

Figure 15–3   Vocal cords and glottis, superior view. **(A)** Position of the vocal cords during breathing. **(B)** Position of the vocal cords during speaking.

of the lungs. Between the pleural membranes is serous fluid, which prevents friction and keeps the two membranes together during breathing.

Alveoli

The functional units of the lungs are the air sacs called **alveoli**. The flat alveolar type I cells that form most of the alveolar walls are simple squamous epithelium. In the spaces between clusters of alveoli is elastic connective tissue, which is important for exhalation. Within the alveoli are macrophages that phagocytize pathogens or other foreign material that may not have been swept out by the ciliated epithelium of the bronchial tree. There are millions of alveoli in each lung, and each alveolus is surrounded by a network of pulmonary capillaries (see Fig 15–4). Recall that capillaries are also made of simple squamous epithelium, so there are only two cells between the air in the alveoli and the blood in the pulmonary capillaries, which permits efficient diffusion of gases (Fig. 15–5).

Each alveolus is lined with a thin layer of tissue fluid, which is essential for the diffusion of gases, because a gas must dissolve in a liquid in order to enter or leave a cell (the earthworm principle—an earthworm breathes through its moist skin, and will suffocate if its skin dries out). Although this tissue fluid is necessary, it creates a potential problem in that it would make the walls of an alveolus stick together

internally. Imagine a plastic bag that is wet inside; its walls would stick together because of the surface tension of the water. This is just what would happen in alveoli, and inflation would be very difficult.

This problem is overcome by **pulmonary surfactant**, a lipoprotein secreted by alveolar type II cells, also called septal cells. Surfactant mixes with the tissue fluid within the alveoli and decreases its surface tension, permitting inflation of the alveoli (see Box 15–2: Hyaline Membrane Disease). Normal inflation of the alveoli in turn permits the exchange of gases, but before we discuss this process, we will first see how air gets into and out of the lungs.

MECHANISM OF BREATHING

Ventilation is the term for the movement of air to and from the alveoli. The two aspects of ventilation are inhalation and exhalation, which are brought about by the nervous system and the respiratory muscles. The respiratory centers are located in the medulla and pons. Their specific functions will be covered in a later section, but it is the medulla that generates impulses to the respiratory muscles.

These muscles are the diaphragm and the external and internal intercostal muscles (Fig. 15–6). The **diaphragm** is a dome-shaped muscle below the lungs; when it contracts, the diaphragm flattens and

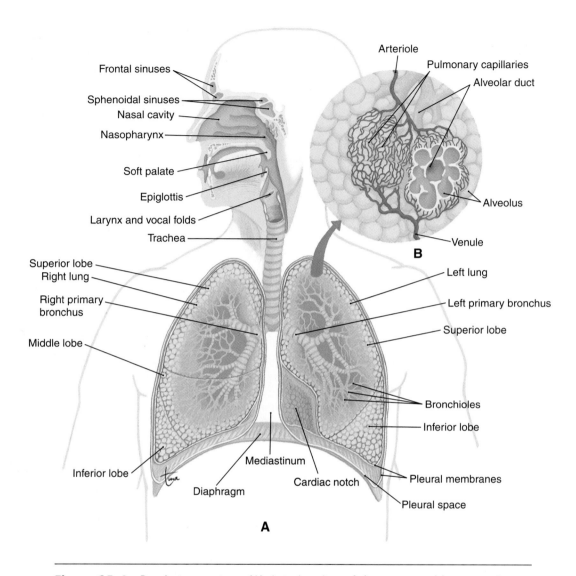

Figure 15–4   Respiratory system. **(A)** Anterior view of the upper and lower respiratory tracts. **(B)** Microscopic view of alveoli and pulmonary capillaries. (The colors represent the vessels, not the oxygen content of the blood within the vessels.)

moves downward. The intercostal muscles are found between the ribs. The **external intercostal muscles** pull the ribs upward and outward, and the **internal intercostal muscles** pull the ribs downward and inward. Ventilation is the result of the respiratory muscles producing changes in the pressure within the alveoli and bronchial tree.

With respect to breathing, the important pressures are these three:

1. **Atmospheric pressure**—the pressure of the air around us. At sea level, atmospheric pressure is 760 mmHg. At higher altitudes, of course, atmospheric pressure is lower.
2. **Intrapleural pressure**—the pressure within the potential pleural space between the parietal pleura and visceral pleura. This is a potential rather than a real space. A thin layer of serous fluid causes the two pleural membranes to adhere

Box 15–1   ASTHMA

Asthma is usually triggered by an infection or allergic reaction that affects the smooth muscle and glands of the bronchioles. Allergens include foods and inhaled substances such as dust and pollen. Wheezing and dyspnea (difficult breathing) characterize an asthma attack, which may range from mild to fatal.

As part of the allergic response, the smooth muscle of the bronchioles constricts. Because there is no cartilage present in their walls, the bronchioles may close completely. The secretion of mucus increases, perhaps markedly, so the already constricted bronchioles may become clogged or completely obstructed with mucus.

Chronic asthma is a predisposing factor for emphysema. When obstructed bronchioles prevent ventilation of alveoli, the walls of the alveoli begin to deteriorate and break down, leaving large cavities that do not provide much surface area for gas exchange.

One possible way to prevent such serious lung damage is to prevent asthma attacks with a medication that blocks the release of IgE antibodies. An allergy is an immune overreaction, and blocking such a reaction would prevent the damaging effects of inflammation.

---

to one another. Intrapleural pressure is always slightly below atmospheric pressure (about 756 mmHg), and is called a *negative* pressure. The elastic lungs are always tending to collapse and pull the visceral pleura away from the parietal pleura. The serous fluid, however, prevents actual separation of the pleural membranes (see Box 15–3: Pneumothorax).

3. **Intrapulmonic pressure**—the pressure within the bronchial tree and alveoli. This pressure fluctuates below and above atmospheric pressure during each cycle of breathing.

INHALATION

Inhalation, also called **inspiration**, is a precise sequence of events that may be described as follows: Motor impulses from the medulla travel along the **phrenic nerves** to the diaphragm and along the **intercostal nerves** to the external intercostal muscles. The diaphragm contracts, moves downward, and expands the chest cavity from top to bottom. The external intercostal muscles pull the ribs up and out, which expands the chest cavity from side to side and front to back.

As the chest cavity is expanded, the parietal pleura expands with it. Intrapleural pressure becomes even more negative as a sort of suction is created between the pleural membranes. The adhesion created by the serous fluid, however, permits the visceral pleura to be expanded too, and this expands the lungs as well.

As the lungs expand, intrapulmonic pressure falls below atmospheric pressure, and air enters the nose and travels through the respiratory passages to the alveoli. Entry of air continues until intrapulmonic pressure is equal to atmospheric pressure; this is a normal inhalation. Of course, inhalation can be continued beyond normal, that is, a deep breath. This requires a more forceful contraction of the respiratory muscles to further expand the lungs, permitting the entry of more air.

EXHALATION

Exhalation may also be called **expiration** and begins when motor impulses from the medulla decrease, and the diaphragm and external intercostal muscles relax. As the chest cavity becomes smaller, the lungs are compressed, and their elastic connective tissue, which was stretched during inhalation, recoils and also compresses the alveoli. As intrapulmonic pressure rises above atmospheric pressure, air is forced out of the lungs until the two pressures are again equal.

Notice that inhalation is an active process that requires muscle contraction, but normal exhalation is a passive process, depending to a great extent on the normal elasticity of healthy lungs. In other words, under normal circumstances we must expend energy to inhale but not to exhale (see Box 15–4: Emphysema).

We can, however, go beyond a normal exhalation and expel more air, such as when talking, singing, or blowing up a balloon. Such a forced exhalation is an active process that requires contraction of other muscles. Contraction of the internal intercostal muscles pulls the ribs down and in and squeezes even more air out of the lungs. Contraction of abdominal muscles, such as the rectus abdominus, compresses the abdominal organs and pushes the diaphragm

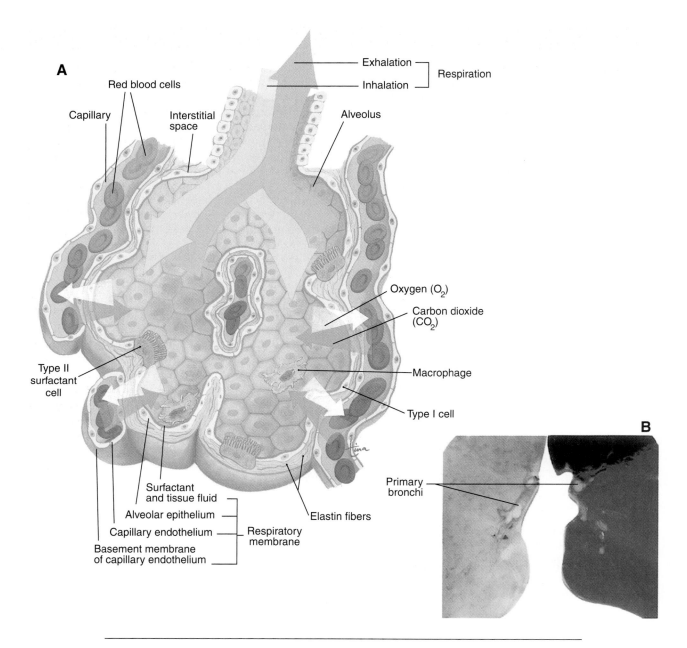

Figure 15–5 **(A)** Alveolar structure showing type I and type II cells, and alveolar macrophages. The respiratory membrane: the structures and substances through which gases must pass as they diffuse from air to blood (oxygen) or from blood to air (CO_2). **(B)** Sections of human lungs embedded in plastic. On the left is a normal adult lung; on the right is a smoker's lung. (Photograph by Dan Kaufman.)

Box 15–2   HYALINE MEMBRANE DISEASE

Hyaline membrane disease is also called respiratory distress syndrome (RDS) of the newborn, and most often affects premature infants whose lungs have not yet produced sufficient quantities of pulmonary surfactant.

The first few breaths of a newborn inflate most of the previously collapsed lungs, and the presence of surfactant permits the alveoli to remain open. The following breaths become much easier, and normal breathing is established.

Without surfactant, the surface tension of the tissue fluid lining the alveoli causes the air sacs to collapse after each breath rather than remain inflated. Each breath, therefore, is difficult, and the newborn must expend a great deal of energy just to breathe.

Premature infants may require respiratory assistance until their lungs are mature enough to produce surfactant. Use of a synthetic surfactant has significantly helped some infants, and because they can breathe more normally, their dependence on respirators is minimized. Still undergoing evaluation are the effects of the long-term use of this surfactant in the most premature babies, who may require it for much longer periods of time.

upward, which also forces more air out of the lungs (see Box 15–5: The Heimlich Maneuver).

EXCHANGE OF GASES

There are two sites of exchange of oxygen and carbon dioxide: the lungs and the tissues of the body. The exchange of gases between the air in the alveoli and the blood in the pulmonary capillaries is called **external respiration**. This term may be a bit confusing at first, because we often think of "external" as being outside the body. In this case, however, "external" means the exchange that involves air from the external environment, though the exchange takes place within the lungs. **Internal respiration** is the exchange of gases between the blood in the systemic capillaries and the tissue fluid (cells) of the body.

The air we inhale (the earth's atmosphere) is approximately 21% oxygen and 0.04% carbon dioxide. Although most (78%) of the atmosphere is nitrogen, this gas is not physiologically available to us, and we simply exhale it. This exhaled air also contains

Figure 15–6 Actions of the respiratory muscles. **(A)** Inhalation: diaphragm contracts downward; external intercostal muscles pull rib cage upward and outward; lungs are expanded. **(B)** Normal exhalation: diaphragm relaxes upward; rib cage falls down and in as external intercostal muscles relax; lungs are compressed.

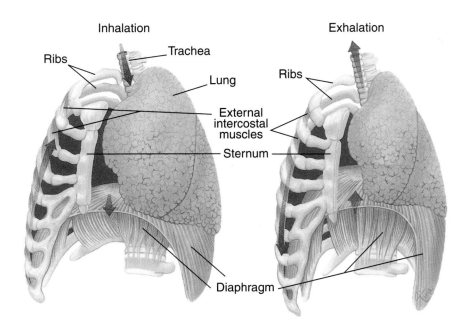

Box 15–3   PNEUMOTHORAX

Pneumothorax is the presence of air in the pleural space, which causes collapse of the lung on that side. Recall that the pleural space is only a potential space because the serous fluid keeps the pleural membranes adhering to one another, and the intrapleural pressure is always slightly below atmospheric pressure. Should air at atmospheric pressure enter the pleural cavity, the suddenly higher pressure outside the lung will contribute to its collapse (the other factor is the normal elasticity of the lungs).

A spontaneous pneumothorax, without apparent trauma, may result from rupture of weakened alveoli on the lung surface. Pulmonary diseases such as emphysema may weaken alveoli

Puncture wounds of the chest wall also allow air into the pleural space, with resulting collapse of a lung. In severe cases, large amounts of air push the heart, great vessels, trachea, and esophagus toward the opposite side (mediastinal shift), putting pressure on the other lung and making breathing difficult. This is called tension pneumothorax, and requires rapid medical intervention to remove the trapped air.

---

about 16% oxygen and 4.5% carbon dioxide, so it is apparent that some oxygen is retained within the body, and the carbon dioxide produced by cells is exhaled.

DIFFUSION OF GASES— PARTIAL PRESSURES

Within the body, a gas will diffuse from an area of greater concentration to an area of lesser concentration. The concentration of each gas in a particular site (alveolar air, pulmonary blood, and so on) is expressed in a value called **partial pressure**. The partial pressure of a gas, measured in mmHg, is the pressure it exerts within a mixture of gases, whether the mixture is actually in a gaseous state or is in a liquid such as blood. The partial pressures of oxygen and carbon dioxide in the atmosphere and in the sites of exchange in the body are listed in Table 15–1. The abbreviation for partial pressure is "P," which is used, for example, on hospital lab slips for blood gases and will be used here.

The partial pressures of oxygen and carbon dioxide at the sites of external respiration (lungs) and internal respiration (body) are shown in Fig. 15–7. Because partial pressure reflects concentration, a gas will diffuse from an area of higher partial pressure to an area of lower partial pressure.

The air in the alveoli has a high PO_2 and a low PCO_2. The blood in the pulmonary capillaries, which has just come from the body, has a low PO_2 and a high PCO_2. Therefore, in external respiration, oxygen diffuses from the air in the alveoli to the blood, and carbon

dioxide diffuses from the blood to the air in the alveoli. The blood that returns to the heart now has a high PO_2 and a low PCO_2 and is pumped by the left ventricle into systemic circulation.

The arterial blood that reaches systemic capillaries has a high PO_2 and a low PCO_2. The body cells and tissue fluid have a low PO_2 and a high PCO_2 because cells continuously use oxygen in cell respiration (energy production) and produce carbon dioxide in this process. Therefore, in internal respiration, oxygen diffuses from the blood to tissue fluid (cells), and carbon dioxide diffuses from tissue fluid to the blood. The blood that enters systemic veins to return to the heart now has a low PO_2 and a high PCO_2 and is pumped by the right ventricle to the lungs to participate in external respiration.

Disorders of gas exchange often involve the lungs, that is, external respiration (see Box 15–6: Pulmonary Edema and Box 15–7: Pneumonia).

TRANSPORT OF GASES IN THE BLOOD

As you already know, most oxygen is carried in the blood bonded to the **hemoglobin** in red blood cells. (Although some oxygen is dissolved in blood plasma, it is not enough to sustain life.) The mineral iron is part of hemoglobin and gives this protein its oxygen-carrying ability.

The oxygen-hemoglobin bond is formed in the lungs where PO_2 is high. This bond, however, is relatively unstable, and when blood passes through

Box 15–4   EMPHYSEMA

Emphysema, a form of chronic obstructive pulmonary disease (COPD), is a degenerative disease in which the alveoli lose their elasticity and cannot recoil. Perhaps the most common (and avoidable) cause is cigarette smoking; other causes are long-term exposure to severe air pollution or industrial dusts, or chronic asthma. Inhaled irritants damage the alveolar walls and cause deterioration of the elastic connective tissue surrounding the alveoli. Macrophages migrate to the damaged areas, and seem to produce an enzyme that contributes to the destruction of the protein elastin. This is an instance of a useful body response (for cleaning up damaged tissue) becoming damaging when it is excessive. As the alveoli break down, larger air cavities are created that are not efficient in gas exchange (see below).

In progressive emphysema, damaged lung tissue is replaced by fibrous connective tissue (scar tissue), which further limits the diffusion of gases. Blood oxygen level decreases, and blood carbon dioxide level increases. Accumulating carbon dioxide decreases the pH of body fluids; this is a respiratory acidosis.

One of the most characteristic signs of emphysema is that the affected person must make an effort to exhale. The loss of lung elasticity makes normal exhalation an active process, rather than the passive process it usually is. The person must expend energy to exhale in order to make room in the lungs for inhaled air. This extra "work" required for exhalation may be exhausting for the person and contribute to the debilitating nature of emphysema.

A   Normal Lung   **B**   Emphysema

Box Figure 15–A   (A) Lung tissue with normal alveoli. (B) Lung tissue in emphysema.

tissues with a low P_{O_2}, the bond breaks, and oxygen is released to the tissues. The lower the oxygen concentration in a tissue, the more oxygen hemoglobin will release. This ensures that active tissues, such as exercising muscles, receive as much oxygen as possible to continue cell respiration. Other factors that increase the release of oxygen from hemoglobin are a high P_{CO_2} (actually a lower pH) and a high temperature, both of which are also characteristic of active tissues (see Box 15–8: Carbon Monoxide).

Carbon dioxide transport is a little more complicated. Some carbon dioxide is dissolved in the plasma, and some is carried by hemoglobin (carbaminohemoglobin), but these account for only 10% to 30% of total CO_2 transport. Most carbon dioxide is carried in the plasma in the form of bicarbonate ions (HCO_3^-). Let us look at the reactions that transform CO_2 into a bicarbonate ion.

When carbon dioxide enters the blood, most diffuses into red blood cells, which contain the

Box 15–5   THE HEIMLICH MANEUVER

The **Heimlich maneuver** has received much well-deserved publicity, and indeed it is a life-saving technique.

If a person is choking on a foreign object (such as food) lodged in the pharynx or larynx, the air in the lungs may be utilized to remove the object. The physiology of this technique is illustrated in the accompanying figure.

The person performing the maneuver stands behind the choking victim and puts both arms around the victim's waist. One hand forms a fist that is placed between the victim's navel and rib cage (below the diaphragm), and the other hand covers the fist. It is important to place hands correctly, in order to avoid breaking the victim's ribs. With both hands, a quick, forceful upward thrust is made and repeated if necessary. This forces the diaphragm upward to compress the lungs and force air out. The forcefully expelled air is often sufficient to dislodge the foreign object.

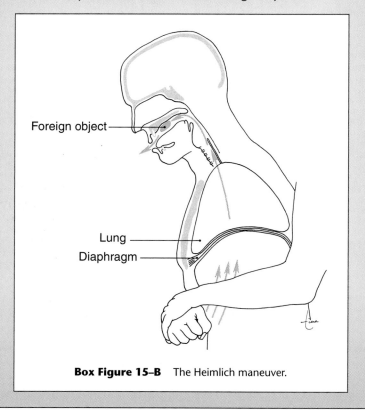

Box Figure 15–B   The Heimlich maneuver.

enzyme **carbonic anhydrase**. This enzyme (which contains zinc) catalyzes the reaction of carbon dioxide and water to form carbonic acid:

$$CO_2 + H_2O \rightarrow H_2CO_3$$

The carbonic acid then dissociates:

$$H_2CO_3 \rightarrow H^+ + HCO_3^-$$

The bicarbonate ions diffuse out of the red blood cells into the plasma, leaving the hydrogen ions (H^+) in the red blood cells. The many H^+ ions would tend to make the red blood cells too acidic, but hemoglobin acts as a buffer to prevent acidosis. To maintain an ionic equilibrium, chloride ions (Cl^-) from the plasma enter the red blood cells; this is called the chloride shift. Where is the CO_2? In the plasma as part of HCO_3^- ions. When the blood reaches the lungs, an area of lower P_{CO_2}, these reactions are reversed, CO_2 is re-formed and diffuses into the alveoli to be exhaled.

Table 15–1 | PARTIAL PRESSURES

Site	Po$_2$ (mmHg)	Pco$_2$ (mmHg)
Atmosphere	160	0.15
Alveolar air	104	40
Pulmonary blood (venous)	40	45
Systemic blood (arterial)	100	40
Tissue fluid	40	50

Partial pressure is calculated as follows:

% of the gas in the mixture × total pressure = Pgas

Example: **O$_2$ in the atmosphere**
21% × 760 mmHg = 160 mmHg (Po$_2$)

Example: **CO$_2$ in the atmosphere**
0.04% × 760 mmHg = 0.15 mmHg (Pco$_2$)

Notice that alveolar partial pressures are not exactly those of the atmosphere. Alveolar air contains significant amounts of water vapor and the CO_2 diffusing in from the blood. Oxygen also diffuses readily from the alveoli into the pulmonary capillaries. Therefore, alveolar Po$_2$ is lower than atmospheric Po$_2$, and alveolar Pco$_2$ is significantly higher than atmospheric Pco$_2$.

PULMONARY VOLUMES

The capacity of the lungs varies with the size and age of the person. Taller people have larger lungs than do shorter people. Also, as we get older our lung capacity diminishes as lungs lose their elasticity and the respiratory muscles become less efficient. For the following pulmonary volumes, the values given are those for healthy young adults. These are also shown in Fig. 15–8.

1. **Tidal volume**—the amount of air involved in one normal inhalation and exhalation. The average tidal volume is 500 ml, but many people often have lower tidal volumes due to shallow breathing.
2. **Minute respiratory volume** (MRV)—the amount of air inhaled and exhaled in 1 minute. MRV is calculated by multiplying tidal volume by the number of respirations per minute (average range: 12 to 20 per minute). If tidal volume is 500 ml and the respiratory rate is 12 breaths per minute, the MRV is 6000 ml, or 6 liters of air per minute, which is average. Shallow breathing usually indicates a smaller than average tidal volume, and would thus require more respirations per minute to obtain the necessary MRV.

3. **Inspiratory reserve**—the amount of air, beyond tidal volume, that can be taken in with the deepest possible inhalation. Normal inspiratory reserve ranges from 2000 to 3000 ml.
4. **Expiratory reserve**—the amount of air, beyond tidal volume, that can be expelled with the most forceful exhalation. Normal expiratory reserve ranges from 1000 to 1500 ml.
5. **Vital capacity**—the sum of tidal volume, inspiratory reserve, and expiratory reserve. Stated another way, vital capacity is the amount of air involved in the deepest inhalation followed by the most forceful exhalation. Average range of vital capacity is 3500 to 5000 ml.
6. **Residual air**—the amount of air that remains in the lungs after the most forceful exhalation; the average range is 1000 to 1500 ml. Residual air is important to ensure that there is some air in the lungs at all times, so that exchange of gases is a continuous process, even between breaths.

Some of the volumes described above can be determined with instruments called spirometers, which measure movement of air. Trained singers and musicians who play wind instruments often have vital capacities much larger than would be expected for their height and age, because their respiratory muscles have become more efficient with "practice." The same is true for athletes who exercise regularly. A person with emphysema, however, must "work" to exhale, and vital capacity and expiratory reserve volume are often much lower than average.

REGULATION OF RESPIRATION

There are two types of mechanisms that regulate breathing: nervous mechanisms and chemical mechanisms. Because any changes in the rate or depth of breathing are ultimately brought about by nerve impulses, we will consider nervous mechanisms first.

NERVOUS REGULATION

The respiratory centers are located in the **medulla** and **pons**, which are parts of the brain stem (see Fig. 15–9). Within the medulla are the inspiration center and expiration center.

The **inspiration center** automatically generates impulses in rhythmic spurts. These impulses travel

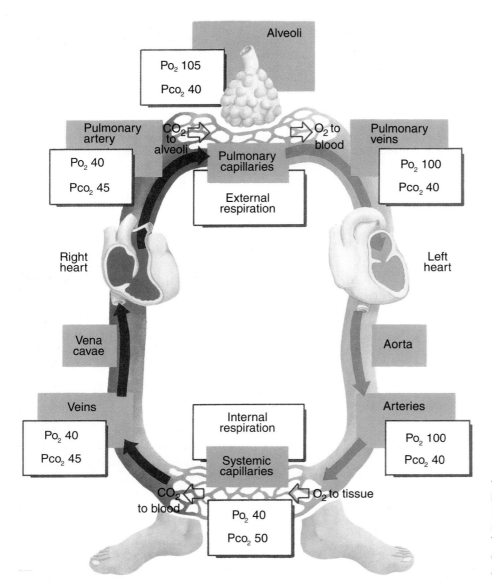

Figure 15–7 External respiration in the lungs and internal respiration in the body. The partial pressures of oxygen and carbon dioxide are shown at each site.

along nerves to the respiratory muscles to stimulate their contraction. The result is inhalation. As the lungs inflate, baroreceptors in lung tissue detect this stretching and generate sensory impulses to the medulla; these impulses begin to depress the inspiration center. This is called the Hering-Breuer inflation reflex, which also helps prevent overinflation of the lungs.

As the inspiration center is depressed, the result is a decrease in impulses to the respiratory muscles, which relax to bring about exhalation. Then the inspiration center becomes active again to begin another cycle of breathing. When there is a need for more forceful exhalations, such as during exercise, the inspiration center activates the **expiration center**,

which generates impulses to the internal intercostal and abdominal muscles.

The two respiratory centers in the pons work with the inspiration center to produce a normal rhythm of breathing. The **apneustic center** prolongs inhalation, and is then interrupted by impulses from the **pneumotaxic center**, which contributes to exhalation. In normal breathing, inhalation lasts 1 to 2 seconds, followed by a slightly longer (2 to 3 seconds) exhalation, producing the normal range of respiratory rate of 12 to 20 breaths per minute.

What has just been described is normal breathing, but variations are possible and quite common. Emotions often affect respiration; a sudden fright may

Box 15–6   PULMONARY EDEMA

Pulmonary edema is the accumulation of fluid in the alveoli. This is often a consequence of congestive heart failure in which the left side of the heart (or the entire heart) is not pumping efficiently. If the left ventricle does not pump strongly, the chamber does not empty as it should and cannot receive all the blood flowing in from the left atrium. Blood flow, therefore, is "congested," and blood backs up in the pulmonary veins and then in the pulmonary capillaries. As blood pressure increases in the pulmonary capillaries, filtration creates tissue fluid that collects in the alveoli.

Fluid-filled alveoli are no longer sites of efficient gas exchange, and the resulting hypoxia leads to the symptoms of **dyspnea** and increased respiratory rate. The most effective treatment is that which restores the pumping ability of the heart to normal.

Box 15–7   PNEUMONIA

Pneumonia is a bacterial infection of the lungs. Although there are many bacteria that can cause pneumonia, the most common one is probably *Streptococcus pneumoniae*. This species is estimated to cause at least 500,000 cases of pneumonia every year in the United States, with 50,000 deaths.

S. pneumoniae is a transient inhabitant of the upper respiratory tract, but in otherwise healthy people, the ciliated epithelium and the immune system prevent infection. Most cases of pneumonia occur in elderly people following a primary infection such as influenza.

When the bacteria are able to establish themselves in the alveoli, the alveolar cells secrete fluid that accumulates in the air sacs. Many neutrophils migrate to the site of infection and attempt to phagocytize the bacteria. The alveoli become filled with fluid, bacteria, and neutrophils (this is called consolidation); this decreases the exchange of gases.

Pneumovax is a vaccine for this type of pneumonia. It contains only the capsules of *S. pneumoniae* and cannot cause the disease. The vaccine is recommended for people over the age of 60 years, and for those with chronic pulmonary disorders or any debilitating disease. It has also been approved for administration to infants.

Box 15–8   CARBON MONOXIDE

Carbon monoxide (CO) is a colorless, odorless gas that is produced during the combustion of fuels such as gasoline, coal, oil, and wood. As you know, CO is a poison that may cause death if inhaled in more than very small quantities or for more than a short period of time.

The reason CO is so toxic is that it forms a very strong and stable bond with the hemoglobin in RBCs. Hemoglobin with CO bonded to it cannot bond to and transport oxygen. The effect of CO, therefore, is to drastically decrease the amount of oxygen carried in the blood. As little as 0.1% CO in inhaled air can saturate half the total hemoglobin with CO.

Lack of oxygen is often apparent in people with light skin as **cyanosis**, a bluish cast to the skin, lips, and nailbeds. This is because hemoglobin is dark red unless something (usually oxygen) is bonded to it. When hemoglobin bonds to CO, however, it becomes a bright, cherry red. This color may be seen in light skin and may be very misleading; the person with CO poisoning is in a severely hypoxic state.

Although CO is found in cigarette smoke, it is present in such minute quantities that it is not lethal. Heavy smokers, however, may be in a mild but chronic hypoxic state because much of their hemoglobin is firmly bonded to CO. As a compensation, RBC production may increase, and a heavy smoker may have a hematocrit over 50%.

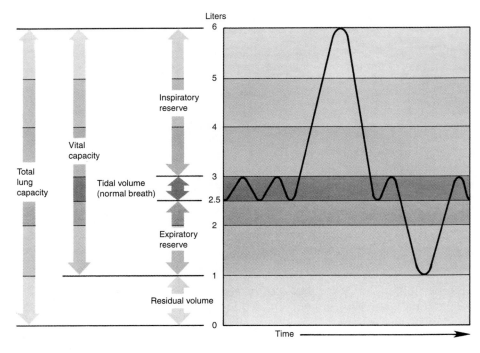

Figure 15–8 Pulmonary volumes. See text for description.

bring about a gasp or a scream, and anger usually increases the respiratory rate. In these situations, impulses from the **hypothalamus** modify the output from the medulla. The **cerebral cortex** enables us to voluntarily change our breathing rate or rhythm to talk, sing, breathe faster or slower, or even to stop breathing for 1 or 2 minutes. Such changes cannot be continued indefinitely, however, and the medulla will eventually resume control.

Coughing and **sneezing** are reflexes that remove irritants from the respiratory passages; the medulla contains the centers for both of these reflexes. Sneezing is stimulated by an irritation of the nasal mucosa, and coughing is stimulated by irritation of the mucosa of the pharynx, larynx, or trachea. The reflex action is essentially the same for both: An inhalation is followed by exhalation beginning with the glottis closed to build up pressure. Then the glottis opens suddenly, and the exhalation is explosive. A cough directs the exhalation out the mouth, while a sneeze directs the exhalation out the nose.

Yet another respiratory reflex is yawning. Most of us yawn when we are tired, but the stimulus for and purpose of yawning are not known with certainty. There are several possibilities, such as lack of oxygen or accumulation of carbon dioxide, but we really do not know. Nor do we know why yawning is contagious, but seeing someone yawn is almost sure to elicit a yawn of one's own. You may even have yawned while reading this paragraph about yawning.

CHEMICAL REGULATION

Chemical regulation refers to the effect on breathing of blood pH and blood levels of oxygen and carbon dioxide. This is shown in Fig. 15–10. **Chemoreceptors** that detect changes in blood gases and pH are located in the carotid and aortic bodies and in the medulla itself.

A decrease in the blood level of oxygen (hypoxia) is detected by the chemoreceptors in the **carotid** and **aortic bodies**. The sensory impulses generated by these receptors travel along the glossopharyngeal and vagus nerves to the medulla, which responds by increasing respiratory rate or depth (or both). This response will bring more air into the lungs so that more oxygen can diffuse into the blood to correct the hypoxic state.

Carbon dioxide becomes a problem when it is present in excess in the blood, because excess CO_2 lowers the pH when it reacts with water to form carbonic acid (a source of H^+ ions). That is, excess CO_2 makes

Figure 15–9   Nervous regulation of respiration. **(A)** Midsagittal section of brain. **(B)** Respiratory centers in medulla and pons. **(C)** Respiratory muscles. See text for description.

the blood or other body fluids less alkaline (or more acidic). The **medulla** contains **chemoreceptors** that are very sensitive to changes in pH, especially decreases. If accumulating CO_2 lowers blood pH, the medulla responds by increasing respiration. This is not for the purpose of inhaling, but rather to exhale more CO_2 to raise the pH back to normal.

Of the two respiratory gases, which is the more important as a regulator of respiration? Our guess might be oxygen, because it is essential for energy production in cell respiration. However, the respiratory system can maintain a normal blood level of oxygen even if breathing decreases to half the normal rate or stops for a few moments. Recall that exhaled

air is 16% oxygen. This oxygen did not enter the blood but was available to do so if needed. Also, the residual air in the lungs supplies oxygen to the blood even if breathing rate slows.

Therefore, carbon dioxide must be the major regulator of respiration, and the reason is that carbon dioxide affects the pH of the blood. As was just mentioned, an excess of CO_2 causes the blood pH to decrease, a process that must not be allowed to continue. Therefore, any increase in blood CO_2 level is quickly compensated for by increased breathing to exhale more CO_2. If, for example, you hold your breath, what is it that makes you breathe again? Have you run out of oxygen? Probably not, for the reasons mentioned

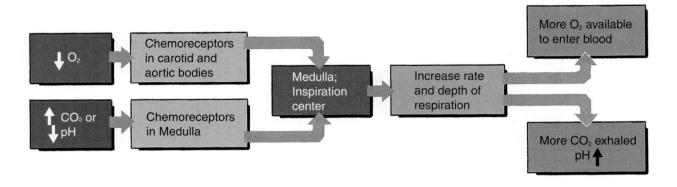

Figure 15–10   Chemical regulation of respiration. See text for description.

above. What has happened is that accumulating CO_2 has lowered blood pH enough to stimulate the medulla to start the breathing cycle again.

In some situations, oxygen does become the major regulator of respiration. People with severe, chronic pulmonary diseases such as emphysema have decreased exchange of both oxygen and carbon dioxide in the lungs. The decrease in pH caused by accumulating CO_2 is corrected by the kidneys, but the blood oxygen level keeps decreasing. Eventually, the oxygen level may fall so low that it does provide a very strong stimulus to increase the rate and depth of respiration.

RESPIRATION AND ACID–BASE BALANCE

As you have just seen, respiration affects the pH of body fluids because it regulates the amount of carbon dioxide in these fluids. Remember that CO_2 reacts with water to form carbonic acid (H_2CO_3), which ionizes into H^+ ions and HCO_3^- ions. The more hydrogen ions present in a body fluid, the lower the pH, and the fewer hydrogen ions present, the higher the pH.

The respiratory system may be the cause of a pH imbalance, or it may help correct a pH imbalance created by some other cause.

RESPIRATORY ACIDOSIS AND ALKALOSIS

Respiratory acidosis occurs when the rate or efficiency of respiration decreases, permitting carbon

dioxide to accumulate in body fluids. The excess CO_2 results in the formation of more H^+ ions, which decrease the pH. Holding one's breath can bring about a mild respiratory acidosis, which will soon stimulate the medulla to initiate breathing again. More serious causes of respiratory acidosis are pulmonary diseases, such as pneumonia and emphysema, or severe asthma. Each of these impairs gas exchange and allows excess CO_2 to remain in body fluids.

Respiratory alkalosis occurs when the rate of respiration increases, and CO_2 is very rapidly exhaled. Less CO_2 decreases H^+ ion formation, which increases the pH. Breathing faster for a few minutes can bring about a mild state of respiratory alkalosis. Babies who cry for extended periods (crying is a noisy exhalation) put themselves in this condition. In general, however, respiratory alkalosis is not a common occurrence. Severe physical trauma and shock, or certain states of mental or emotional anxiety, may be accompanied by hyperventilation and also result in respiratory alkalosis. In addition, traveling to a higher altitude (less oxygen in the atmosphere) may cause a temporary increase in breathing rate before compensation occurs (increased rate of RBC production—see Chapter 11).

RESPIRATORY COMPENSATION

If a pH imbalance is caused by something other than a change in respiration, it is called a metabolic acidosis or alkalosis. In either case, the change in pH stimulates a change in respiration that may help restore the pH of body fluids to normal.

Metabolic acidosis may be caused by untreated diabetes mellitus (ketoacidosis), kidney disease, or severe diarrhea. In such situations, the H^+ ion concentration of body fluids is increased. Respiratory compensation involves an increase in the rate and depth of respiration to exhale more CO_2 to decrease H^+ ion formation, which will raise the pH toward the normal range.

Metabolic alkalosis is not a common occurrence but may be caused by ingestion of excessive amounts of alkaline medications such as those used to relieve gastric disturbances. Another possible cause is vomiting of stomach contents only. In such situations, the H^+ ion concentration of body fluids is decreased. Respiratory compensation involves a decrease in respiration to retain CO_2 in the body to increase H^+ ion formation, which will lower the pH toward the normal range.

Respiratory compensation for an ongoing metabolic pH imbalance cannot be complete, because there are limits to the amounts of CO_2 that may be exhaled or retained. At most, respiratory compensation is only about 75% effective. A complete discussion of acid–base balance is found in Chapter 19.

AGING AND THE RESPIRATORY SYSTEM

Perhaps the most important way to help your respiratory system age gracefully is not to smoke. In the absence of chemical assault, respiratory function does diminish but usually remains adequate. The respiratory muscles, like all skeletal muscles, weaken with age. Lung tissue loses its elasticity and alveoli are lost as their walls deteriorate. All of this results

in decreased ventilation and lung capacity, but the remaining capacity is usually sufficient for ordinary activities. The cilia of the respiratory mucosa deteriorate with age, and the alveolar macrophages are not as efficient, which make elderly people more prone to pneumonia, a serious pulmonary infection.

Chronic alveolar hypoxia from diseases such as emphysema or chronic bronchitis may lead to pulmonary hypertension, which in turn overworks the right ventricle of the heart. Systemic hypertension often weakens the left ventricle of the heart, leading to congestive heart failure and pulmonary edema, in which excess tissue fluid collects in the alveoli and decreases gas exchange. Though true at any age, the interdependence of the respiratory and circulatory systems is particularly apparent in elderly people.

SUMMARY

As you have learned, respiration is much more than the simple mechanical actions of breathing. Inhalation provides the body with the oxygen that is necessary for the production of ATP in the process of cell respiration. Exhalation removes the CO_2 that is a product of cell respiration. Breathing also regulates the level of CO_2 within the body, and this contributes to the maintenance of the acid–base balance of body fluids. Although the respiratory gases do not form structural components of the body, their contributions to the chemical level of organization are essential to the functioning of the body at every level.

STUDY OUTLINE

The respiratory system moves air into and out of the lungs, which are the site of exchange for O_2 and CO_2 between the air and the blood. The functioning of the respiratory system is directly dependent on the proper functioning of the circulatory system.
1. The upper respiratory tract consists of those parts outside the chest cavity.
2. The lower respiratory tract consists of those parts within the chest cavity.

Nose—made of bone and cartilage covered with skin
1. Hairs inside the nostrils block the entry of dust.

Nasal Cavities—within the skull; separated by the nasal septum (see Fig. 15–1)
1. Nasal mucosa is ciliated epithelium with goblet cells; surface area is increased by the conchae.
2. Nasal mucosa warms and moistens the incoming air; dust and microorganisms are trapped on mucus and swept by the cilia to the pharynx.

3. Olfactory receptors respond to vapors in inhaled air.
4. Paranasal sinuses in the maxillae, frontal, sphenoid, and ethmoid bones open into the nasal cavities: functions are to lighten the skull and provide resonance for the voice.

Pharynx—posterior to nasal and oral cavities (see Fig. 15–1)

1. Nasopharynx—above the level of the soft palate, which blocks it during swallowing; a passageway for air only. The eustachian tubes from the middle ears open into it. The adenoid is a lymph nodule on the posterior wall.
2. Oropharynx—behind the mouth; a passageway for both air and food. Palatine tonsils are on the lateral walls.
3. Laryngopharynx—a passageway for both air and food; opens anteriorly into the larynx and posteriorly into the esophagus.

Larynx—the voice box and the airway between the pharynx and trachea (see Fig. 15–2)

1. Made of nine cartilages; the thyroid cartilage is the largest and most anterior.
2. The epiglottis is the uppermost cartilage; covers the larynx during swallowing.
3. The vocal cords are lateral to the glottis, the opening for air (see Fig. 15–3).
4. During speaking, the vocal cords are pulled across the glottis and vibrated by exhaled air, producing sounds that may be turned into speech.
5. The cranial nerves for speaking are the vagus and accessory.

Trachea—extends from the larynx to the primary bronchi (see Fig. 15–4)

1. Sixteen to 20 C-shaped cartilages in the tracheal wall keep the trachea open.
2. Mucosa is ciliated epithelium with goblet cells; cilia sweep mucus, trapped dust, and microorganisms upward to the pharynx.

Bronchial Tree—extends from the trachea to the alveoli (see Fig. 15–4)

1. The right and left primary bronchi are branches of the trachea; one to each lung.
2. Secondary bronchi: to the lobes of each lung (three right, two left)

3. Bronchioles—no cartilage in their walls.

Pleural Membranes—serous membranes of the thoracic cavity

1. Parietal pleura lines the chest wall.
2. Visceral pleura covers the lungs.
3. Serous fluid between the two layers prevents friction and keeps the membranes together during breathing.

Lungs—on either side of the heart in the chest cavity; extend from the diaphragm below up to the level of the clavicles

1. The rib cage protects the lungs from mechanical injury.
2. Hilus—indentation on the medial side: primary bronchus and pulmonary artery and veins enter (also bronchial vessels).

Alveoli—the sites of gas exchange in the lungs

1. Made of alveolar type I cells, simple squamous epithelium; thin to permit diffusion of gases.
2. Surrounded by pulmonary capillaries, which are also made of simple squamous epithelium (see Fig. 15–4).
3. Elastic connective tissue between alveoli is important for normal exhalation.
4. A thin layer of tissue fluid lines each alveolus; essential to permit diffusion of gases (see Fig. 15–5).
5. Alveolar type II cells produce pulmonary surfactant that mixes with the tissue fluid lining to decrease surface tension to permit inflation of the alveoli.
6. Alveolar macrophages phagocytize foreign material.

Mechanism of Breathing

1. Ventilation is the movement of air into and out of the lungs: inhalation and exhalation.
2. Respiratory centers are in the medulla and pons.
3. Respiratory muscles are the diaphragm and external and internal intercostal muscles (see Fig. 15–6).
   - Atmospheric pressure is air pressure: 760 mmHg at sea level.
   - Intrapleural pressure is within the potential pleural space; always slightly below atmospheric pressure ("negative").
   - Intrapulmonic pressure is within the bronchial tree and alveoli; fluctuates during breathing.

Inhalation (inspiration)

1. Motor impulses from medulla travel along phrenic nerves to diaphragm, which contracts and moves down. Impulses are sent along intercostal nerves to external intercostal muscles, which pull ribs up and out.
2. The chest cavity is expanded and expands the parietal pleura.
3. The visceral pleura adheres to the parietal pleura and is also expanded and in turn expands the lungs.
4. Intrapulmonic pressure decreases, and air rushes into the lungs.

Exhalation (expiration)

1. Motor impulses from the medulla decrease, and the diaphragm and external intercostal muscles relax.
2. The chest cavity becomes smaller and compresses the lungs.
3. The elastic lungs recoil and further compress the alveoli.
4. Intrapulmonic pressure increases, and air is forced out of the lungs. Normal exhalation is passive.
5. Forced exhalation: contraction of the internal intercostal muscles pulls the ribs down and in; contraction of the abdominal muscles forces the diaphragm upward.

Exchange of Gases

1. External respiration is the exchange of gases between the air in the alveoli and the blood in the pulmonary capillaries.
2. Internal respiration is the exchange of gases between blood in the systemic capillaries and tissue fluid (cells).
3. Inhaled air (atmosphere) is 21% O_2 and 0.04% CO_2. Exhaled air is 16% O_2 and 4.5% CO_2.
4. Diffusion of O_2 and CO_2 in the body occurs because of pressure gradients (see Table 15–1). A gas will diffuse from an area of higher partial pressure to an area of lower partial pressure.
5. External respiration: Po_2 in the alveoli is high, and Po_2 in the pulmonary capillaries is low, so O_2 diffuses from the air to the blood. Pco_2 in the alveoli is low, and Pco_2 in the pulmonary capillaries is high, so CO_2 diffuses from the blood to the air and is exhaled (see Fig. 15–7).
6. Internal respiration: Po_2 in the systemic capillaries is high, and Po_2 in the tissue fluid is low, so O_2 diffuses from the blood to the tissue fluid and cells. Pco_2 in the systemic capillaries is low, and Pco_2 in

the tissue fluid is high, so CO_2 diffuses from the tissue fluid to the blood (see Fig. 15–7).

Transport of Gases in the Blood

1. Oxygen is carried by the iron of hemoglobin (Hb) in the RBCs. The O_2-Hb bond is formed in the lungs where the Po_2 is high.
2. In tissues, Hb releases much of its O_2; the important factors are low Po_2 in tissues, high Pco_2 in tissues, and a high temperature in tissues.
3. Most CO_2 is carried as HCO_3^- ions in blood plasma. CO_2 enters the RBCs and reacts with H_2O to form carbonic acid (H_2CO_3). Carbonic anhydrase is the enzyme that catalyzes this reaction. H_2CO_3 dissociates to H^+ ions and HCO_3^- ions. The HCO_3^- ions leave the RBCs and enter the plasma; Hb buffers the H^+ ions that remain in the RBCs. Cl^- ions from the plasma enter the RBCs to maintain ionic equilibrium (the chloride shift).
4. When blood reaches the lungs, CO_2 is re-formed, diffuses into the alveoli, and is exhaled.

Pulmonary Volumes (see Fig. 15–8)

1. Tidal volume—the amount of air in one normal inhalation and exhalation.
2. Minute respiratory volume—the amount of air inhaled and exhaled in 1 minute.
3. Inspiratory reserve—the amount of air beyond tidal in a maximal inhalation.
4. Expiratory reserve—the amount of air beyond tidal in the most forceful exhalation.
5. Vital capacity—the sum of tidal volume, inspiratory and expiratory reserves.
6. Residual volume—the amount of air that remains in the lungs after the most forceful exhalation; provides for continuous exchange of gases.

Nervous Regulation of Respiration (see Fig. 15–9)

1. The medulla contains the inspiration center and expiration center.
2. Impulses from the inspiration center to the respiratory muscles cause their contraction; the chest cavity is expanded.
3. Baroreceptors in lung tissue detect stretching and send impulses to the medulla to depress the inspiration center. This is the Hering-Breuer inflation reflex, which also prevents overinflation of the lungs.

4. The expiration center is stimulated by the inspiration center when forceful exhalations are needed.

5. In the pons: the apneustic center prolongs inhalation, and the pneumotaxic center helps bring about exhalation. These centers work with the inspiration center in the medulla to produce a normal breathing rhythm.

6. The hypothalamus influences changes in breathing in emotional situations. The cerebral cortex permits voluntary changes in breathing.

7. Coughing and sneezing remove irritants from the upper respiratory tract; the centers for these reflexes are in the medulla.

Chemical Regulation of Respiration (see Fig. 15–10)

1. Decreased blood O_2 is detected by chemoreceptors in the carotid body and aortic body. Response: increased respiration to take more air into the lungs.

2. Increased blood CO_2 level is detected by chemoreceptors in the medulla. Response: increased respiration to exhale more CO_2.

3. CO_2 is the major regulator of respiration because excess CO_2 decreases the pH of body fluids ($CO_2 + H_2O \rightarrow H_2CO_3 \rightarrow H^+ + HCO_3^-$). Excess H^+ ions lower pH.

4. Oxygen becomes a major regulator of respiration when blood level is very low, as may occur with severe, chronic pulmonary disease.

Respiration and Acid–Base Balance

1. Respiratory acidosis: a decrease in the rate or efficiency of respiration permits excess CO_2 to accumulate in body fluids, resulting in the formation of excess H^+ ions, which lower pH. Occurs in severe pulmonary disease.

2. Respiratory alkalosis: an increase in the rate of respiration increases the CO_2 exhaled, which decreases the formation of H^+ ions and raises pH. Occurs during hyperventilation or when first at a high altitude.

3. Respiratory compensation for metabolic acidosis: increased respiration to exhale CO_2 to decrease H^+ ion formation to raise pH to normal.

4. Respiratory compensation for metabolic alkalosis: decreased respiration to retain CO_2 to increase H^+ ion formation to lower pH to normal.

REVIEW QUESTIONS

1. State the three functions of the nasal mucosa. (p. 326)

2. Name the three parts of the pharynx; state whether each is an air passage only or an air and food passage. (pp. 326–327)

3. Name the tissue that lines the larynx and trachea, and describe its function. State the function of the cartilage of the larynx and trachea. (p. 328)

4. Name the pleural membranes, state the location of each, and describe the functions of serous fluid. (pp. 328–329)

5. Name the tissue of which the alveoli and pulmonary capillaries are made, and explain the importance of this tissue in these locations. Explain the function of pulmonary surfactant. (p. 329)

6. Name the respiratory muscles, and describe how they are involved in normal inhalation and exhalation. Define these pressures and relate them to a cycle of breathing: atmospheric pressure, intrapulmonic pressure. (pp. 329–331)

7. Describe external respiration in terms of partial pressures of oxygen and carbon dioxide. (p. 334)

8. Describe internal respiration in terms of partial pressures of oxygen and carbon dioxide. (p. 334)

9. Name the cell, protein, and mineral that transport oxygen in the blood. State the three factors that increase the release of oxygen in tissues. (pp. 334–335)

10. Most carbon dioxide is transported in what part of the blood, and in what form? Explain the function of hemoglobin with respect to carbon dioxide transport. (pp. 335–336)

11. Name the respiratory centers in the medulla and pons, and explain how each is involved in a breathing cycle. (pp. 337–338)

12. State the location of chemoreceptors affected by a low blood oxygen level; describe the body's response to hypoxia and its purpose. State the location of chemoreceptors affected by a high blood CO_2 level; describe the body's response and its purpose. (pp. 340–341)

13. For respiratory acidosis and alkalosis: state a cause and explain what happens to the pH of body fluids. (p. 342)

14. Explain how the respiratory system may compensate for metabolic acidosis or alkalosis. For an ongoing pH imbalance, what is the limit of respiratory compensation? (pp. 342–343)

FOR FURTHER THOUGHT

1. Name four types of tissues that contribute to the functioning of the lungs, and describe the physical characteristics of each that are important. Name two types of cells that are also important to the functioning of the lungs.

2. As recently as 40 years ago (the early 1960s) it was believed that mouth-to-mouth resuscitation was not really helpful to another person. What mistaken belief about the air we exhale contributed to that thinking, and what are the facts?

3. You are making a list of vital organs, organs we cannot live without. Should you include the larynx on your list? Explain why or why not.

4. At a construction site, a hole caved in and buried a workman up to his shoulders in wet sand. The foreman told the trapped man that a crane would be there in 20 minutes to pull him out, but another worker said they couldn't wait, and had to dig *now*. He was right. Why is this a life-threatening emergency?

5. A patient's blood pH is 7.34, and his respirations are 32 per minute. What acid–base situation is this patient in? State your reasoning step-by-step.

6. Mrs. D is in the emergency room because of severe abdominal pain that may be appendicitis. Her blood pH is 7.47 and her respirations are 34 per minute. What acid–base situation is Mrs. D in? State your reasoning step-by-step.

CHAPTER 16

Student Objectives

- Describe the general functions of the digestive system, and name its major divisions.
- Explain the difference between mechanical and chemical digestion, and name the end products of digestion.
- Describe the structure and functions of the teeth and tongue.
- Explain the functions of saliva.
- Describe the location and function of the pharynx and esophagus.
- Describe the structure and function of each of the four layers of the alimentary tube.
- Describe the location, structure, and function of the stomach, liver, gallbladder, pancreas, and small intestine.
- Describe absorption in the small intestine.
- Describe the location and functions of the large intestine.
- Explain the functions of the normal flora of the colon.
- Describe the functions of the liver.

The Digestive System

New Terminology

Alimentary tube (AL-i-**MEN**-tah-ree TOOB)

Chemical digestion (**KEM**-i-kuhl dye-**JES**-chun)

Common bile duct (**KOM**-mon BYL DUKT)

Defecation reflex (DEF-e-**KAY**-shun)

Duodenum (dew-**AH**-den-um)

Emulsify (e-**MULL**-si-fye)

Enamel (e-**NAM**-uhl)

Essential amino acids (e-**SEN**-shul ah-**ME**-noh **ASS**-ids)

External anal sphincter (eks-**TER**-nuhl **AY**-nuhl **SFINK**-ter)

Ileocecal valve (ILL-ee-oh-**SEE**-kuhl VALV)

Internal anal sphincter (in-**TER**-nuhl **AY**-nuhl **SFINK**-ter)

Lower esophageal sphincter (e-SOF-uh-**JEE**-uhl **SFINK**-ter)

Mechanical digestion (muh-**KAN**-i-kuhl dye-**JES**-chun)

Non-essential amino acids (NON-e-**SEN**-shul ah-**ME**-noh **ASS**-ids)

Normal flora (**NOR**-muhl **FLOOR**-ah)

Periodontal membrane (PER-ee-oh-**DON**-tal)

Pyloric sphincter (pye-**LOR**-ik **SFINK**-ter)

Rugae (**ROO**-gay)

Villi (**VILL**-eye)

Related Clinical Terminology

Appendicitis (uh-PEN-di-**SIGH**-tis)

Diverticulitis (DYE-ver-TIK-yoo-**LYE**-tis)

Gastric ulcer (**GAS**-trik **UL**-ser)

Hepatitis (HEP-uh-**TIGH**-tis)

Lactose intolerance (**LAK**-tohs in-**TAHL**-er-ense)

Lithotripsy (LITH-oh-**TRIP**-see)

Paralytic ileus (**PAR**-uh-LIT-ik **ILL**-ee-us)

Peritonitis (per-i-toh-**NIGH**-tis)

Pyloric stenosis (pye-**LOR**-ik ste-**NOH**-sis)

*Terms that appear in **bold type** in the chapter text are defined in the glossary, which begins on page 521.*

A hurried breakfast when you are late for work or school . . . Thanksgiving dinner . . . going on a diet to lose 5 pounds . . . what do these experiences all have in common? Food. We may take food for granted, celebrate with it, or wish we wouldn't eat quite so much of it. Although food is not as immediate a need for human beings as is oxygen, it is a very important part of our lives. Food provides the raw materials or nutrients that cells use to reproduce and to build new tissue. The energy needed for cell reproduction and tissue building is released from food in the process of cell respiration. In fact, a supply of nutrients from regular food intake is so important that the body can even store any excess for use later. Those "extra 5 pounds" are often stored fat in adipose tissue.

The food we eat, however, is not in a form that our body cells can use. A turkey sandwich, for example, consists of complex proteins, fats, and carbohydrates. The function of the **digestive system** is to change these complex organic nutrient molecules into simple organic and inorganic molecules that can then be absorbed into the blood or lymph to be transported to cells. In this chapter we will discuss the organs of digestion and the contribution each makes to digestion and absorption.

DIVISIONS OF THE DIGESTIVE SYSTEM

The two divisions of the digestive system are the alimentary tube and the accessory organs (Fig. 16–1). The **alimentary tube** extends from the mouth to the anus. It consists of the oral cavity, pharynx, esophagus, stomach, small intestine, and large intestine. Digestion takes place within the oral cavity, stomach, and small intestine; most absorption of nutrients takes place in the small intestine. Undigestible material, primarily cellulose, is eliminated by the large intestine (also called the colon).

The **accessory organs** of digestion are the teeth, tongue, salivary glands, liver, gallbladder, and pancreas. Digestion does not take place *within* these organs, but each contributes something *to* the digestive process.

TYPES OF DIGESTION

The food we eat is broken down in two complementary processes: mechanical digestion and chemical digestion. **Mechanical digestion** is the physical breaking up of food into smaller pieces. Chewing is an example of this. As food is broken up, more of its surface area is exposed for the action of digestive enzymes. Enzymes are discussed in Chapter 2. The work of the digestive enzymes is the **chemical digestion** of broken up food particles, in which complex chemical molecules are changed into much simpler chemicals that the body can utilize. Such enzymes are specific with respect to the fat, protein, or carbohydrate food molecules each can digest. For example, protein-digesting enzymes work only on proteins, not on carbohydrates or fats. Each enzyme is produced by a particular digestive organ and functions at a specific site. However, the enzyme's site of action may or may not be its site of production. These digestive enzymes and their functions are discussed in later sections.

END PRODUCTS OF DIGESTION

Before we describe the actual organs of digestion, let us see where the process of digestion will take us, or rather, will take our food. The three types of complex organic molecules found in food are carbohydrates, proteins, and fats. Each of these complex molecules is digested to a much more simple substance that the body can then use. Carbohydrates, such as starches and disaccharides, are digested to monosaccharides such as glucose, fructose, and galactose. Proteins are digested to amino acids, and fats are digested to fatty acids and glycerol. Also part of food, and released during digestion, are vitamins, minerals, and water.

We will now return to the beginning of the alimentary tube and consider the digestive organs and the process of digestion.

ORAL CAVITY

Food enters the **oral cavity** (or **buccal cavity**) by way of the mouth. The boundaries of the oral cavity are the hard and soft palates, superiorly; the cheeks, laterally; and the floor of the mouth, inferiorly. Within the oral cavity are the teeth and tongue and the openings of the ducts of the salivary glands.

TEETH

The function of the **teeth** is, of course, chewing. This is the process that mechanically breaks food into smaller pieces and mixes it with saliva. An individual

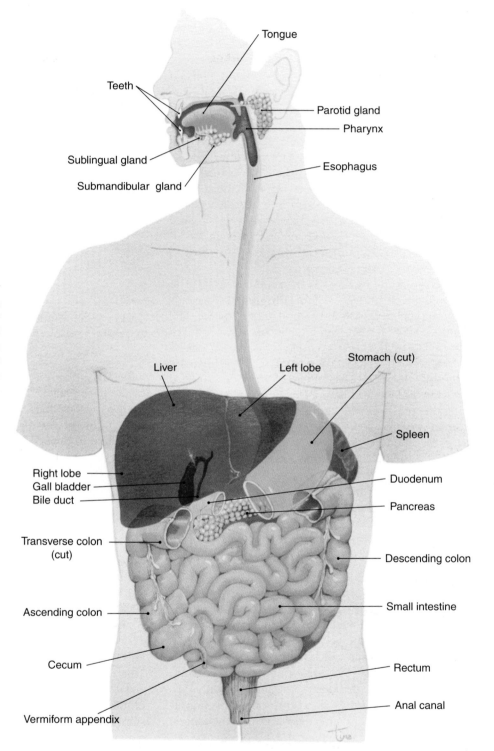

Figure 16–1 The digestive organs shown in anterior view of the trunk and left lateral view of the head. (The spleen is not a digestive organ but is included to show its location relative to the stomach, pancreas, and colon.)

develops two sets of teeth: deciduous and permanent. The **deciduous teeth** begin to erupt through the gums at about 6 months of age, and the set of 20 teeth is usually complete by the age of 2 years. These teeth are gradually lost throughout childhood and replaced by the **permanent teeth**, the first of which are molars that emerge around the age of 6 years. A complete set of permanent teeth consists of 32 teeth; the types of teeth are incisors, canines, premolars, and molars. The wisdom teeth are the third molars on either side of each jawbone. In some people, the wisdom teeth may not emerge from the jawbone because there is no room for them along the gum line. These wisdom teeth are said to be impacted and may put pressure on the roots of the second molars. In such cases, extraction of a wisdom tooth may be necessary to prevent damage to other teeth.

The structure of a tooth is shown in Fig. 16–2. The crown is visible above the gum **(gingiva)**. The root is enclosed in a socket in the mandible or maxillae. The periodontal membrane lines the socket and produces a bone-like cement that anchors the tooth. The outermost layer of the crown is **enamel**, which is made by cells called ameloblasts. Enamel provides a hard chewing surface and is more resistant to decay than are other parts of the tooth. Within the enamel is **dentin**, which is very similar to bone and is produced by cells called odontoblasts. Dentin also forms the roots of a tooth. The innermost portion of a tooth is the **pulp cavity**, which contains blood vessels and nerve endings of the trigeminal nerve (5th cranial). Erosion of the enamel and dentin layers by bacterial acids (dental caries or cavities) may result in bacterial invasion of the pulp cavity and a very painful toothache.

TONGUE

The **tongue** is made of skeletal muscle that is innervated by the hypoglossal nerves (12th cranial). On the upper surface of the tongue are small projections called **papillae**, many of which contain taste buds (see also Chapter 9). The sensory nerves for taste are also cranial nerves: the facial (7th) and glossopharyngeal (9th). As you know, the sense of taste is important because it makes eating enjoyable, but the tongue has other functions as well.

Chewing is efficient because of the action of the tongue in keeping the food between the teeth and mixing it with saliva. Elevation of the tongue is the first step in swallowing. This is a voluntary action, in

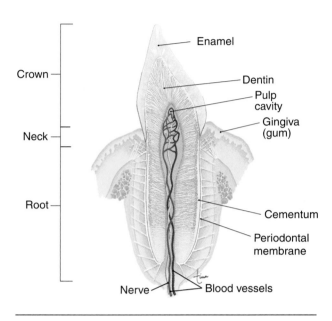

Figure 16–2   Tooth structure. Longitudinal section of a tooth showing internal structure.

which the tongue contracts and meets the resistance of the hard palate. The mass of food, called a bolus, is thus pushed backward toward the pharynx. The remainder of swallowing is a reflex, which is described in the section on the pharynx.

SALIVARY GLANDS

The digestive secretion in the oral cavity is **saliva**, produced by three pairs of **salivary glands**, which are shown in Fig. 16–3. The **parotid glands** are just below and in front of the ears. The **submandibular** (also called submaxillary) glands are at the posterior corners of the mandible, and the **sublingual** glands are below the floor of the mouth. Each gland has at least one duct that takes saliva to the oral cavity.

Secretion of saliva is continuous, but the amount varies in different situations. The presence of food (or anything else) in the mouth increases saliva secretion. This is a parasympathetic response mediated by the facial and glossopharyngeal nerves. The sight or smell of food also increases secretion of saliva. Sympathetic stimulation in stress situations decreases secretion, making the mouth dry and swallowing difficult.

Saliva is mostly water, which is important to dissolve food for tasting and to moisten food for swallowing. The digestive enzyme in saliva is salivary amylase, which breaks down starch molecules to

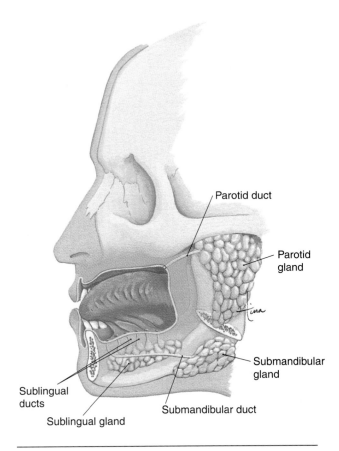

Figure 16–3 shows labels: Parotid duct, Parotid gland, Submandibular gland, Submandibular duct, Sublingual gland, Sublingual ducts.

Figure 16–3 The salivary glands shown in left lateral view.

the swallowing reflex. The reflex center for swallowing is in the medulla, which coordinates the many actions that take place: constriction of the pharynx, cessation of breathing, elevation of the soft palate to block the nasopharynx, elevation of the larynx and closure of the epiglottis, and peristalsis of the esophagus. As you can see, swallowing is rather complicated, but because it is a reflex we don't have to think about making it happen correctly. Talking or laughing while eating, however, may interfere with the reflex and cause food to go into the "wrong pipe," the larynx. When that happens, the cough reflex is usually effective in clearing the airway.

ESOPHAGUS

The **esophagus** is a muscular tube that takes food from the pharynx to the stomach; no digestion takes place here. Peristalsis of the esophagus propels food in one direction and ensures that food gets to the stomach even if the body is horizontal or upside down. At the junction with the stomach, the lumen (cavity) of the esophagus is surrounded by the **lower esophageal sphincter** (LES or cardiac sphincter), a circular smooth muscle. The LES relaxes to permit food to enter the stomach, then contracts to prevent the backup of stomach contents. If the LES does not close completely, gastric juice may splash up into the esophagus; this is a painful condition we call gastroesophageal reflux, or heartburn.

STRUCTURAL LAYERS OF THE ALIMENTARY TUBE

Before we continue with our discussion of the organs of digestion, we will first examine the typical structure of the alimentary tube. When viewed in cross-section, the alimentary tube has four layers (Fig. 16–4): the mucosa, submucosa, external muscle layer, and serosa. Each layer has a specific structure, and its functions contribute to the functioning of the organs of which it is a part.

MUCOSA

The **mucosa**, or lining, of the alimentary tube is made of epithelial tissue, areolar connective tissue, and two thin layers of smooth muscle. In the esophagus the epithelium is stratified squamous epithelium;

shorter chains of glucose molecules, or to maltose, a disaccharide. Most of us, however, do not chew our food long enough for the action of salivary amylase to be truly effective. As you will see, another amylase from the pancreas is also available to digest starch. Table 16–1 summarizes the functions of digestive secretions.

PHARYNX

As described in the last chapter, the oropharynx and laryngopharynx are food passageways connecting the oral cavity to the esophagus. No digestion takes place in the pharynx. Its only related function is swallowing, the mechanical movement of food. When the bolus of food is pushed backward by the tongue, the constrictor muscles of the pharynx contract as part of

Table 16–1 | THE PROCESS OF DIGESTION

Organ	Enzyme or Other Secretion	Function	Site of Action
Salivary glands	• Amylase	• Converts starch to maltose	Oral cavity
Stomach	• Pepsin	• Converts proteins to polypeptides	Stomach
	• HCl	• Changes pepsinogen to pepsin; maintains pH 1–2; destroys pathogens	Stomach
Liver	• Bile salts	• Emulsify fats	Small intestine
Pancreas	• Amylase	• Converts starch to maltose	Small Intestine
	• Trypsin	• Converts polypeptides to peptides	Small Intestine
	• Lipase	• Converts emulsified fats to fatty acids and glycerol	Small Intestine
Small intestine	• Peptidases	• Convert peptides to amino acids	Small Intestine
	• Sucrase	• Converts sucrose to glucose and fructose	Small Intestine
	• Maltase	• Converts maltose to glucose (2)	Small Intestine
	• Lactase	• Converts lactose to glucose and galactose	Small Intestine

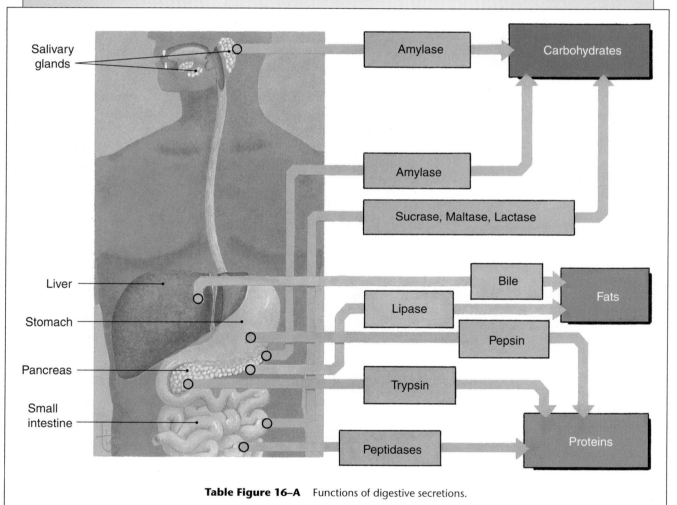

Table Figure 16–A   Functions of digestive secretions.

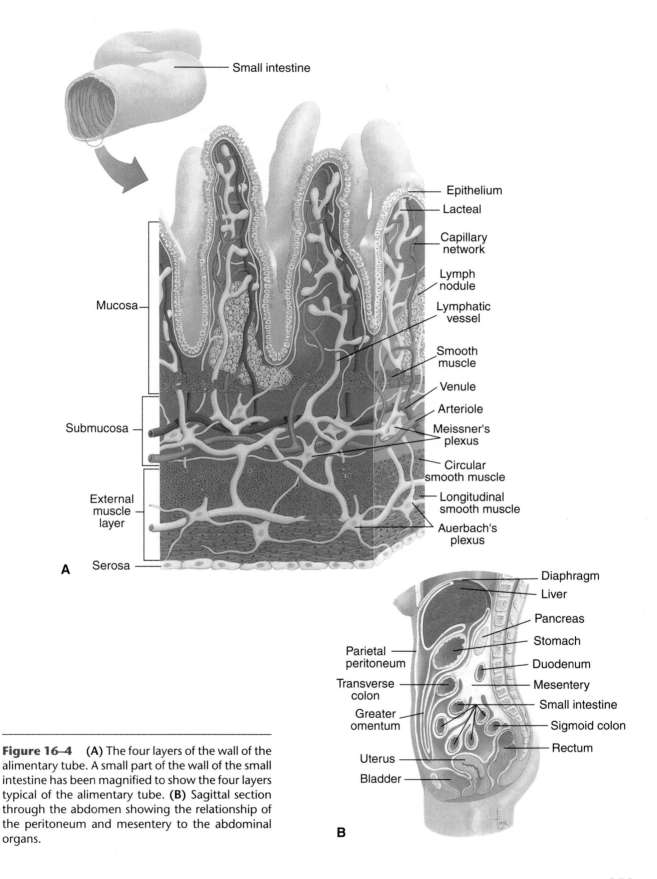

Small intestine

Epithelium

Lacteal

Capillary
network

Lymph
nodule

Lymphatic
vessel

Smooth
muscle

Venule

Arteriole

Meissner's
plexus

Circular
smooth muscle

Longitudinal
smooth muscle

Auerbach's
plexus

Mucosa

Submucosa

External
muscle
layer

Serosa

A

Diaphragm

Liver

Pancreas

Stomach

Duodenum

Mesentery

Small intestine

Sigmoid colon

Rectum

Parietal
peritoneum

Transverse
colon

Greater
omentum

Uterus

Bladder

B

Figure 16–4 **(A)** The four layers of the wall of the alimentary tube. A small part of the wall of the small intestine has been magnified to show the four layers typical of the alimentary tube. **(B)** Sagittal section through the abdomen showing the relationship of the peritoneum and mesentery to the abdominal organs.

in the stomach and intestines it is simple columnar epithelium. The epithelium secretes mucus, which lubricates the passage of food, and also secretes the digestive enzymes of the stomach and small intestine. Just below the epithelium, within the areolar connective tissue, are lymph nodules that contain lymphocytes to produce antibodies, and macrophages to phagocytize bacteria or other foreign material that get through the epithelium. The thin layers of smooth muscle create folds in the mucosa, and ripples, so that all of the epithelial cells are in touch with the contents of the organ. In the stomach and small intestine this is important for absorption.

SUBMUCOSA

The **submucosa** is made of areolar connective tissue with many blood vessels and lymphatic vessels. Many millions of nerve fibers are also present, part of what is called the **enteric nervous system**, or the "brain of the gut," which extends the entire length of the alimentary tube. The nerve networks in the submucosa are called **Meissner's plexus** (or submucosal plexus), and they innervate the mucosa to regulate secretions. Parasympathetic impulses increase secretions, whereas sympathetic impulses decrease secretions. Sensory neurons are also present to the smooth muscle (a stretched or cramping gut is painful), as are motor neurons to blood vessels, to regulate vessel diameter and blood flow.

EXTERNAL MUSCLE LAYER

The external muscle layer typically contains two layers of smooth muscle: an inner, circular layer and an outer, longitudinal layer. Variations from the typical do occur, however. In the esophagus, this layer is striated muscle in the upper third, which gradually changes to smooth muscle in the lower portions. The stomach has three layers of smooth muscle, rather than two.

Contractions of this muscle layer help break up food and mix it with digestive juices. The one-way contractions of **peristalsis** move the food toward the anus. **Auerbach's plexus** (or myenteric plexus) is the portion of the enteric nervous system in this layer, and some of its millions of neurons are autonomic. Sympathetic impulses decrease contractions and peristalsis, whereas parasympathetic impulses increase contractions and peristalsis, promoting normal digestion. The parasympathetic nerves are the

vagus (10th cranial) nerves; they truly live up to the meaning of *vagus,* which is "wanderer."

SEROSA

Above the diaphragm, for the esophagus, the serosa, the outermost layer, is fibrous connective tissue. Below the diaphragm, the serosa is the **mesentery** or visceral peritoneum, a serous membrane. Lining the abdominal cavity is the parietal peritoneum, usually simply called the **peritoneum**. The peritoneum-mesentery is actually one continuous membrane (see Fig. 16–4). The serous fluid between the peritoneum and mesentery prevents friction when the alimentary tube contracts and the organs slide against one another.

The above descriptions are typical of the layers of the alimentary tube. As noted, variations are possible, and any important differences are mentioned in the sections that follow on specific organs.

STOMACH

The **stomach** is located in the upper left quadrant of the abdominal cavity, to the left of the liver and in front of the spleen. Although part of the alimentary tube, the stomach is not a tube, but rather a sac that extends from the esophagus to the small intestine. Because it is a sac, the stomach is a reservoir for food, so that digestion proceeds gradually and we do not have to eat constantly. Both mechanical and chemical digestion take place in the stomach.

The parts of the stomach are shown in Fig. 16–5. The cardiac orifice is the opening of the esophagus, and the fundus is the portion above the level of this opening. The body of the stomach is the large central portion, bounded laterally by the greater curvature and medially by the lesser curvature. The pylorus is adjacent to the duodenum of the small intestine, and the pyloric sphincter surrounds the junction of the two organs. The fundus and body are mainly storage areas, whereas most digestion takes place in the pylorus.

When the stomach is empty, the mucosa appears wrinkled or folded. These folds are called **rugae;** they flatten out as the stomach is filled and permit expansion of the lining without tearing it. The **gastric pits** are the glands of the stomach and consist of

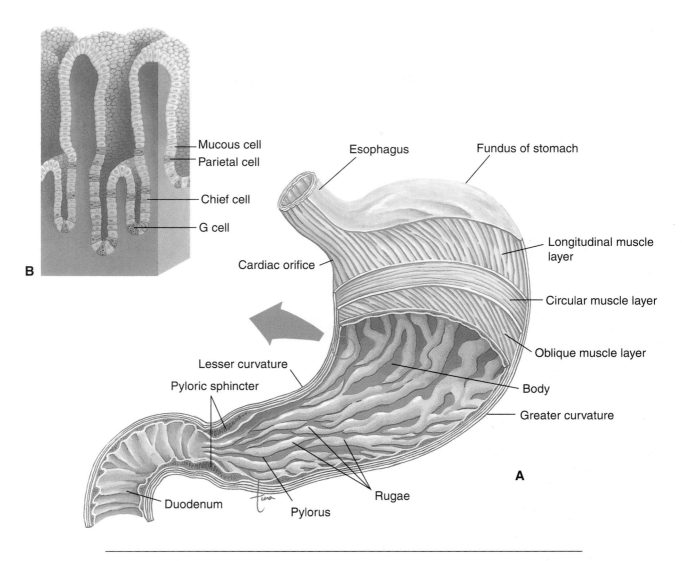

Figure 16–5 **(A)** The stomach in anterior view. The stomach wall has been sectioned to show the muscle layers and the rugae of the mucosa. **(B)** Gastric pits (glands) showing the types of cells present. See text for functions.

several types of cells; their collective secretions are called gastric juice. **Mucous cells** secrete mucus, which coats the stomach lining and helps prevent erosion by the gastric juice. **Chief cells** secrete **pepsinogen**, an inactive form of the enzyme **pepsin. Parietal cells** secrete hydrochloric acid (HCl), which converts pepsinogen to pepsin, which then begins the digestion of proteins to polypeptides. Hydrochloric acid also gives gastric juice its pH of 1 to 2. This very acidic pH is necessary for pepsin to

function and also kills most microorganisms that enter the stomach. The parietal cells also secrete intrinsic factor, which is necessary for the absorption of vitamin B_{12}. Enteroendocrine cells called G cells secrete the hormone gastrin.

Gastric juice is secreted in small amounts at the sight or smell of food. This is a parasympathetic response that ensures that some gastric juice will be present in the stomach when food arrives. The presence of food in the stomach causes the G cells to secrete gastrin, a hormone that stimulates the secretion of greater amounts of gastric juice.

The external muscle layer of the stomach consists of three layers of smooth muscle: circular, longitudinal, and oblique layers. These three layers are innervated by the myenteric plexuses of the enteric nervous system. Stimulatory impulses are carried from the CNS by the vagus nerves (10th cranial), and provide for very efficient mechanical digestion to change food into a thick liquid called chyme. The pyloric sphincter is usually contracted when the stomach is churning food; it relaxes at intervals to permit small amounts of chyme to pass into the duodenum. This sphincter then contracts again to prevent the backup of intestinal contents into the stomach (see Box 16–1: Disorders of the Stomach).

SMALL INTESTINE

The **small intestine** is about 1 inch (2.5 cm) in diameter and approximately 20 feet (6 m) long and extends from the stomach to the cecum of the large intestine.

Within the abdominal cavity, the large intestine encircles the coils of the small intestine (see Fig. 16–1).

The **duodenum** is the first 10 inches (25 cm) of the small intestine. The common bile duct enters the duodenum at the ampulla of Vater (or hepatopancreatic ampulla). The **jejunum** is about 8 feet long, and the **ileum** is about 11 feet in length. In a living person, however, the small intestine is always contracted and is therefore somewhat shorter.

Digestion is completed in the small intestine, and the end products of digestion are absorbed into the blood and lymph. The mucosa (see Fig. 16–4) has simple columnar epithelium that includes cells with microvilli and goblet cells that secrete mucus. Enteroendocrine cells secrete the hormones of the small intestine. Lymph nodules called Peyer's patches are especially abundant in the ileum to destroy absorbed pathogens. The external muscle layer has the typical circular and longitudinal smooth muscle layers that mix the chyme with digestive secretions and propel the chyme toward the colon. Stimulatory impulses to the enteric nerves of these muscle layers are carried by the vagus nerves. The waves of peri-

---

Box 16–1 DISORDERS OF THE STOMACH

Vomiting is the expulsion of stomach and intestinal contents through the esophagus and mouth. Stimuli include irritation of the stomach, motion sickness, food poisoning, or diseases such as meningitis. The vomiting center is in the medulla, which coordinates the simultaneous contraction of the diaphragm and the abdominal muscles. This squeezes the stomach and upper intestine, expelling their contents. As part of the reflex, the lower esophageal sphincter relaxes, and the glottis closes. If the glottis fails to close, as may happen in alcohol or drug intoxication, aspiration of vomitus may occur and result in fatal obstruction of the respiratory passages.

Pyloric stenosis means that the opening of the pyloric sphincter is narrowed, and emptying of the stomach is impaired. This is most often a congenital disorder caused by hypertrophy of the pyloric sphincter. For reasons unknown, this condition is more common in male infants than in female infants. When the stomach does not empty efficiently, its internal pressure increases. Vomiting relieves the pressure; this is a classic symptom of pyloric steno-

sis. Correcting this condition requires surgery to widen the opening in the sphincter.

A **gastric ulcer** is an erosion of the mucosa of the stomach. Because the normal stomach lining is adapted to resist the corrosive action of gastric juice, ulcer formation is the result of oversecretion of HCl or undersecretion of mucus.

As erosion reaches the submucosa, small blood vessels are ruptured and bleed. If vomiting occurs, the vomitus has a "coffee-ground" appearance due to the presence of blood acted on by gastric juice. A more serious complication is perforation of the stomach wall, with leakage of gastric contents into the abdominal cavity, and **peritonitis.**

The bacterium called *Helicobacter pylori* is the cause of most gastric ulcers. For many patients, a few weeks of antibiotic therapy to eradicate this bacterium has produced rapid healing of their ulcers. This bacterium also seems to be responsible for virtually all cases of stomach cancer.

The medications that decrease the secretion of HCl are useful for ulcer patients not helped by antibiotics.

stalsis, however, can take place without stimulation by the central nervous system; the enteric nervous system can function independently and promote normal peristalsis.

There are three sources of digestive secretions that function within the small intestine: the liver, the pancreas, and the small intestine itself. We will return to the small intestine after considering these other organs.

LIVER

The **liver** (Fig. 16–6) consists of two large lobes, right and left, and fills the upper right and center of the abdominal cavity, just below the diaphragm. The structural unit of the liver is the **liver lobule**, a roughly hexagonal column of liver cells (hepatocytes). Between adjacent lobules are branches of the hepatic artery and portal vein. The capillaries of a lobule are sinusoids, large and very permeable vessels between the rows of liver cells. The sinusoids receive blood from both the hepatic artery and portal vein, and it is with this mixture of blood that the liver cells carry out their functions. The hepatic artery brings oxygenated blood, and the portal vein brings blood from the digestive organs and spleen (see Fig. 13-7). Each lobule has a central vein. The central veins of all the lobules unite to form the hepatic veins, which take blood out of the liver to the inferior vena cava.

The cells of the liver have many functions (which are discussed in a later section), but their only digestive function is the production of **bile**. Bile enters the small bile ducts, called bile canaliculi, on the liver cells, which unite to form larger ducts and finally merge to form the **hepatic duct**, which takes bile out of the liver (Fig. 16–6). The hepatic duct unites with the cystic duct of the gallbladder to form the **common bile duct**, which takes bile to the duodenum.

Bile is mostly water and has an excretory function in that it carries bilirubin and excess cholesterol to the intestines for elimination in feces. The digestive function of bile is accomplished by **bile salts**, which **emulsify** fats in the small intestine. Emulsification means that large fat globules are broken into smaller globules. This is mechanical, not chemical, digestion; the fat is still fat but now has more surface area to facilitate chemical digestion.

Production of bile is stimulated by the hormone **secretin**, which is produced by the duodenum when food enters the small intestine. Table 16–2 summarizes the regulation of secretion of all digestive secretions.

GALLBLADDER

The **gallbladder** is a sac about 3 to 4 inches (7.5 to 10 cm) long located on the undersurface of the right lobe of the liver. Bile in the hepatic duct of the liver flows through the **cystic duct** into the gallbladder (see Fig. 16–6), which stores bile until it is needed in the small intestine. The gallbladder also concentrates bile by absorbing water (see Box 16–2: Gallstones).

When fatty foods enter the duodenum, the enteroendocrine cells of the duodenal mucosa secrete the hormone **cholecystokinin**. It is this hormone that stimulates contraction of the smooth muscle in the wall of the gallbladder, which forces bile into the cystic duct, then into the common bile duct, and on into the duodenum.

PANCREAS

The **pancreas** is located in the upper left abdominal quadrant between the curve of the duodenum and the spleen and is about 6 inches (15 cm) in length. The endocrine functions of the pancreas were discussed in Chapter 10, so only the exocrine functions will be considered here. The exocrine glands of the pancreas are called acini (singular: acinus) (Fig. 16–7). They produce enzymes that are involved in the digestion of all three types of complex food molecules.

The pancreatic enzyme **amylase** digests starch to maltose. You may recall that this is the "backup" enzyme for salivary amylase, though pancreatic amylase is responsible for most digestion of starch. **Lipase** converts emulsified fats to fatty acids and glycerol. The emulsifying or fat-separating action of bile salts increases the surface area of fats so that lipase works effectively. Trypsinogen is an inactive enzyme that is changed to active **trypsin** in the duodenum. Trypsin digests polypeptides to shorter chains of amino acids.

The pancreatic enzyme juice is carried by small ducts that unite to form larger ducts, then finally the main **pancreatic duct**. An accessory duct may also be present. The main pancreatic duct emerges from

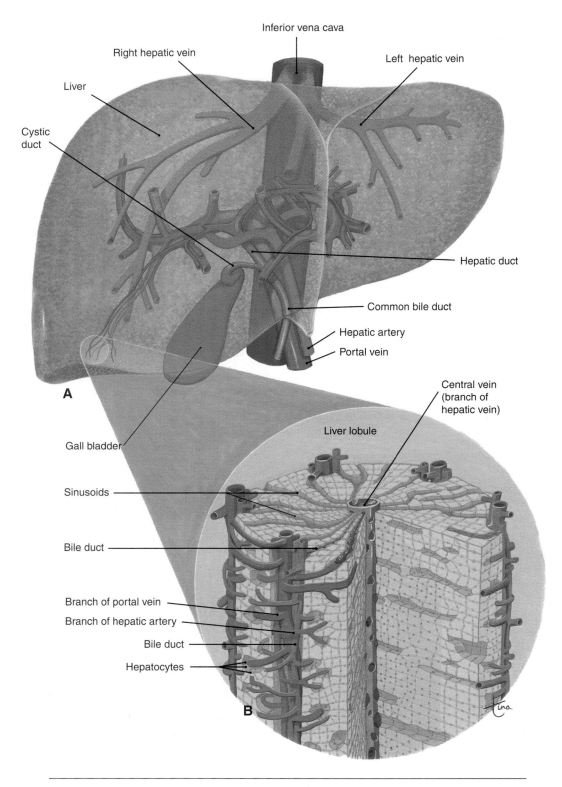

Figure 16–6   **(A)** The liver and gallbladder with blood vessels and bile ducts. **(B)** Magnified view of one liver lobule. See text for description.

Table 16–2	REGULATION OF DIGESTIVE SECRETIONS	

Secretion	Nervous Regulation	Chemical Regulation
Saliva	Presence of food in mouth or sight of food; parasympathetic impulses along 7th and 9th cranial nerves	• None
Gastric juice	Sight or smell of food; parasympathetic impulses along 10th cranial nerves	• Gastrin—produced by the G cells of the gastric mucosa when food is present in the stomach
Bile		
Secretion by the liver	None	• Secretin—produced by the enteroendocrine cells of the duodenum when chyme enters
Contraction of the gallbladder	None	• Cholecystokinin—produced by the enteroendocrine cells of the duodenum when chyme enters
Enzyme pancreatic juice	None	• Cholecystokinin—from the duodenum
Bicarbonate pancreatic juice	None	• Secretin—from the duodenum
Intestinal juice	Presence of chyme in the duodenum; parasympathetic impulses along 10th cranial nerves	• None

the medial side of the pancreas and joins the common bile duct to the duodenum (Fig. 16–7).

The pancreas also produces a **bicarbonate juice** (containing sodium bicarbonate), which is alkaline. Because the gastric juice that enters the duodenum is very acidic, it must be neutralized to prevent damage to the duodenal mucosa. This neutralizing is accomplished by the sodium bicarbonate in pancreatic juice, and the pH of the duodenal chyme is raised to about 7.5.

Secretion of pancreatic juice is stimulated by the hormones secretin and cholecystokinin, which are produced by the duodenal mucosa when chyme enters the small intestine. **Secretin** stimulates the production of bicarbonate juice by the pancreas, and **cholecystokinin** stimulates the secretion of the pancreatic enzymes.

COMPLETION OF DIGESTION AND ABSORPTION

SMALL INTESTINE

The secretion of the epithelium of the intestinal glands (or crypts of Lieberkühn) is stimulated by the presence of food in the duodenum. The intestinal enzymes are the peptidases and sucrase, maltase, and lactase. **Peptidases** complete the digestion of protein by breaking down short polypeptide chains to amino acids. **Sucrase, maltase**, and **lactase**, respectively, digest the disaccharides sucrose, maltose, and lactose to monosaccharides.

The enteroendocrine cells of the intestinal glands secrete the hormones of the small intestine. Secretion is stimulated by food entering the duodenum.

A summary of the digestive secretions and their functions is found in Table 16–1. Regulation of these secretions is shown in Table 16–2.

ABSORPTION

Most absorption of the end products of digestion takes place in the small intestine (although the stomach does absorb water and alcohol). The process of absorption requires a large surface area, which is provided by several structural modifications of the small intestine; these are shown in Fig. 16–8. **Plica circulares**, or circular folds, are macroscopic folds of the mucosa and submucosa, somewhat like accordion pleats. The mucosa is further folded into projections called **villi**, which give the inner surface of the intestine a velvet-like appearance. Each columnar cell (except the mucus-secreting goblet cells) of the villi

Box 16–2   GALLSTONES

One of the functions of the gallbladder is to concentrate bile by absorbing water. If the bile contains a high concentration of cholesterol, absorption of water may lead to precipitation and the formation of cholesterol crystals. These crystals are **gallstones**.

If the gallstones are small, they will pass through the cystic duct and common bile duct to the duodenum without causing symptoms. If large, however, the gallstones cannot pass out of the gallbladder, and may cause mild to severe pain that often radiates to the right shoulder. Obstructive jaundice may occur if bile backs up into the liver and bilirubin is reabsorbed into the blood.

There are several possible treatments for gallstones. Medications that dissolve gallstones work slowly, over the course of several months, and are useful if biliary obstruction is not severe. An instrument that generates shock waves (called a lithotripter) may be used to pulverize the stones into smaller pieces that may easily pass into the duodenum; this procedure is called **lithotripsy**. Surgery to remove the gallbladder (cholecystectomy) is required in some cases. The hepatic duct is then connected directly to the common bile duct, and dilute bile flows into the duodenum. Following such surgery, the patient should avoid meals high in fats.

---

also has **microvilli** on its free surface. Microvilli are microscopic folds of the cell membrane, and are collectively called the **brush border**. All of these folds greatly increase the surface area of the intestinal lining. It is estimated that if the intestinal mucosa could be flattened out, it would cover more than 2000 square feet (half a basketball court).

The absorption of nutrients takes place from the lumen of the intestine into the vessels within the villi. Refer to Fig. 16–8 and notice that within each villus is a **capillary network** and a **lacteal**, which is a dead-end lymph capillary. Water-soluble nutrients are absorbed into the blood in the capillary networks. Monosaccharides, amino acids, positive ions, and the water-soluble vitamins (vitamin C and the B vitamins) are absorbed by active transport. Negative ions may be absorbed by either passive or active transport mechanisms. Water is absorbed by osmosis following the absorption of minerals, especially sodium. Certain nutrients have additional special requirements for their absorption: For example, vitamin B_{12} requires the intrinsic factor produced by the parietal cells of the gastric mucosa, and the efficient absorption of calcium ions requires parathyroid hormone and vitamin D.

Fat-soluble nutrients are absorbed into the lymph in the lacteals of the villi. Bile salts are necessary for the efficient absorption of fatty acids and the fat-soluble vitamins (A, D, E, K). Once absorbed, fatty acids are recombined with glycerol to form triglycerides. These triglycerides then form globules that include cholesterol and protein; these lipid–protein complexes are called **chylomicrons**. In the form of chylomicrons, most absorbed fat is transported by the lymph and eventually enters the blood in the left subclavian vein.

Blood from the capillary networks in the villi does not return directly to the heart but first travels through the portal vein to the liver. You may recall the importance of portal circulation, discussed in Chapter 13. This pathway enables the liver to regulate the blood levels of glucose and amino acids, store certain vitamins, and remove potential poisons from the blood (see Box 16–3: Disorders of the Intestines).

LARGE INTESTINE

The **large intestine**, also called the **colon**, is approximately 2.5 inches (6.3 cm) in diameter and 5 feet (1.5 m) in length. It extends from the ileum of the small intestine to the anus, the terminal opening. The parts of the colon are shown in Fig. 16–9. The **cecum** is the first portion, and at its junction with the ileum is the **ileocecal valve**, which is not a sphincter but serves the same purpose. After undigested food (which is now mostly cellulose) and water pass from the ileum into the cecum, closure of the ileocecal valve prevents the backflow of fecal material.

Attached to the cecum is the **appendix**, a small, dead-end tube with abundant lymphatic tissue. The appendix seems to be a **vestigial organ**, that is, one whose size and function seem to be reduced. Although there is abundant lymphatic tissue in the wall of the appendix, the possibility that the appendix is concerned with immunity is not known with

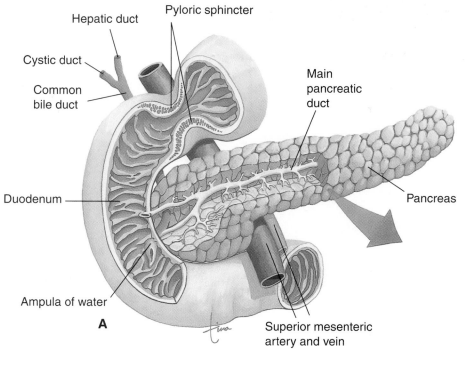

Hepatic duct

Pyloric sphincter

Cystic duct

Common bile duct

Main pancreatic duct

Duodenum

Pancreas

Ampula of water

A

Superior mesenteric artery and vein

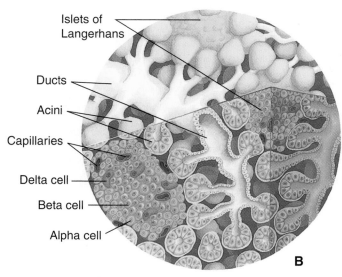

Islets of Langerhans

Ducts

Acini

Capillaries

Delta cell

Beta cell

Alpha cell

B

Figure 16–7 **(A)** The pancreas, sectioned to show the pancreatic ducts. The main pancreatic duct joins the common bile duct. **(B)** Microscopic section showing acini with their ducts and several islets of Langerhans.

certainty. **Appendicitis** refers to inflammation of the appendix, which may occur if fecal material becomes impacted within it. This usually necessitates an **appendectomy**, the surgical removal of the appendix.

The remainder of the colon consists of the ascending, transverse, and descending colon, which encircle the small intestine; the sigmoid colon, which turns medially and downward; the rectum; and the anal canal. The rectum is about 6 inches long, and the anal

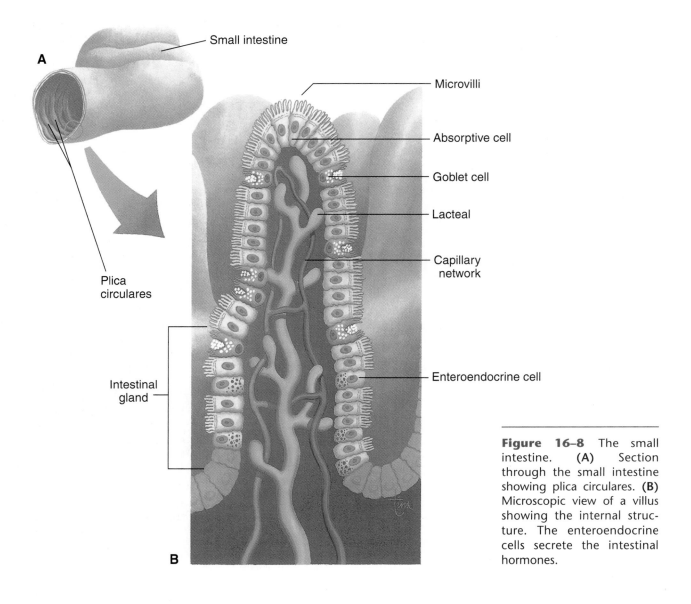

A

Small intestine

Microvilli

Absorptive cell

Goblet cell

Lacteal

Capillary network

Enteroendocrine cell

Plica circulares

Intestinal gland

B

Figure 16–8 The small intestine. **(A)** Section through the small intestine showing plica circulares. **(B)** Microscopic view of a villus showing the internal structure. The enteroendocrine cells secrete the intestinal hormones.

canal is the last inch of the colon that surrounds the anus. Clinically, however, the terminal end of the colon is usually referred to as the rectum.

No digestion takes place in the colon. The only secretion of the colonic mucosa is mucus, which lubricates the passage of fecal material. The longitudinal smooth muscle layer of the colon is in three bands called **taeniae coli**. The rest of the colon is "gathered" to fit these bands. This gives the colon a puckered appearance; the puckers or pockets are called **haustra**, which provide for more surface area within the colon.

The functions of the colon are the absorption of water, minerals, and vitamins and the elimination of undigestible material. About 80% of the water that enters the colon is absorbed (400 to 800 ml per day). Positive and negative ions are also absorbed. The vitamins absorbed are those produced by the **normal flora**, the trillions of bacteria that live in the colon. Vitamin K is produced and absorbed in amounts usually sufficient to meet a person's daily need. Other vitamins produced in smaller amounts include riboflavin, thiamin, biotin, and folic acid. Everything absorbed by the colon circulates first to the liver by

Box 16–3   DISORDERS OF THE INTESTINES

Duodenal ulcers are erosions of the duodenal wall caused by the gastric juice that enters from the stomach. The most serious consequences are bleeding and perforation.

Paralytic ileus is the cessation of contraction of the smooth muscle layer of the intestine. This is a possible complication of abdominal surgery, but it may also be the result of peritonitis or inflammation elsewhere in the abdominal cavity. In the absence of peristalsis, intestinal obstruction may occur. Bowel movements cease, and vomiting occurs to relieve the pressure within the alimentary tube. Treatment involves suctioning the intestinal contents to eliminate any obstruction and allow the intestine to regain its normal motility.

Lactose intolerance is the inability to digest lactose because of deficiency of the enzyme lactase. Lactase deficiency may be congenital, a consequence of prematurity, or acquired later in life. The delayed form is quite common among people of African or Asian ancestry, and in part is probably genetic. When lactose, or milk sugar, is not digested, it undergoes fermentation in the intestine. Symptoms include diarrhea, abdominal pain, bloating, and flatulence (gas formation).

Salmonella food poisoning is caused by bacteria in the genus *Salmonella*. These are part of the intestinal flora of animals, and animal foods such as meat and eggs may be sources of infection. These bacteria are not normal for people, and they cause the intestines to secrete large amounts of fluid. Symptoms include diarrhea, abdominal cramps, and vomiting and usually last only a few days. For elderly or debilitated people, however, salmonella food poisoning may be very serious or even fatal.

Diverticula are small outpouchings through weakened areas of the intestinal wall. They are more likely to occur in the colon than in the small intestine and may exist for years without causing any symptoms. The presence of diverticula is called **diverticulosis**. Inflammation of diverticula is called **diverticulitis**, which is usually the result of entrapment of feces and bacteria. Symptoms include abdominal pain and tenderness and fever. If uncomplicated, diverticulitis may be treated with antibiotics and modifications in diet. The most serious complication is perforation of diverticula, allowing fecal material into the abdominal cavity, causing peritonitis. A diet high in fiber is believed to be an important aspect of prevention, to provide bulk in the colon and prevent weakening of its wall.

---

way of portal circulation. Yet another function of the normal colon flora is to inhibit the growth of pathogens (see Box 16–4: Infant Botulism).

ELIMINATION OF FECES

Feces consist of cellulose and other undigestible material, dead and living bacteria, and water. Elimination of feces is accomplished by the **defecation reflex**, a spinal cord reflex that may be controlled voluntarily. The rectum is usually empty until peristalsis of the colon pushes feces into it. These waves of peristalsis tend to occur after eating, especially when food enters the duodenum. The wall of the rectum is stretched by the entry of feces, and this is the stimulus for the defecation reflex.

Stretch receptors in the smooth muscle layer of the rectum generate sensory impulses that travel to the sacral spinal cord. The returning motor impulses cause the smooth muscle of the rectum to contract. Surrounding the anus is the **internal anal sphincter**, which is made of smooth muscle. As part of the

reflex this sphincter relaxes, permitting defecation to take place.

The **external anal sphincter** is made of skeletal muscle and surrounds the internal anal sphincter (Fig. 16–10). If defecation must be delayed, the external sphincter may be voluntarily contracted to close the anus. The awareness of the need to defecate passes as the stretch receptors of the rectum adapt. These receptors will be stimulated again when the next wave of peristalsis reaches the rectum (see Box 16–5: Fiber).

OTHER FUNCTIONS OF THE LIVER

The **liver** is a remarkable organ, and only the brain is capable of a greater variety of functions. The liver cells (hepatocytes) produce many enzymes that catalyze many different chemical reactions. These reactions are the functions of the liver. As blood flows through the sinusoids (capillaries) of the liver (see Fig. 16–6),

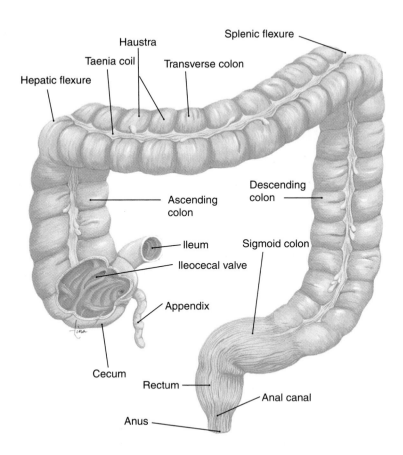

Hepatic flexure
Taenia coil
Haustra
Transverse colon
Splenic flexure
Ascending colon
Descending colon
Ileum
Ileocecal valve
Sigmoid colon
Appendix
Cecum
Rectum
Anal canal
Anus

Figure 16–9 The large intestine shown in anterior view. The term *flexure* means a turn or bend.

materials are removed by the liver cells, and the products of the liver cells are secreted into the blood. Some of the liver functions will already be familiar to you. Others are mentioned again and discussed in more detail in the next chapter. Because the liver has such varied effects on so many body systems, we will use the categories below to summarize the liver functions.

1. Carbohydrate metabolism—As you know, the liver regulates the blood glucose level. Excess glucose is converted to glycogen (glycogenesis) when

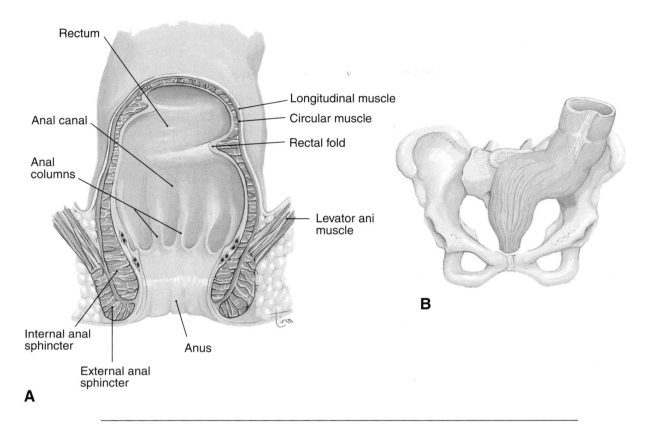

Figure 16–10   **(A)** Internal and external anal sphincters shown in a frontal section through the lower rectum and anal canal. **(B)** Position of rectum and anal canal relative to pelvic bone.

Box 16–5   FIBER

Fiber is a term we use to refer to the organic materials in the cell walls of plants. These are mainly cellulose and pectins. The role of dietary fiber and possible benefits that a high-fiber diet may provide are currently the focus of much research. It is important to differentiate what is known from what is, at present, merely speculation.

Many studies have shown that populations (large groups of people) who consume high-fiber diets tend to have a lower frequency of certain diseases. These include diverticulitis, colon cancer, coronary artery disease, diabetes, and hypertension. Such diseases are much more common among populations whose diets are low in vegetables, fruits, and whole grains, and high in meat, dairy products, and processed foods.

Claims that high-fiber diets directly lower blood levels of cholesterol and fats are not yet supported by definitive clinical or experimental studies. One possible explanation may be that a person whose diet consists largely of high-fiber foods simply eats less of foods high in cholesterol and fats, and this is the reason for their lower blood levels of fats and cholesterol.

Should people try to make great changes in their diets? Probably not, not if they are careful to limit fat intake and to include significant quantities of vegetables and fruits. Besides the possible benefits of fiber, unprocessed plant foods provide important amounts of vitamins and minerals.

blood glucose is high; the hormones insulin and cortisol facilitate this process. During hypoglycemia or stress situations, glycogen is converted back to glucose (glycogenolysis) to raise the blood glucose level. Epinephrine and glucagon are the hormones that facilitate this process.

The liver also changes other monosaccharides to glucose. Fructose and galactose, for example, are end products of the digestion of sucrose and lactose. Because most cells, however, cannot readily use fructose and galactose as energy sources, they are converted by the liver to glucose, which is easily used by cells.

2. Amino acid metabolism—The liver regulates blood levels of amino acids based on tissue needs for protein synthesis. Of the 20 different amino acids needed for the production of human proteins, the liver is able to synthesize 12, called the **non-essential amino acids**. The chemical process by which this is done is called **transamination**, the transfer of an amino group (NH_2) from an amino acid present in excess to a free carbon chain that forms a complete, new amino acid molecule. The other eight amino acids, which the liver cannot synthesize, are called the **essential amino acids**. In this case, "essential" means that the amino acids must be supplied by our food, because the liver cannot manufacture them. Similarly, "non-essential" means that the amino acids do not have to be supplied in our food because the liver *can* make them. All 20 amino acids are required in order to make our body proteins.

Excess amino acids, those not needed right away for protein synthesis, cannot be stored. However, they do serve another useful purpose. By the process of **deamination**, which also occurs in the liver, the NH_2 group is removed from an amino acid, and the remaining carbon chain may be converted to a simple carbohydrate molecule or to fat. Thus, excess amino acids are utilized for energy production: either for immediate energy or for the potential energy stored as fat in adipose tissue. The NH_2 groups that were detached from the original amino acids are combined to form urea, a waste product that will be removed from the blood by the kidneys and excreted in urine.

3. Lipid metabolism—The liver forms lipoproteins, which as their name tells us, are molecules of lipids and proteins, for the transport of fats in the blood to other tissues. The liver also synthesizes cholesterol and excretes excess cholesterol into bile to be eliminated in feces.

Fatty acids are a potential source of energy, but in order to be used in cell respiration they must be broken down to smaller molecules. In the process of **beta-oxidation**, the long carbon chains of fatty acids are split into two-carbon molecules called acetyl groups, which are simple carbohydrates. These acetyl groups may be used by the liver cells to produce ATP or may be combined to form ketones to be transported in the blood to other cells. These other cells then use the ketones to produce ATP in cell respiration.

4. Synthesis of plasma proteins—This is a liver function that you will probably remember from Chapter 11. The liver synthesizes many of the proteins that circulate in the blood. **Albumin**, the most abundant plasma protein, helps maintain blood volume by pulling tissue fluid into capillaries.

The **clotting factors** are also produced by the liver. These, as you recall, include prothrombin, fibrinogen, and Factor 8, which circulate in the blood until needed in the chemical clotting mechanism. The liver also synthesizes alpha and beta **globulins**, which are proteins that serve as carriers for other molecules, such as fats, in the blood.

5. Formation of bilirubin—This is another familiar function: The liver contains fixed macrophages that phagocytize old RBCs. Bilirubin is then formed from the heme portion of the hemoglobin. The liver also removes from the blood the bilirubin formed in the spleen and red bone marrow, and excretes it into bile to be eliminated in feces.

6. Phagocytosis by **Kupffer cells**—The fixed macrophages of the liver are called Kupffer cells (or stellate reticuloendothelial cells). Besides destroying old RBCs, Kupffer cells phagocytize pathogens or other foreign material that circulate through the liver. Many of the bacteria that get to the liver come from the colon. These bacteria are part of the normal flora of the colon but would be very harmful elsewhere in the body. The bacteria that enter the blood with the water absorbed by the colon are carried to the liver by way of portal circulation. The Kupffer cells in the liver phagocytize and destroy these bacteria, removing them from the blood before the blood returns to the heart.

7. Storage—The liver stores the fat-soluble vitamins A, D, E, and K, and the water-soluble vitamin B_{12}. Up to a 6- to 12-month supply of vitamins A and D

may be stored, and liver is an excellent dietary source of these vitamins.

Also stored by the liver are the minerals iron and copper. You already know that iron is needed for hemoglobin and myoglobin and enables these proteins to bond to oxygen. Copper (as well as iron) is part of some of the proteins needed for cell respiration, and is part of some of the enzymes necessary for hemoglobin synthesis.

8. Detoxification—The liver is capable of synthesizing enzymes that will detoxify harmful substances, that is, change them to less harmful ones. Alcohol, for example, is changed to acetate, which is a two-carbon molecule (an acetyl group) that can be used in cell respiration.

Medications are all potentially toxic, but the liver produces enzymes that break them down or change them. When given in a proper dosage, a medication exerts its therapeutic effect but is then changed to less active substances that are usually excreted by the kidneys. An overdose of a drug means that there is too much of it for the liver to detoxify in a given time, and the drug will remain in the body with possibly harmful effects. This is why alcohol should never be consumed when taking medication. Such a combination may cause the liver's detoxification ability to be overworked and ineffective, with the result that both the alcohol and the medication will remain toxic for a longer time. Barbiturates taken as sleeping pills after consumption of alcohol have too often proved fatal for just this reason.

Ammonia is a toxic substance produced by the bacteria in the colon. Because it is soluble in water, some ammonia is absorbed into the blood, but it is carried first to the liver by portal circulation. The liver converts ammonia to urea, a less toxic substance, before the ammonia can circulate and damage other organs, especially the brain. The urea formed is excreted by the kidneys (see Box 16–6: Hepatitis).

Box 16–6   HEPATITIS

Hepatitis is inflammation of the liver caused by any of several viruses. The most common of these hepatitis viruses have been designated A, B, and C, although there are others. Symptoms of hepatitis include anorexia, nausea, fatigue, and possibly jaundice. Severity of disease ranges from very mild (even asymptomatic) to fatal. Hundreds of thousands of cases of hepatitis occur in the United States every year, and although liver inflammation is common to all of them, the three hepatitis viruses have different modes of transmission and different consequences for affected people.

Hepatitis A is an intestinal virus that is spread by the fecal–oral route. Food contaminated by the hands of people with mild cases is the usual vehicle of transmission, although shellfish harvested from water contaminated with human sewage are another possible source of this virus. Hepatitis A is most often mild, recovery provides lifelong immunity, and the carrier state is not known to occur. A vaccine is available, but people who have been exposed to hepatitis A may receive gamma globulin by injection to prevent the disease.

Hepatitis B is contracted by exposure to the body fluids of an infected person; these fluids include blood and semen. Hepatitis B may be severe or even fatal, and approximately 10% of those who recover become carriers of the virus. Possible consequences of the carrier state are chronic hepatitis progressing to cirrhosis or primary liver cancer. Of equal importance, carriers are sources of the virus for others, especially their sexual partners.

A vaccine is available for hepatitis B, and although it is expensive, health-care workers who have contact with blood, even occasionally, should receive it. Other potential recipients of the vaccine are the sexual partners of carriers. Pediatricians now consider this vaccine one of the standard ones for infants.

The **hepatitis C** virus is also present in body fluids and is spread by blood or mucous membrane contact. Most people develop chronic disease, but many may remain asymptomatic for years after being infected. With active disease the virus can and does cause liver failure. The only therapy then is a liver transplant.

It is important for health-care personnel, and their patients, to know that these types of hepatitis are not spread by blood transfusions. Donated blood is tested for all three viruses.

AGING AND THE DIGESTIVE SYSTEM

Many changes can be expected in the aging digestive system. The sense of taste becomes less acute, less saliva is produced, and there is greater likelihood of periodontal disease and loss of teeth. Secretions are reduced throughout the digestive system, and the effectiveness of peristalsis diminishes. Indigestion may become more frequent, especially if the LES loses its tone, and there is a greater chance of peptic ulcer. In the colon, diverticula may form; these are bubble-like outpouchings of the weakened wall of the colon that may be asymptomatic or become infected. Sluggish peristalsis contributes to constipation, which in turn may contribute to the formation of hemorrhoids. The risk of oral cancer or colon cancer also increases with age.

The liver usually continues to function adequately even well into old age, unless damaged by pathogens such as the hepatitis viruses or by toxins such as alcohol. There is a greater tendency for gallstones to form, perhaps necessitating removal of the gallbladder. In the absence of specific diseases, the pancreas usually functions well, although acute pancreatitis of unknown cause is somewhat more likely in elderly people.

SUMMARY

The processes of the digestion of food and the absorption of nutrients enable the body to use complex food molecules for many purposes. Much of the food we eat literally becomes part of us. The body synthesizes proteins and lipids for the growth and repair of tissues and produces enzymes to catalyze all of the reactions that contribute to homeostasis. Some of our food provides the energy required for growth, repair, movement, sensation, and thinking. In the next chapter we will discuss the chemical basis of energy production from food and consider the relationship of energy production to the maintenance of body temperature.

STUDY OUTLINE

Function of the Digestive System—to break down food into simple chemicals that can be absorbed into the blood and lymph and utilized by cells

Divisions of the Digestive System
1. Alimentary tube—oral cavity, pharynx, esophagus, stomach, small intestine, large intestine. Digestion takes place in the oral cavity, stomach, and small intestine.
2. Accessory organs—salivary glands, teeth and tongue, liver and gallbladder, pancreas. Each contributes to digestion.

Types of Digestion
1. Mechanical—breaks food into smaller pieces to increase the surface area for the action of enzymes.
2. Chemical—enzymes break down complex organics into simpler organics and inorganics; each enzyme is specific for the food it will digest.

End Products of Digestion
1. Carbohydrates are digested to monosaccharides.

2. Fats are digested to fatty acids and glycerol.
3. Proteins are digested to amino acids.
4. Other end products are vitamins, minerals, and water.

Oral Cavity—food enters by way of the mouth
1. Teeth and tongue break up food and mix it with saliva.
2. Tooth structure (see Fig. 16–2)—enamel covers the crown and provides a hard chewing surface; dentin is within the enamel and forms the roots; the pulp cavity contains blood vessels and endings of the trigeminal nerve; the periodontal membrane produces cement to anchor the tooth in the jawbone.
3. The tongue is skeletal muscle innervated by the hypoglossal nerves. Papillae on the upper surface contain taste buds (facial and glossopharyngeal nerves). Functions: taste, keeps food between the teeth when chewing, elevates to push food backward for swallowing.

4. Salivary glands—parotid, submandibular, and sublingual (see Fig. 16–3); ducts take saliva to the oral cavity.

5. Saliva—amylase digests starch to maltose; water dissolves food for tasting and moistens food for swallowing; lysozyme inhibits the growth of bacteria (see Tables 16–1 and 16–2).

Pharynx—food passageway from the oral cavity to the esophagus

1. No digestion takes place.
2. Contraction of pharyngeal muscles is part of swallowing reflex, regulated by the medulla.

Esophagus—food passageway from pharynx to stomach

1. No digestion takes place.
2. Lower esophageal sphincter (LES) at junction with stomach prevents backup of stomach contents.

Structural Layers of the Alimentary Tube (see Fig. 16–4)

1. Mucosa (lining)—made of epithelial tissue that produces the digestive secretions; lymph nodules contain macrophages to phagocytize pathogens that penetrate the mucosa; thin layer of smooth muscle to ripple the epithelium.
2. Submucosa—areolar connective tissue with blood vessels and lymphatic vessels; Meissner's plexus is a nerve network that innervates the mucosa, part of the enteric nervous system that extends the entire length of the alimentary tube.
3. External muscle layer—typically an inner circular layer and an outer longitudinal layer of smooth muscle; function is mechanical digestion and peristalsis; innervated by Auerbach's plexus, part of the enteric nervous system; sympathetic impulses decrease motility; parasympathetic impulses increase motility.
4. Serosa—outermost layer; above the diaphragm is fibrous connective tissue; below the diaphragm is the mesentery (serous). The peritoneum (serous) lines the abdominal cavity; serous fluid prevents friction between the serous layers.

Stomach—in upper left abdominal quadrant; a muscular sac that extends from the esophagus to the small intestine (see Fig. 16–5)

1. Reservoir for food; begins the digestion of protein.

2. Gastric juice is secreted by gastric pits (see Tables 16–1 and 16–2).
3. The pyloric sphincter at the junction with the duodenum prevents backup of intestinal contents.

Liver—consists of two lobes in the upper right and center of the abdominal cavity (see Figs. 16–1 and 16–6)

1. Functional unit is the hexagonal liver lobule: liver cells, sinusoids, branches of the hepatic artery and portal vein, and bile ducts.
2. The only digestive secretion is bile; the hepatic duct takes bile out of the liver and unites with the cystic duct of the gallbladder to form the common bile duct to the duodenum.
3. Bile salts emulsify fats, a type of mechanical digestion (see Table 16–1).
4. Excess cholesterol and bilirubin are excreted by the liver into bile.

Gallbladder—on undersurface of right lobe of liver (see Fig. 16–6)

1. Stores and concentrates bile until needed in the duodenum (see Table 16–2).
2. The cystic duct joins the hepatic duct to form the common bile duct.

Pancreas—in upper left abdominal quadrant between the duodenum and the spleen (see Fig. 16–1)

1. Pancreatic juice is secreted by acini, carried by pancreatic duct to the common bile duct to the duodenum (see Fig. 16–7).
2. Enzyme pancreatic juice contains enzymes for the digestion of all three food types (see Tables 16–1 and 16–2).
3. Bicarbonate pancreatic juice neutralizes HCl from the stomach in the duodenum.

Small Intestine—coiled within the center of the abdominal cavity (see Fig. 16–1); extends from stomach to colon

1. Duodenum—first 10 inches; the common bile duct brings in bile and pancreatic juice. Jejunum (8 feet) and ileum (11 feet).
2. Enzymes secreted by the intestinal glands complete digestion (see Tables 16–1 and 16–2). Surface area for absorption is increased by plica circulares, villi,

and microvilli (see Fig. 16–8); microvilli are the brush border.

3. The villi contain capillary networks for the absorption of water-soluble nutrients: monosaccharides, amino acids, vitamin C and the B vitamins, minerals, and water. Blood from the small intestine goes to the liver first by way of portal circulation.

4. The villi contain lacteals (lymph capillaries) for the absorption of fat-soluble nutrients: vitamins A, D, E, and K, fatty acids and glycerol, which are combined to form chylomicrons. Lymph from the small intestine is carried back to the blood in the left subclavian vein.

Large Intestine (colon)—extends from the small intestine to the anus

1. Colon—parts (see Fig. 16–9): cecum, ascending colon, transverse colon, descending colon, sigmoid colon, rectum, anal canal.

2. Ileocecal valve—at the junction of the cecum and ileum; prevents backup of fecal material into the small intestine.

3. Colon—functions: absorption of water, minerals, vitamins; elimination of undigestible material.

4. Normal flora—the bacteria of the colon; produce vitamins, especially vitamin K, and inhibit the growth of pathogens.

5. Defecation reflex—stimulus: stretching of the rectum when peristalsis propels feces into it. Sensory impulses go to the sacral spinal cord, and motor impulses return to the smooth muscle of the rectum, which contracts. The internal anal sphincter relaxes to permit defecation. Voluntary control

is provided by the external anal sphincter, made of skeletal muscle (see Fig. 16–10).

Liver—other functions

1. Carbohydrate metabolism—excess glucose is stored in the form of glycogen and converted back to glucose during hypoglycemia; fructose and galactose are changed to glucose.

2. Amino acid metabolism—the non-essential amino acids are synthesized by transamination; excess amino acids are changed to carbohydrates or fats by deamination; the amino groups are converted to urea and excreted by the kidneys.

3. Lipid metabolism—formation of lipoproteins for transport of fats in the blood; synthesis of cholesterol; excretion of excess cholesterol into bile; beta-oxidation of fatty acids to form two-carbon acetyl groups for energy use.

4. Synthesis of plasma proteins—albumin to help maintain blood volume; clotting factors for blood clotting; alpha and beta globulins as carrier molecules.

5. Formation of bilirubin—old RBCs are phagocytized, and bilirubin is formed from the heme and put into bile to be eliminated in feces.

6. Phagocytosis by Kupffer cells—fixed macrophages; phagocytize old RBCs and bacteria, especially bacteria absorbed by the colon.

7. Storage—vitamins: B_{12}, A, D, E, K, and the minerals iron and copper.

8. Detoxification—liver enzymes change potential poisons to less harmful substances; examples of toxic substances are alcohol, medications, and ammonia absorbed by the colon.

REVIEW QUESTIONS

1. Name the organs of the alimentary tube, and describe the location of each. Name the accessory digestive organs, and describe the location of each. (pp. 350, 352, 353, 356, 358, 359, 362)

2. Explain the purpose of mechanical digestion, and give two examples. Explain the purpose of chemical digestion, and give two examples. (pp. 350, 354)

3. Name the end products of digestion, and explain how each is absorbed in the small intestine. (pp. 350, 362)

4. Explain the function of teeth and tongue, salivary amylase, enamel of teeth, lysozyme, and water of saliva. (pp. 350, 352)

5. Describe the function of the pharynx, esophagus, and lower esophageal sphincter. (p. 353)

6. Name and describe the four layers of the alimentary tube. (pp. 353, 356)

7. State the two general functions of the stomach and the function of the pyloric sphincter. Explain the function of pepsin, HCl, and mucus. (pp. 356–357)

8. Describe the general functions of the small intestine, and name the three parts. Describe the structures that increase the surface area of the small intestine. (pp. 358, 361, 362)

9. Explain how the liver, gallbladder, and pancreas contribute to digestion. (pp. 359, 361)

10. Describe the internal structure of a villus, and explain how structure is related to absorption. (p. 362)

11. Name the parts of the large intestine, and describe the function of the ileocecal valve. (pp. 362, 364)

12. Describe the functions of the colon and of the normal flora of the colon. (p. 364)

13. With respect to the defecation reflex, explain the stimulus, the part of the CNS directly involved, the effector muscle, the function of the internal anal sphincter, and the voluntary control possible. (p. 365)

14. Name the vitamins and minerals stored in the liver. Name the fixed macrophages of the liver, and explain their function. (pp. 368–369)

15. Describe how the liver regulates blood glucose level. Explain the purpose of the processes of deamination and transamination. (p. 368)

16. Name the plasma proteins produced by the liver, and state the function of each. (p. 368)

17. Name the substances excreted by the liver into bile. (p. 368)

FOR FURTHER THOUGHT

1. The colon does not have villi as part of its mucosa. Explain why villi are not necessary.

2. Food remains in the stomach for several hours. Passage of food through the small intestine also requires several hours. These two organs have very different shapes. Explain why they are able to retain food for so long, for efficient digestion and absorption.

3. Diarrhea can be unpleasant, but does have a purpose. Explain, and state the disadvantages as well.

4. Explain how a spinal cord transection at the level of T10 will affect the defecation reflex.

5. You have seen the word *enteric* (or *entero*) several times in this chapter. What does it mean? Define each of these: enteric bacilli, enterovirus, Enterococcus.

6. The word *symbiosis* indicates two different kinds of living things, and literally means "together-life." Our own alimentary tube is a perfect example. Explain, and state the advantages to each living thing.

CHAPTER 17

Chapter Outline

Student Objectives

- State the normal range of human body temperature.
- Explain how cell respiration produces heat and the factors that affect heat production.
- Describe the pathways of heat loss through the skin and respiratory tract.
- Explain why the hypothalamus is called the "thermostat" of the body.
- Describe the mechanisms to increase heat loss.
- Describe the mechanisms to conserve heat.
- Explain how a fever is caused and its advantages and disadvantages.
- Define metabolism, anabolism, and catabolism.
- Describe what happens to a glucose molecule during the three stages of cell respiration.
- State what happens to each of the products of cell respiration.
- Explain how amino acids and fats may be used for energy production.
- Describe the synthesis uses for glucose, amino acids, and fats.

Body Temperature and Metabolism

Student Objectives (Continued)

- Explain what is meant by metabolic rate and kilocalories.
- Describe the factors that affect a person's metabolic rate.

New Terminology

Anabolism (an-**AB**-uh-lizm)
Catabolism (kuh-**TAB**-uh-lizm)
Coenzyme (ko-**EN**-zime)
Conduction (kon-**DUK**-shun)
Convection (kon-**VEK**-shun)
Cytochromes (**SIGH**-toh-krohms)
Endogenous pyrogen (en-**DOJ**-en-us **PYE**-roh-jen)
Fever (**FEE**-ver)
Glycolysis (gly-**KAHL**-ah-sis)
Kilocalorie (KILL-oh-**KAL**-oh-ree)
Krebs cycle (KREBS **SIGH**-kuhl)
Metabolism (muh-**TAB**-uh-lizm)
Minerals (**MIN**-er-als)
Pyrogen (**PYE**-roh-jen)
Radiation (RAY-dee-**AY**-shun)
Vitamins (**VY**-tah-mins)

Related Clinical Terminology

Antipyretic (AN-tigh-pye-**RET**-ik)
Basal metabolic rate (**BAY**-zuhl met-ah-**BAHL**-ik RAYT)
Frostbite (**FRAWST**-bite)
Heat exhaustion (HEET eks-**ZAWS**-chun)
Heat stroke (HEET STROHK)
Hypothermia (HIGH-poh-**THER**-mee-ah)

*Terms that appear in **bold type** in the chapter text are defined in the glossary, which begins on page 521.*

During every moment of our lives, our cells are breaking down food molecules to obtain ATP for energy-requiring cellular processes. Naturally, we are not aware of the process of cell respiration, but we may be aware of one of the products—energy in the form of heat. The human body is indeed warm, and its temperature is regulated very precisely. Though we cannot stand barefoot on the ice of Antarctica for months in winter, as penguins do, we can adapt to and survive a wide range of environmental temperatures.

This chapter discusses the regulation of body temperature and also discusses **metabolism**, which is the total of all reactions that take place within the body. These reactions include the energy-releasing ones of cell respiration and energy-requiring ones such as protein synthesis, or DNA synthesis for mitosis. As you will see, body temperature and metabolism are inseparable.

BODY TEMPERATURE

The normal range of human body temperature is 96.5 to 99.5°F (36 to 38°C), with an average of 98.6°F (37°C). (A 1992 study suggested a slightly lower average temperature: 98.2°F or 36.8°C. Whether these values will replace the more "traditional" average temperatures remains to be seen. Thus far, they have not.) Within a 24-hour period, an individual's temperature fluctuates 1 to 2°F, with the lowest temperatures occurring during sleep.

At either end of the age spectrum, however, temperature regulation may not be as precise as it is in older children or younger adults. Infants have more surface area (skin) relative to volume and are likely to lose heat more rapidly. In the elderly, the mechanisms that maintain body temperature may not function as efficiently as they once did, and changes in environmental temperature may not be compensated for as quickly or effectively. This is especially important to remember when caring for patients who are very young or very old.

HEAT PRODUCTION

Cell respiration, the process that releases energy from food to produce ATP, also produces heat as one of its energy products. Although cell respiration takes place constantly, many factors influence the rate of this process:

1. The hormone **thyroxine** (and T_3), produced by the thyroid gland, increases the rate of cell respiration and heat production. The secretion of thyroxine is regulated by the body's rate of energy production, the metabolic rate itself (see Chapter 10 for the feedback mechanism involving the hypothalamus and anterior pituitary gland). When the metabolic rate decreases, the thyroid gland is stimulated to secrete more thyroxine. As thyroxine increases the rate of cell respiration, a negative feedback mechanism inhibits further secretion until metabolic rate decreases again. Thus, thyroxine is secreted whenever there is a need for increased cell respiration and is probably the most important regulator of day-to-day energy production.

2. In stress situations, **epinephrine** and norepinephrine are secreted by the adrenal medulla, and the **sympathetic** nervous system becomes more active. Epinephrine increases the rate of cell respiration, especially in organs such as the heart, skeletal muscles, and liver. Sympathetic stimulation also increases the activity of these organs. The increased production of ATP to meet the demands of the stress situation also means that more heat will be produced.

3. Organs that are normally active (producing ATP) are significant sources of heat when the body is at rest. The skeletal muscles, for example, are usually in a state of slight contraction called muscle tone. Because even slight contraction requires ATP, the muscles are also producing heat. This amounts to about 25% of the total body heat at rest and much more during exercise when more ATP is produced.

The liver is another organ that is continually active, producing ATP to supply energy for its many functions. As a result, the liver produces as much as 20% of the total body heat at rest. The heat produced by these active organs is dispersed throughout the body by the blood. As the relatively cooler blood flows through organs such as the muscles and liver, the heat they produce is transferred to the blood, warming it. The warmed blood circulates to other areas of the body, distributing this heat.

4. The intake of food also increases heat production, because the metabolic activity of the digestive tract is increased. Heat is generated as the digestive organs produce ATP for peristalsis and for the synthesis of digestive enzymes.

Table 17–1	FACTORS THAT AFFECT HEAT PRODUCTION
Factor	**Effect**
Thyroxine	• The most important regulator of day-to-day metabolism; increases use of foods for ATP production, thereby increasing heat production
Epinephrine and sympathetic stimulation	• Important in stress situations; increases the metabolic activity of many organs; increases ATP and heat production
Skeletal muscles	• Normal muscle tone requires ATP; the heat produced is about 25% of the total body heat at rest
Liver	• Always metabolically active; produces as much as 20% of total body heat at rest
Food intake	• Increases activity of the GI tract; increases ATP and heat production
Higher body temperature	• Increases metabolic rate, which increases heat production, which further increases metabolic rate and heat production; may become detrimental during high fevers

5. Changes in body temperature also have an effect on metabolic rate and heat production. This becomes clinically important when a person has a **fever**, an abnormally high body temperature. The higher temperature increases the metabolic rate, which increases heat production and elevates body temperature further. Thus, a high fever may trigger a vicious cycle of ever-increasing heat production. Fever is discussed later in this chapter.

The factors that affect heat production are summarized in Table 17–1.

HEAT LOSS

The pathways of heat loss from the body are the skin, respiratory tract, and to a lesser extent, the urinary and digestive tracts.

Heat Loss through the Skin

Because the skin covers the body, most body heat is lost from the skin to the environment. When the environment is cooler than body temperature (as it usually is), heat loss is unavoidable. The amount of heat that is lost is determined by blood flow through the skin and by the activity of sweat glands.

Blood flow through the skin influences the amount of heat lost by the processes of radiation, conduction, and convection. **Radiation** means that heat from the body is transferred to cooler objects not touching the skin, much as a radiator warms the contents of a room (radiation starts to become less effective when the environmental temperature rises above 88°F). **Conduction** is the loss of heat to cooler air or objects, such as clothing, that touch the skin. **Convection** means that air currents move the warmer air away from the skin surface and facilitate the loss of heat; this is why a fan makes us feel cooler on hot days. Loss of heat by convection also gives us the "wind chill factor" we hear about in winter. A cold day that is windy will feel colder than a cold day when the air is still, because the wind blows the slightly warmer air surrounding the body away, replacing it with colder air.

As you may recall from Chapter 5, the temperature of the skin and the subsequent loss of heat are determined by blood flow through the skin. The arterioles in the dermis may constrict or dilate to decrease or increase blood flow. In a cold environment, **vasoconstriction** decreases blood flow through the dermis and thereby decreases heat loss. In a warm environment, **vasodilation** in the dermis increases blood flow to the body surface and loss of heat to the environment.

The other mechanism by which heat is lost from the skin is sweating. The **eccrine sweat glands** secrete sweat (water) onto the skin surface, and excess body heat evaporates the sweat. Think of running water into a hot frying pan; the pan is rapidly cooled as its heat vaporizes the water. Although sweating is not quite as dramatic (no visible formation of steam), the principle is just the same.

Sweating is most efficient when the humidity of the surrounding air is low. Humidity is the percentage of the maximum amount of water vapor the atmosphere can contain. A humidity reading of 90% means that the air is already 90% saturated with water vapor and can hold little more. In such a situation, sweat does not readily evaporate, but rather, remains on the skin even as more sweat is secreted. If the humidity is 40%, however, the air can hold a great deal more water vapor, and sweat evaporates quickly from the skin

Box 17–1   HEAT-RELATED DISORDERS

Heat exhaustion is caused by excessive sweating with loss of water and salts, especially NaCl. The affected person feels very weak, and the skin is usually cool and clammy (moist). Body temperature is normal or slightly below normal, the pulse is often rapid and weak, and blood pressure may be low because of fluid loss. Other symptoms may include dizziness, vomiting, and muscle cramps. Treatment involves rest and consumption of salty fluids or fruit juices (in small amounts at frequent intervals).

Heat stroke is a life-threatening condition that may affect elderly or chronically ill people on hot, humid days, or otherwise healthy people who exercise too strenuously during such weather. High humidity makes sweating an ineffective mechanism of heat loss, but in high heat the sweating process continues. As fluid loss increases, sweating stops to preserve body fluid, and body temperature rises rapidly (over 105°F, possibly as high as 110°F).

The classic symptom of heat stroke is hot, dry skin. The affected person often loses consciousness, reflecting the destructive effect of such a high body temperature on the brain. Treatment should involve hospitalization so that IV fluids may be administered and body temperature lowered under medical supervision. A first-aid measure would be the application of cool (not ice cold) water to as much of the skin as possible. Fluids should never be forced on an unconscious person, because the fluid may be aspirated into the respiratory tract.

---

surface, removing excess body heat. In air that is completely dry, a person may tolerate a temperature of 200°F for nearly 1 hour.

Although sweating is a very effective mechanism of heat loss, it does have a disadvantage in that it requires the loss of water in order to also lose heat. Water loss during sweating may rapidly lead to dehydration, and the water lost must be replaced by drinking fluids (see Box 17–1: Heat-Related Disorders).

Small amounts of heat are also lost in what is called "insensible water loss." Because the skin is not like a plastic bag, but is somewhat permeable to water, a small amount of water diffuses through the skin and is evaporated by body heat. Compared to sweating, however, insensible water loss is a minor source of heat loss.

Heat Loss through the Respiratory Tract

Heat is lost from the respiratory tract as the warmth of the respiratory mucosa evaporates some water from the living epithelial surface. The water vapor formed is exhaled, and a small amount of heat is lost.

Animals such as dogs that do not have numerous sweat glands often pant in warm weather. Panting is the rapid movement of air into and out of the upper respiratory passages, where the warm surfaces evaporate large amounts of water. In this way the animal may lose large amounts of heat.

Heat Loss through the Urinary and Digestive Tracts

When excreted, urine and feces are at body temperature, and their elimination results in a very small amount of heat loss. The pathways of heat loss are summarized in Table 17–2.

REGULATION OF BODY TEMPERATURE

The **hypothalamus** is responsible for the regulation of body temperature and is considered the "thermostat" of the body. As the thermostat, the hypothalamus maintains the "setting" of body temperature by balancing heat production and heat loss to keep the body at the set temperature.

In order to do this, the hypothalamus must receive information about the temperature within the body and about the environmental temperature. Specialized neurons of the hypothalamus detect changes in the temperature of the blood that flows through the brain. The temperature receptors in the skin provide information about the external temperature changes to which the body is exposed. The hypothalamus then integrates this sensory information and promotes the necessary responses to maintain body temperature within the normal range.

Mechanisms to Increase Heat Loss

In a warm environment or during exercise, the body temperature tends to rise, and greater heat loss is

Table 17–2 | PATHWAYS OF HEAT LOSS

Pathway	Mechanism
Skin (major pathway)	• Radiation and conduction—heat is lost from the body to cooler air or objects. • Convection—air currents move warm air away from the skin. • Sweating—excess body heat evaporates sweat on the skin surface.
Respiratory tract (secondary pathway)	• Evaporation—body heat evaporates water from the respiratory mucosa, and water vapor is exhaled.
Urinary tract (minor pathway)	• Urination—urine is at body temperature when eliminated.
Digestive tract (minor pathway)	• Defecation—feces are at body temperature when eliminated.

needed. This is accomplished by vasodilation in the dermis and an increase in sweating. Vasodilation brings more warm blood close to the body surface, and heat is lost to the environment. However, if the environmental temperature is close to or higher than body temperature, this mechanism becomes ineffective. The second mechanism is increased sweating, in which excess body heat evaporates the sweat on the skin surface. As mentioned previously, sweating becomes inefficient when the atmospheric humidity is high.

On hot days, heat production may also be decreased by a decrease in muscle tone. This is why we may feel very sluggish on hot days; our muscles are even less slightly contracted than usual and are slower to respond.

Mechanisms to Conserve Heat

In a cold environment, heat loss from the body is unavoidable but may be minimized to some extent. Vasoconstriction in the dermis shunts blood away from the body surface, so that more heat is kept in the core of the body. Sweating decreases, and will stop completely if the temperature of the hypothalamus falls below about 98.6°F.

If these mechanisms are not sufficient to prevent the body temperature from dropping, more heat may be produced by increasing muscle tone. When this greater muscle tone becomes noticeable and rhythmic, it is called shivering and may increase heat production by as much as five times the normal.

People also have behavioral responses to cold, and these too are important to prevent heat loss. Such things as putting on a sweater or going indoors reflect our awareness of the discomfort of being cold. For people (we do not have thick fur as do some other mammals), these voluntary activities are of critical importance to the prevention of excessive heat loss when it is very cold (see Box 17–2: Cold-Related Disorders).

FEVER

A fever is an abnormally high body temperature and may accompany infectious diseases, extensive physical trauma, cancer, or damage to the CNS. The substances that may cause a fever are called **pyrogens**. Pyrogens include bacteria, foreign proteins, and chemicals released during inflammation. These inflammatory chemicals are called **endogenous pyrogens**. *Endogenous* means "generated from within." It is believed that pyrogens chemically affect the hypothalamus and "raise the setting" of the hypothalamic thermostat. The hypothalamus will then stimulate responses by the body to raise body temperature to this higher setting.

Let us use as a specific example a child who has a strep throat. The bacterial and endogenous pyrogens reset the hypothalamic thermostat upward, to 102°F. At first, the body is "colder" than the setting of the hypothalamus, and the heat conservation and production mechanisms are activated. The child feels cold and begins to shiver (chills). Eventually, sufficient heat is produced to raise the body temperature to the hypothalamic setting of 102°F. At this time, the child will feel neither too warm nor too cold, because the body temperature is what the hypothalamus wants.

As the effects of the pyrogens diminish, the hypothalamic setting decreases, perhaps close to normal again, 99°F. Now the child will feel warm, and the heat-loss mechanisms will be activated. Vasodilation in the skin and sweating will occur until the body temperature drops to the new hypothalamic setting. This is sometimes referred to as the "crisis," but actually the crisis has passed, because sweating indicates that the body temperature is returning to normal. The

Box 17–2   COLD-RELATED DISORDERS

Frostbite is the freezing of part of the body. Fingers, toes, the nose, and ears are most often affected by prolonged exposure to cold, because these areas have little volume in proportion to their surface.

At first the skin tingles, then becomes numb. If body fluids freeze, ice crystals may destroy capillaries and tissues (because water expands when it freezes), and blisters form. In the most severe cases gangrene develops, that is, tissue dies because of lack of oxygen.

Treatment of frostbite includes rewarming the affected area. If skin damage is apparent, it should be treated as if it were a burn injury.

Hypothermia is an abnormally low body temperature (below 95°F) that is most often the result of prolonged exposure to cold. Although the affected person certainly feels cold at first, this sensation may pass and be replaced by confusion, slurred speech, drowsiness, and lack of coordination. At this stage, people often do not realize the seriousness of their condition, and if outdoors (ice skating or skiing) may not seek a warmer environment. In progressive hypothermia, breathing and heart rate slow, and coma and death follow.

Other people at greater risk for hypothermia include the elderly, whose temperature-regulating mechanisms are no longer effective, and quadriplegics, who have no sensation of cold in the body. For both of these groups, heat production is or may be low because of inactivity of skeletal muscles.

Artificial hypothermia may be induced during some types of cardiovascular or neurological surgery. This carefully controlled lowering of body temperature decreases the metabolic rate and need for oxygen and makes possible prolonged surgery without causing extensive tissue death in the patient.

---

sequence of temperature changes during a fever is shown in Fig. 17–1.

You may be wondering if a fever serves a useful purpose. For low fevers that are the result of infection, the answer seems to be yes. White blood cells increase their activity at moderately elevated temperatures, and the metabolism of some pathogens is inhibited. Thus, a fever may be beneficial in that it may shorten the duration of an infection by accelerating the destruction of the pathogen.

High fevers, however, may have serious consequences. A fever increases the metabolic rate, which increases heat production, which in turn raises body temperature even more. This is a positive feedback mechanism that will continue until an external event (such as aspirin or death of the pathogens) acts as a brake. When the body temperature rises above 106°F, the hypothalamus begins to lose its ability to regulate temperature. The proteins of cells, especially the enzymes, are also damaged by such high temperatures. Enzymes become denatured, that is, lose their shape and do not catalyze the reactions necessary within cells. As a result, cells begin to die. This is most serious in the brain, because neurons cannot be replaced, and is the cause of brain damage that may follow a prolonged high fever. The effects of changes in body temperature on the hypothalamus are shown in Fig. 17–2.

A medication such as aspirin is called an **antipyretic** because it lowers a fever, probably by affecting the hypothalamic thermostat. To help lower a high fever, the body may be cooled by sponging with cool water. The excessive body heat will cause this external water to evaporate, thus reducing temperature. A very high fever requires medical attention.

METABOLISM

The term **metabolism** encompasses all of the reactions that take place in the body. Everything that happens within us is part of our metabolism. The reactions of metabolism may be divided into two major categories: anabolism and catabolism.

Anabolism means synthesis or "formation" reactions, the bonding together of smaller molecules to form larger ones. The synthesis of hemoglobin by cells of the red bone marrow, synthesis of glycogen by liver cells, and synthesis of fat to be stored in adipose tissue are all examples of anabolism. Such reactions require energy, usually in the form of ATP.

Catabolism means decomposition, the breaking of bonds of larger molecules to form smaller molecules. Cell respiration is a series of catabolic reactions that break down food molecules to carbon dioxide and water. During catabolism, energy is often released and

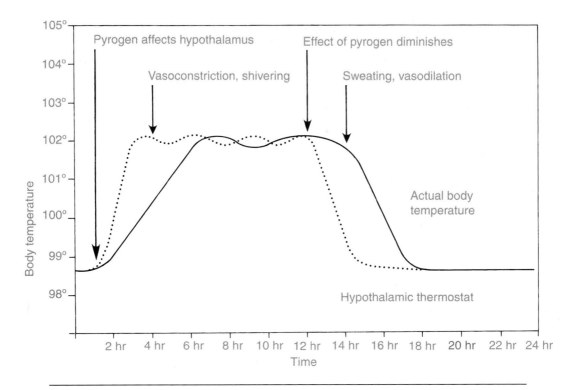

Figure 17–1 Changes in body temperature during an episode of fever. The body temperature (*solid line*) changes lag behind the changes in the hypothalamic thermostat (*dotted line*) but eventually reach whatever the thermostat has called for.

used to synthesize ATP (the heat energy released was discussed in the previous section). The ATP formed during catabolism is then used for energy-requiring anabolic reactions.

Most of our anabolic and catabolic reactions are catalyzed by enzymes. Enzymes are proteins that enable reactions to take place rapidly at body temperature (see Chapter 2 to review the Active Site Theory of enzyme functioning). The body has thousands of enzymes, and each is specific, that is, will catalyze only one type of reaction. As you read the discussions that follow, keep in mind the essential role of enzymes.

CELL RESPIRATION

You are already familiar with the summary reaction of cell reaction,

$$C_6H_{12}O_6 + O_2 \rightarrow CO_2 + H_2O + ATP + Heat$$
(glucose)

the purpose of which is to produce ATP. Glucose contains potential energy, and when it is broken down to CO_2 and H_2O, this energy is released in the forms of ATP and heat. The oxygen that is required comes from breathing, and the CO_2 formed is circulated to the lungs to be exhaled. The water formed is called metabolic water, and helps to meet our daily need for water. Energy in the form of heat gives us a body temperature, and the ATP formed is used for energy-requiring reactions. Synthesis of ATP means that energy is used to bond a free phosphate molecule to ADP (adenosine diphosphate). ADP and free phosphates are present in cells after ATP has been broken down for energy-requiring processes.

The breakdown of glucose summarized above is not quite that simple, however, and involves a complex series of reactions. Glucose is taken apart "piece by piece," with the removal of hydrogens and the splitting of carbon–carbon bonds. This releases the energy of glucose gradually, so that a significant portion (about 40%) is available to synthesize ATP.

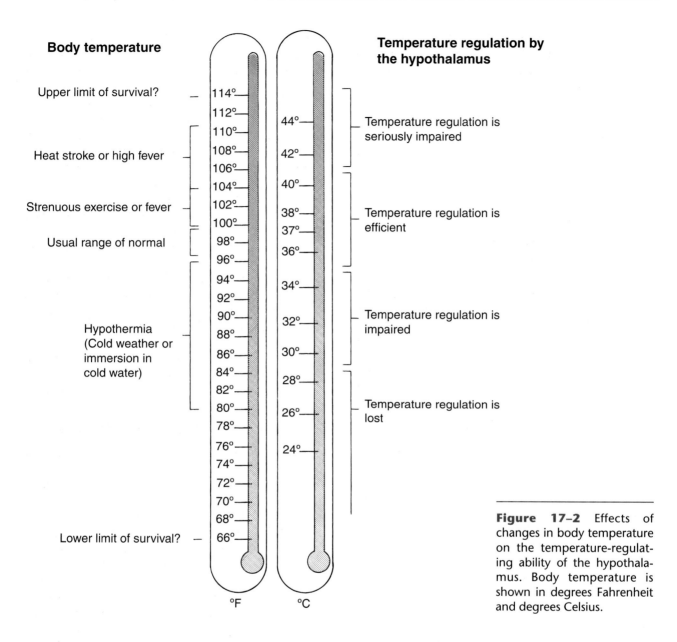

Body temperature

Upper limit of survival? — 114°

112°
110°
Heat stroke or high fever — 108°
106°
104°
Strenuous exercise or fever — 102°
100°
Usual range of normal — 98°
96°
94°
92°
90°
Hypothermia
(Cold weather or 88°
immersion in 86°
cold water) 84°
82°
80°
78°
76°
74°
72°
70°
68°
Lower limit of survival? — 66°

°F

44°
42°
40°
38°
37°
36°
34°
32°
30°
28°
26°
24°

°C

Temperature regulation by the hypothalamus

Temperature regulation is seriously impaired

Temperature regulation is efficient

Temperature regulation is impaired

Temperature regulation is lost

Figure 17–2 Effects of changes in body temperature on the temperature-regulating ability of the hypothalamus. Body temperature is shown in degrees Fahrenheit and degrees Celsius.

Cell respiration of glucose involves three major stages: glycolysis, the Krebs citric acid cycle, and the cytochrome (or electron) transport system. Although the details of each stage are beyond the scope of this book, we will summarize the most important aspects of each, and then relate to them the use of amino acids and fats for energy.

Glycolysis

The enzymes for the reactions of **glycolysis** are found in the cytoplasm of cells, and oxygen is not required (glycolysis is an anaerobic process). Refer now to Fig. 17–3 as you read the following. In glycolysis, a six-carbon glucose molecule is broken down to two three-carbon molecules of pyruvic acid. Two molecules of ATP are necessary to start the process. The energy they supply is called energy of activation and is necessary to make glucose unstable enough to begin to break down. As a result of these reactions, enough energy is released to synthesize four molecules of ATP, for a net gain of two ATP molecules per glucose molecule. Also during glycolysis, two pairs of hydrogens are removed by NAD, a carrier molecule that contains the vitamin **niacin**. Two NAD molecules thus become 2NADH$_2$, and these attached hydrogen pairs will be transported to the cytochrome transport system (stage 3).

If no oxygen is present in the cell, as may happen in muscle cells during exercise, pyruvic acid is converted to lactic acid, which causes muscle fatigue. If oxygen *is* present, however, pyruvic acid continues into the next stage, the Krebs citric acid cycle (or, more simply, the Krebs cycle).

Krebs Citric Acid Cycle

The enzymes for the **Krebs cycle** (or citric acid cycle) are located in the mitochondria of cells. This second stage of cell respiration is aerobic, meaning that oxygen is required. In a series of reactions, a pyruvic acid molecule is "taken apart," and its carbons are converted to CO_2. The first CO_2 molecule is removed by an enzyme that contains the vitamin **thiamine**. This leaves a two-carbon molecule called an acetyl group, which combines with a molecule called coenzyme A to form acetyl coenzyme A (acetyl CoA). As acetyl CoA continues in the Krebs cycle, two more carbons are removed as CO_2, and more pairs of hydrogens are picked up by NAD and FAD (another carrier molecule that contains the vitamin **riboflavin**). NADH$_2$ and FADH$_2$ will carry their hydrogens to the cytochrome transport system.

During the Krebs cycle, a small amount of energy is released, enough to synthesize one molecule of ATP (two per glucose). Notice also that a four-carbon molecule (oxaloacetic acid) is regenerated after the formation of CO_2. This molecule will react with the next acetyl CoA, which is what makes the Krebs cycle truly a self-perpetuating cycle. The results of the stages of cell respiration are listed in Table 17–3. Before you continue, you may wish to look at that table to see just where the process has gotten thus far.

Cytochrome Transport System

Cytochromes are proteins that contain either **iron** or **copper** and are found in the mitochondria of cells. The pairs of hydrogens that were once part of glucose are brought to the cytochromes by the carrier molecules NAD and FAD. Each hydrogen atom is then split into its proton (H$^+$ ion) and its electron. The electrons of the hydrogens are passed from one cytochrome to the next, and finally to oxygen. The reactions of the electrons with the cytochromes release most of the

energy that was contained in the glucose molecule, enough to synthesize 34 molecules of ATP. As you can see, most of the ATP produced in cell respiration comes from this third stage.

Finally, and very importantly, each oxygen atom that has gained two electrons (from the cytochromes) reacts with two of the H$^+$ ions (protons) to form water. The formation of metabolic water contributes to the necessary intracellular fluid, and also prevents acidosis. If H$^+$ ions accumulated, they would rapidly lower the pH of the cell. This does not happen, however, because the H$^+$ ions react with oxygen to form water, and a decrease in pH is prevented.

The summary of the three stages of cell respiration in Table 17–3 also includes the vitamins and minerals that are essential for this process. An important overall concept is the relationship between eating and breathing. Eating provides us with a potential energy source (often glucose) and with necessary vitamins and minerals. However, to release the energy from food, we must breathe. This is *why* we breathe. The oxygen we inhale is essential for the completion of cell respiration, and the CO_2 produced is exhaled.

Proteins and Fats as Energy Sources

Although glucose is the preferred energy source for cells, proteins and fats also contain potential energy and are alternative energy sources in certain situations.

As you know, proteins are made of the smaller molecules called **amino acids**, and the primary use for the amino acids we obtain from food is the synthesis of new proteins. Excess amino acids, however, those not needed immediately for protein synthesis, may be used for energy production. In the liver, excess amino acids are **deaminated**, that is, the amino group (NH$_2$) is removed. The remaining portion is converted to a molecule that will fit into the Krebs cycle. For example, a deaminated amino acid may be changed to a three-carbon pyruvic acid or to a two-carbon acetyl group. When these molecules enter the Krebs cycle, the results are just the same as if they had come from glucose. This is diagrammed in Fig. 17–3.

Fats are made of glycerol and fatty acids, which are the end products of fat digestion. These molecules may also be changed to ones that will take part in the Krebs cycle, and the reactions that change them usually take place in the liver. Glycerol is a three-carbon molecule that can be converted to the three-carbon pyruvic acid, which enters the Krebs cycle.

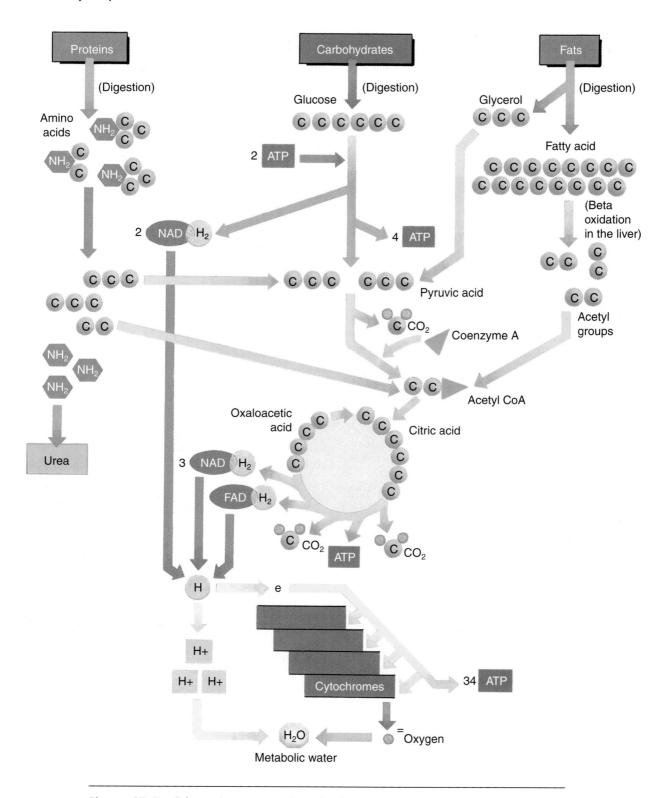

Figure 17–3 Schematic representation of cell respiration. The breakdown of glucose is shown in the center, amino acids on the left, and fatty acids and glycerol on the right. See text for description.

| Table 17–3 | SUMMARY OF CELL RESPIRATION |

Stage	Molecules That Enter the Process	Results	Vitamins or Minerals Needed
Glycolysis (cytoplasm)	Glucose—ATP needed as energy of activation	• 2 ATP (net) • 2 $NADH_2$ (to cytochrome transport system) • 2 pyruvic acid (aerobic: to Krebs cycle; anaerobic: lactic acid formation)	• Niacin (part of NAD)
Krebs citric acid cycle (mitochondria)	Pyruvic acid—from glucose or glycerol or excess amino acids *or* Acetyl CoA—from fatty acids or excess amino acids	• CO_2 (exhaled) • ATP (2 per glucose) • 3 $NADH_2$ and 1 $FADH_2$ (to cytochrome transport system) • A 4-carbon molecule is regenerated for the next cycle	• Thiamine (for removal of CO_2) • Niacin (part of NAD) • Riboflavin (part of FAD) • Pantothenic acid (part of coenzyme A)
Cytochrome transport system (mitochondria)	$NADH_2$ and $FADH_2$—from glycolysis or the Krebs cycle	• 34 ATP • Metabolic water	• Iron and copper (part of some cytochromes)

In the process of beta-oxidation, the long carbon chains of fatty acids are split into two-carbon acetyl groups, which enter a later step in the Krebs cycle (see Fig. 17–3).

Both amino acids and fatty acids may be converted by the liver to **ketones**, which are two- or four-carbon molecules such as acetone and acetoacetic acid. Although body cells can use ketones in cell respiration, they do so slowly. In situations in which fats or amino acids have become the primary energy sources, a state called **ketosis** may develop; this is described in Box 17–3: Ketosis. Excess amino acids may also be converted to glucose; this is important to supply the brain when dietary intake of carbohydrates is low. The effects of hormones on the metabolism of food are summarized in Table 17–4.

Energy Available from the Three Nutrient Types

The potential energy in food is measured in units called **Calories** or **kilocalories**. A calorie (lowercase "c") is the amount of energy needed to raise the temperature of 1 gram of water 1°C. A kilocalorie or Calorie (capital "C") is 1000 times that amount of energy.

| Box 17–3 | KETOSIS |

When fats and amino acids are to be used for energy, they are often converted by the liver to ketones. Ketones are organic molecules such as acetone that may be changed to acetyl CoA and enter the Krebs cycle. Other cells are able to use ketones as an energy source, but they do so slowly. When ketones are produced in small amounts, as they usually are between meals, the blood level does not rise sharply.

A state of **ketosis** exists when fats and proteins become the primary energy sources, and ketones accumulate in the blood faster than cells can utilize them. Because ketones are organic acids, they lower the pH of the blood. As the blood ketone level rises, the kidneys excrete ketones, but they must also excrete more water as a solvent, which leads to dehydration.

Ketosis is clinically important in diabetes mellitus, starvation, and eating disorders such as anorexia nervosa. Diabetics whose disease is poorly controlled may progress to **ketoacidosis**, a form of metabolic acidosis that may lead to confusion, coma, and death. Reversal of this state requires a carbohydrate energy source and the insulin necessary to utilize it.

Table 17–4 HORMONES THAT REGULATE METABOLISM

Hormone (gland)	Effects
Thyroxine (thyroid gland)	• Increases use of all three food types for energy (glucose, fats, amino acids) • Increases protein synthesis
Growth hormone (anterior pituitary)	• Increases amino acid transport into cells • Increases protein synthesis • Increases use of fats for energy
Insulin (pancreas)	• Increases glucose transport into cells and use for energy • Increases conversion of glucose to glycogen in liver and muscles • Increases transport of amino acids and fatty acids into cells to be used for synthesis (*not* energy production)
Glucagon (pancreas)	• Increases conversion of glycogen to glucose • Increases use of amino acids and fats for energy
Cortisol (adrenal cortex)	• Increases conversion of glucose to glycogen in liver • Increases use of amino acids and fats for energy • Decreases protein synthesis except in liver and GI tract
Epinephrine (adrenal medulla)	• Increases conversion of glycogen to glucose • Increases use of fats for energy

One gram of carbohydrate yields about 4 kilocalories. A gram of protein also yields about 4 kilocalories. A gram of fat, however, yields 9 kilocalories, and a gram of alcohol yields 7 kilocalories. This is why a diet high in fat is more likely to result in weight gain if the calories are not expended in energy-requiring activities.

You may have noticed that calorie content is part of the nutritional information on food labels. Here, however, the term *calorie* actually means Calorie or kilocalories but is used for the sake of simplicity.

SYNTHESIS USES OF FOODS

Besides being available for energy production, each of the three food types is used in anabolic reactions to synthesize necessary materials for cells and tissues.

Glucose

Glucose is the raw material for the synthesis of another important monosaccharide, the **pentose sugars** that are part of nucleic acids. Deoxyribose is the five-carbon sugar found in DNA, and ribose is found in RNA. This function of glucose is very important, for without the pentose sugars our cells could neither produce new chromosomes for cell division nor carry out the process of protein synthesis.

Any glucose in excess of immediate energy needs or the need for pentose sugars is converted to **glycogen** in the liver and skeletal muscles. Glycogen is then an energy source during states of hypoglycemia or during exercise.

Amino Acids

As mentioned previously, the primary uses for amino acids are the synthesis of the **non-essential amino acids** by the liver and the synthesis of new **proteins** in all tissues. By way of review, we can mention some proteins with which you are already familiar: keratin and melanin in the epidermis; collagen in the dermis, tendons, and ligaments; myosin, actin, and myoglobin in muscle cells; hemoglobin in RBCs; antibodies produced by WBCs; prothrombin and fibrinogen for clotting; albumin to maintain blood volume; pepsin and amylase for digestion; growth hormone and insulin; and the thousands of enzymes needed to catalyze reactions within the body.

The amino acids we obtain from the proteins in our food are used by our cells to synthesize all of these proteins in the amounts needed by the body. Only when the body's needs for new proteins have been met are amino acids used for energy production.

Fatty Acids and Glycerol

The end products of fat digestion that are not needed immediately for energy production may be stored as fat (triglycerides) in **adipose tissue**. Most adipose tissue is found subcutaneously and is potential energy for times when food intake decreases. Notice in Table 17–4 that insulin promotes fat synthesis and storage. One theory of weight gain proposes that a diet high in sugars and starches stimulates the secretion of so much insulin that fat can only be stored, not taken out of storage and used for energy.

Fatty acids and glycerol are also used for the synthesis of **phospholipids**, which are essential components of all cell membranes. Myelin, for example, is a phospholipid of the membranes of Schwann cells, which form the myelin sheath of peripheral neurons.

The liver can synthesize most of the fatty acids needed by the body. Two exceptions are linoleic acid and linolenic acid, which are **essential fatty acids** and must be obtained from the diet. Linoleic acid is part of lecithin, which in turn is part of all cell membranes. Vegetable oils are good sources of these essential fatty acids.

When fatty acids are broken down in the process of beta-oxidation, the resulting acetyl groups may also be used for the synthesis of **cholesterol**, a steroid. This takes place primarily in the liver, although all cells are capable of synthesizing cholesterol for their cell membranes. The liver uses cholesterol to synthesize bile salts for the emulsification of fats in digestion. The **steroid hormones** are also synthesized from cholesterol. Cortisol and aldosterone are produced by the adrenal cortex; estrogen and progesterone by the ovaries, and testosterone by the testes.

VITAMINS AND MINERALS

Vitamins are organic molecules needed in very small amounts for normal body functioning. Some vitamins are **coenzymes**, that is, they are necessary for the functioning of certain enzymes. Others are antioxidant vitamins, including vitamins C, E, and beta-carotene (a precursor for vitamin A). Antioxidants prevent damage from **free radicals**, which are molecules that contain an unpaired electron and are highly reactive. The reactions of free radicals can damage DNA, cell membranes, and the cell organelles. Free radicals are formed during some normal body reactions, but smoking and exposure to pollution will increase their formation. Antioxidant vitamins combine with free radicals before they can react with cellular components. Plant foods are good sources of these vitamins. Table 17–5 summarizes some important metabolic and nutritional aspects of the vitamins we need.

Minerals are simple inorganic chemicals and have a variety of functions, many of which you are already familiar with. Table 17–6 lists some important

aspects of minerals. We will return to the minerals as part of our study of fluid–electrolyte balance in Chapter 19.

METABOLIC RATE

Although the term **metabolism** is used to describe all of the chemical reactions that take place within the body, **metabolic rate** is usually expressed as an amount of heat production. This is because many body processes that utilize ATP also produce heat. These processes include the contraction of skeletal muscle, the pumping of the heart, and the normal breakdown of cellular components. Therefore, it is possible to quantify heat production as a measure of metabolic activity.

As mentioned previously, the energy available from food is measured in kilocalories (kcal). Kilocalories are also the units used to measure the energy expended by the body. During sleep, for example, energy expended by a 150-pound person is about 60 to 70 kcal per hour. Getting up and preparing breakfast increases energy expenditure to 80 to 90 kcal per hour. For mothers with several small children, this value may be significantly higher. Clearly, greater activity results in greater energy expenditure.

The energy required for merely living (lying quietly in bed) is the **basal metabolic rate** (BMR). See Box 17–4: Metabolic Rate for a formula to estimate your own metabolic rate. A number of factors affect the metabolic rate of an active person:

1. Exercise—Contraction of skeletal muscle increases energy expenditure and raises metabolic rate (see Box 17–5: Weight Loss).
2. Age—Metabolic rate is highest in young children and decreases with age. The energy requirements for growth and the greater heat loss by a smaller body contribute to the higher rate in children. After growth has stopped, metabolic rate decreases about 2% per decade. If a person becomes less active, the total decrease is almost 5% per decade.
3. Body configuration of adults—Tall, thin people usually have higher metabolic rates than do short, stocky people of the same weight. This is so because the tall, thin person has a larger surface area (proportional to weight) through which heat is continuously lost. The metabolic rate, therefore, is slightly higher to compensate for the greater heat loss. The variance of surface-to-weight ratios for

Table 17–5 | VITAMINS

Vitamin	Functions	Food Sources	Comment
Water Soluble			
Thiamine (B$_1$)	• Conversion of pyruvic acid to acetyl CoA in cell respiration • Synthesis of pentose sugars • Synthesis of acetylcholine	• Meat, eggs, legumes, green leafy vegetables, grains	Rapidly destroyed by heat
Riboflavin (B$_2$)	• Part of FAD in cell respiration	• Meat, milk, cheese, grains	Small amounts produced by GI bacteria
Niacin (nicotinamide)	• Part of NAD in cell respiration • Metabolism of fat for energy	• Meat, fish, grains, legumes	
Pyridoxine (B$_6$)	• Part of enzymes needed for amino acid metabolism and protein synthesis, nucleic acid synthesis, synthesis of antibodies	• Meat, fish, grains, yeast, yogurt	Small amounts produced by GI bacteria
B$_{12}$ (cyanocobalamin)	• Synthesis of DNA, especially in RBC production • Metabolism of amino acids for energy	• Liver, meat, fish, eggs, milk, cheese	Contains cobalt; intrinsic factor required for absorption
Biotin	• Synthesis of nucleic acids • Metabolism of fatty acids and amino acids	• Yeast, liver, eggs	Small amounts produced by GI bacteria
Folic acid (folacin)	• Synthesis of DNA, especially in blood cell production	• Liver, grains, legumes, leafy green vegetables	Small amounts produced by GI bacteria
Pantothenic acid	• Part of coenzyme A in cell respiration, use of amino acids and fats for energy	• Meat, fish, grains, legumes, vegetables	Small amounts produced by GI bacteria
Vitamin C (ascorbic acid)	• Synthesis of collagen, especially for wound healing • Metabolism of amino acids • Absorption of iron • An antioxidant— prevents cellular damage from free radicals	• Citrus fruits, tomatoes, potatoes	Rapidly destroyed by heat
Fat Soluble			
Vitamin A	• Synthesis of rhodopsin • Calcification of growing bones • Maintenance of epithelial tissues	• Yellow and green vegetables, liver, milk, eggs	Stored in liver; bile salts required for absorption
Vitamin D	• Absorption of calcium and phosphorus in the small intestine	• Fortified milk, egg yolks, fish liver oils	Produced in skin exposed to UV rays; stored in liver; bile salts required for absorption
Vitamin E	• An antioxidant—prevents destruction of cell membranes • Contributes to wound healing and detoxifying ability of the liver	• Nuts, wheat germ, seed oils	Stored in liver and adipose tissue; bile salts required for absorption
Vitamin K	• Synthesis of prothrombin and other clotting factors	• Liver, spinach, cabbage	Large amounts produced by GI bacteria; bile salts required for absorption; stored in liver

Table 17–6   MINERALS

Mineral	Functions	Food Sources	Comment
Calcium	• Formation of bones and teeth • Neuron and muscle functioning • Blood clotting	• Milk, cheese, yogurt, shellfish, leafy green vegetables	Vitamin D required for absorption; stored in bones
Phosphorus	• Formation of bones and teeth • Part of DNA, RNA, and ATP • Part of phosphate buffer system	• Milk, cheese, fish, meat	Vitamin D required for absorption; stored in bones
Sodium	• Contributes to osmotic pressure of body fluids • Nerve impulse transmission and muscle contraction • Part of bicarbonate buffer system	• Table salt, almost all foods	Most abundant cation (+) in extracellular fluid
Potassium	• Contributes to osmotic pressure of body fluids • Nerve impulse transmission and muscle contraction	• Virtually all foods	Most abundant cation (+) in intracellular fluid
Chlorine	• Contributes to osmotic pressure of body fluids • Part of HCl in gastric juice	• Table salt	Most abundant anion (–) in extracellular fluid
Iron	• Part of hemoglobin and myoglobin • Part of some cytochromes in cell respiration	• Meat, shellfish, dried apricots, legumes, eggs	Stored in liver
Iodine	• Part of thyroxine and T_3	• Iodized salt, seafood	
Sulfur	• Part of some amino acids • Part of thiamine and biotin	• Meat, eggs	Insulin and keratin require sulfur
Magnesium	• Formation of bone • Metabolism of ATP–ADP	• Green vegetables, legumes, seafood, milk	Part of chlorophyll in green plants
Manganese	• Formation of urea • Synthesis of fatty acids and cholesterol	• Legumes, grains, nuts, leafy green vegetables	Some stored in liver
Copper	• Synthesis of hemoglobin • Part of some cytochromes in cell respiration • Synthesis of melanin	• Liver, seafood, grains, nuts, legumes	Stored in liver
Cobalt	• Part of vitamin B_{12}	• Liver, meat, fish	Vitamin B_{12} stored in liver
Zinc	• Part of carbonic anhydrase needed for CO_2 transport • Part of peptidases needed for protein digestion • Necessary for normal taste sensation • Involved in wound healing	• Meat, seafood, grains, legumes	

different body configurations is illustrated in Fig. 17–4.

4. Sex hormones—Testosterone increases metabolic activity to a greater degree than does estrogen, giving men a slightly higher metabolic rate than women. Also, men tend to have more muscle, an active tissue, whereas women tend to have more fat, a relatively inactive tissue.

5. Sympathetic stimulation—In stress situations, the metabolism of many body cells is increased. Also

Box 17–4   METABOLIC RATE

To estimate your own **basal metabolic rate** (BMR), calculate kilocalories (kcal) used per hour as follows:

> For women: use the factor of 0.9 kcal per kilogram (kg) of body weight
> For men: use the factor of 1.0 kcal per kg of body weight
> Then multiply kcal/hour by 24 hours to determine kcal per day.

Example: A **120-pound woman**

1. Change pounds to kilograms:
   120 lb at 2.2 lb/kg = 55 kg
2. Multiply kg weight by the BMR factor:
   55 kg × 0.9 kcal/kg/hr = 49.5 kcal/hr
3. Multiply kcal/hr by 24:
   49.5 kcal/hr × 24 = 1188 kcal/day*
   *This is an approximate BMR, about 1200 kcal/day

Example: **A 160-pound man**

1. 160 lb at 2.2 lb/kg = 73 kg
2. 73 kg × 1.0 kcal/kg/hr = 73 kcal/hr
3. 73 kcal/hr × 24 = 1752 kcal/day

To approximate the amount of energy actually expended during an average day (24 hours), the following percentages may be used:

> Sedentary activity: add 40% to 50% of the BMR to the BMR
> Light activity: add 50% to 65% of the BMR to the BMR
> Moderate activity: add 65% to 75% of the BMR to the BMR
> Strenuous activity: add 75% to 100% of the BMR to the BMR

Using our example of the 120-pound woman with a BMR of 1200 kcal/day:

> Sedentary: 1680 to 1800 kcal/day
> Light: 1800 to 1980 kcal/day
> Moderate: 1980 to 2100 kcal/day
> Strenuous: 2100 to 2400 kcal/day

Box 17–5   WEIGHT LOSS

Although diet books are often found on the bestseller lists, there is no magic method that will result in weight loss. Losing weight depends on one simple fact: calorie expenditure in activity must exceed calorie intake in food (the term **calorie** here will be used to mean kilocalorie).

In order to lose 1 pound of body fat, which consists of fat, water, and protein, 3500 calories of energy must be expended. Although any form of exercise requires calories, the more strenuous the exercise, the more calories expended. Some examples are shown below.

Most food packaging contains nutritional information, including the calories per serving of the food. Keeping track of daily caloric intake is an important part of a decision to try to lose weight. It is also important to remember that sustained loss of fat usually does not exceed 1 to 2 pounds per week. In part this is so because as calorie intake decreases, the metabolic rate decreases. There will also be loss of some body protein so that amino acids can be converted to glucose to supply the brain.

A sensible weight-loss diet will include carbohydrate to supply energy needs, will have sufficient protein (40 to 45 grams per day), and will be low in animal fat. Including vegetables and fruits will supply vitamins, minerals, and fiber.

Activity	Calories per 10 minutes (average for a 150-lb person)	Activity	Calories per 10 minutes (average for a 150-lb person
Walking slowly	30	Running (8 mph)	120
Walking briskly	45	Cycling (10 mph)	70
Walking up stairs	170	Cycling (15 mph)	115
Dancing (slow)	40	Swimming	100
Dancing (fast)	65		

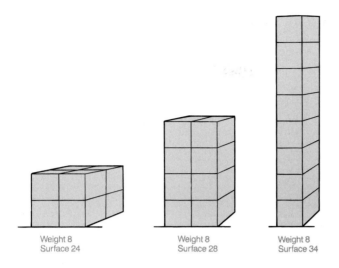

Figure 17–4 Surface-to-weight ratios. Imagine that the three shapes are people who all weigh the same amount. The "tall, thin person" on the right has about 50% more surface area than does the "short, stocky person" on the left. The more surface area (where heat is lost), the higher the metabolic rate.

Weight 8
Surface 24

Weight 8
Surface 28

Weight 8
Surface 34

contributing to this are the hormones epinephrine and norepinephrine. As a result, metabolic rate increases.

6. Decreased food intake—If the intake of food decreases for a prolonged period of time, metabolic rate also begins to decrease. It is as if the body's metabolism is "slowing down" to conserve whatever energy sources may still be available. (See also Box 17–6: Leptin and Body-Mass Index.)
7. Climate—People who live in cold climates may have metabolic rates 10% to 20% higher than people who live in tropical regions. This is believed to be due to the variations in the secretion of thyroxine, the hormone most responsible for regulation of metabolic rate. In a cold climate, the necessity for greater heat production brings about an increased secretion of thyroxine and a higher metabolic rate.

AGING AND METABOLISM

As mentioned in the previous section, metabolic rate decreases with age. Elderly people who remain active, however, can easily maintain a metabolic rate (energy production) adequate for their needs as long as their general health is good.

Sensitivity to external temperature changes may decrease with age, and the regulation of body temperature is no longer as precise. Sweat glands are not as

---

Box 17–6   LEPTIN AND BODY-MASS INDEX

The 1994 discovery of the hormone leptin was reported to the general public in 1995, along with speculation that leptin could become an anti-obesity medication. Leptin is a protein produced by fat cells, and signals the hypothalamus to release a chemical that acts as an appetite suppressant. It seems to inform the brain of how much stored fat the body has, and is therefore involved in the regulation of body weight.

Another likely role for leptin is as a contributor to the onset of puberty, especially in females. Girls who are very thin, with little body fat, tend to have a later first menstrual period than girls with average body fat, and a certain level of body fat is necessary for continued ovulation. Leptin may be the chemical mediator of this information.

The most recent research indicates that leptin directly decreases fat storage in cells, and improves

the efficiency of the pancreatic cells that produce insulin. What was first believed to be a simple chemical signal has proved to be much more complex.

A good measure of leanness or fatness is the **body-mass index.**

To calculate: Multiple weight in pounds by 703.
Divide by height in inches.
Divide again by height in inches = body-mass index
Example: A person five foot six weighing 130 pounds.
$130 \times 703 = 91,390$
$91,390 \div 66 = 1385$
$1385 \div 66 = 20.98$

The optimal body-mass index is considered to be 21. Any index over 25 is considered overweight.

active, and prolonged high environmental temperatures are a real danger for elderly people.

SUMMARY

Food is needed for the synthesis of new cells and tissues, or is utilized to produce the energy required for such synthesis reactions. As a consequence of metabolism, heat energy is released to provide a constant body temperature and permit the continuation of metabolic activity. The metabolic pathways described in this chapter are only a small portion of the body's total metabolism. Even this simple presentation, however, suggests the great chemical complexity of the functioning human being.

STUDY OUTLINE

Body Temperature
1. Normal range is 96.5 to 99.5°F (36 to 38°C), with an average of 98.6°F (37°C).
2. Normal fluctuation in 24 hours is 1 to 2°F.
3. Temperature regulation in infants and the elderly is not as precise as it is at other ages.

Heat Production
Heat is one of the energy products of cell respiration. Many factors affect the total heat actually produced (see Table 17–1).
1. Thyroxine from the thyroid gland—the most important regulator of daily heat production. As metabolic rate decreases, more thyroxine is secreted to increase the rate of cell respiration.
2. Stress—sympathetic impulses and epinephrine and norepinephrine increase the metabolic activity of many organs, increasing the production of ATP and heat.
3. Active organs continuously produce heat. Skeletal muscle tone produces 25% of the total body heat at rest. The liver provides up to 20% of the resting body heat.
4. Food intake increases the activity of the digestive organs and increases heat production.
5. Changes in body temperature affect metabolic rate. A fever increases the metabolic rate, and more heat is produced; this may become detrimental during very high fevers.

Heat Loss (see Table 17–2)
1. Most heat is lost through the skin.
2. Blood flow through the dermis determines the amount of heat that is lost by radiation, conduction, and convection.
3. Vasodilation in the dermis increases blood flow and heat loss; radiation and conduction are effective only if the environment is cooler than the body.
4. Vasoconstriction in the dermis decreases blood flow and conserves heat in the core of the body.
5. Sweating is a very effective heat loss mechanism; excess body heat evaporates sweat on the skin surface; sweating is most effective when the atmospheric humidity is low.
6. Sweating also has a disadvantage in that water is lost and must be replaced to prevent serious dehydration.
7. Heat is lost from the respiratory tract by the evaporation of water from the warm respiratory mucosa; water vapor is part of exhaled air.
8. A very small amount of heat is lost as urine and feces are excreted at body temperature.

Regulation of Heat Loss
1. The hypothalamus is the thermostat of the body and regulates body temperature by balancing heat production and heat loss.
2. The hypothalamus receives information from its own neurons (blood temperature) and from the temperature receptors in the dermis.
3. Mechanisms to increase heat loss are vasodilation in the dermis and increased sweating. Decreased muscle tone will decrease heat production.
4. Mechanisms to conserve heat are vasoconstriction in the dermis and decreased sweating. Increased muscle tone (shivering) will increase heat production.

Fever—an abnormally elevated body temperature
1. Pyrogens are substances that cause a fever: bacteria, foreign proteins, or chemicals released during inflammation (endogenous pyrogens).

2. Pyrogens raise the setting of the hypothalamic thermostat; the person feels cold and begins to shiver to produce heat.

3. When the pyrogen has been eliminated, the hypothalamic setting returns to normal; the person feels warm, and sweating begins to lose heat to lower the body temperature.

4. A low fever may be beneficial because it increases the activity of WBCs and inhibits the activity of some pathogens.

5. A high fever may be detrimental because enzymes are denatured at high temperatures. This is most critical in the brain, where cells that die cannot be replaced.

Metabolism—all the reactions within the body

1. Anabolism—synthesis reactions that usually require energy in the form of ATP.

2. Catabolism—decomposition reactions that often release energy in the form of ATP.

3. Enzymes catalyze most anabolic and catabolic reactions.

Cell Respiration—the breakdown of food molecules to release their potential energy and synthesize ATP

1. Glucose + oxygen yields CO_2 + H_2O + ATP + heat.

2. The breakdown of glucose involves three stages: glycolysis, Krebs cycle, and the cytochrome transport system (see Table 17–3 and Fig. 17–3).

3. The oxygen necessary comes from breathing.

4. The water formed becomes part of intracellular fluid; CO_2 is exhaled; ATP is used for energy-requiring reactions; heat provides a body temperature.

Proteins and Fats—as energy sources (see Table 17–4 for hormonal regulation)

1. Excess amino acids are deaminated in the liver and converted to pyruvic acid or acetyl groups to enter the Krebs cycle. Amino acids may also be converted to glucose to supply the brain (Fig. 17–3).

2. Glycerol is converted to pyruvic acid to enter the Krebs cycle.

3. Fatty acids, in the process of beta-oxidation in the liver, are split into acetyl groups to enter the Krebs cycle; ketones are formed for transport to other cells (see Fig. 17–3).

Energy Available from Food

1. Energy is measured in kilocalories (Calories): kcal.

2. There are 4 kcal per gram of carbohydrate, 4 kcal per gram of protein, 9 kcal per gram of fat. With reference to food, kilocalories may be called calories.

Synthesis Uses of Foods

1. Glucose—used to synthesize the pentose sugars for DNA and RNA; used to synthesize glycogen to store energy in liver and muscles.

2. Amino acids—used to synthesize new proteins and the non-essential amino acids; essential amino acids must be obtained in the diet.

3. Fatty acids and glycerol—used to synthesize phospholipids for cell membranes, triglycerides for fat storage in adipose tissue, and cholesterol and other steroids; essential fatty acids must be obtained in the diet.

4. Vitamins and minerals—see Tables 17–5 and 17–6.

Metabolic Rate—the heat production by the body; measured in kcal

1. Basal metabolic rate (BMR) is the energy required to maintain life (see Box 17–4); several factors influence the metabolic rate of an active person.

2. Age—metabolic rate is highest in young children and decreases with age.

3. Body configuration—more surface area proportional to weight (tall and thin) means a higher metabolic rate.

4. Sex hormones—men usually have a higher metabolic rate than do women; men have more muscle proportional to fat than do women.

5. Sympathetic stimulation—metabolic activity increases in stress situations.

6. Decreased food intake—metabolic rate decreases to conserve available energy sources.

7. Climate—people who live in cold climates usually have higher metabolic rates because of a greater need for heat production.

REVIEW QUESTIONS

1. State the normal range of human body temperature in °F and °C. (p. 376)

2. State the summary equation of cell respiration, and state what happens to (or the purpose of) each of the products. (p. 381)

3. Describe the role of each in heat production: thyroxine, skeletal muscles, stress situations, and the liver. (p. 376)

4. Describe the two mechanisms of heat loss through the skin, and explain the role of blood flow. Describe how heat is lost through the respiratory tract. (pp. 377–378)

5. Explain the circumstances when sweating and vasodilation in the dermis are not effective mechanisms of heat loss. (p. 377)

6. Name the part of the brain that regulates body temperature, and explain what is meant by a thermostat. (p. 378)

7. Describe the responses by the body to a warm environment and to a cold environment. (pp. 378–379)

8. Explain how pyrogens are believed to cause a fever, and give two examples of pyrogens. (p. 379)

9. Define metabolism, anabolism, catabolism, kilocalorie, and metabolic rate. (pp. 380, 385, 387)

10. Name the three stages of the cell respiration of glucose and state where in the cell each takes place and whether or not oxygen is required. (pp. 382–383)

11. For each, state the molecules that enter the process and the results of the process: glycolysis, Krebs cycle, and cytochrome transport system. (pp. 384–385)

12. Explain how fatty acids, glycerol, and excess amino acids are used for energy production in cell respiration. (pp. 383, 385)

13. Describe the synthesis uses for glucose, amino acids, and fatty acids. (pp. 386–387)

14. Describe four factors that affect the metabolic rate of an active person. (pp. 387, 391)

15. If lunch consists of 60 grams of carbohydrate, 15 grams of protein, and 10 grams of fat, how many kilocalories are provided by this meal? (p. 386)

FOR FURTHER THOUGHT

1. For many people, iceberg lettuce is the vegetable eaten most often. What does lettuce provide? What does lettuce lack, compared to vegetables such as broccoli?

2. Fourteen-year-old Donna has just decided that eating meat is "gross," and that she will be a vegetarian. What difficulties are there with such a diet; that is, what nutrients may be lacking? How may they be obtained?

3. Studies with animals have shown that caloric restriction may prolong life by protecting the brain from some effects of aging. The animals' diet was about half the usual calories they would consume. For people, 1250–1500 calories per day would be restrictive (compared to the 2000 calories or more that many of us in North America consume). Would it be worth it for a life span

of 110 years? Describe the problems with such a diet.

4. Every summer small children are left alone in cars "just for a few minutes," while a parent does an errand. The result may be tragic—severe brain damage or death of the child from heat stroke. Explain why small children are so susceptible to heat.

5. Remember the *Titanic*, which sank in April of 1912? There were not enough lifeboats for everyone, and many people were in the water of the North Atlantic. They did have life jackets, and did not drown, but many were dead within half an hour. Explain why.

6. An elderly person and a quadriplegic person may each have difficulties during cold weather. Explain how the problem is a little different for each.

CHAPTER 18

The Urinary System

CHAPTER 18

Student Objectives

- Describe the location and general function of each organ of the urinary system.
- Name the parts of a nephron and the important blood vessels associated with them.
- Explain how the following are involved in urine formation: glomerular filtration, tubular reabsorption, tubular secretion, and blood flow through the kidney.
- Describe the mechanisms of tubular reabsorption, and explain the importance of tubular secretion.
- Describe how the kidneys help maintain normal blood volume and blood pressure.
- Name and state the functions of the hormones that affect the kidneys.
- Describe how the kidneys help maintain normal pH of blood and tissue fluid.
- Describe the urination reflex, and explain how voluntary control is possible.
- Describe the characteristics of normal urine.

The Urinary System

New Terminology

Bowman's capsule (**BOW**-manz **KAP**-suhl)

Detrusor muscle (de-**TROO**-ser)

External urethral sphincter (yoo-**REE**-thruhl **SFINK**-ter)

Glomerular filtration rate (gloh-**MER**-yoo-ler fill–**TRAY**-shun RAYT)

Glomerulus (gloh-**MER**-yoo-lus)

Internal urethral sphincter (yoo-**REE**-thruhl **SFINK**-ter)

Juxtaglomerular cells (JUKS-tah-gloh-**MER**-yoo-ler SELLS)

Micturition (MIK-tyoo-**RISH**-un)

Nephron (**NEFF**-ron)

Nitrogenous wastes (nigh-**TRAH**-jen-us)

Peritubular capillaries (PER-ee-**TOO**-byoo-ler)

Renal corpuscle (**REE**-nuhl **KOR**-pus'l)

Renal filtrate (**REE**-nuhl **FILL**-trayt)

Renal tubule (**REE**-nuhl **TOO**-byoo'l)

Retroperitoneal (RE-troh-PER-i-toh-**NEE**-uhl)

Specific gravity (spe-**SIF**-ik **GRA**-vi-tee)

Threshold level (**THRESH**-hold **LE**-vuhl)

Trigone (**TRY**-gohn)

Ureter (**YOOR**-uh-ter)

Urethra (yoo-**REE**-thrah)

Urinary bladder (**YOOR**-i-NAR-ee **BLA**-der)

Related Clinical Terminology

Cystitis (sis-**TIGH**-tis)

Dysuria (dis-**YOO**-ree-ah)

Hemodialysis (HEE-moh-dye-**AL**-i-sis)

Nephritis (ne-**FRY**-tis)

Oliguria (AH-li-**GYOO**-ree-ah)

Polyuria (PAH-li-**YOO**-ree-ah)

Renal calculi (**REE**-nuhl **KAL**-kew-lye)

Renal failure (**REE**-nuhl **FAYL**-yer)

Uremia (yoo-**REE**-me-ah)

*Terms that appear in **bold type** in the chapter text are defined in the glossary, which begins on page 521.*

The first successful human organ transplant was a kidney transplant performed in 1953. Because the donor and recipient were identical twins, rejection was not a problem. Thousands of kidney transplants have been performed since then, and the development of immunosuppressive medications has permitted many people to live normal lives with donated kidneys. Although a person usually has two kidneys, it is clear that one kidney can carry out the complex work required to maintain homeostasis of the body fluids.

The urinary system consists of two kidneys, two ureters, the urinary bladder, and the urethra (Fig. 18–1). The formation of urine is the function of the kidneys, and the rest of the system is responsible for eliminating the urine.

Body cells produce waste products such as urea, creatinine, and ammonia, which must be removed from the blood before they accumulate to toxic levels. As the kidneys form urine to excrete these waste products, they also accomplish several other important functions:

1. Regulation of the volume of blood by excretion or conservation of water
2. Regulation of the electrolyte content of the blood by the excretion or conservation of minerals
3. Regulation of the acid–base balance of the blood by excretion or conservation of ions such as H^+ ions or HCO_3^- ions
4. Regulation of all of the above in tissue fluid

The process of urine formation, therefore, helps maintain the normal composition, volume, and pH of both blood and tissue fluid by removing those substances that would upset the normal constancy and balance of these extracellular fluids.

KIDNEYS

The two **kidneys** are located in the upper abdominal cavity on either side of the vertebral column, behind the peritoneum (retroperitoneal). The upper portions of the kidneys rest on the lower surface of the diaphragm and are enclosed and protected by the lower rib cage (see Fig. 18–1). The kidneys are embedded in adipose tissue that acts as a cushion and is in turn covered by a fibrous connective tissue membrane called the **renal fascia**, which helps hold the kidneys in place (see Box 18–1: Floating Kidney).

Each kidney has an indentation called the **hilus** on its medial side. At the hilus, the renal artery enters the kidney, and the renal vein and ureter emerge. The renal artery is a branch of the abdominal aorta, and the renal vein returns blood to the inferior vena cava (see Fig. 18–1). The ureter carries urine from the kidney to the urinary bladder.

INTERNAL STRUCTURE OF THE KIDNEY

In a coronal or frontal section of the kidney, three areas can be distinguished (Fig. 18–2). The lateral and middle areas are tissue layers, and the medial area at the hilus is a cavity. The outer tissue layer is called the **renal cortex**; it is made of renal corpuscles and convoluted tubules. These are parts of the nephron and are described in the next section. The inner tissue layer is the **renal medulla**, which is made of loops of Henle and collecting tubules (also parts of the nephron). The renal medulla consists of wedge-shaped pieces called **renal pyramids**. The tip of each pyramid is its apex or papilla.

The third area is the **renal pelvis**; this is not a layer of tissues, but rather a cavity formed by the expansion of the ureter within the kidney at the hilus. Funnel-shaped extensions of the renal pelvis, called **calyces** (singular: **calyx**), enclose the papillae of the renal pyramids. Urine flows from the renal pyramids into the calyces, then to the renal pelvis and out into the ureter.

THE NEPHRON

The **nephron** is the structural and functional unit of the kidney. Each kidney contains approximately 1 million nephrons. It is in the nephrons, with their associated blood vessels, that urine is formed. Each nephron has two major portions: a renal corpuscle and a renal tubule. Each of these major parts has further subdivisions, which are shown with their blood vessels in Fig. 18–3.

Renal Corpuscle

A **renal corpuscle** consists of a glomerulus surrounded by a Bowman's capsule. The **glomerulus** is a capillary network that arises from an **afferent arteriole** and empties into an **efferent arteriole**. The diameter of the efferent arteriole is smaller than that of the afferent arteriole, which helps maintain a fairly high blood pressure in the glomerulus.

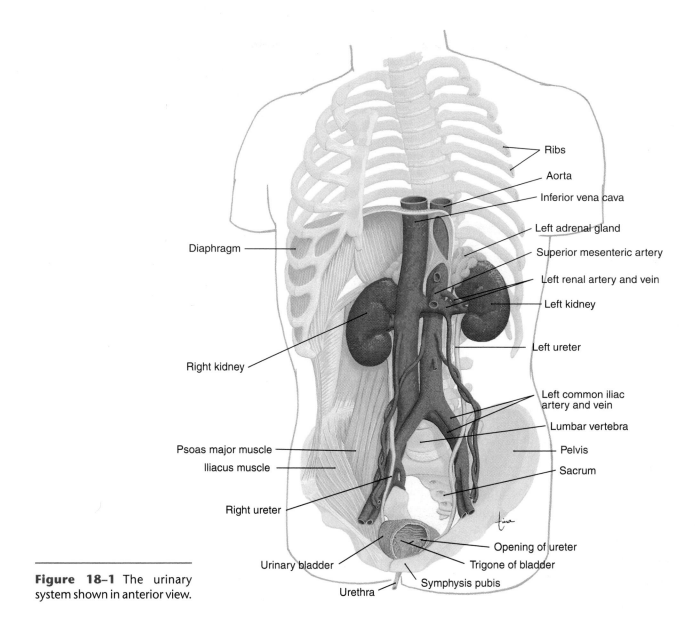

Figure 18–1 The urinary system shown in anterior view.

Bowman's capsule (or glomerular capsule) is the expanded end of a renal tubule; it encloses the glomerulus. The inner layer of Bowman's capsule is made of podocytes; the name means "foot cells," and the "feet" of the podocytes are on the surface of the glomerular capillaries. The arrangement of podocytes creates pores, spaces between adjacent "feet," which make this layer very permeable. The outer layer of Bowman's capsule has no pores and is not permeable. The space between the inner and outer layers of Bowman's capsule contains renal filtrate, the fluid that

is formed from the blood in the glomerulus and will eventually become urine.

Renal Tubule

The **renal tubule** continues from Bowman's capsule and consists of the following parts: **proximal convoluted tubule** (in the renal cortex), **loop of Henle** (or loop of the nephron, in the renal medulla), and **distal convoluted tubule** (in the renal cortex). The distal convoluted tubules from several nephrons empty into a **collecting tubule**. Several collecting tubules then unite to form a papillary duct that empties urine into a calyx of the renal pelvis.

Cross-sections of the parts of the renal tubule are shown in Fig. 18–3. Notice how thin the walls of the tubule are, and also the microvilli in the proximal convoluted tubule. These anatomic characteristics provide for efficient exchanges of materials, as you will see.

All parts of the renal tubule are surrounded by **peritubular capillaries**, which arise from the efferent arteriole. The peritubular capillaries will receive the materials reabsorbed by the renal tubules; this is described in the section on urine formation.

BLOOD VESSELS OF THE KIDNEY

The pathway of blood flow through the kidney is an essential part of the process of urine formation. Blood from the abdominal aorta enters the **renal artery**, which branches extensively within the kidney into smaller arteries (see Fig. 18–2). The smallest arteries give rise to afferent arterioles in the renal cortex (see Fig. 18–3). From the afferent arterioles, blood flows into the glomeruli (capillaries), to efferent arterioles, to peritubular capillaries, to veins within the kidney, to the **renal vein**, and finally to the inferior vena cava. Notice that in this pathway there are two sets of capillaries, and recall that it is in capillaries that exchanges take place between the blood and surrounding tissues. Therefore, in the kidneys there are two sites of exchange. The exchanges that take place between the nephrons and the capillaries of the kidneys will form urine from blood plasma.

In Fig. 18–3 are two views of a vascular cast of a kidney; the shape of the blood vessels has been preserved in red plastic. You can see how dense the vasculature of a kidney is, and most of these vessels are capillaries.

FORMATION OF URINE

The formation of urine involves three major processes. The first is glomerular filtration, which takes place in the renal corpuscles. The second and third are tubular reabsorption and tubular secretion, which take place in the renal tubules.

GLOMERULAR FILTRATION

You may recall that filtration is the process in which blood pressure forces plasma and dissolved material out of capillaries. In **glomerular filtration**, blood pressure forces plasma, dissolved substances, and small proteins out of the glomeruli and into Bowman's capsules. This fluid is no longer plasma but is called **renal filtrate**.

The blood pressure in the glomeruli, compared to that in other capillaries, is relatively high, about 60 mmHg. The pressure in Bowman's capsule is very low, and its inner layer is very permeable, so that approximately 20% to 25% of the blood that enters glomeruli becomes renal filtrate in Bowman's capsules. The blood cells and larger proteins are too large to be forced out of the glomeruli, so they remain in the blood. Waste products are dissolved in blood plasma, so they pass into the renal filtrate. Useful materials such as nutrients and minerals are also dissolved in plasma and are also present in renal filtrate. Filtration is not selective with respect to usefulness; it is selective only with respect to size. Therefore, renal filtrate is very much like blood plasma, except that there is far less protein, and no blood cells are present.

The **glomerular filtration rate** (GFR) is the amount of renal filtrate formed by the kidneys in 1 minute, and averages 100 to 125 ml per minute. GFR may be altered if the rate of blood flow through the

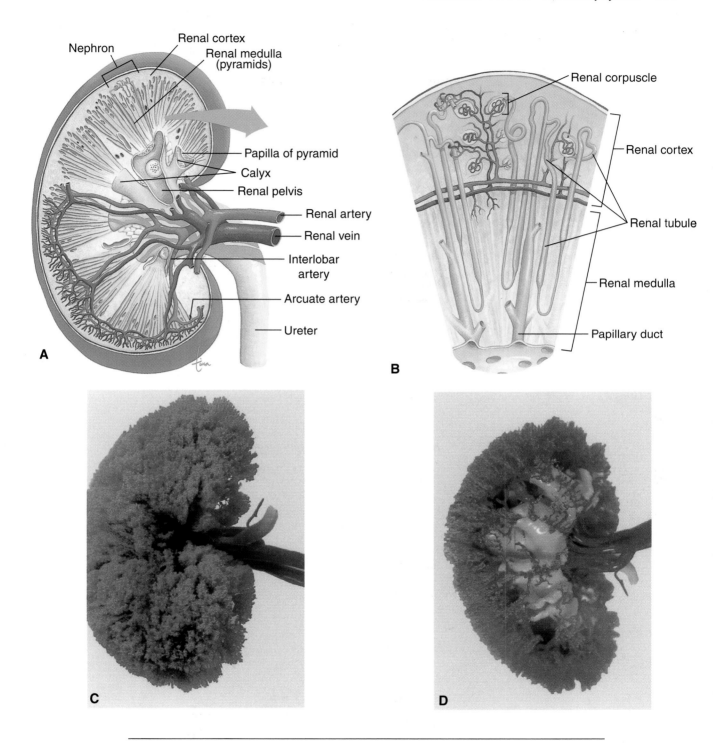

Figure 18–2 **(A)** Frontal section of the right kidney showing internal structure and blood vessels. **(B)** The magnified section of the kidney shows several nephrons. **(C)** Vascular cast of a kidney in lateral view. Red plastic fills the blood vessels. **(D)** Vascular cast in medial view. Blood vessels have been removed; yellow plastic fills the renal pelvis. (Photographs C and D by Dan Kaufman.)

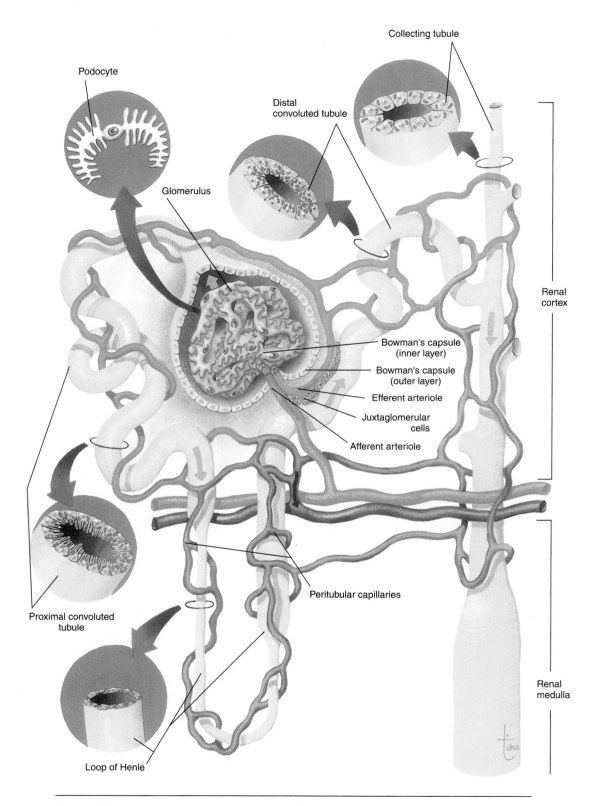

Figure 18–3 A nephron with its associated blood vessels. Portions of the nephron have been magnified. The arrows indicate the direction of blood flow and flow of renal filtrate. See text for description.

Box 18–2   RENAL FAILURE AND HEMODIALYSIS

Renal failure, the inability of the kidneys to function properly, may be the result of three general causes, which may be called prerenal, intrinsic renal, and postrenal.

Prerenal means that the problem is "before" the kidneys, that is, in the blood flow to the kidneys. Any condition that decreases blood flow to the kidneys may result in renal damage and failure. Examples are severe hemorrhage or very low blood pressure following a heart attack (MI).

Intrinsic renal means that the problem is in the kidneys themselves. Bacterial infections of the kidneys or exposure to chemicals (certain antibiotics) may cause this type of damage. Polycystic kidney disease is a genetic disorder in which the kidney tubules dilate and become nonfunctional. Severe damage may not be apparent until age 40 to 60 years but may then progress to renal failure.

Postrenal means that the problem is "after" the kidneys, somewhere in the rest of the urinary tract. Obstruction of urine flow may be caused by kidney stones, a twisted ureter, or prostatic hypertrophy.

Treatment of renal failure involves correcting the specific cause, if possible. If not possible, and kidney damage is permanent, the person is said to have chronic renal failure. **Hemodialysis** is the use of an artificial kidney machine to do what the patient's nephrons can no longer do. The patient's blood is passed through minute tubes surrounded by fluid (dialysate) with the same chemical composition as plasma. Waste products and excess minerals diffuse out of the patient's blood into the fluid of the machine.

Although hemodialysis does prolong life for those with chronic renal failure, it does not fully take the place of functioning kidneys. The increasing success rate of kidney transplants, however, does indeed provide the possibility of a normal life for people with chronic renal failure.

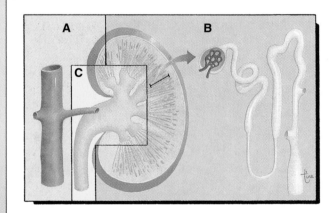

Box Figure 18–A   Causes of renal failure. **(A)** Prerenal. **(B)** Intrinsic renal. **(C)** Postrenal.

kidney changes. If blood flow increases, the GFR increases, and more filtrate is formed. If blood flow decreases (as may happen following a severe hemorrhage), the GFR decreases, less filtrate is formed, and urinary output decreases (see Box 18–2: Renal Failure and Hemodialysis).

TUBULAR REABSORPTION

Tubular reabsorption takes place from the renal tubules into the peritubular capillaries. In a 24-hour period, the kidneys form 150 to 180 liters of filtrate, and normal urinary output in that time is 1 to 2 liters. Therefore, it becomes apparent that most of the renal filtrate does not become urine. Approximately 99% of the filtrate is reabsorbed back into the blood in the peritubular capillaries. Only about 1% of the filtrate will enter the renal pelvis as urine.

Most reabsorption and secretion (about 65%) take place in the proximal convoluted tubules, whose cells have **microvilli** that greatly increase their surface area. The distal convoluted tubules and collecting tubules are also important sites for the reabsorption of water (Fig. 18–4).

Mechanisms of Reabsorption

1. **Active transport**—the cells of the renal tubule use ATP to transport most of the useful materials from the filtrate to the blood. These useful materials include glucose, amino acids, vitamins, and positive ions.

   For many of these substances, the renal tubules have a **threshold level** of reabsorption. This means that there is a limit to how much the tubules can remove from the filtrate. For example, if the filtrate level of glucose is normal (reflecting a normal blood glucose level), the tubules will reabsorb all of the glucose, and none will be found in the urine. If, however, the blood glucose level is above normal, the amount of glucose in the filtrate will also be above normal and will exceed the threshold level of reabsorption. In this situation, therefore, some glucose will be present in urine.

   The reabsorption of Ca^{+2} ions is increased by parathyroid hormone (PTH). The parathyroid glands secrete PTH when the blood calcium level decreases. The reabsorption of Ca^{+2} ions by the kidneys is one of the mechanisms by which the blood calcium level is raised back to normal.

   The hormone aldosterone, secreted by the adrenal cortex, increases the reabsorption of Na^+ ions and the excretion of K^+ ions. Besides regulating the blood levels of sodium and potassium, aldosterone also affects the volume of blood.

2. **Passive transport**—many of the negative ions that are returned to the blood are reabsorbed following the reabsorption of positive ions, because unlike charges attract.

3. **Osmosis**—the reabsorption of water follows the reabsorption of minerals, especially sodium ions. The hormones that affect reabsorption of water are discussed in the next section.

4. **Pinocytosis**—small proteins are too large to be reabsorbed by active transport. They become adsorbed to the membranes of the cells of the proximal convoluted tubules. The cell membrane then sinks inward and folds around the protein to take it in. Normally all proteins in the filtrate are reabsorbed; none is found in urine.

TUBULAR SECRETION

This mechanism also changes the composition of urine. In **tubular secretion**, substances are actively secreted from the blood in the peritubular capillaries into the filtrate in the renal tubules. Waste products such as ammonia and some creatinine, and the metabolic products of medications may be secreted into the filtrate to be eliminated in urine. Hydrogen ions (H^+) may be secreted by the tubule cells to help maintain the normal pH of blood.

HORMONES THAT INFLUENCE REABSORPTION OF WATER

Aldosterone is secreted by the adrenal cortex in response to a high blood potassium level, to a low blood sodium level, or to a decrease in blood pressure. When aldosterone stimulates the reabsorption of Na^+ ions, water follows from the filtrate back to the blood. This helps maintain normal blood volume and blood pressure.

You may recall that the antagonist to aldosterone is **atrial natriuretic hormone** (ANH), which is secreted by the atria of the heart when the atrial walls are stretched by high blood pressure or greater blood volume. ANH decreases the reabsorption of Na^+ ions by the kidneys; these remain in the filtrate, as does water, and are excreted. By increasing the elimination of sodium and water, ANH lowers blood volume and blood pressure.

Antidiuretic hormone (ADH) is released by the posterior pituitary gland when the amount of water in the body decreases. Under the influence of ADH, the distal convoluted tubules and collecting tubules are able to reabsorb more water from the renal filtrate. This helps maintain normal blood volume and blood pressure, and also permits the kidneys to produce urine that is more concentrated than body fluids. Producing a concentrated urine is essential to prevent excessive water loss while still excreting all the substances that must be eliminated.

If the amount of water in the body increases, however, the secretion of ADH diminishes, and the kidneys will reabsorb less water. Urine then becomes dilute, and water is eliminated until its concentration in the body returns to normal. This may occur following ingestion of excessive quantities of fluids.

Figure 18–4 Schematic representation of glomerular filtration, tubular reabsorption, and tubular secretion. The renal tubule has been uncoiled, and the peritubular capillaries are shown adjacent to the tubule.

Table 18–1	EFFECTS OF HORMONES ON THE KIDNEYS
Hormone (gland)	**Function**
Antidiuretic hormone (ADH) (posterior pituitary)	• Increases reabsorption of water from the filtrate to the blood.
Parathyroid hormone (PTH) (parathyroid glands)	• Increases reabsorption of Ca^{+2} ions from filtrate to the blood and excretion of phosphate ions into the filtrate.
Aldosterone (adrenal cortex)	• Increases reabsorption of Na^+ ions from the filtrate to the blood and excretion of K^+ ions into the filtrate. Water is reabsorbed following the reabsorption of sodium.
Atrial natriuretic hormone (ANH) (atria of heart)	• Decreases reabsorption of Na^+ ions, which remain in the filtrate. More sodium and water are eliminated in urine.

SUMMARY OF URINE FORMATION

1. The kidneys form urine from blood plasma. Blood flow through the kidneys is a major factor in determining urinary output.
2. Glomerular filtration is the first step in urine formation. Filtration is not selective in terms of usefulness of materials; it is selective only in terms of size. High blood pressure in the glomeruli forces plasma, dissolved materials, and small proteins into Bowman's capsules; the fluid is now called renal filtrate.
3. Tubular reabsorption is selective in terms of usefulness. Nutrients such as glucose, amino acids, and vitamins are reabsorbed by active transport and may have renal threshold levels. Positive ions are reabsorbed by active transport and negative ions most often by passive transport. Water is reabsorbed by osmosis, and small proteins are reabsorbed by pinocytosis.

    Reabsorption takes place from the filtrate in the renal tubules to the blood in the peritubular capillaries.
4. Tubular secretion takes place from the blood in the peritubular capillaries to the filtrate in the renal tubules and can ensure that wastes such as creatinine or excess H^+ ions are actively put into the filtrate to be excreted.
5. Hormones such as aldosterone, ANH, and ADH influence the reabsorption of water and help maintain normal blood volume and blood pressure. The secretion of ADH determines whether a concentrated or dilute urine will be formed.
6. Waste products remain in the renal filtrate and are excreted in urine. The effects of hormones on the kidneys are summarized in Table 18–1 and illustrated in Fig. 18–5.

THE KIDNEYS AND ACID–BASE BALANCE

The kidneys are the organs most responsible for maintaining the pH of blood and tissue fluid within normal ranges. They have the greatest ability to compensate for the pH changes that are a normal part of body metabolism or the result of disease, and to make the necessary corrections.

This regulatory function of the kidneys is complex, but at its simplest it may be described as follows. If body fluids are becoming too acidic, the kidneys will secrete more H^+ ions into the renal filtrate and will return more HCO_3^- ions to the blood. This will help raise the pH of the blood back to normal. The reactions involved in such a mechanism are shown in Fig. 18–6, and we will return to it later. First, however, let us briefly consider how the kidneys will compensate for body fluids that are becoming too alkaline. You might expect the kidneys to do just the opposite of what is described above, and that is just what happens. The kidneys will return H^+ ions to the blood and excrete HCO_3^- ions in urine. This will help lower the pH of the blood back to normal.

Because the natural tendency is for body fluids to become more acidic, let us look at the pH-raising mechanism in more detail (see Fig. 18–6). The cells of the renal tubules can secrete H^+ ions or ammonia in exchange for Na^+ ions, and by doing so, influence the reabsorption of other ions. Hydrogen ions are

Figure 18–5 Effects of hormones on the kidneys.

obtained from the reaction of CO_2 and water (or other processes). An amine group from an amino acid is combined with a H^+ ion to form ammonia.

The tubule cell secretes the H^+ ion and the ammonia into the renal filtrate, and two Na^+ ions are reabsorbed in exchange. In the filtrate, the H^+ ion and ammonia form NH_4^+ (an ammonium radical), which reacts with a chloride ion (Cl^-) to form NH_4Cl (ammonium chloride) that is excreted in urine.

As the Na^+ ions are returned to the blood in the peritubular capillaries, HCO_3^- ions follow. Notice what has happened: Two H^+ ions have been excreted in urine, and two Na^+ ions and two HCO_3^- ions have been returned to the blood. As reactions like these take place, the body fluids are prevented from becoming too acidic.

Another mechanism used by the cells of the kidney tubules to regulate pH is the phosphate buffer system, which is described in Chapter 19.

OTHER FUNCTIONS OF THE KIDNEYS

In addition to the functions described thus far, the kidneys have other functions, some of which are not directly related to the formation of urine. These func-

Peritubular capillary

Renal tubule

Filtrate

Blood

Urine

Figure 18–6 Renal regulation of acid–base balance. The cells of the renal tubule secrete H^+ ions and ammonia into the filtrate and return Na^+ ions and HCO_3^- ions to the blood in the peritubular capillaries. See text for further description.

tions are secretion of renin (which does influence urine formation), production of erythropoietin, and activation of vitamin D.

1. **Secretion of renin**—When blood pressure decreases, the **juxtaglomerular** (*juxta* means "next to") cells in the walls of the afferent arterioles secrete the enzyme **renin**. Renin then initiates the renin-angiotensin mechanism to raise blood pressure. This was first described in Chapter 13, and the sequence of events is presented in Table 18–2. The end product of this mechanism is **angiotensin II**, which causes vasoconstriction and increases the secretion of aldosterone, both of which help raise blood pressure.

   A normal blood pressure is essential to normal body functioning. Perhaps the most serious change is a sudden, drastic decrease in blood pressure, as would follow a severe hemorrhage. In response to

Table 18–2	THE RENIN-ANGIOTENSIN MECHANISM

Sequence

1. Decreased blood pressure stimulates the kidneys to secrete renin.
2. Renin splits the plasma protein angiotensinogen (synthesized by the liver) to angiotensin I.
3. Angiotensin I is converted to angiotensin II by an enzyme found primarily in lung tissue.
4. Angiotensin II causes vasoconstriction and stimulates the adrenal cortex to secrete aldosterone.

such a decrease, the kidneys will decrease filtration and urinary output and will initiate the formation of angiotensin II. In these ways the kidneys help ensure that the heart has enough blood to pump to maintain cardiac output and blood pressure.

Box 18–3   ERYTHROPOIETIN

Anemia is one of the most debilitating consequences of renal failure, one that hemodialysis cannot reverse. Diseased kidneys stop producing erythropoietin, a natural stimulus for RBC production. Recently, however, erythropoietin has been produced by genetic engineering and is available for hemodialysis patients. In the past, their anemia could only be treated with transfusions, which exposed these patients to possible immunologic complications of repeated exposure to donated blood or to viral diseases such as hepatitis C (before 1990). The synthetic erythropoietin eliminates such risks. Others who benefit from this medication are cancer patients and AIDS patients with severe anemia.

2. **Secretion of erythropoietin**—This hormone is secreted whenever the blood oxygen level decreases (a state of hypoxia). Erythropoietin stimulates the red bone marrow to increase the rate of RBC production. With more RBCs in circulation, the oxygen-carrying capacity of the blood is greater, and the hypoxic state may be corrected (see also Box 18–3: Erythropoietin).

3. **Activation of vitamin D**—This vitamin exists in several structural forms that are converted to **calciferol** (D_2) by the kidneys. Calciferol is the most active form of vitamin D, which increases the absorption of calcium and phosphate in the small intestine.

ELIMINATION OF URINE

The ureters, urinary bladder, and urethra do not change the composition or amount of urine, but are responsible for the periodic elimination of urine.

URETERS

Each **ureter** extends from the hilus of a kidney to the lower, posterior side of the urinary bladder (see Fig. 18–1). Like the kidneys, the ureters are retroperitoneal, that is, behind the peritoneum of the dorsal abdominal cavity.

The smooth muscle in the wall of the ureter contracts in peristaltic waves to propel urine toward the urinary bladder. As the bladder fills, it expands and compresses the lower ends of the ureters to prevent backflow of urine.

URINARY BLADDER

The **urinary bladder** is a muscular sac below the peritoneum and behind the pubic bones. In women, the bladder is inferior to the uterus; in men, the bladder is superior to the prostate gland. The bladder is a reservoir for accumulating urine, and it contracts to eliminate urine.

The mucosa of the bladder is **transitional epithelium**, which permits expansion without tearing the lining. When the bladder is empty, the mucosa appears wrinkled; these folds are **rugae**, which also permit expansion. On the floor of the bladder is a triangular area called the **trigone**, which has no rugae and does not expand. The points of the triangle are the openings of the two ureters and that of the urethra (Fig. 18–7).

The smooth muscle layer in the wall of the bladder is called the **detrusor muscle**. It is a muscle in the form of a sphere; when it contracts it becomes a smaller sphere, and its volume diminishes. Around the opening of the urethra the muscle fibers of the detrusor form the **internal urethral sphincter** (or sphincter of the bladder), which is involuntary.

URETHRA

The urethra (see Fig. 18–7) carries urine from the bladder to the exterior. The **external urethral sphincter** is made of the surrounding skeletal muscle of the pelvic floor, and is under voluntary control.

In women, the urethra is 1 to 1.5 inches (2.5 to 4 cm) long and is anterior to the vagina. In men, the urethra is 7 to 8 inches (17 to 20 cm) long. The first part just outside the bladder is called the prostatic urethra because it is surrounded by the prostate gland. The next inch is the membranous urethra, around which is the external urethral sphincter. The longest portion is the cavernous urethra (or spongy or penile urethra), which passes through the cavernous (or erectile) tissue of the penis. The male urethra carries semen as well as urine.

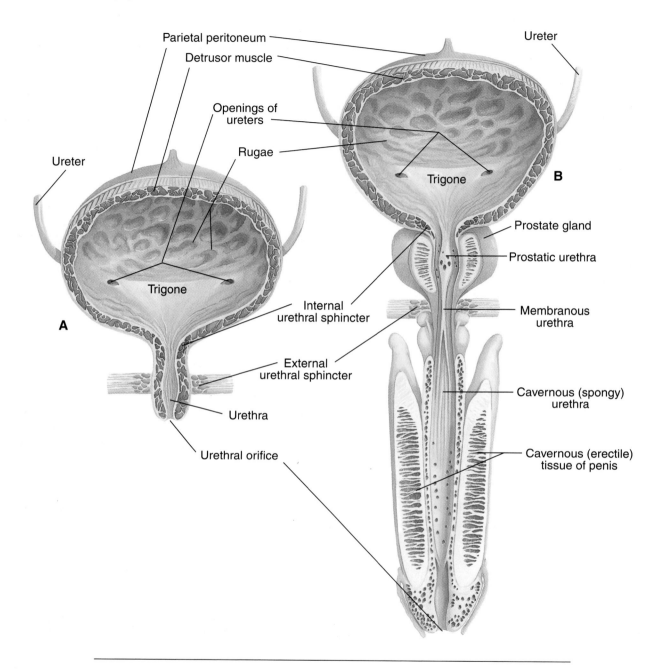

Figure 18–7 **(A)** Frontal section of female urinary bladder and urethra. **(B)** Frontal section of male urinary bladder and urethra.

THE URINATION REFLEX

Urination may also be called **micturition** or **voiding**. This reflex is a spinal cord reflex over which voluntary control may be exerted. The stimulus for the reflex is stretching of the detrusor muscle of the bladder. The bladder can hold as much as 800 ml of urine, or even more, but the reflex is activated long before the maximum is reached.

When urine volume reaches 200 to 400 ml, the stretching is sufficient to generate sensory impulses that travel to the sacral spinal cord. Motor impulses return along parasympathetic nerves to the detrusor muscle, causing contraction. At the same time, the internal urethral sphincter relaxes. If the external urethral sphincter is voluntarily relaxed, urine flows into the urethra, and the bladder is emptied.

Urination can be prevented by voluntary contraction of the external urethral sphincter. However, if the bladder continues to fill and be stretched, voluntary control is eventually no longer possible.

CHARACTERISTICS OF URINE

The characteristics of urine include the physical and chemical aspects that are often evaluated as part of a urinalysis. Some of these are described in this section, and others are included in Appendix D: Normal Values for Some Commonly Used Urine Tests.

Amount—normal urinary output per 24 hours is 1 to 2 liters. There are many factors that can significantly change output. Excessive sweating or loss of fluid through diarrhea will decrease urinary output (**oliguria**) to conserve body water. Excessive fluid intake will increase urinary output (**polyuria**). Consumption of alcohol will also increase output because alcohol inhibits the secretion of ADH, and the kidneys will reabsorb less water.

Color—the typical yellow color of urine (from urochrome, a breakdown product of bile) is often referred to as "straw" or "amber." Concentrated urine is a deeper yellow (amber) than is dilute urine. Freshly voided urine is also clear rather than cloudy.

Specific gravity—the normal range is 1.010 to 1.025; this is a measure of the dissolved materials in urine.

The specific gravity of distilled water is 1.000, meaning that there are no solutes present. Therefore, the higher the specific gravity number, the more dissolved material is present. Someone who has been exercising strenuously and has lost body water in sweat will usually produce less urine, which will be more concentrated and have a higher specific gravity.

The specific gravity of the urine is an indicator of the concentrating ability of the kidneys: The kidneys must excrete the waste products that are constantly formed in as little water as possible.

pH—the pH range of urine is between 4.6 and 8.0, with an average value of 6.0. Diet has the greatest influence on urine pH. A vegetarian diet will result in a more alkaline urine, whereas a high-protein diet will result in a more acidic urine.

Constituents—urine is approximately 95% water, which is the solvent for waste products and salts. Salts are not considered true waste products because they may well be utilized by the body when needed, but excess amounts will be excreted in urine (see Box 18–4: Kidney Stones).

Nitrogenous wastes—as their name indicates, all of these wastes contain nitrogen. Urea is formed by liver cells when excess amino acids are deaminated to be used for energy production. Creatinine comes from the metabolism of creatine phosphate, an energy source in muscles. Uric acid comes from the metabolism of nucleic acids, that is, the breakdown of DNA and RNA. Although these are waste products, there is always a certain amount of each in the blood. Box 18–5: Blood Tests and Kidney Function describes the relationship between blood levels of these waste products and kidney function.

Box 18–4 KIDNEY STONES

Kidney stones, or **renal calculi**, are crystals of the salts that are normally present in urine. A very high concentration of salts in urine may trigger precipitation of the salt and formation of crystals, which can range in size from microscopic to 10 to 20 mm in diameter. The most common type of kidney stone is made of calcium salts; a less common type is made of uric acid.

Kidney stones are most likely to form in the renal pelvis. Predisposing factors include decreased fluid intake or overingestion of minerals (as in mineral supplements), both of which lead to the formation of a very concentrated urine.

The entry of a kidney stone into a ureter may cause intense pain (renal colic) and bleeding. Obstruction of a ureter by a stone may cause backup of urine and possible kidney damage. Treatments include surgery to remove the stone, or lithotripsy, the use of shock waves to crush the stone into pieces small enough to be eliminated without damage to the urinary tract.

Box 18–5 BLOOD TESTS AND KIDNEY FUNCTION

Waste products are normally present in the blood, and the concentration of each varies within a normal range. As part of the standard lab work called blood chemistry, the levels of the three nitrogenous waste products are determined (urea, creatinine, and uric acid).

If blood levels of these three substances are within normal ranges, it may be concluded that the kidneys are excreting these wastes at normal rates. If, however, these blood levels are elevated, one possible cause is that kidney function has been impaired.

Of the three, the creatinine level is probably the most reliable indicator of kidney functioning. Blood urea nitrogen (BUN) may vary considerably in certain situations not directly related to the kidneys. For example, BUN may be elevated as a consequence of a high-protein diet or of starvation when body protein is being broken down at a faster rate than normal. Uric acid levels may also vary according to diet. However, elevated blood levels of all three nitrogenous wastes usually indicate impaired glomerular filtration.

Other non-nitrogenous waste products include small amounts of urobilin from the hemoglobin of old RBCs (see Fig. 11–4), and may include the metabolic products of medications. Table 18–3 summarizes the characteristics of urine.

When a substance not normally found in urine does appear there, there is a reason for it. The reason may be quite specific or more general. Table 18–4 lists some abnormal constituents of urine and possible reasons for each (see Box 18–6: Urinary Tract Infections).

AGING AND THE URINARY SYSTEM

With age, the number of nephrons in the kidneys decreases, often to half the original number by the age of 70 to 80, and the kidneys lose some of their concentrating ability. The glomerular filtration rate also decreases, partly as a consequence of arteriosclerosis and diminished renal blood flow. Despite these changes, excretion of nitrogenous wastes usually remains adequate.

The urinary bladder decreases in size and the tone of the detrusor muscle decreases. These changes may lead to a need to urinate more frequently. Urinary incontinence (the inability to control voiding) is *not* an inevitable consequence of aging, and can be prevented or minimized. Elderly people are, however, more at risk for infections of the urinary tract, especially if voiding leaves residual urine in the bladder.

Table 18–3 | CHARACTERISTICS OF NORMAL URINE

Characteristic	Description
Amount	• 1–2 liters per 24 hours; highly variable depending on fluid intake and water loss through the skin and GI tract
Color	• Straw or amber; darker means more concentrated; should be clear, not cloudy
Specific gravity	• 1.010–1.025; a measure of the dissolved material in urine; the lower the value, the more dilute the urine
pH	• Average 6; range 4.6–8.0; diet has the greatest effect on urine pH
Composition	• 95% water; 5% salts and waste products
Nitrogenous wastes	• Urea—from amino acid metabolism • Creatinine—from muscle metabolism • Uric acid—from nucleic acid metabolism

Table 18–4 | ABNORMAL CONSTITUENTS IN URINE

Characteristic	Reason(s)
Glycosuria (the presence of glucose)	As long as blood glucose levels are within normal limits, filtrate levels will also be normal and will not exceed the threshold level for reabsorption. In an untreated diabetic, for example, blood glucose is too high; therefore the filtrate glucose level is too high. The kidneys reabsorb glucose up to their threshold level, but the excess remains in the filtrate and is excreted in urine.
Proteinuria (the presence of protein)	Most plasma proteins are too large to be forced out of the glomeruli, and the small proteins that enter the filtrate are reabsorbed by pinocytosis. The presence of protein in the urine indicates that the glomeruli have become too permeable, as occurs in some types of kidney disease.
Hematuria (the presence of blood—RBCs)	The presence of RBCs in urine may also indicate that the glomeruli have become too permeable. Another possible cause might be bleeding somewhere in the urinary tract. Pinpointing the site of bleeding would require specific diagnostic tests.
Bacteriuria (the presence of bacteria)	Bacteria give urine a cloudy rather than clear appearance; WBCs may be present also. The presence of bacteria means that there is an infection somewhere in the urinary tract. Further diagnostic tests would be needed to determine the precise location.
Ketonuria (the presence of ketones)	Ketones are formed from fats and proteins that are used for energy production. A trace of ketones in urine is normal. Higher levels of ketones indicate an increased use of fats and proteins for energy. This may be the result of malfunctioning carbohydrate metabolism (as in diabetes mellitus) or simply the result of a high-protein diet.

Box 18–6   URINARY TRACT INFECTIONS

Infections may occur anywhere in the urinary tract and are most often caused by the microbial agents of sexually transmitted diseases (see Chapter 20) or by the bacteria that are part of the normal flora of the colon. In women especially, the urinary and anal openings are in close proximity, and colon bacteria on the skin of the perineum may invade the urinary tract. The use of urinary catheters in hospitalized or bed-ridden patients may also be a factor if sterile technique is not carefully followed.

Cystitis is inflammation of the urinary bladder. Symptoms include frequency of urination, painful voiding, and low back pain. **Nephritis** (or pyelonephritis) is inflammation of the kidneys. Although this may be the result of a systemic bacterial infection, nephritis is a common complication of untreated lower urinary tract infections such as cystitis. Possible symptoms are fever and flank pain (in the area of the kidneys). Untreated nephritis may result in severe damage to nephrons and progress to renal failure.

SUMMARY

The kidneys are the principal regulators of the internal environment of the body. The composition of all body fluids is either directly or indirectly regulated by the kidneys as they form urine from blood plasma. The kidneys are also of great importance in the regulation of the pH of the body fluids. These topics are the subject of the next chapter.

STUDY OUTLINE

The urinary system consists of two kidneys, two ureters, the urinary bladder, and the urethra.

1. The kidneys form urine to excrete waste products and to regulate the volume, electrolytes, and pH of blood and tissue fluid.
2. The other organs of the system are concerned with elimination of urine.

Kidneys (see Fig. 18–1)

1. Retroperitoneal on either side of the backbone in the upper abdominal cavity; partially protected by the lower rib cage.
2. Adipose tissue and the renal fascia cushion the kidneys and help hold them in place.
3. Hilus—an indentation on the medial side; renal artery enters, renal vein and ureter emerge.

Kidney—internal structure (see Fig. 18–2)

1. Renal cortex—outer tissue layer, made of renal corpuscles and convoluted tubules.
2. Renal medulla (pyramids)—inner tissue layer, made of loops of Henle and collecting tubules.
3. Renal pelvis—a cavity formed by the expanded end of the ureter within the kidney at the hilus; extensions around the papillae of the pyramids are called calyces, which collect urine.

The Nephron—the functional unit of the kidney (see Fig. 18–3); 1 million per kidney

1. Renal corpuscle—consists of a glomerulus surrounded by a Bowman's capsule.
   - Glomerulus—a capillary network between an afferent arteriole and an efferent arteriole.
   - Bowman's capsule—the expanded end of a renal tubule that encloses the glomerulus; inner layer is made of podocytes, has pores, and is very permeable; contains renal filtrate (potential urine).
2. Renal tubule—consists of the proximal convoluted tubule, loop of Henle, distal convoluted tubule, and collecting tubule. Collecting tubules unite to form papillary ducts that empty urine into the calyces of the renal pelvis.
   - Peritubular capillaries—arise from the efferent arteriole and surround all parts of the renal tubule.

Blood Vessels of the Kidney (see Figs. 18–1, 18–2, and 18–3)

1. Pathway: abdominal aorta → renal artery → small arteries in the kidney → afferent arterioles → glomeruli → efferent arterioles → peritubular capillaries → small veins in the kidney → renal vein → inferior vena cava.
2. Two sets of capillaries provide for two sites of exchanges between the blood and tissues in the process of urine formation.

Formation of Urine (see Fig. 18–4)

1. Glomerular filtration—takes place from the glomerulus to Bowman's capsule. High blood pressure (60 mmHg) in the glomerulus forces plasma, dissolved materials, and small proteins out of the blood and into Bowman's capsule. The fluid is now called filtrate. Filtration is selective only in terms of size; blood cells and large proteins remain in the blood.
2. GFR is 100 to 125 ml per minute. Increased blood flow to the kidney increases GFR; decreased blood flow decreases GFR.
3. Tubular reabsorption—takes place from the filtrate in the renal tubule to the blood in the peritubular capillaries; 99% of the filtrate is reabsorbed; only 1% becomes urine.
   - Active transport—reabsorption of glucose, amino acids, vitamins, and positive ions; threshold level is a limit to the quantity that can be reabsorbed.
   - Passive transport—most negative ions follow the reabsorption of positive ions.
   - Osmosis—water follows the reabsorption of minerals, especially sodium.
   - Pinocytosis—small proteins are engulfed by proximal tubule cells.
4. Tubular secretion—takes place from the blood in the peritubular capillaries to the filtrate in the renal tubule; creatinine and other waste products may be secreted into the filtrate to be excreted in urine; secretion of H^+ ions helps maintain pH of blood.
5. Hormones that affect reabsorption—aldosterone, atrial natriuretic hormone, antidiuretic hormone, and parathyroid hormone—see Table 18–1 and Fig. 18–5.

The Kidneys and Acid–Base Balance

1. The kidneys have the greatest capacity to compensate for normal and abnormal pH changes.
2. If the body fluids are becoming too acidic, the kidneys excrete H^+ ions and return HCO_3^- ions to the blood (see Fig. 18–6).
3. If the body fluids are becoming too alkaline, the kidneys return H^+ ions to the blood and excrete HCO_3^- ions.

Other Functions of the Kidneys

1. Secretion of renin by juxtaglomerular cells when blood pressure decreases (see Table 18–2). Angiotensin II causes vasoconstriction and increases secretion of aldosterone.
2. Secretion of erythropoietin in response to hypoxia; stimulates RBM to increase rate of RBC production.
3. Activation of vitamin D—conversion of inactive forms to the active form.

Elimination of Urine—the function of the ureters, urinary bladder, and urethra

Ureters (see Figs. 18–1 and 18–7)

1. Each extends from the hilus of a kidney to the lower posterior side of the urinary bladder.
2. Peristalsis of smooth muscle layer propels urine toward bladder.

Urinary Bladder (see Figs. 18–1 and 18–7)

1. A muscular sac below the peritoneum and behind the pubic bones; in women, below the uterus; in men, above the prostate gland.

2. Mucosa—transitional epithelial tissue folded into rugae; permit expansion without tearing.
3. Trigone—triangular area on bladder floor; no rugae, does not expand; bounded by openings of ureters and urethra.
4. Detrusor muscle—the smooth muscle layer, a spherical muscle; contracts to expel urine (reflex).
5. Internal urethral sphincter—involuntary; formed by detrusor muscle fibers around the opening of the urethra.

Urethra—takes urine from the bladder to the exterior (see Fig. 18–7)

1. In women—1 to 1.5 inches long; anterior to vagina.
2. In men—7 to 8 inches long; passes through the prostate gland and penis.
3. Has the external urethral sphincter: skeletal muscle of pelvic floor (voluntary).

The Urination Reflex—also called micturition or voiding

1. Stimulus: stretching of the detrusor muscle by accumulating urine.
2. Sensory impulses to spinal cord, motor impulses return to detrusor muscle, which contracts; internal urethral sphincter relaxes.
3. The external urethral sphincter provides voluntary control.

Characteristics of Urine (see Table 18–3)

Abnormal Constituents of Urine (see Table 18–4)

REVIEW QUESTIONS

1. Describe the location of the kidneys, ureters, urinary bladder, and urethra. (pp. 398, 409)

2. Name the three areas of the kidney, and state what each consists of. (p. 398)

3. Name the two major parts of a nephron. State the general function of nephrons. (p. 398)

4. Name the parts of a renal corpuscle. What process takes place here? Name the parts of a renal tubule. What processes take place here? (pp. 398–400)

5. State the mechanism of tubular reabsorption of each of the following: (p. 404)
   a. Water
   b. Glucose
   c. Small proteins
   d. Positive ions
   e. Negative ions
   f. Amino acids
   g. Vitamins

   Also explain what is meant by a threshold level of reabsorption.

6. Explain the importance of tubular secretion. (p. 404)

7. Describe the pathway of blood flow through the kidney from the abdominal aorta to the inferior vena cava. (p. 400)

8. Name the two sets of capillaries in the kidney, and state the processes that take place in each. (pp. 400, 403)

9. Name the hormone that has each of these effects on the kidneys: (pp. 406–407)
   a. Promotes reabsorption of Na^+ ions
   b. Promotes direct reabsorption of water
   c. Promotes reabsorption of Ca^{+2} ions
   d. Promotes excretion of K^+ ions
   e. Decreases reabsorption of Na^+ ions

10. In what circumstances will the kidneys excrete H^+ ions? What ions will be returned to the blood? How will this affect the pH of blood? (p. 406)

11. In what circumstances do the kidneys secrete renin, and what is its purpose? (p. 408)

12. In what circumstances do the kidneys secrete erythropoietin, and what is its purpose? (p. 409)

13. Describe the function of the ureters and that of the urethra. (p. 409)

14. With respect to the urinary bladder, describe the function of rugae and the detrusor muscle. (p. 409)

15. Describe the urination reflex in terms of stimulus, part of the CNS involved, effector muscle, internal urethral sphincter, and voluntary control. (pp. 410–411)

16. Describe the characteristics of normal urine in terms of appearance, amount, pH, specific gravity, and composition. (p. 411)

17. State the source of each of the nitrogenous waste products: creatinine, uric acid, and urea. (p. 411)

FOR FURTHER THOUGHT

1. The functioning of the kidneys may be likened to cleaning your room by throwing everything out the window, then going outside to retrieve what you wish to keep, such as jammies and slippers. Imagine the contents of a room, liken them to the materials in the blood (you yourself are a kidney), and describe what happens to each, and why.

2. Explain why fatty acids are not found in urine. Under what circumstances are water-soluble vitamins (such as vitamin C) found in urine?

3. Explain how a spinal cord transection at the level of T 11 will affect the urination reflex.

4. As part of his yearly physical for the college football team, 20-year-old Patrick has a urinalysis, which shows a high level of ketones. He is not diabetic, and is not ill. What might cause the high urine level of ketones? What test that is part of

blood chemistry (for nitrogenous wastes) would help confirm this?

5. A patient being evaluated for food poisoning has a blood pH of 7.33, a urine pH of 4.5, and a respiratory rate of 28 per minute. What kind of pH imbalance is this? Explain your reasoning step by step.

6. Erythropoietin, called EPO, has become a drug used illegally by some athletes. Which athletes, that is, in what kind of sports? What benefits are they hoping for? What part of a CBC would indicate that an athlete is taking EPO? Explain.

7. After a 4-hour workout on a hot June day, the high school track coach tells her group to keep drinking plenty of water. The girls assure their coach that they will know just how to determine if they are sufficiently hydrated that evening, that they have their color scheme memorized. What do they mean?

CHAPTER 19

Fluid–Electrolyte and Acid–Base Balance

CHAPTER 19

Chapter Outline

Water Compartments

Water Intake and Output
Regulation of Water Intake and Output

Electrolytes
Electrolytes in Body Fluids
Intake, Output, and Regulation

Acid–Base Balance
Buffer Systems
    Bicarbonate buffer system
    Phosphate buffer system
    Protein buffer system
Respiratory Mechanisms
    Respiratory acidosis and alkalosis
    Respiratory compensation for metabolic pH
    changes
Renal Mechanisms
Effects of pH Changes

Aging and Fluid and pH Regulation

Box 19–1	EDEMA	
Box 19–2	ELECTROLYTE IMBALANCES	

Student Objectives

- Describe the water compartments and the name for the water in each.
- Explain how water moves between compartments.
- Explain the regulation of the intake and output of water.
- Name the major electrolytes in body fluids, and state their functions.
- Explain the regulation of the intake and output of electrolytes.
- Describe the three buffer systems in body fluids.
- Explain why the respiratory system has an effect on pH, and describe respiratory compensating mechanisms.
- Explain the renal mechanisms for pH regulation of extracellular fluid.
- Describe the effects of acidosis and alkalosis.

Fluid–Electrolyte and Acid–Base Balance

New Terminology

Amine group (ah-**MEEN)**
Anions (**AN**-eye-ons)
Carboxyl group (kar-**BAHK**-sul)
Cations (**KAT**-eye-ons)
Electrolytes (ee-**LEK**-troh-lites)
Osmolarity (ahs-moh-**LAR**-i-tee)
Osmoreceptors (AHS-moh-re-**SEP**-ters)

Related Clinical Terminology

Edema (uh-**DEE**-muh)
Hypercalcemia (HIGH-per-kal-**SEE**-me-ah)
Hyperkalemia (HIGH-per-kuh-**LEE**-me-ah)
Hypernatremia (HIGH-per-nuh-**TREE**-me-ah)
Hypocalcemia (HIGH-poh-kal-**SEE**-me-ah)
Hypokalemia (HIGH-poh-kuh-**LEE**-me-ah)
Hyponatremia (HIGH-poh-nuh-**TREE**-me-ah)

*Terms that appear in **bold type** in the chapter text are defined in the glossary, which begins on page 521.*

People are watery creatures. More precisely, we are salt-watery creatures, though not as salty as the oceans. Water, the fluid medium of the human body, makes up 55% to 75% of the total body weight. Electrolytes are the positive and negative ions present in body fluids. In previous chapters we have called these salts or, in some cases, trace elements. Many of these ions are minerals that are already familiar to you. They each have specific functions in body fluids, and some of them are also involved in the maintenance of the normal pH of the body fluids. In this chapter we will first discuss fluid–electrolyte balance, then review and summarize the mechanisms involved in acid–base balance.

WATER COMPARTMENTS

Most of the water of the body, about two-thirds of the total water volume, is found within individual cells and is called **intracellular fluid** (ICF). The remaining third is called **extracellular fluid** (ECF) and includes blood plasma, lymph, tissue fluid, and the specialized fluids such as cerebrospinal fluid, synovial fluid, aqueous humor, and serous fluid.

Water constantly moves from one fluid site in the body to another by the processes of filtration and osmosis. These fluid sites are called **water compart-**

ments (Fig. 19–1). The chambers of the heart and all of the blood vessels form one compartment, and the water within is called plasma. By the process of filtration in capillaries, some plasma is forced out into tissue spaces (another compartment) and is then called tissue fluid. When tissue fluid enters cells by the process of osmosis, it has moved to still another compartment and is called intracellular fluid. The tissue fluid that enters lymph capillaries is in yet another compartment and is called lymph.

The other process (besides filtration) by which water moves from one compartment to another is osmosis, which, you may recall, is the diffusion of water through a semi-permeable membrane. Water will move through cell membranes from the area of its greater concentration to the area of its lesser concentration. Another way of expressing this is to say that water will diffuse to an area with a greater concentration of dissolved material. The concentration of electrolytes present in the various water compartments determines just how osmosis will take place. Therefore, if water is in balance in all of the compartments, the electrolytes are also in balance. Although water and ions are constantly moving, their relative proportions in the compartments remain constant; this is fluid–electrolyte homeostasis, and its maintenance is essential for life (see Box 19–1: Edema).

Figure 19–1 Water compartments. The name given to water in each of its locations is indicated.

Box 19–1   EDEMA

Edema is an abnormal increase in the amount of tissue fluid, which may be localized or systemic. Sometimes edema is inapparent, and sometimes it is apparent as swelling.

Localized edema follows injury and inflammation of a body part. Spraining an ankle, for example, damages tissues that then release histamine. Histamine increases the permeability of capillaries, and more tissue fluid is formed. As tissue fluid accumulates, the ankle may become swollen.

Systemic edema is the result of an imbalance between the movement of water out of and into capillaries, that is, between filtration and osmosis. Excessive filtration will occur when capillary pressure rises. This may be caused by venous obstruction due to blood clots or by congestive heart failure. Edema of this type is often apparent in the lower extremities

(pulmonary edema was described in Chapter 15).

Systemic bacterial infections may increase capillary permeability, and loss of plasma to tissue spaces is one aspect of septicemia. In this situation, however, the edema is of secondary importance to the hypotension, which may be life-threatening.

Insufficient osmosis, the return of tissue fluid into capillaries, is a consequence of a decrease in plasma proteins, especially albumin. This may occur in severe liver diseases such as cirrhosis, kidney disease involving loss of protein in urine, malnutrition, or severe burn injuries.

Because edema is a symptom rather than a disease, treatment is aimed at correcting the specific cause. If that is not possible, the volume of tissue fluid may be diminished by a low-salt diet and the use of diuretics.

WATER INTAKE AND OUTPUT

Most of the water the body requires comes from the ingestion of liquids; this amount averages 1600 ml per day. The food we eat also contains water. Even foods we think of as somewhat dry, such as bread, contain significant amounts of water. The daily water total from food averages 700 ml. The last source of water, about 200 ml per day, is the metabolic water that is a product of cell respiration. The total intake of water per day, therefore, is about 2500 ml, or 2.5 liters.

Most of the water lost from the body is in the form of urine produced by the kidneys; this averages 1500 ml per day. About 500 ml per day is lost in the form of sweat, another 300 ml per day is in the form of water vapor in exhaled air, and another 200 ml per day is lost in feces. The total output of water is thus about 2500 ml per day.

Naturally, any increase in water output must be compensated for by an increase in intake. Someone who exercises strenuously, for example, may lose 1 to 2 liters of water in sweat and must replace that water by drinking more fluids. In a healthy individual, water intake equals water output, even though the amounts of each may vary greatly from the averages used above (Fig. 19–2 and Table 19–1).

REGULATION OF WATER INTAKE AND OUTPUT

The hypothalamus in the brain contains **osmoreceptors** that detect changes in the osmolarity of body fluids. **Osmolarity** is the concentration of dissolved materials present in a fluid. Dehydration raises the osmolarity of the blood; that is, there is less water in proportion to the amount of dissolved materials. Another way to express this is to simply say that the blood is now a more concentrated solution. When dehydrated, we feel the sensation of thirst, characterized by dryness of the mouth and throat, as less saliva is produced. Thirst is an uncomfortable sensation, and we drink fluids to relieve it. The water we drink is readily absorbed by the mucosa of the stomach and small intestine and has the effect of decreasing the osmolarity of the blood. In other words, we can say that the water we just drank is causing the blood to become a more dilute solution, and, as the serum osmolarity returns to normal, the sensation of thirst diminishes.

As you may recall, the hypothalamus is also involved in water balance because of its production of antidiuretic hormone (ADH), which is stored in the posterior pituitary gland. In a state of dehydration, the hypothalamus stimulates the release of ADH from the posterior pituitary. Antidiuretic hormone then

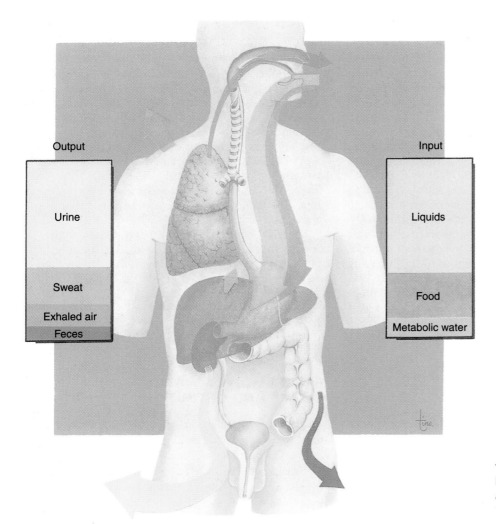

Output

Urine

Sweat

Exhaled air

Feces

Input

Liquids

Food

Metabolic water

Figure 19–2 Water intake and output. See text and Table 19–1 for description.

Table 19–1	WATER INTAKE AND OUTPUT

Form	Average Amount per 24 Hours (ml)
Intake	
Liquids	1600
Food	700
Metabolic water	200
Output	
Urine	1500
Sweat (and insensible water loss)	500
Exhaled air (water vapor)	300
Feces	200

increases the reabsorption of water by the kidney tubules. Water is returned to the blood to preserve blood volume, and urinary output decreases.

The hormone aldosterone, from the adrenal cortex, also helps regulate water output. Aldosterone increases the reabsorption of Na^+ ions by the kidney tubules, and water from the renal filtrate follows the Na^+ ions back to the blood. Aldosterone is secreted when the Na^+ ion concentration of the blood decreases or whenever there is a significant decrease in blood pressure (the renin-angiotensin mechanism).

Several other factors may also contribute to water loss. These include excessive sweating, hemorrhage, diarrhea or vomiting, severe burns, and fever. In these circumstances, the kidneys will conserve water, but water must also be replaced by increased consumption. Following hemorrhage or during certain disease states, fluids may also be replaced by intravenous administration.

A less common occurrence is that of too much water in the body. This may happen following over-consumption of fluids. The osmolarity of the blood decreases, and there is too much water in proportion to electrolytes (or, the blood is too dilute). This condition may become symptomatic, and is called water intoxication. Symptoms are dizziness, abdominal cramps, nausea, and lethargy. Convulsions are possible in severe cases, and fluids must be restricted until the kidneys can excrete the excess water. A hormone that will contribute to that is atrial natriuretic hormone (ANH), which is secreted by the atria when blood volume or blood pressure increases. ANH then decreases the reabsorption of Na^+ ions by the kidneys, which increases urinary output of sodium and water. Also, secretion of ADH will diminish, which will contribute to a greater urinary output that will return the blood osmolarity to normal.

ELECTROLYTES

Electrolytes are chemicals that dissolve in water and dissociate into their positive and negative ions. Most electrolytes are the inorganic salts, acids, and bases found in all body fluids.

Most organic compounds are non-electrolytes, that is, they do not ionize when in solution. Glucose, for example, dissolves in water but does not ionize; it remains as intact glucose molecules. Some proteins, however, do form ionic bonds and when in solution dissociate into ions.

Positive ions are called **cations**. Examples are Na^+, K^+, Ca^{+2}, Mg^{+2}, Fe^{+2}, and H^+. Negative ions are called **anions**, and examples are Cl^-, HCO_3^-, SO_4^{-2} (sulfate), HPO_4^{-2} (phosphate), and protein anions.

Electrolytes help create the osmolarity of body fluids and, therefore, help regulate the osmosis of water between water compartments. Some electrolytes are involved in acid–base regulatory mechanisms, or they are part of structural components of tissues or part of enzymes.

ELECTROLYTES IN BODY FLUIDS

The three principal fluids in the body are intracellular fluid and the extracellular fluids plasma and tissue fluid. The relative concentrations of the most important electrolytes in these fluids are depicted in Fig. 19–3. The major differences may be summarized as follows. In intracellular fluid, the most abundant cation is K^+, the most abundant anion is HPO_4^{-2}, and protein anions are also abundant. In both tissue fluid and plasma, the most abundant cation is Na^+, and the most abundant anion is Cl^-. Protein anions form a significant part of plasma but not of tissue fluid. The functions of the major electrolytes are described in Table 19–2.

INTAKE, OUTPUT, AND REGULATION

Electrolytes are part of the food and beverages we consume, are absorbed by the GI tract into the blood, and become part of body fluids. Hormones regulate the ECF concentrations of some electrolytes. Aldosterone increases the reabsorption of Na^+ ions and the excretion of K^+ ions by the kidneys. The blood sodium level is thereby raised, and the blood potassium level is lowered. Atrial natriuretic hormone (ANH) increases the excretion of Na^+ ions by the kidneys and lowers the blood sodium level. Parathyroid hormone (PTH) and calcitonin regulate the blood levels of calcium and phosphate. PTH increases the reabsorption of these minerals from bones, and increases their absorption from food in the small intestine (vitamin D is also necessary). Calcitonin promotes the removal of calcium and phosphate from the blood to form bone matrix.

Electrolytes are lost in urine, sweat, and feces. Urine contains the electrolytes that are not reabsorbed by the kidney tubules; the major one of these is Na^+ ions. Other electrolytes are present in urine when their concentrations in the blood exceed the body's need for them.

The most abundant electrolytes in sweat are Na^+ ions and Cl^- ions. Electrolytes lost in feces are those that are not absorbed in either the small intestine or colon.

Some of the major imbalances of electrolyte levels are described in Box 19–2: Electrolyte Imbalances.

ACID–BASE BALANCE

You have already learned quite a bit about the regulation of the pH of body fluids in the chapters on chemistry, the respiratory system, and the urinary

Figure 19–3 Electrolyte concentrations in intracellular fluid, tissue fluid, and plasma. Concentrations are expressed in milliequivalents per liter. See text for summary of major differences among these fluids.

system. In this section, we will put all of that information together. You may first wish to review the pH scale, described in Chapter 2.

The normal pH range of blood is 7.35 to 7.45. The pH of tissue fluid is similar but can vary slightly above or below this range. The intracellular fluid has a pH range of 6.8 to 7.0. Notice that these ranges of pH are quite narrow; they must be maintained in order for enzymatic reactions and other processes to proceed normally.

Maintenance of acid–base homeostasis is accomplished by the buffer systems in body fluids, respirations, and the kidneys.

BUFFER SYSTEMS

The purpose of a **buffer system** is to prevent drastic changes in the pH of body fluids by chemically reacting with strong acids or bases that would otherwise greatly change the pH. A buffer system consists of a weak acid and a weak base. These molecules react with strong acids or bases that may be produced and change them to substances that do not have a great effect on pH.

Bicarbonate Buffer System

The two components of this buffer system are carbonic acid (H_2CO_3), a weak acid, and sodium bicarbonate ($NaHCO_3$), a weak base. Each of these molecules participates in a specific type of reaction.

If a potential pH change is created by a strong acid, the following reaction takes place:

$$\underset{\text{(strong acid)}}{HCl} + NaHCO_3 \rightarrow NaCl + \underset{\text{(weak acid)}}{H_2CO_3}$$

The strong acid has reacted with the sodium bicarbonate to produce a salt (NaCl) that has no effect on pH and a weak acid that has little effect on pH.

If a potential pH change is created by a strong base, the following reaction takes place:

Table 19–2 MAJOR ELECTROLYTES

Electrolyte	Plasma Level mEq/L*	ICF Level mEq/L	Functions
Sodium (Na⁺)	136–142	10	• Creates much of the osmotic pressure of ECF; the most abundant cation in ECF • Essential for electrical activity of neurons and muscle cells
Potassium (K⁺)	3.8–5.0	141	• Creates much of the osmotic pressure in ICF; the most abundant cation in ICF • Essential for electrical activity of neurons and muscle cells
Calcium (Ca⁺²)	4.6–5.5	1	• Most (98%) is found in bones and teeth • Maintains normal excitability of neurons and muscle cells • Essential for blood clotting
Magnesium (Mg⁺²)	1.3–2.1	58	• Most (50%) is found in bone • More abundant in ICF than in ECF • Essential for ATP production and activity of neurons and muscle cells
Chloride (Cl⁻)	95–103	4	• Most abundant anion in ECF; diffuses easily into and out of cells; helps regulate osmotic pressure • Part of HCl in gastric juice
Bicarbonate (HCO₃⁻)	28	10	• Part of the bicarbonate buffer system
Phosphate (HPO₄⁻²)	1.7–2.6	75	• Most (85%) is found in bones and teeth • Primarily an ICF anion • Part of DNA, RNA, ATP, phospholipids • Part of phosphate buffer system
Sulfate (SO₄⁻²)	1	2	• Part of some amino acids and proteins

* The concentration of an ion is often expressed in milliequivalents per liter, abbreviated mEq/L, which is the number of electrical charges in each liter of solution.

Box 19–2   ELECTROLYTE IMBALANCES

IMBALANCES OF SODIUM

Hyponatremia—a consequence of excessive sweating, diarrhea, or vomiting. Characterized by dizziness, confusion, weakness, low BP, shock.

Hypernatremia—a consequence of excessive water loss or sodium ingestion. Characterized by loss of ICF and extreme thirst and agitation.

IMBALANCES OF POTASSIUM

Hypokalemia—a consequence of vomiting or diarrhea or kidney disease. Characterized by fatigue, confusion, possible cardiac failure.

Hyperkalemia—a consequence of acute renal failure or Addison's disease. Characterized by weakness, abnormal sensations, cardiac arrhythmias, and possible cardiac arrest.

IMBALANCES OF CALCIUM

Hypocalcemia—a consequence of hypoparathyroidism or decreased calcium intake. Characterized by muscle spasms leading to tetany.

Hypercalcemia—a consequence of hyperparathyroidism. Characterized by muscle weakness, bone fragility, and possible kidney stones.

$$NaOH + H_2CO_3 \rightarrow H_2O + NaHCO_3$$
(strong base)   (weak base)

The strong base has reacted with the carbonic acid to produce water, which has no effect on pH and a weak base that has little effect on pH.

The bicarbonate buffer system is important in both the blood and tissue fluid. During normal metabolism, these fluids tend to become more acidic, so more sodium bicarbonate than carbonic acid is needed. The usual ratio of these molecules to each other is about 20 to 1 ($NaHCO_3$ to H_2CO_3).

Phosphate Buffer System

The two components of this buffer system are sodium dihydrogen phosphate (NaH_2PO_4), a weak acid, and sodium monohydrogen phosphate (Na_2HPO_4), a weak base. Let us use specific reactions to show how this buffer system works.

If a potential pH change is created by a strong acid, the following reaction takes place:

$$HCl + Na_2HPO_4 \rightarrow NaCl + NaH_2PO_4$$
(strong acid)   (weak acid)

The strong acid has reacted with the sodium monohydrogen phosphate to produce a salt that has no effect on pH and a weak acid that has little effect on pH.

If a potential pH change is created by a strong base, the following reaction takes place:

$$NaOH + NaH_2PO_4 \rightarrow H_2O + Na_2HPO_4$$
(strong base)   (weak base)

The strong base has reacted with the sodium dihydrogen phosphate to form water, which has no effect on pH and a weak base that has little effect on pH.

The phosphate buffer system is important in the regulation of the pH of the blood by the kidneys. The cells of the kidney tubules can remove excess hydrogen ions by forming NaH_2PO_4, which is excreted in urine. The retained Na^+ ions are returned to the blood in the peritubular capillaries, along with bicarbonate ions (Fig. 19–4).

Protein Buffer System

This buffer system is the most important one in the intracellular fluid. You may recall from Chapter 15 that hemoglobin buffers the hydrogen ions formed during CO_2 transport. The amino acids that make up proteins each have a **carboxyl group** (COOH) and an **amine**

(or amino) **group** (NH_2) and may act as either acids or bases.

The carboxyl group may act as an acid because it can donate a hydrogen ion (H^+) to the fluid to counteract increasing alkalinity:

$$
NH_2-\overset{\overset{\displaystyle H}{|}}{\underset{\underset{\displaystyle R}{|}}{C}}-COOH \rightarrow NH_2-\overset{\overset{\displaystyle H}{|}}{\underset{\underset{\displaystyle R}{|}}{C}}-COO^- + H^+
$$

The amine group may act as a base because it can pick up an excess hydrogen ion from the fluid to counteract increasing acidity:

$$
COOH-\overset{\overset{\displaystyle H}{|}}{\underset{\underset{\displaystyle R}{|}}{C}}-NH_2 \rightarrow COOH-\overset{\overset{\displaystyle H}{|}}{\underset{\underset{\displaystyle R}{|}}{C}}-NH_3^+
$$

The buffer systems react within a fraction of a second to prevent drastic pH changes. However, they have the least capacity to prevent great changes in pH because a limited number of molecules of these buffers are present in body fluids. When an ongoing cause is disrupting the normal pH, the respiratory and renal mechanisms will also be needed.

RESPIRATORY MECHANISMS

The respiratory system affects pH because it regulates the amount of CO_2 present in body fluids. As you know, the respiratory system may be the cause of a pH imbalance or may help correct a pH imbalance from some other cause.

Respiratory Acidosis and Alkalosis

Respiratory acidosis is caused by anything that decreases the rate or efficiency of respiration. Severe pulmonary diseases are possible causes of respiratory acidosis. When CO_2 cannot be exhaled as fast as it is formed during cell respiration, excess CO_2 results in the formation of excess H^+ ions, as shown in this reaction:

$$CO_2 + H_2O \rightarrow H_2CO_3 \rightarrow H^+ + HCO_3^-$$

The excess H^+ ions lower the pH of body fluids.

Respiratory alkalosis is far less common but is the result of breathing more rapidly, which increases the amount of CO_2 exhaled. Because there are fewer CO_2 molecules in the body fluids, fewer H^+ ions are formed, and pH tends to rise.

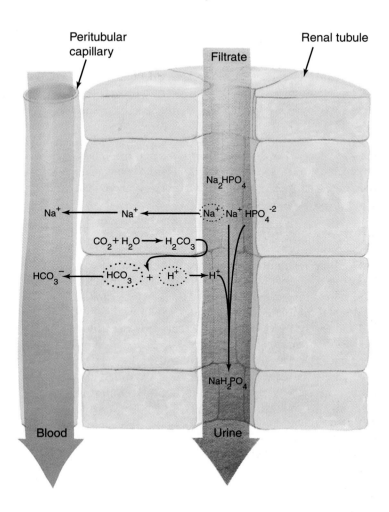

Figure 19–4 The phosphate buffer system. The reactions are shown in a kidney tubule. See text for description

Respiratory Compensation for Metabolic pH Changes

Changes in pH caused by other than a respiratory disorder are called metabolic acidosis or alkalosis. In either case, the respiratory system may help prevent a drastic change in pH.

Metabolic acidosis may be caused by kidney disease, uncontrolled diabetes mellitus, excessive diarrhea or vomiting, or the use of some diuretics. When excess H^+ ions are present in body fluids, pH begins to decrease, and this stimulates the respiratory centers in the medulla. The response is to increase the rate of breathing to exhale more CO_2 to decrease H^+ ion formation. This helps raise the pH back toward the normal range.

Metabolic alkalosis is not common, but may be caused by the overuse of antacid medications or the vomiting of stomach contents only. As the pH of body fluids begins to rise, breathing slows and decreases the amount of CO_2 exhaled. The CO_2 retained within

the body increases the formation of H^+ ions, which will help lower the pH back toward the normal range.

The respiratory system responds quickly to prevent drastic changes in pH, usually within 1 to 3 minutes. For an ongoing metabolic pH imbalance, however, the respiratory mechanism does not have the capacity to fully compensate. In such cases, respiratory compensation is only 50% to 75% effective.

RENAL MECHANISMS

As just discussed in Chapter 18, the kidneys help regulate the pH of extracellular fluid by excreting or conserving H^+ ions and by reabsorbing (or not) Na^+ ions and HCO_3^- ions. One mechanism was depicted in Fig. 18–5, and another, involving the phosphate buffer system, is shown in Fig. 19–4.

The kidneys have the greatest capacity to buffer an ongoing pH change. Although the renal mechanisms do not become fully functional for several hours to days, once they do they continue to be effective far

Table 19–3	pH CHANGES	
Change	**Possible Causes**	**Compensation**
Metabolic acidosis	• Kidney disease, ketosis, diarrhea, or vomiting	• Increased respirations to exhale CO_2
Metabolic alkalosis	• Overingestion of bicarbonate medications, gastric suctioning	• Decreased respirations to retain CO_2
Respiratory acidosis	• Decreased rate or efficiency of respiration: emphysema, asthma, pneumonia, paralysis of respiratory muscles	• Kidneys excrete H^+ ions and reabsorb Na^+ ions and HCO_3^- ions
Respiratory alkalosis	• Increased rate of respiration: anxiety, high altitude	• Kidneys retain H^+ ions and excrete Na^+ ions and HCO_3^- ions

longer than respiratory mechanisms. Let us use as an example a patient with untreated diabetes mellitus who is in ketoacidosis, a metabolic acidosis. As acidic ketones accumulate in the blood, the capacity of the ECF buffer systems is quickly exhausted. Breathing rate then increases, and more CO_2 is exhaled to decrease H^+ ion formation and raise the pH of ECF. There is, however, a limit to how much the respiratory rate can increase, but the renal buffering mechanisms will then become effective. At this time it is the kidneys that are keeping the patient alive by preventing acidosis from reaching a fatal level. Even the kidneys have limits, however, and the cause of the acidosis must be corrected to prevent death.

EFFECTS OF pH CHANGES

A state of **acidosis** is most detrimental to the central nervous system, causing depression of impulse transmission at synapses. A person in acidosis becomes confused and disoriented, then lapses into a coma.

Alkalosis has the opposite effect and affects both the central and peripheral nervous system. Increased synaptic transmission, even without stimuli, is first indicated by irritability and muscle twitches. Progressive alkalosis is characterized by severe muscle spasms and convulsions.

The types of pH changes are summarized in Table 19–3.

AGING AND FLUID AND pH REGULATION

Changes in fluid balance or pH in elderly people are often the result of disease or damage to particular organs. A weak heart (congestive heart failure) that cannot pump efficiently allows blood to back up in circulation. In turn, this may cause edema, an abnormal collection of fluid. Edema may be systemic (often apparent in the lower legs) if the right ventricle is weak, or pulmonary if the left ventricle is failing.

The sense of thirst may not be as acute in elderly people, who may become severely dehydrated by the time they feel thirsty. An important behavioral consideration is that elderly people who fear urinary incontinence may decrease their intake of fluids.

Deficiencies of minerals in elderly people may be the result of poor nutrition or a side effect of some medications, especially those for hypertension that increase urinary output. Disturbances in pH may be caused by chronic pulmonary disease, diabetes, or kidney disease.

STUDY OUTLINE

Fluid–Electrolyte Balance

1. Water makes up 55% to 75% of the total body weight.

2. Electrolytes are the ions found in body fluids; most are minerals.

Water Compartments (see Fig. 19–1)

1. Intracellular fluid (ICF)—water within cells; about two-thirds of total body water.
2. Extracellular fluid (ECF)—water outside cells; includes plasma, lymph, tissue fluid, and specialized fluids.
3. Water constantly moves from one compartment to another. Filtration: plasma becomes tissue fluid. Osmosis: tissue fluid becomes plasma, or lymph, or ICF.
4. Osmosis is regulated by the concentration of electrolytes in body fluids (osmolarity). Water will diffuse through membranes to areas of greater electrolyte concentration.

Water Intake (see Fig. 19–2)

1. Fluids, food, metabolic water—see Table 19–1.

Water Output (see Fig. 19–2)

1. Urine, sweat, exhaled air, feces—see Table 19–1.
2. Any variation in output must be compensated for by a change in input.

Regulation of Water Intake and Output

1. Hypothalamus contains osmoreceptors that detect changes in osmolarity of body fluids.
2. Dehydration stimulates the sensation of thirst, and fluids are consumed to relieve it.
3. ADH released from the posterior pituitary increases the reabsorption of water by the kidneys.
4. Aldosterone secreted by the adrenal cortex increases the reabsorption of Na^+ ions by the kidneys; water is then reabsorbed by osmosis.
5. If there is too much water in the body, secretion of ADH decreases, and urinary output increases.
6. If blood volume increases, ANH promotes loss of Na^+ ions and water in urine.

Electrolytes

1. Chemicals that dissolve in water and dissociate into ions; most are inorganic.
2. Cations are positive ions such as Na^+ and K^+.
3. Anions are negative ions such as Cl^- and HCO_3^-.
4. By creating osmotic pressure, electrolytes regulate the osmosis of water between compartments.

Electrolytes in Body Fluids (see Fig. 19–3 and Table 19–2)

1. ICF—principal cation is K^+; principal anion is HPO_4^{-2}; protein anions are also abundant.
2. Plasma—principal cation is Na^+; principal anion is Cl^-; protein anions are significant.
3. Tissue fluid—same as plasma except that protein anions are insignificant.

Intake, Output, and Regulation

1. Intake—electrolytes are part of food and beverages.
2. Output—urine, sweat, feces.
3. Hormones involved: aldosterone—Na^+ and K^+; ANH—Na^+; PTH and calcitonin—Ca^{+2} and HPO_4^{-2}.

Acid–Base Balance

1. Normal pH Ranges—blood: 7.35 to 7.45; ICF: 6.8 to 7.0; tissue fluid: similar to blood.
2. Normal pH of body fluids is maintained by buffer systems, respirations, and the kidneys.

Buffer Systems

1. Each consists of a weak acid and a weak base; react with strong acids or bases to change them to substances that do not greatly affect pH. React within a fraction of a second, but have the least capacity to prevent pH changes.
2. Bicarbonate buffer system—see text for reactions; important in both blood and tissue fluid; base to acid ratio is 20 to 1.
3. Phosphate buffer system—see Fig. 19–4 and text for reactions; important in ICF and in the kidneys.
4. Protein buffer system—amino acids may act as either acids or bases. See text for reactions; important in ICF.

Respiratory Mechanisms

1. The respiratory system affects pH because it regulates the amount of CO_2 in body fluids.
2. May be the cause of a pH change or help compensate for a metabolic pH change—see Table 19–3.
3. Respiratory compensation is rapidly effective (within a few minutes), but limited in capacity if the pH imbalance is ongoing.

Renal Mechanisms

1. The kidneys have the greatest capacity to buffer pH changes, but they may take several hours to days to become effective (see Table 19–3).
2. Reactions: see Figs. 18–5 and 19–4.
3. Summary of reactions: in response to acidosis, the kidneys will excrete H^+ ions and retain Na^+ ions and HCO_3^- ions; in response to alkalosis, the kidneys will retain H^+ ions and excrete Na^+ ions and HCO_3^- ions.

Effects of pH Changes

1. Acidosis—depresses synaptic transmission in the CNS; result is confusion, coma, and death.

2. Alkalosis—increases synaptic transmission in the CNS and PNS; result is irritability, muscle spasms, and convulsions.

REVIEW QUESTIONS

1. Name the major water compartments and the name for water in each of them. Name three specialized body fluids and state the location of each. (p. 420)

2. Explain how water moves between compartments; name the processes. (p. 420)

3. Describe the three sources of water for the body and the relative amounts of each. (p. 421)

4. Describe the pathways of water output. Which is the most important? What kinds of variations are possible in water output. (p. 421)

5. Name the hormones that affect fluid volume, and state the function of each. (pp. 421–423)

6. Define electrolyte, cation, anion, osmosis, and osmolarity. (pp. 421, 423)

7. Name the major electrolytes in plasma, tissue fluid, and intracellular fluid, and state their functions. (pp. 423, 425)

8. Explain how the bicarbonate buffer system will react to buffer a strong acid. (pp. 424, 426)

9. Explain how the phosphate buffer system will react to buffer a strong acid. (p. 426)

10. Explain why an amino acid may act as either an acid or a base. (p. 426)

11. Describe the respiratory compensation for metabolic acidosis and for metabolic alkalosis. (p. 427)

12. If the body fluids are becoming too acidic, what ions will the kidneys excrete? What ions will the kidneys return to the blood? (p. 427)

13. Which of the pH regulatory mechanisms works most rapidly? Most slowly? Which of these mechanisms has the greatest capacity to buffer an ongoing pH change? Which mechanism has the least capacity? (pp. 426–428)

14. Describe the effects of acidosis and alkalosis. (p. 428)

FOR FURTHER THOUGHT

1. Men tend to be more watery than women. The reason has to do with two tissues, one of which is more watery than the other. What are these tissues that are usually present in different proportions in men and women? Explain your answer.

2. Mrs. T, age 82, tells her visiting nurse that she has trouble walking around her house because her feet and ankles are swollen. The nurse makes a doctor's appointment for Mrs. T., and says the problem may be her heart. Explain.

3. Ms. H, age 18, is on a diet that advises eight 8-ounce glasses of water a day. Ms. H thinks that if eight glasses are good, perhaps 12 glasses would be better, because "water is good for you." What can you tell her? Is water always good?

4. Mr. C has what he calls "acid indigestion," and takes chewable tablets to try to relieve it. He admits that the fruit flavors of the tablets often have him "popping them like candy" all day. He is visiting his doctor because he says his muscles feel "jumpy." What would you expect to find for blood pH, respirations per minute, and urine pH? Explain your answers.

CHAPTER 20

The Reproductive Systems

CHAPTER 20

Chapter Outline

Student Objectives

- Describe the process of meiosis. Define diploid and haploid.
- Describe the differences between spermatogenesis and oogenesis.
- Name the hormones necessary for the formation of gametes, and state the function of each.
- Describe the location and functions of the testes.
- Explain the functions of the epididymis, ductus deferens, ejaculatory duct, and urethra.
- Explain the functions of the seminal vesicles, prostate gland, and bulbourethral glands.
- Describe the composition of semen, and explain why its pH must be alkaline.
- Name the parts of a sperm cell, and state the function of each.
- Describe the functions of the ovaries, fallopian tubes, uterus, and vagina.
- Describe the structure and function of the myometrium and endometrium.
- Describe the structure of the mammary glands and the functions of the hormones involved in lactation.
- Describe the menstrual cycle in terms of the hormones involved and the changes in the ovaries and endometrium.

The Reproductive Systems

New Terminology

Cervix (**SIR**-viks)
Ductus deferens (**DUK**-tus **DEF**-er-enz)
Endometrium (EN-doh-**MEE**-tree-uhm)
Fallopian tube (fuh-**LOH**-pee-an TOOB)
Graafian follicle (**GRAF**-ee-uhn **FAH**-li-kuhl)
Inguinal canal (**IN**-gwi-nuhl ka-**NAL**)
Menopause (**MEN**-ah-paws)
Menstrual cycle (**MEN**-stroo-uhl **SIGH**-kuhl)
Myometrium (MY-oh-**MEE**-tree-uhm)
Oogenesis (OH-oh-**JEN**-e-sis)
Prostate gland (**PRAHS**-tayt)
Seminiferous tubules (sem-i-**NIFF**-er-us)
Spermatogenesis (SPER-ma-toh-**JEN**-e-sis)
Vulva (**VUHL**-vah)
Zygote (**ZYE**-goht)

Related Clinical Terminology

Amenorrhea (ay-MEN-uh-**REE**-ah)
Down syndrome (DOWN **SIN**-drohm)
Ectopic pregnancy (ek-**TOP**-ik **PREG**-nun-see)
In vitro fertilization (IN **VEE**-troh FER-ti-li-**ZAY**-shun)
Mammography (mah-**MOG**-rah-fee)
Prostatic hypertrophy (prahs-**TAT**-ik high-**PER**-truh-fee)
Trisomy (**TRY**-suh-mee)
Tubal ligation (**TOO**-buhl lye-**GAY**-shun)
Vasectomy (va-**SEK**-tuh-me)

*Terms that appear in **bold type** in the chapter text are defined in the glossary, which begins on page 521.*

The purpose of the male and female **reproductive systems** is to continue the human species by the production of offspring. How dry and impersonal that sounds, until we remember that each of us is a continuation of our species and that many of us in turn will have our own children. Although some other animals care for their offspring in organized families or societies, the human species is unique, because of cultural influences, in the attention we give to reproduction and to family life.

Yet like other animals, the actual production and growth of offspring is a matter of our anatomy and physiology. The male and female reproductive systems produce **gametes**, that is, sperm and egg cells, and ensure the union of gametes in fertilization following sexual intercourse. In women, the uterus provides the site for the developing embryo/fetus until it is sufficiently developed to survive outside the womb.

This chapter describes the organs of reproduction and the role of each in the creation of new life or the functioning of the reproductive system as a whole. First, however, we will discuss the formation of gametes.

MEIOSIS

The cell division process of **meiosis** produces the gametes, sperm or egg cells. In meiosis, one cell with the diploid number of chromosomes (46 for people) divides twice to form four cells, each with the haploid number of chromosomes. Haploid means half the usual diploid number, so for people the haploid number is 23. Although the process of meiosis is essentially the same in men and women, there are important differences.

SPERMATOGENESIS

Spermatogenesis is the process of meiosis as it takes place in the testes, the site of sperm production. Within each testis are **seminiferous tubules** that contain spermatogonia, or sperm-generating cells. These divide first by mitosis to produce primary spermatocytes (Fig. 20–1). As you may recall from Chapter 10, gamete formation is regulated by hormones. Follicle-stimulating hormone (FSH) from the anterior pituitary gland initiates sperm production, and testosterone, secreted by the testes when stimulated by luteinizing hormone (LH) from the anterior pituitary, promotes the maturation of sperm. Inhibin, also produced by the testes, decreases the secretion of FSH. As you can see in Fig. 20–1, for each primary spermatocyte that undergoes meiosis, four functional sperm cells are produced.

Sperm production begins at **puberty** (10 to 14 years of age), and millions of sperm are formed each day in the testes. Although sperm production diminishes with advancing age, there is usually no complete cessation, as there is of egg production in women at menopause.

OOGENESIS

Oogenesis is the process of meiosis for egg cell formation; it begins in the ovaries and is also regulated by hormones. FSH initiates the growth of **ovarian follicles**, each of which contains an oogonium, or egg-generating cell (Fig. 20–2). This hormone also stimulates the follicle cells to secrete estrogen, which promotes the maturation of the ovum. Notice that for each primary oocyte that undergoes meiosis, only one functional egg cell is produced. The other three cells produced are called polar bodies. They have no function, and will simply deteriorate. A mature ovarian follicle actually contains the secondary oocyte; the second meiotic division will take place if and when the egg is fertilized.

The production of ova begins at puberty (10 to 14 years of age) and continues until **menopause** (45 to 55 years of age), when the ovaries atrophy and no longer respond to pituitary hormones. During this 30- to 40-year span, egg production is cyclical, with a mature ovum being produced approximately every 28 days (the menstrual cycle is discussed later in this chapter). Actually, *several* follicles usually begin to develop during each cycle. However, the rupturing (ovulation) of the first follicle to mature stops the growth of the others.

The process of meiosis is like other human processes in that "mistakes" may sometimes occur. One of these, trisomy, is discussed in Box 20–1: Trisomy and Down Syndrome

The haploid egg and sperm cells produced by meiosis each have 23 chromosomes. When fertilization occurs, the nuclei of the egg and sperm merge, and the fertilized egg **(zygote)** has 46 chromosomes, the diploid number. Thus, meiosis maintains the diploid number of the human species by reducing the number of chromosomes by half in the formation of gametes.

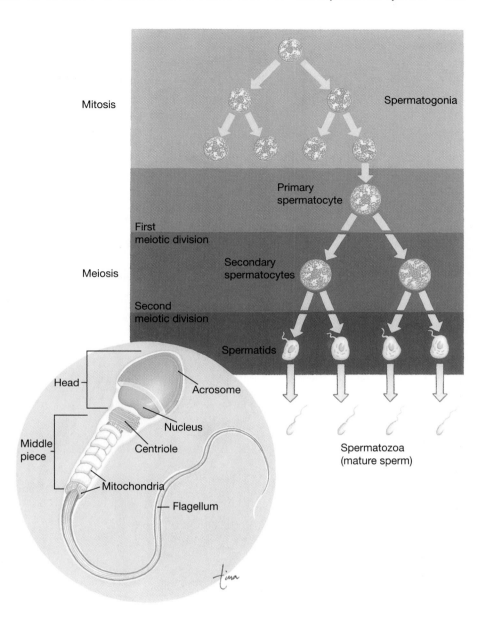

Figure 20–1 Spermatogenesis. The process of mitosis and meiosis are shown. For each primary spermatocyte that undergoes meiosis, four functional sperm cells are formed. The structure of a mature sperm cell is also shown.

MALE REPRODUCTIVE SYSTEM

The male reproductive system consists of the testes and a series of ducts and glands. Sperm are produced in the testes and are transported through the reproductive ducts: epididymis, ductus deferens, ejaculatory duct, and urethra (Fig. 20–3). The reproductive glands produce secretions that become part of semen, the fluid that is ejaculated from the urethra. These glands are the seminal vesicles, prostate gland, and bulbourethral glands.

TESTES

The **testes** are located in the **scrotum**, a sac of skin between the upper thighs. The temperature within the scrotum is about 96°F, slightly lower than body temperature, which is necessary for the production of viable sperm. In the male fetus, the testes develop near the kidneys, then descend into the scrotum just before birth. **Cryptorchidism** is the condition in which the testes fail to descend, and the result is sterility unless the testes are surgically placed in the scrotum.

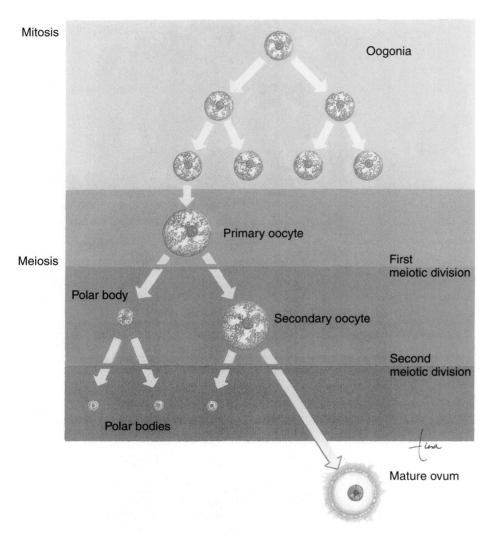

Mitosis

Oogonia

Meiosis

Primary oocyte

First
meiotic division

Polar body

Secondary oocyte

Second
meiotic division

Polar bodies

Mature ovum

Figure 20–2 Oogenesis. The processes of mitosis and meiosis are shown. For each primary oocyte that undergoes meiosis, only one functional ovum is formed.

Each testis is about 1.5 inches long by 1 inch wide (4 cm × 2.5 cm) and is divided internally into lobes (Fig. 20–4). Each lobe contains several **seminiferous tubules**, in which spermatogenesis takes place. Among the spermatogonia of the seminiferous tubules are **sustentacular (Sertoli) cells**, which produce the hormone **inhibin** when stimulated by testosterone. Between the loops of the seminiferous tubules are **interstitial cells**, which produce **testosterone** when stimulated by luteinizing hormone (LH) from the anterior pituitary gland. Besides its role in the maturation of sperm, testosterone is also responsible for the male secondary sex characteristics, which begin to develop at puberty (Table 20–1).

A sperm cell consists of several parts, which are shown in Fig. 20–1. The head contains the 23 chromosomes. On the tip of the head is the **acrosome**, which contains enzymes to digest the membrane of an egg cell. Within the middle piece are mitochondria that produce ATP. The **flagellum** provides motility, the capability of the sperm cell to move. It is the beating of the flagellum that requires energy from ATP.

Sperm from the seminiferous tubules enter a tubular network called the rete testis, then enter the epididymis, the first of the reproductive ducts.

EPIDIDYMIS

The **epididymis** (plural: epididymides) is a tube about 20 feet (6 m) long that is coiled on the posterior surface of each testis (see Fig. 20–4). Within the epididymis the sperm complete their maturation, and

Box 20–1   TRISOMY AND DOWN SYNDROME

Trisomy means the presence of three (rather than the normal two) of a particular chromosome in the cells of an individual. This may occur because of non-disjunction (nonseparation) of a chromosome pair during the second meiotic division, usually in an egg cell. The egg cell has two of a particular chromosome, and if fertilized by a sperm, will then contain three of that chromosome, and a total of 47 chromosomes.

Most trisomies are probably lethal, that is, the affected embryo will quickly die, even before the woman realizes she is pregnant. When an embryo-fetus survives and a child is born with a trisomy, there are always developmental defects present.

The severity of trisomies may be seen in two of the more rarely occurring ones: Trisomy 13 and Trisomy 18, each of which occurs about once for every 5000 live births. Both of these trisomies are characterized by severe mental and physical retardation, heart defects, deafness, and bone abnormalities. Affected infants usually die within their first year.

Down syndrome (Trisomy 21) is the most common trisomy, with a frequency of about one per 650 live births. Children with Down syndrome are mentally retarded, but there is a great range of mental ability in this group. Physical characteristics include a skin fold above each eye, short stature, poor muscle tone, and heart defects. Again, the degree of severity is highly variable.

Women over the age of 35 are believed to be at greater risk of having a child with Down syndrome. The reason may be that as egg cells age the process of meiosis is more likely to proceed incorrectly.

---

their flagella become functional. Smooth muscle in the wall of the epididymis propels the sperm into the ductus deferens.

DUCTUS DEFERENS

Also called the **vas deferens**, the **ductus deferens** extends from the epididymis in the scrotum on its own side into the abdominal cavity through the **inguinal canal**. This canal is an opening in the abdominal wall for the **spermatic cord**, a connective tissue sheath that contains the ductus deferens, testicular blood vessels, and nerves. Because the inguinal canal is an opening in a muscular wall, it is a natural "weak spot," and it is the most common site of hernia formation in men.

Once inside the abdominal cavity, the ductus deferens extends upward over the urinary bladder, then down the posterior side to join the ejaculatory duct on its own side (see Fig. 20–3). The smooth muscle layer of the ductus deferens contracts in waves of peristalsis as part of ejaculation (see Box 20–2: Contraception).

EJACULATORY DUCTS

Each of the two **ejaculatory ducts** receives sperm from the ductus deferens and the secretion of the seminal vesicle on its own side. Both ejaculatory ducts empty into the single urethra (see Fig. 20–3).

SEMINAL VESICLES

The paired **seminal vesicles** are posterior to the urinary bladder (see Fig. 20–3). Their secretion contains fructose to provide an energy source for sperm and is alkaline to enhance sperm motility. The duct of each seminal vesicle joins the ductus deferens on that side to form the ejaculatory duct.

PROSTATE GLAND

A muscular gland just below the urinary bladder, the **prostate gland** surrounds the first inch of the urethra as it emerges from the bladder (see Fig. 20–3). The glandular tissue of the prostate secretes an alkaline fluid that helps maintain sperm motility. The smooth muscle of the prostate gland contracts during **ejaculation** to contribute to the expulsion of semen from the urethra (see Box 20–3: Prostatic Hypertrophy).

BULBOURETHRAL GLANDS

Also called Cowper's glands, the **bulbourethral glands** are located below the prostate gland and empty into the urethra. Their alkaline secretion coats the interior of the urethra just before ejaculation, which will neutralize any acidic urine that might be present.

You have probably noticed that all of the secretions of the male reproductive glands are alkaline. This is important because the cavity of the female vagina has an acidic pH created by the normal flora, the natural

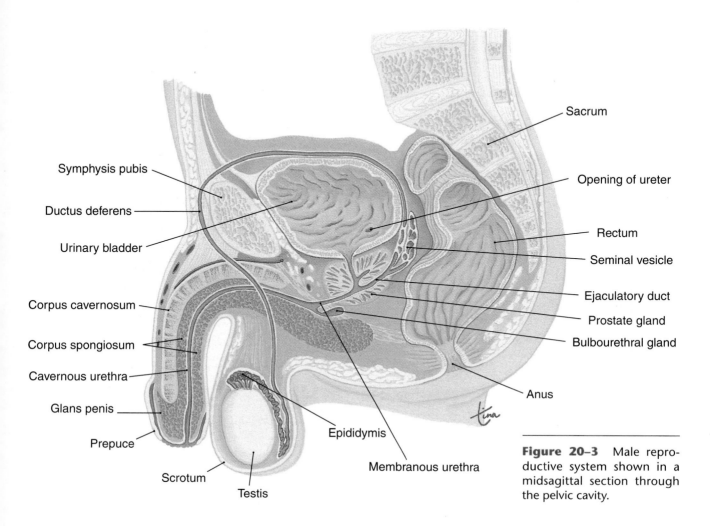

Symphysis pubis

Ductus deferens

Urinary bladder

Corpus cavernosum

Corpus spongiosum

Cavernous urethra

Glans penis

Prepuce

Scrotum

Testis

Epididymis

Membranous urethra

Sacrum

Opening of ureter

Rectum

Seminal vesicle

Ejaculatory duct

Prostate gland

Bulbourethral gland

Anus

Figure 20–3 Male reproductive system shown in a midsagittal section through the pelvic cavity.

bacterial population of the vagina. The alkalinity of seminal fluid helps neutralize the acidic vaginal pH and permits sperm motility in what might otherwise be an unfavorable environment.

URETHRA—PENIS

The **urethra** is the last of the ducts through which semen travels, and its longest portion is enclosed within the penis. The **penis** is an external genital organ; its distal end is called the glans penis and is covered with a fold of skin called the prepuce or foreskin. **Circumcision** is the surgical removal of the foreskin. This is a common procedure performed on male infants, although there is considerable medical debate as to whether circumcision truly has a useful purpose.

Within the penis are three masses of cavernous (erectile) tissue (see Fig. 20–3). Each consists of a framework of smooth muscle and connective tissue that contains blood sinuses, which are large, irregular vascular channels.

When blood flow through these sinuses is minimal, the penis is flaccid. During sexual stimulation, the arteries to the penis dilate, the sinuses fill with blood, and the penis becomes erect and firm. The dilation of penile arteries and the resulting erection are brought about by parasympathetic impulses. The erect penis is capable of penetrating the female vagina to deposit sperm. The culmination of sexual stimulation is ejaculation, a sympathetic response which is brought about by peristalsis of all of the reproductive ducts, and contraction of the prostate gland and the muscles of the pelvic floor.

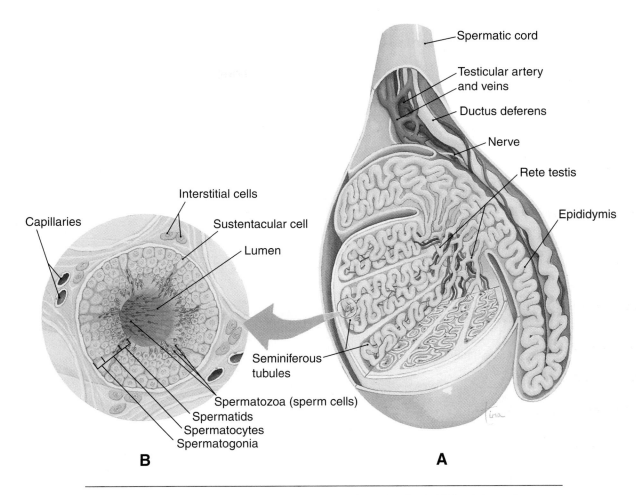

Figure 20–4   **(A)** Midsagittal section of portion of a testis; the epididymis is on the posterior side of the testis. **(B)** Cross-section through a seminiferous tubule showing development of sperm.

SEMEN

Semen consists of sperm and the secretions of the seminal vesicles, prostate gland, and bulbourethral glands; its average pH is about 7.4. During ejaculation, approximately 2 to 4 ml of semen is expelled. Each milliliter of semen contains about 100 million sperm cells.

FEMALE REPRODUCTIVE SYSTEM

The female reproductive system consists of the paired ovaries and fallopian tubes, the single uterus and vagina, and the external genital structures (Fig. 20–5). Egg cells (ova) are produced in the ovaries and travel through the fallopian tubes to the uterus. The uterus is the site for the growth of the embryo-fetus.

OVARIES

The **ovaries** are a pair of oval structures about 1.5 inches (4 cm) long on either side of the uterus in the pelvic cavity (Fig. 20–6). The ovarian ligament extends from the medial side of an ovary to the uterine wall, and the broad ligament is a fold of the peritoneum that covers the ovaries. These ligaments help keep the ovaries in place.

Within an ovary are several hundred thousand **primary follicles**, which are present at birth. During a woman's childbearing years, only 300 to 400 of these follicles will produce mature ova. As with

Table 20–1 | HORMONES OF MALE REPRODUCTION

Hormone	Secreted by	Functions
FSH	Anterior pituitary	• Initiates production of sperm in the testes
LH (ICSH)	Anterior pituitary	• Stimulates secretion of testosterone by the testes
Testosterone*	Testes (interstitial cells)	• Promotes maturation of sperm • Initiates development of the secondary sex characteristics: —growth of the reproductive organs —growth of the larynx —growth of facial and body hair —increased protein synthesis, especially in skeletal muscles
Inhibin	Testes (sustentacular cells)	• Decreases secretion of FSH to maintain constant rate of spermatogenesis

* In both sexes, testosterone (from the adrenal cortex in women) contributes to sex drive and muscle-protein synthesis.

Box 20–2   CONTRACEPTION

There are several methods of contraception, or birth control; some are more effective than others.

Sterilization—Sterilization in men involves a relatively simple procedure called a **vasectomy**. The ductus (vas) deferens is accessible in the scrotum, in which a small incision is made on either side. The ductus is then sutured and cut. Although sperm are still produced in the testes, they cannot pass the break in the ductus, and they simply die and are reabsorbed.

Sterilization in women is usually accomplished by **tubal ligation**, the suturing and severing of the fallopian tubes. Usually this can be done by way of a small incision in the abdominal wall. Ova cannot pass the break in the tube, nor can sperm pass from the uterine side to fertilize an ovum.

When done properly, these forms of surgical sterilization are virtually 100% effective.

Oral contraceptives ("the pill")—Birth control pills contain progesterone and estrogen in varying proportions. They prevent ovulation by inhibiting the secretion of FSH and LH from the anterior pituitary gland. When taken according to sched-ule, birth control pills are about 98% effective. Some women report side effects such as headaches, weight gain, and nausea. Women who use this method of contraception should not smoke, because smoking seems to be associated with abnormal clotting and a greater risk of heart attack or stroke.

Barrier methods—These include the condom, diaphragm, and cervical cap, which prevent sperm from reaching the uterus and fallopian tubes. The use of a spermicide (sperm-killing chemical) increases the effectiveness of these methods. A condom is a latex or rubber sheath that covers the penis and collects and contains ejaculated semen. Leakage is possible, however, and the condom is considered 80% to 90% effective. This is the only contraceptive method that decreases the spread of sexually transmitted diseases.

The diaphragm and cervical cap are plastic structures that are inserted into the vagina to cover the cervix. They are about 80% effective. These methods should not be used, however, by women with vaginal infections or abnormal Pap smears or who have had toxic shock syndrome.

sperm production in men, the supply of potential gametes far exceeds what is actually needed, but this helps ensure the continuation of the human species.

Each primary ovarian follicle contains an oocyte, a potential ovum or egg cell. Surrounding the oocyte are the follicle cells, which secrete estrogen. Maturation of a follicle, requiring FSH and estrogen, was described previously in the section on oogenesis. A mature follicle may also be called a **graafian follicle**, and the hormone LH from the anterior pituitary gland causes ovulation, that is, rupture of the mature follicle with release of the ovum. At this time, other devel-

Box 20–3   PROSTATIC HYPERTROPHY

Prostatic hypertrophy is enlargement of the prostate gland. Benign prostatic hypertrophy is a common occurrence in men over the age of 60 years. The enlarged prostate compresses the urethra within it and may make urination difficult or result in urinary retention. A prostatectomy is a surgical procedure to remove part or all of the prostate. A possible consequence is that ejaculation may be impaired. Many experimental surgical procedures are now undergoing clinical trials to determine if they are more likely to preserve sexual function. Other research involves the use of new medications to shrink enlarged prostate tissue.

Cancer of the prostate is the second most common cancer among men (lung cancer is first). Most cases occur in men over the age of 50 years. Treatment may include surgery to remove the prostate, radiation therapy, or hormone therapy to reduce the patient's level of testosterone.

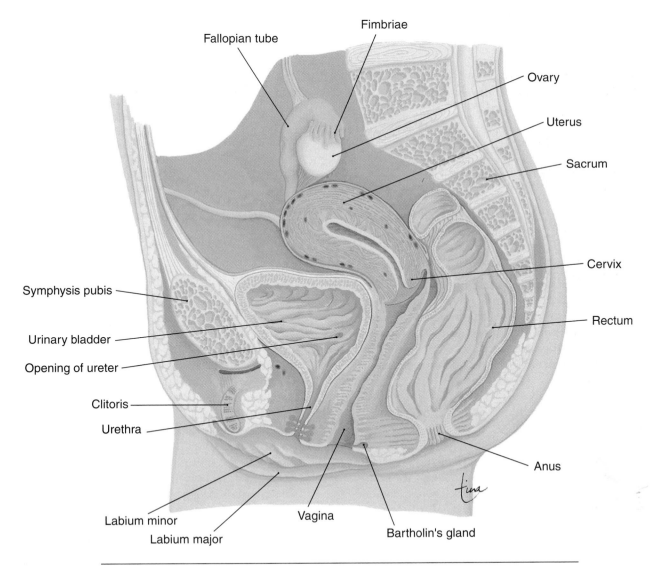

Figure 20–5   Female reproductive system shown in a midsagittal section through the pelvic cavity.

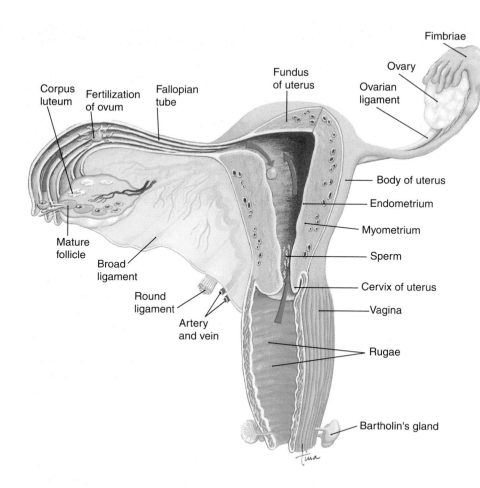

Corpus luteum

Fertilization of ovum

Fallopian tube

Fundus of uterus

Fimbriae

Ovary

Ovarian ligament

Body of uterus

Endometrium

Myometrium

Sperm

Cervix of uterus

Vagina

Rugae

Bartholin's gland

Mature follicle

Broad ligament

Round ligament

Artery and vein

Figure 20–6   Female reproductive system shown in anterior view. The left ovary has been sectioned to show the developing follicles. The left fallopian tube has been sectioned to show fertilization. The uterus and vagina have been sectioned to show internal structures. Arrows indicate the movement of the ovum toward the uterus and the movement of sperm from the vagina toward the fallopian tube.

oping follicles begin to deteriorate; these are called **atretic follicles** and have no further purpose. Under the influence of LH, the ruptured follicle becomes the **corpus luteum** and begins to secrete progesterone as well as estrogen. Hormones produced in smaller amounts by the corpus luteum are inhibin and relaxin.

FALLOPIAN TUBES

There are two fallopian tubes (also called uterine tubes or oviducts); each is about 4 inches (10 cm) long. The lateral end of a fallopian tube encloses an ovary, and the medial end opens into the uterus. The end of the tube that encloses the ovary has **fimbriae**, fringe-like projections that create currents in the fluid surrounding the ovary to pull the ovum into the fallopian tube.

Because the ovum has no means of self-locomotion (as do sperm), the structure of the fallopian tube

ensures that the ovum will be kept moving toward the uterus. The smooth muscle layer of the tube contracts in peristaltic waves that help propel the ovum (or zygote, as you will see in a moment). The mucosa is extensively folded and is made of ciliated epithelial tissue. The sweeping action of the cilia also moves the ovum toward the uterus.

Fertilization usually takes place in the fallopian tube. If not fertilized, an ovum dies within 24 to 48 hours and disintegrates, either in the tube or the uterus. If fertilized, the ovum becomes a zygote and is swept into the uterus; this takes about 4 to 5 days (see Box 20–4: *In Vitro* Fertilization).

Sometimes the zygote will not reach the uterus but will still continue to develop. This is called an **ectopic pregnancy**; *ectopic* means in an abnormal site. The developing embryo may become implanted in the fallopian tube, the ovary itself, or even elsewhere in the abdominal cavity. An ectopic pregnancy usually does not progress very long, because these other sites

In vitro **fertilization** is fertilization outside the body, usually in a glass dish. A woman who wishes to conceive by this method is given FSH to stimulate the simultaneous development of several ovarian follicles. LH may then be given to stimulate simultaneous ovulation. The ova are removed by way of a small incision in the abdominal wall and are placed in a solution containing the sperm of the woman's partner (or an anonymous donor). After fertilization and the first mitotic divisions of cleavage, the very early embryo is placed in the woman's uterus.

It is also possible to mix the removed ova with sperm and return them almost immediately to the woman's fallopian tube. Development then proceeds as if the ova had been fertilized naturally.

Since the birth of the first "test tube baby" in 1978, many thousands of babies have been born following *in vitro* fertilization. The techniques are not always successful, and repeated attempts can be very expensive.

are not specialized to provide a placenta or to expand to accommodate the growth of a fetus, as the uterus is. The spontaneous termination of an ectopic pregnancy is usually the result of bleeding in the mother, and surgery may be necessary to prevent maternal death from circulatory shock. Occasionally an ectopic pregnancy does go to full term and produces a healthy baby; such an event is a credit to the adaptability of the human body and to the advances of medical science.

UTERUS

The **uterus** is shaped like an upside-down pear, about 3 inches long by 2 inches wide (7.5 × 5 cm), superior to the urinary bladder and between the two ovaries in the pelvic cavity (see Fig. 20–5). The broad ligament also covers the uterus (see Fig. 20–6). During pregnancy the uterus increases greatly in size, contains the placenta to nourish the embryo-fetus, and expels the baby at the end of gestation.

The parts and layers of the uterus are shown in Fig. 20–6. The **fundus** is the upper portion above the entry of the fallopian tubes, and the **body** is the large central portion. The narrow, lower end of the uterus is the **cervix**, which opens into the vagina.

The outermost layer of the uterus, the serosa or epimetrium, is a fold of the peritoneum. The **myometrium** is the smooth muscle layer; during pregnancy these cells increase in size to accommodate the growing fetus and contract for labor and delivery at the end of pregnancy.

The lining of the uterus is the **endometrium**, which itself consists of two layers. The **basilar layer**, adjacent to the myometrium, is vascular but very thin and is a permanent layer. The **functional layer** is regenerated and lost during each menstrual cycle. Under the influence of estrogen and progesterone from the ovaries, the growth of blood vessels thickens the functional layer in preparation for a possible embryo. If fertilization does not occur, the functional layer sloughs off in menstruation. During pregnancy, the endometrium forms the maternal portion of the placenta.

VAGINA

The **vagina** is a muscular tube about 4 inches (10 cm) long that extends from the cervix to the vaginal orifice in the **perineum** (pelvic floor). It is posterior to the urethra and anterior to the rectum (see Fig. 20–5). The vaginal opening is usually partially covered by a thin membrane called the **hymen**, which is ruptured by the first sexual intercourse or by the use of tampons during the menstrual period.

The functions of the vagina are to receive sperm from the penis during sexual intercourse, to serve as the exit for the menstrual blood flow, and to serve as the birth canal at the end of pregnancy.

The vaginal mucosa after puberty is stratified squamous epithelium, which is relatively resistant to pathogens. The normal flora (bacteria) of the vagina creates an acidic pH that helps inhibit the growth of pathogens (see Box 20–5: Sexually Transmitted Diseases [STDs]).

EXTERNAL GENITALS

The female external genital structures may also be called the **vulva** (Fig. 20–7), and include the clitoris,

Box 20–5   SEXUALLY TRANSMITTED DISEASES (STDs)

Gonorrhea—caused by the bacterium *Neisseria gonorrhoeae*. Infected men have urethritis with painful and frequent urination and pus in the urine. Women are often asymptomatic, and the bacteria may spread from the cervix to other reproductive organs (pelvic inflammatory disease [PID]). The use of antibiotics in the eyes of all newborns has virtually eliminated neonatal conjunctivitis acquired from an infected mother. Gonorrhea can be treated with antibiotics, but resistant strains of the bacteria complicate treatment. Despite this, the number of reported cases of gonorrhea has been decreasing in recent years.

Syphilis—caused by the bacterium *Treponema pallidum*. Although syphilis can be cured with penicillin, it is a disease that may be ignored by the person who has it because the symptoms may seem minor and often do not last long. If untreated, however, syphilis may cause severe or even fatal damage to the nervous system and heart. In the last few years the number of reported cases of syphilis has been decreasing, and the CDC has hopes of eradicating syphilis in the United States.

Genital herpes—caused by the virus Herpes simplex (usually type 2). Painful lesions in the geni-

tal area are the primary symptom. Although the lesions heal within 5 to 9 days, recurrences are possible, perhaps triggered by physiological stresses such as illness. Although herpes is not curable at present, medications have proved useful in suppressing recurrences. It is estimated that 2 million new cases of genital herpes occur every year.

Neonatal herpes is infection of a newborn during passage through the birth canal. The infant's immune system is too immature to control the herpes virus, and this infection may be fatal or cause brain damage. A pregnant woman with a history of genital herpes may choose to have the baby delivered by cesarean section to avoid this possible outcome.

Chlamydial infection—caused by the very simple bacterium *Chlamydia trachomatis*. This is one of the most prevalent STDs in the United States, with estimates of 4 million new cases yearly. Infected men may have urethritis or epididymitis. Women often have no symptoms at first but may develop PID that increases the risk of ectopic pregnancy. Infants born to infected women may develop conjunctivitis or pneumonia. Chlamydial infection can be successfully treated with antibiotics such as erythromycin or azithromycin.

labia majora and minora, and the Bartholin's glands (see Fig. 20–5).

The **clitoris** is a small mass of erectile tissue anterior to the urethral orifice. The only function of the clitoris is sensory, it responds to sexual stimulation, and its vascular sinuses become filled with blood.

The mons pubis is a pad of fat over the pubic symphysis, covered with skin and pubic hair. Extending posteriorly from the mons are the **labia majora** (lateral) and **labia minora** (medial), which are paired folds of skin. The area between the labia minora is called the vestibule and contains the openings of the

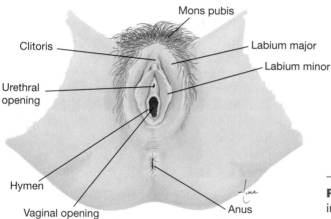

Figure 20–7   Female external genitals (vulva) shown in inferior view of the perineum.

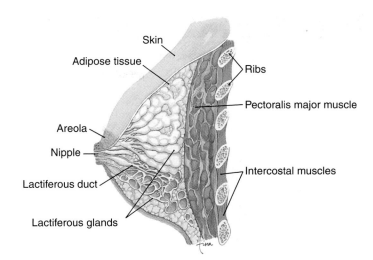

Skin

Adipose tissue

Ribs

Pectoralis major muscle

Areola

Nipple

Intercostal muscles

Lactiferous duct

Lactiferous glands

Figure 20–8 Mammary gland shown in a midsagittal section.

urethra and vagina. The labia cover these openings and prevent drying of their mucous membranes.

Bartholin's glands, also called vestibular glands (see Figs. 20–5 and 20–6), are within the floor of the vestibule; their ducts open onto the mucosa at the vaginal orifice. The secretion of these glands keeps the mucosa moist and lubricates the vagina during sexual intercourse.

MAMMARY GLANDS

The **mammary glands** are structurally related to the skin but functionally related to the reproductive system because they produce milk for the nourishment of offspring. Enclosed within the breasts, the mammary glands are anterior to the pectoralis major muscles; their structure is shown in Fig. 20–8.

The glandular tissue is surrounded by adipose tissue. The **alveolar glands** produce milk after pregnancy; the milk enters lactiferous ducts which converge at the nipple. The skin around the nipple is a pigmented area called the areola.

The formation of milk is under hormonal control. During pregnancy, high levels of estrogen and progesterone prepare the glands for milk production. **Prolactin** from the anterior pituitary gland causes the actual synthesis of milk after pregnancy. The sucking of the infant on the nipple stimulates the hypothalamus to send nerve impulses to the posterior pituitary gland, which secretes **oxytocin** to cause the release of milk. The effects of these hormones on the mammary glands are summarized in Table 20–2 (see also Box 20–6: Mammography).

THE MENSTRUAL CYCLE

The **menstrual cycle** includes the activity of the hormones of the ovaries and anterior pituitary gland

Table 20–2	HORMONE EFFECTS ON THE MAMMARY GLANDS	
Hormone	**Secreted by**	**Functions**
Estrogen	• Ovary (follicle) • Placenta	• Promotes growth of duct system
Progesterone	• Ovary (corpus luteum) • Placenta	• Promotes growth of secretory cells
Prolactin	• Anterior pituitary	• Promotes production of milk after birth
Oxytocin	• Posterior pituitary (hypothalamus)	• Promotes release of milk

and the resultant changes in the ovaries and uterus. These are all incorporated into Fig. 20–9, which may look complicated at first, but refer to it as you read the following.

Notice first the four hormones involved: **FSH** and **LH** from the anterior pituitary gland, **estrogen** from the ovarian follicle, and **progesterone** from the corpus luteum. The fluctuations of these hormones are shown as they would occur in an average 28-day cycle. A cycle may be described in terms of three phases: menstrual phase, follicular phase, and luteal phase.

1. **Menstrual phase**—The loss of the functional layer of the endometrium is called **menstruation** or the menses. Although this is actually the end of a menstrual cycle, the onset of menstruation is easily pinpointed and is, therefore, a useful starting point. Menstruation may last 2 to 8 days, with an average of 3 to 6 days. At this time, secretion of FSH is increasing, and several ovarian follicles begin to develop.
2. **Follicular phase**—FSH stimulates growth of ovarian follicles and secretion of estrogen by the follicle cells. The secretion of LH is also increasing but more slowly. FSH and estrogen promote the growth and maturation of the ovum, and estrogen stimulates the growth of blood vessels in the endometrium to regenerate the functional layer.

   This phase ends with ovulation, when a sharp increase in LH causes rupture of a mature ovarian follicle.
3. **Luteal phase**—Under the influence of LH, the ruptured follicle becomes the corpus luteum and

begins to secrete progesterone as well as estrogen. Progesterone stimulates further growth of blood vessels in the functional layer of the endometrium and promotes the storage of nutrients such as glycogen.

As progesterone secretion increases, LH secretion decreases, and if the ovum is not fertilized, the secretion of progesterone also begins to decrease. Without progesterone, the endometrium cannot be maintained and begins to slough off in menstruation. FSH secretion begins to increase (as estrogen and progesterone decrease), and the cycle begins again.

Also secreted by the corpus luteum during a cycle are the hormones inhibin and relaxin. **Inhibin** inhibits the secretion of FSH, and perhaps LH as well, from the anterior pituitary gland. **Relaxin** is believed to inhibit contractions of the myometrium (as does progesterone), which would help make implantation of the early embryo successful.

The 28-day cycle shown in Fig. 20–9 is average. Women may have cycles of anywhere from 23 to 35 days, the normal range. Women who engage in strenuous exercise over prolonged periods of time may experience **amenorrhea**, that is, cessation of menses. This seems to be related to reduction of body fat. Apparently the reproductive cycle ceases if a woman does not have sufficient reserves of energy for herself and a developing fetus. The exact mechanism by which this happens is not completely understood at present (see Box 17–6). Amenorrhea may also accompany states of physical or emotional stress, anorexia nervosa, or various endocrine disorders.

The functions of the hormones of female reproduction are summarized in Table 20–3.

AGING AND THE REPRODUCTIVE SYSTEMS

For women there is a definite end to reproductive capability; this is called the menopause and usually occurs between the ages of 45 and 55. Estrogen secretion decreases; ovulation and menstrual cycles become irregular and finally cease. The decrease in estrogen has other effects as well. Loss of bone matrix may lead to osteoporosis and fractures; an increase in blood cholesterol makes women more likely to develop coronary artery disease; drying of the vaginal

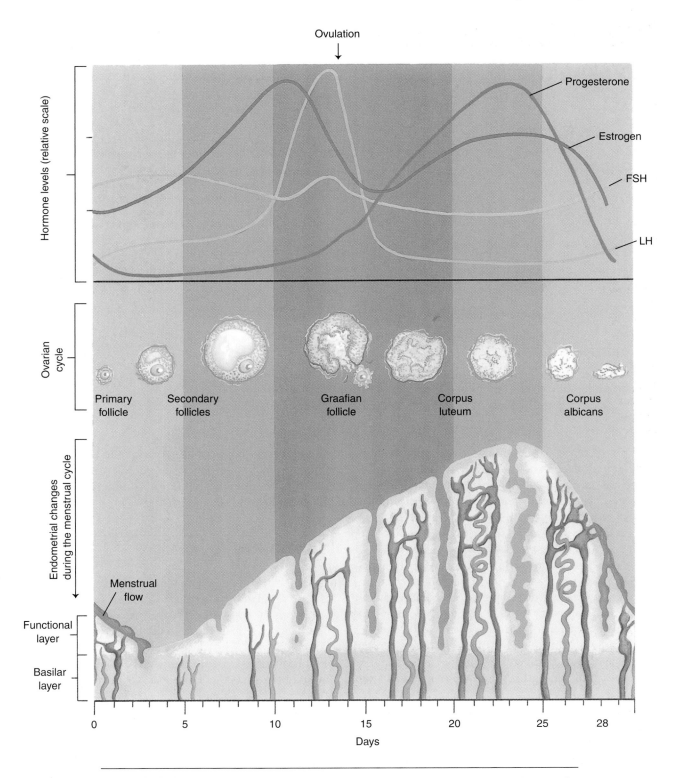

Figure 20–9   The menstrual cycle. The levels of the important hormones are shown relative to one another throughout the cycle. Changes in the ovarian follicle are depicted. The relative thickness of the endometrium is also shown.

Table 20–3	HORMONES OF FEMALE REPRODUCTION	
Hormone	**Secreted by**	**Functions**
FSH	Anterior pituitary	• Initiates development of ovarian follicles • Stimulates secretion of estrogen by follicle cells
LH	Anterior pituitary	• Causes ovulation • Converts the ruptured ovarian follicle into the corpus luteum • Stimulates secretion of progesterone by the corpus luteum

Estrogen*	Ovary (follicle)
	Placenta during pregnancy
		• Promotes maturation of ovarian follicles
		• Promotes growth of blood vessels in the endometrium
		• Initiates development of the secondary sex characteristics:
		  —growth of the uterus and other reproductive organs
		  —growth of the mammary ducts and fat deposition in the breasts
		  —broadening of the pelvic bone
		  —subcutaneous fat deposition in hips and thighs

Progesterone	Ovary (corpus luteum) Placenta during pregnancy	• Promotes further growth of blood vessels in the endometrium and storage of nutrients • Inhibits contractions of the myometrium
Inhibin	Ovary (corpus luteum)	• Inhibits secretion of FSH
Relaxin	Ovary (corpus luteum) Placenta during pregnancy	• Inhibits contractions of the myometrium to facilitate implantation • Promotes stretching of ligaments of the pubic symphysis

* Estrogen has effects on organs such as bones and blood vessels in both men and women. Estrogen is produced in fat tissue in the breasts and hips. In men, testosterone is converted to estrogen in the brain.

mucosa increases susceptibility to vaginal infections. Estrogen replacement therapy may delay some of these consequences of menopause, but there are risks involved, and women should be fully informed of them before starting such therapy. The likelihood of breast cancer also increases with age, and women over age 50 should consider having a mammogram to serve as a baseline, then one at least every other year.

For most men, testosterone secretion continues throughout life, as does sperm production, though both diminish with advancing age. Perhaps the most common reproductive problem for older men is prostatic hypertrophy, enlargement of the prostate gland. As the urethra is compressed, urination becomes difficult, and residual urine in the bladder increases the chance of urinary tract infection. Prostate hypertrophy is usually benign, but cancer of the prostate is one of the more common cancers in elderly men.

SUMMARY

The production of male or female gametes is a process that is regulated by hormones. When fertilization of an ovum by a sperm cell takes place, the zygote, or fertilized egg, has the potential to become a new human being. The development of the zygote to embryo-fetus to newborn infant is also dependent on hormones and is the subject of our next chapter.

STUDY OUTLINE

Reproductive Systems—purpose is to produce gametes (egg and sperm), to ensure fertilization, and in women to provide a site for the embryo-fetus

Meiosis—the cell division process that produces gametes

1. One cell with the diploid number of chromosomes (46) divides twice to form four cells, each with the haploid number of chromosomes (23).
2. Spermatogenesis takes place in the testes; a continuous process from puberty throughout life; each cell produces four functional sperm (see Fig. 20–1). FSH and testosterone are directly necessary (see Table 20–1).
3. Oogenesis takes place in the ovaries; the process is cyclical (every 28 days) from puberty until menopause; each cell produces one functional ovum and three non-functional polar bodies (see Fig. 20–2). FSH, LH, and estrogen, are necessary (see Table 20–3).

Male Reproductive System—consists of the testes and the ducts and glands that contribute to the formation of semen (see Fig. 20–3)

1. Testes (paired)—located in the scrotum between the upper thighs; temperature in the scrotum is 96°F to permit production of viable sperm. Sperm are produced in seminiferous tubules (see Fig. 20–4 and Table 20–1). A sperm cell consists of the head that contains 23 chromosomes, the middle piece that contains mitochondria, the flagellum for motility, and the acrosome on the tip of the head to digest the membrane of the egg cell (see Fig. 20–1).
2. Epididymis (paired)—a long coiled tube on the posterior surface of each testis (see Fig. 20–4). Sperm complete their maturation here.
3. Ductus deferens (paired)—extends from the epididymis into the abdominal cavity through the inguinal canal, over and down behind the urinary bladder to join the ejaculatory duct (see Fig. 20–3). Smooth muscle in the wall contracts in waves of peristalsis.
4. Ejaculatory ducts (paired)—receive sperm from the ductus deferens and the secretions from the seminal vesicles (see Fig. 20–3); empty into the urethra.

5. Seminal vesicles (paired)—posterior to urinary bladder; duct of each opens into ejaculatory duct (see Fig. 20–3). Secretion contains fructose to nourish sperm and is alkaline to enhance sperm motility.
6. Prostate gland (single)—below the urinary bladder, encloses the first inch of the urethra (see Fig. 20–3); secretion is alkaline to maintain sperm motility; smooth muscle contributes to the force required for ejaculation.
7. Bulbourethral glands (paired)—below the prostate gland; empty into the urethra (see Fig. 20–3); secretion is alkaline to line the urethra prior to ejaculation.
8. Urethra (single)—within the penis; carries semen to exterior (see Fig. 20–3). The penis contains three masses of erectile tissue that have blood sinuses. Sexual stimulation and parasympathetic impulses cause dilation of the penile arteries and an erection. Ejaculation of semen involves peristalsis of all male ducts and contraction of the prostate gland and pelvic floor.
9. Semen—composed of sperm and the secretions of the seminal vesicles, prostate gland, and bulbourethral glands. The alkaline pH (7.4) neutralizes the acidic pH of the female vagina.

Female Reproductive System—consists of the ovaries, fallopian tubes, uterus, vagina, and external genitals

1. Ovaries (paired)—located on either side of the uterus (see Fig. 20–6). Egg cells are produced in ovarian follicles; each ovum contains 23 chromosomes. Ovulation of a graafian follicle is stimulated by LH (see Table 20–3).
2. Fallopian tubes (paired)—each extends from an ovary to the uterus (see Fig. 20–6); fimbriae sweep the ovum into the tube; ciliated epithelial tissue and peristalsis of smooth muscle propel the ovum toward the uterus; fertilization usually takes place in the fallopian tube.
3. Uterus (single)—superior to the urinary bladder and between the two ovaries (see Fig. 20–5). Myometrium is the smooth muscle layer that contracts for delivery (see Fig. 20–6). Endometrium is the lining which may become the placenta; basilar layer is permanent; functional layer is lost

in menstruation and regenerated. Parts: upper fundus, central body, and lower cervix.

4. Vagina (single)—extends from the cervix to the vaginal orifice (see Figs. 20–5 and 20–6). Receives sperm during intercourse; serves as exit for menstrual blood and as the birth canal during delivery. Normal flora provide an acidic pH that inhibits the growth of pathogens.

5. External genitals (see Figs. 20–5 and 20–7)—also called the vulva. The clitoris is a small mass of erectile tissue that responds to sexual stimulation; labia majora and minora are paired folds of skin that enclose the vestibule and cover the urethral and vaginal openings; Bartholin's glands open into the vaginal orifice and secrete mucus.

Mammary Glands—anterior to the pectoralis major muscles, surrounded by adipose tissue (see Fig. 20–8)

1. Alveolar glands produce milk; lactiferous ducts converge at the nipple.
2. Hormonal regulation—see Table 20–2.

The Menstrual Cycle—average is 28 days; includes the hormones FSH, LH, estrogen, and progesterone, and changes in the ovaries and endometrium (see Fig. 20–9 and Table 20–3)

1. Menstrual phase—loss of the endometrium.
2. Follicular phase—several ovarian follicles develop; ovulation is the rupture of a mature follicle; blood vessels grow in the endometrium.
3. Luteal phase—the ruptured follicle becomes the corpus luteum; the endometrium continues to develop.
4. If fertilization does not occur, decreased progesterone results in the loss of the endometrium in menstruation.

REVIEW QUESTIONS

1. Describe spermatogenesis and oogenesis in terms of site, number of functional cells produced by each cell that undergoes meiosis, and timing of the process. (p. 434)

2. Describe the functions of FSH, LH, inhibin, and testosterone in spermatogenesis. Describe the functions of FSH and estrogen in oogenesis. (p. 434)

3. Describe the locations of the testes and epididymides, and explain their functions. (pp. 435–437)

4. Name all the ducts, in order, that sperm travel through from the testes to the urethra. (p. 435)

5. Name the male reproductive glands, and state how each contributes to the formation of semen. (pp. 437–438)

6. Explain how the structure of cavernous tissue permits erection of the penis. Name the structures that bring about ejaculation. (p. 438)

7. State the function of each part of a sperm cell: head, middle piece, flagellum, and acrosome. (p. 436)

8. Describe the location of the ovaries, and name the hormones produced by the ovaries. (pp. 439–442)

9. Explain how an ovum or zygote is kept moving through the fallopian tube. (p. 442)

10. Describe the function of myometrium, basilar layer of the endometrium, and functional layer of the endometrium. Name the hormones necessary for growth of the endometrium. (p. 443)

11. State the functions of the vagina, labia majora and minora, and Bartholin's glands. (pp. 444–445)

12. Name the parts of the mammary glands, and state the function of each. (p. 445)

13. Name the hormone that has each of these effects on the mammary glands: (p. 445)
    a. Causes release of milk
    b. Promotes growth of the ducts
    c. Promotes growth of the secretory cells
    d. Stimulates milk production

14. Name the phase of the menstrual cycle in which each takes place: (p. 446)
    a. Rupture of a mature follicle
    b. Loss of the endometrium
    c. Final development of the endometrium
    d. The corpus luteum develops
    e. Several ovarian follicles begin to develop

FOR FURTHER THOUGHT

1. Compare meiosis to mitosis in terms of number of divisions, number of cells produced, number of chromosomes in each cell, and purpose of the cells produced.

2. An ovum is released by a mature ovarian follicle, but the subsequent corpus luteum does not secrete progesterone. If the ovum is fertilized, is implantation possible? Is a full-term pregnancy possible? Explain your answers.

3. A sexually transmitted disease such as gonorrhea is usually symptomatic for men, but quite often women do not have symptoms. Explain the consequences of this, and to whom those consequences apply.

4. Some textbooks or articles speak of the genitourinary system or the urogenital system. Is this terminology correct for everyone? For anyone? If it is correct for some, describe what the two systems share anatomically.

5. The reproductive system may seem a bit isolated from other body systems in that its purpose is to create new life, not just maintain existing life. But there are significant relationships between the reproductive system and other body systems. Name three organ systems that the reproductive system especially depends upon, and briefly explain that dependence. Then name two systems whose anatomy or physiology is influenced by the hormones of the reproductive system, and describe these influences.

CHAPTER 21

Chapter Outline

Human Development
Fertilization
Implantation
Embryo and Embryonic Membranes
Placenta and Umbilical Cord
    Placental hormones
Parturition and Labor
The Infant at Birth

Genetics
Chromosomes and Genes
Genotype and Phenotype
Inheritance: Dominant–Recessive
Inheritance: Multiple Alleles
Inheritance: Sex-Linked Traits

Box 21–1	TWINS
Box 21–2	FETAL DIAGNOSIS
Box 21–3	CONGENITAL FETAL INFECTIONS
Box 21–4	FETAL ALCOHOL SYNDROME
Box 21–5	PREMATURE BIRTH
Box 21–6	APGAR SCORE
Box 21–7	SOLUTION TO GENETICS QUESTION

Student Objectives

- Describe the process of fertilization and cleavage to the blastocyst stage.
- Explain when, where, and how implantation of the embryo occurs.
- Describe the functions of the embryonic membranes.
- Describe the structure and functions of the placenta and umbilical cord.
- Name and explain the functions of the placental hormones.
- State the length of the average gestation period, and describe the stages of labor.
- Describe the major changes in the infant at birth.
- Describe some important maternal changes during pregnancy.
- Explain homologous chromosomes, autosomes, sex chromosomes, and genes.
- Define alleles, genotype, phenotype, homozygous, and heterozygous.
- Explain the following patterns of inheritance: dominant–recessive, multiple alleles, and sex-linked traits.

Human Development and Genetics

New Terminology

Alleles (uh-**LEELZ**)
Amnion (**AM**-nee-on)
Amniotic fluid (**AM**-nee-AH-tik **FLOO**-id)
Autosomes (**AW**-toh-sohms)
Cleavage (**KLEE**-vije)
Embryo (**EM**-bree-oh)
Genotype (**JEE**-noh-type)
Gestation (jes-**TAY**-shun)
Heterozygous (HET-er-oh-**ZYE**-gus)
Homologous pair (hoh-**MAHL**-ah-gus PAYR)
Homozygous (HOH-moh-**ZYE**-gus)
Implantation (IM-plan-**TAY**-shun)
Labor (**LAY**-ber)
Parturition (PAR-tyoo-**RISH**-uhn)
Phenotype (**FEE**-noh-type)
Sex chromosome (SEKS **KROH**-muh-sohm)

Related Clinical Terminology

Amniocentesis (AM-nee-oh-sen-**TEE**-sis)
Apgar score (**APP**-gar SKOR)
Cesarean section (se-**SAR**-ee-an **SEK**-shun)
Chorionic villus sampling (KOR-ee-**ON**-ik **VILL**–us)
Congenital (kon-**JEN**-i-tuhl)
Fetal alcohol syndrome (**FEE**-tuhl **AL**-koh-hol)
Teratogen (te-**RAH**-toh-jen)

*Terms that appear in **bold type** in the chapter text are defined in the glossary, which begins on page 521.*

How often have we heard comments like "She has her mother's eyes" or "That nose is just like his father's"—because people cannot resist comparing a newborn to its parents. Although a child may not resemble either parent, there is a sound basis for such comparisons, because the genetic makeup and many of the traits of a child are the result of the chromosomes inherited from mother and father.

In this chapter, we will cover some of the fundamentals of genetics and inheritance. First, however, we will look at the development of a fertilized egg into a functioning human being.

HUMAN DEVELOPMENT

During the 40 weeks of gestation, the embryo-fetus is protected and nourished in the uterus of the mother. A human being begins life as one cell, a fertilized egg called a zygote, which develops into an individual human being consisting of billions of cells organized into the body systems with whose functions you are now quite familiar.

FERTILIZATION

Although millions of sperm are deposited in the vagina during sexual intercourse, only one will fertilize an ovum. As the sperm swim through the fluid of the uterus and fallopian tube, they undergo a final metabolic change, called **capacitation**. This change involves the **acrosome**, which becomes more fragile and begins to secrete its enzymes. When sperm and egg make contact, these enzymes will digest the layers of cells and membrane around an ovum.

Once a sperm nucleus enters the ovum, changes in the egg cell membrane block the entry of other sperm. The nucleus of the ovum completes the second meiotic division, and the nuclei of ovum and sperm fuse, restoring the diploid number of chromosomes in the zygote.

The human diploid number of 46 chromosomes is actually 23 pairs of chromosomes; 23 from the sperm and 23 from the egg. These 23 pairs consist of 22 pairs of **autosomes** (designated by the numerals 1 through 22) and one pair of **sex chromosomes**. Women have the sex chromosomes XX, and men have the sex chromosomes XY. Figure 21–1 shows the inheritance of gender. The Y chromosome has a gene that triggers the development of male gonads in the embryo. In the absence of the Y chromosome, the embryo will develop as a female.

IMPLANTATION

Fertilization usually takes place within the fallopian tube, and the zygote begins to divide even as it is being swept toward the uterus. These are mitotic divisions and are called **cleavage**. Refer to Fig. 21–2 as you read the following.

The single-cell zygote divides into a two-cell stage, four-cell stage, eight-cell stage, and so on. Three days after fertilization there are 16 cells, which continue to divide to form a solid sphere of cells called a **morula** (see Box 21–1: Twins). As mitosis proceeds, this sphere becomes hollow and is called a **blastocyst**, which is still about the same size as the original zygote.

A fluid-filled blastocyst consists of an outer layer of cells called the **trophoblast** and an inner cell mass that contains the potential embryo. It is the blastocyst stage that becomes **implanted** in the uterine wall, about 7 to 8 days after fertilization. The trophoblast secretes enzymes to digest the surface of the endometrium, creating a small crater into which the blastocyst sinks. The trophoblast will become the **chorion**, the embryonic membrane that will form the fetal portion of the placenta. Following implantation, the inner cell mass will grow to become the embryo and other membranes.

The cells of the inner cell mass are embryonic stem cells. In these cells, all of the DNA has the potential for being switched on, that is, the potential exists for a cell to develop into any of the 200 kinds of human cells that will be present at birth. As the cells continue to divide and become more numerous, some DNA will be switched off in each cell, genes will become inactive, and the possibilities for the specialization of each cell will be narrowed down. The "switches" are chemicals, most of which are unknown at present. A great deal of research is focusing on discovering the stimuli that turn a stem cell into a muscle cell rather than a nerve cell or skin cell, and so on.

EMBRYO AND EMBRYONIC MEMBRANES

An **embryo** is the developing human individual from the time of implantation until the eighth week of gestation. Several stages of early embryonic development are shown in Fig. 21–3. At approximately 12 days, the **embryonic disc** (the potential person) is

Figure 21–1   Inheritance of gender. Each ovum contains 22 autosomes and an X chromosome. Each sperm contains 22 autosomes and either an X chromosome or a Y chromosome.

simply a plate of cells within the blastocyst. As cells keep dividing, the plate of cells begins to fold. At 14 days twinning is believed to be no longer possible. Very soon thereafter, three primary layers, or germ layers, begin to develop: the **ectoderm, mesoderm**, and **endoderm**. This is a major step in the specialization of the embryo cells, because different sets of genes are switched off for each of the three layers, while the genes appropriate for the layer remain switched on. Each cell is now committed to a particular layer, and can no longer "go back," that is, become a cell of either of the other two layers.

Each primary layer develops further; its cells become more specialized as more and more genes in each cell are switched off. With the active genes, those that remain switched on, the cells in each layer are thereby committed to develop into specific organs or parts of organs. *Ecto* means "outer"; the epidermis is derived from ectoderm, and in some of these cells the gene for producing keratin is active. *Meso* means "middle"; the skeletal muscles develop from mesoderm, and in these cells the genes for producing myosin and actin are active. *Endo* means "inner"; the

stomach lining is derived from endoderm, and in these cells, the gene for producing pepsinogen is active. Table 21–1 lists some other structures derived from each of the primary germ layers.

At 20 days, the **embryonic membranes** can be clearly distinguished from the embryo itself. The **yolk sac** does not contain nutrient yolk, as it does for bird and reptile embryos. It is, however, the site for the formation of the first blood cells and the cells that will become spermatogonia or oogonia. As the embryo grows, the yolk sac membrane is incorporated into the umbilical cord.

The **amnion** is a thin membrane that eventually surrounds the embryo and contains **amniotic fluid**. This fluid provides a cushion for the fetus against mechanical injury as the mother moves. When the fetal kidneys become functional, they excrete urine into the amniotic fluid. Also in this fluid are cells that have sloughed off the fetus; this is clinically important in the procedure called amniocentesis (see Box 21–2: Fetal Diagnosis). The rupture of the amnion (sometimes called the "bag of waters") is usually an indication that labor has begun.

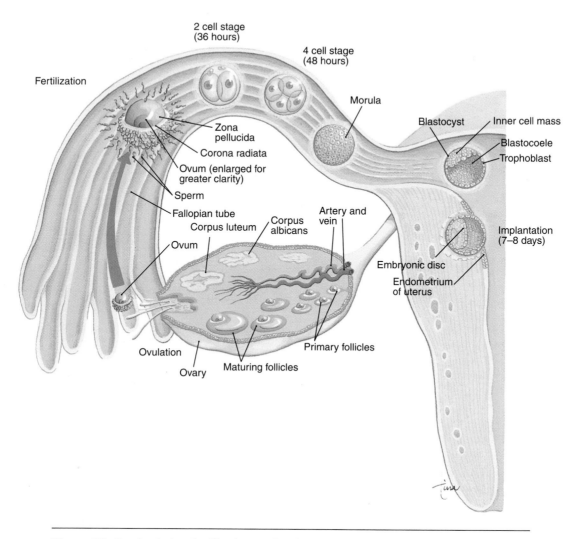

Figure 21–2   Ovulation, fertilization, and early embryonic development. Fertilization takes place in the fallopian tube, and the embryo has reached the blastocyst stage when it becomes implanted in the endometrium of the uterus.

Box 21–1   TWINS

Fraternal twins are the result of two separate ova fertilized by separate sperm. This may occur when two ovarian follicles reach maturity and rupture at the same time. Fraternal twins may be of the same sex or different sexes. Even if of the same sex, however, they are as genetically different as any siblings might be.

Identical twins are the result of the splitting of the very early embryo before the cells start to become specialized. For example, if a 16-cell stage becomes separated into two groups of eight cells each, each group will usually continue to develop in the usual way. Another possible cause is the development of two inner cell masses within the blastocyst. This, too, is before significant specialization has taken place, and each inner cell mass may develop into a complete individual. Twins of this type may be called monozygotic, meaning that they have come from one fertilized egg. Identical twins are always of the same sex, are very much alike in appearance, and in other respects are genetically identical.

Figure 21–3 Embryonic development at 12 days (after fertilization), 14 days, 20 days, and 4 to 5 weeks. By 5 weeks, the embryo has distinct parts but does not yet look definitely human. See text for description of embryonic membranes.

The **chorion** is the name given to the trophoblast as it develops further. Once the embryo has become implanted in the uterus, small projections called **chorionic villi** begin to grow into the endometrium. These will contain the fetal blood vessels that become the fetal portion of the placenta.

At about 4 to 5 weeks of development, the embryo shows definite form. The head is apparent, the heart is beating, and limb buds are visible. The period of embryonic growth continues until the 8th week. At

this time, all of the organ systems have been established. They will continue to grow and mature until the end of gestation. The period of fetal growth extends from the 9th through the 40th week. Table 21–2 lists some of the major aspects of development in the growth of the embryo-fetus. The fetus at 16 weeks is depicted in Fig. 21–4 (see Box 21–3: Congenital Fetal Infections, and Box 21–4: Fetal Alcohol Syndrome). Maternal changes during pregnancy are summarized in Table 21–3.

Table 21–1 | STRUCTURES DERIVED FROM THE PRIMARY GERM LAYERS

Layer	Structures Derived*
Ectoderm	• Epidermis; hair and nail follicles; sweat glands • Nervous system; pituitary gland; adrenal medulla • Lens and cornea; internal ear • Mucosa of oral and nasal cavities; salivary glands
Mesoderm	• Dermis; bone and cartilage • Skeletal muscles; cardiac muscle; most smooth muscle • Kidneys and adrenal cortex • Bone marrow and blood; lymphatic tissue; lining of blood vessels
Endoderm	• Mucosa of esophagus, stomach, and intestines • Epithelium of respiratory tract, including lungs • Liver and mucosa of gallbladder • Thyroid gland; pancreas

* These are representative lists, not all-inclusive ones. Keep in mind also that most organs are combinations of tissues from each of the three germ layers. Related structures are grouped together.

PLACENTA AND UMBILICAL CORD

The **placenta** is made of both fetal and maternal tissue. The chorion of the embryo and the endometrium of the uterus contribute, and the placenta is formed by the third month of gestation (12 weeks).

The mature placenta is a flat disc about 7 inches (17 cm) in diameter.

The structure of a small portion of the placenta is shown in Fig. 21–5. Notice that the fetal blood vessels are within maternal blood sinuses, but there is no direct connection between fetal and maternal vessels.

Box 21–2   FETAL DIAGNOSIS

Several procedures are currently available to determine certain kinds of abnormalities in a fetus or to monitor development.

Ultrasound (or Fetal Ultrasonography)

This is a non-invasive procedure; high-frequency sound waves are transmitted through the abdominal wall into the uterus. The reflected sound waves are converted to an image called a sonogram. This method is used to confirm multiple pregnancies, fetal age or position, or to detect fetal abnormalities such as heart defects or malformations of other organs.

Amniocentesis

This procedure is usually performed at 16 to 18 weeks of gestation. A hypodermic needle is inserted through the wall of the abdomen into the amniotic sac, and about 10 to 20 ml of amniotic fluid is removed. Within this fluid are fetal cells, which can be cultured so that their chromosomes may be examined. Through such examination and biochem-

ical tests, a number of genetic diseases or chromosome abnormalities may be detected. Because women over the age of 35 years are believed to have a greater chance of having a child with Down syndrome, amniocentesis is often recommended for this age group. A family history of certain genetic diseases is another reason a pregnant woman may wish to have this procedure.

Chorionic Villus Sampling (CVS)

In this procedure, a biopsy catheter is inserted through the vagina and cervix to collect a small portion of the chorionic villi. These cells are derived from the fetus but are not part of the fetus itself. The information obtained is the same as that for amniocentesis, but CVS may be performed earlier in pregnancy, at about 8 weeks. Although there is a risk that the procedure may cause a miscarriage, CVS is considered comparable in safety to amniocentesis. It is important to remember that no invasive procedure is without risks.

Table 21–2	GROWTH OF THE EMBRYO–FETUS	
Month of Gestation (end)	**Aspects of Development**	**Approximate Overall Size in Inches**
1	• Heart begins to beat; limb buds form; backbone forms; facial features not distinct	0.25
2	• Calcification of bones begins; fingers and toes are apparent on limbs; facial features more distinct; body systems are established	1.25–1.5
3	• Facial features distinct but eyes are still closed; nails develop on fingers and toes; ossification of skeleton continues; fetus is distinguishable as male or female	3
4	• Head still quite large in proportion to body, but the arms and legs lengthen; hair appears on head; body systems continue to develop	5–7
5	• Skeletal muscles become active ("quickening" may be felt by the mother); body grows more rapidly than head; body is covered with fine hair (lanugo)	10–12
6	• Eyelashes and eyebrows form; eyelids open; skin is quite wrinkled; pulmonary surfactant is first produced	11–14
7	• Head and body approach normal infant proportions; deposition of subcutaneous fat makes skin less wrinkled	13–17
8	• Testes of male fetus descend into scrotum; more subcutaneous fat is deposited; production of pulmonary surfactant is sufficient to permit breathing if birth is premature	16–18
9	• Lanugo is shed; nails are fully developed; cranial bones are ossified with fontanels present; lungs are more mature	19–21

Normally, the blood of the fetus does not mix with that of the mother. The placenta has two functions: to serve as the site of exchanges between maternal and fetal blood and to produce hormones to maintain pregnancy. We will consider the exchanges first.

The fetus is dependent upon the mother for oxygen and nutrients and for the removal of waste products. The **umbilical cord** connects the fetus to the placenta. Within the cord are two umbilical arteries that carry blood from the fetus to the placenta and one umbilical vein that returns blood from the placenta to the fetus.

When blood in the umbilical arteries enters the placenta, CO_2 and waste products in the fetal capillaries diffuse into the maternal blood sinuses. Oxygen diffuses from the maternal blood sinuses into the fetal capillaries; nutrients enter the fetal blood by diffusion and active transport mechanisms. This oxygen- and nutrient-rich blood then flows through the umbilical vein back to the fetus. Circulation within the fetus was described in Chapter 13.

When the baby is delivered at the end of gestation, the umbilical cord is cut. The placenta then detaches from the uterine wall and is delivered as the **afterbirth**.

Placental Hormones

The first hormone secreted by the placenta is **human chorionic gonadotropin** (hCG), which is produced by the chorion of the early embryo. The function of hCG is to stimulate the corpus luteum in the maternal ovary, so that it will continue to secrete estrogen and progesterone. The secretion of progesterone is particularly important to prevent contractions of the myometrium, which would otherwise result in miscarriage of the embryo. Once hCG enters maternal circulation, it is excreted in urine, which is the basis for many pregnancy tests. Tests for hCG in maternal blood are even more precise and can determine whether a pregnancy has occurred even before a menstrual period is missed.

16 weeks

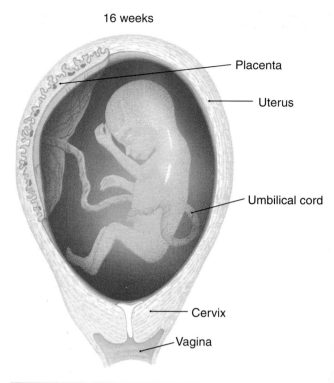

Placenta

Uterus

Umbilical cord

Cervix

Vagina

Figure 21–4   Fetal development at 16 weeks.

The corpus luteum is a small structure, however, and cannot secrete sufficient amounts of estrogen and progesterone to maintain a full-term pregnancy. The placenta itself begins to secrete **estrogen** and **progesterone** within a few weeks, and the levels of these hormones increase until birth. As the placenta takes over, the secretion of hCG decreases, and the corpus luteum becomes non-functional. During pregnancy, estrogen and progesterone inhibit the anterior pituitary secretion of FSH and LH, so no other ovarian follicles develop. These placental hormones also prepare the mammary glands for lactation.

The placenta also secretes **relaxin**, which helps inhibit contractions of the myometrium. Relaxin also permits stretching of the ligaments of the pubic symphysis so that this joint will give a little, if necessary, during birth.

PARTURITION AND LABOR

Parturition is the rather formal term for birth, and **labor** is the sequence of events that occurs during birth. The average gestation period is 40 weeks (280

days), with a range of 37 to 42 weeks (see Box 21–5: Premature Birth). Toward the end of gestation, the placental secretion of progesterone decreases while estrogen level remains high, and the myometrium begins to contract weakly at irregular intervals. At this time the fetus is often oriented head down within the uterus (Fig. 21–6). Labor itself may be divided into three stages.

First stage—dilation of the cervix. As the uterus contracts, the amniotic sac is forced into the cervix, which dilates (widens) the cervical opening. At the end of this stage, the amniotic sac breaks (rupture of the "bag of waters") and the fluid leaves through the vagina, which may now be called the **birth canal**. This stage lasts an average of 8 to 12 hours but may vary considerably.

Second stage—delivery of the infant. More powerful contractions of the uterus are brought about by **oxytocin** released by the posterior pituitary gland and perhaps by the placenta itself. This stage may be prolonged by several factors. If the fetus is positioned other than head down, delivery may be difficult. This is called a breech birth and may necessitate a **cesarean section** (C-section), which is delivery of the fetus through a surgical incision in the abdominal wall and uterus. For some women, the central opening in the pelvic bone may be too small to permit a vaginal delivery. Fetal distress, as determined by fetal monitoring of heartbeat for example, may also require a cesarean section.

Third stage—delivery of the placenta (afterbirth). Continued contractions of the uterus expel the placenta and membranes, usually within 10 minutes after delivery of the infant. There is some bleeding at this time, but the uterus rapidly decreases in size, and the contractions compress the endometrium to close the ruptured blood vessels at the former site of the placenta. This is important to prevent severe maternal hemorrhage.

THE INFANT AT BIRTH

Immediately after delivery, the umbilical cord is clamped and cut, and the infant's nose and mouth are aspirated to remove any fluid that might interfere with breathing (see Box 21–6: Apgar Score). Now the infant is independent of the mother, and the most rapid changes occur in the respiratory and circulatory systems.

As the level of CO_2 in the baby's blood increases, the respiratory center in the medulla is stimulated and

Box 21–3   CONGENITAL FETAL INFECTIONS

A **teratogen** is anything that may cause developmental abnormalities in an embryo-fetus. Several infectious microorganisms are known to be teratogenic; they may cross the placenta from maternal blood to fetal blood and damage the fetus.

Congenital rubella syndrome—the virus of German measles (rubella) is perhaps the best known of the infectious teratogens. If a woman acquires rubella during pregnancy, there is a 20% chance that her fetus will be affected. Consequences for the fetus may be death (stillborn), heart defects, deafness, or mental retardation. Women who have never had rubella should consider receiving the vaccine before they begin to have children. In this way, congenital rubella syndrome is completely prevented.

Congenital varicella syndrome—chickenpox (*Herpes varicella*) is a viral disease that most people have during childhood. If a pregnant woman acquires chickenpox, however, the virus may cross the placenta. Consequences for the fetus include malformed limbs, cutaneous scars, blindness, and mental retardation. Although this is not a common congenital syndrome, women who have never had chickenpox should be educated about it.

Congenital syphilis—syphilis is a sexually transmitted disease caused by a bacterium (*Trepo-nema pallidum*). These bacteria may cross the placenta after the fourth month of gestation. Consequences of early infection of the fetus are death, malformations of bones and teeth, or cataracts. If infection occurs toward the end of gestation, the child may be born with syphilis. This is most often apparent as a rash on the skin and mucous membranes. Syphilis in adults can be cured by penicillin; prevention of congenital syphilis depends upon good prenatal care for women who may be infected. The centers for Disease Control and Prevention has a goal of eradicating syphilis in the United States, which would eliminate fetal infection.

Congenital toxoplasmosis—this condition is caused by the protozoan parasite *Toxoplasma gondii*. For most healthy people, toxoplasmosis has no symptoms at all; it is a harmless infection. Because cats and some other mammals are also hosts for this parasite, pregnant women may acquire infection from contact with cat feces or by eating rare beef or lamb. Consequences for the fetus are death, mental retardation, or blindness. Retinal infection may only become apparent during childhood or adolescence. Prevention now depends upon education of pregnant women to avoid potential sources of infection.

Box 21–4   FETAL ALCOHOL SYNDROME

Fetal alcohol syndrome is the term for a group of characteristics present in infants who were exposed to alcohol during their fetal life. Alcohol is a toxin for adults and even more so for fetal tissues that are immature and growing rapidly. Either alcohol or its toxic intermediate product (acetaldehyde) may pass from maternal to fetal circulation and impair fetal development.

Consequences for infants include low birth weight, small head with facial abnormalities, heart defects, malformation of other organs, and irritability and agitation. The infant often grows slowly, both physically and mentally, and mental retardation is also a possible outcome.

Because there is no way to reverse the damage done by intrauterine exposure to alcohol, the best course is prevention. Education is very important; women should be aware of the consequences their consumption of alcohol may have for a fetus.

brings about inhalation to expand and inflate the lungs. Full expansion of the lungs may take up to 7 days following birth, and the infant's respiratory rate may be very rapid at this time, as high as 40 respirations per minute.

Breathing promotes greater pulmonary circulation, and the increased amount of blood returning to the left atrium closes the flap of the **foramen ovale**. The **ductus arteriosus** begins to constrict, apparently in response to the higher blood oxygen level. Full closure of the ductus arteriosus may take up to 3 months.

The **ductus venosus** no longer receives blood from the umbilical vein and begins to constrict within

Table 21–3	MATERNAL CHANGES DURING PREGNANCY
Aspect	**Change**
Weight	• Gain of 2–3 pounds for each month of gestation
Uterus	• Enlarges considerably and displaces abdominal organs upward
Thyroid gland	• Increases secretion of thyroxine, which increases metabolic rate
Skin	• Appearance of striae (stretch marks) on abdomen
Circulatory system	• Heart rate increases, as do stroke volume and cardiac output; blood volume increases; varicose veins may develop in the legs and anal canal
Digestive system	• Nausea and vomiting may occur in early pregnancy (morning sickness); constipation may occur in later pregnancy
Urinary system	• Kidney activity increases; frequency of urination often increases in later pregnancy (bladder is compressed by uterus)
Respiratory system	• Respiratory rate increases; lung capacity decreases as diaphragm is forced upward by compressed abdominal organs in later pregnancy
Skeletal system	• Lordosis may occur with increased weight at front of abdomen; sacroiliac joints and pubic symphysis become more flexible prior to birth

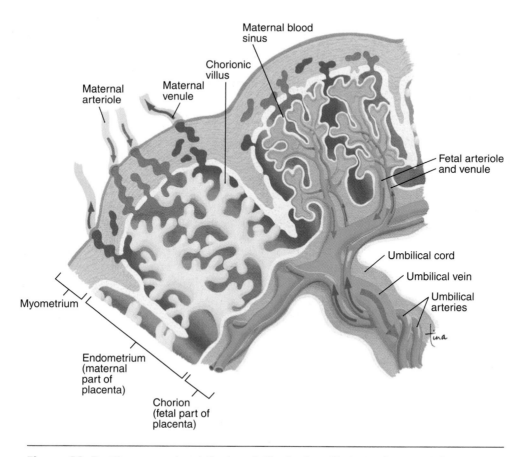

Figure 21–5   Placenta and umbilical cord. The fetal capillaries in chorionic villi are within the maternal blood sinuses. Arrows indicate the direction of blood flow in maternal and fetal vessels.

Box 21–5   PREMATURE BIRTH

A premature birth is the spontaneous delivery of an infant before the end of the gestation period, or the intentional delivery (for reasons concerning the health of the mother or fetus) before that time. A premature infant is one that weighs less than 2500 grams (5.5 pounds).

In terms of gestation time, an 8-month-old infant has a very good chance of surviving if good medical care is available. Infants of 7 months or less have respiratory distress, because their lungs have not yet produced enough surfactant to permit inflation of the alveoli. This is hyaline membrane disease, which was described in Chapter 15.

Infants as young as 24 weeks have been successfully treated and eventually sent home with their parents. Whether there will be any long-term detrimental effects of their very premature births will only be known in time.

Medical science may have reached its maximum capability in this area. In a fetus of 20 weeks, the cells of the alveoli and the cells of the pulmonary capillaries are just not close enough to each other to permit gas exchange. At present there is no medical intervention that can overcome this anatomic fact.

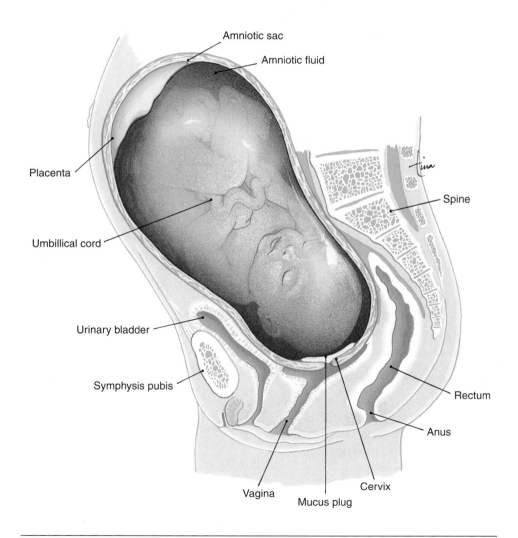

Figure 21–6   Full-term fetus positioned head down within the uterus.

Box 21–6   APGAR SCORE

The Apgar score is an overall assessment of an infant and is usually made 1 minute after birth (may be repeated at 5 minutes if the first score is low). The highest possible score is 10. Infants who score less than 5 require immediate medical attention.

Characteristic	Description	Score
Hearbeat	• Over 100 bpm	2
	• Below 100 bpm	1
	• No heartbeat	0
Respiration	• Strong, vigorous cry	2
	• Weak cry	1
	• No respiratory effort	0
Muscle tone	• Spontaneous, active motion	2
	• Some motion	1
	• No muscle tone	0
Reflex response to stimulation of sole of the foot	• A cry in response	2
	• A grimace in response	1
	• No response	0
Color	• Healthy coloration	2
	• Cyanotic extremities	1
	• Cyanosis of trunk and extremities	0

a few minutes after birth. Within a few weeks the ductus venosus becomes a non-functional ligament.

The infant's liver is not fully mature at birth and may be unable to excrete bilirubin efficiently. This may result in jaundice, which may occur in as many as half of all newborns. Such jaundice is not considered serious unless there is another possible cause, such as Rh incompatibility (see Chapter 11).

GENETICS

Genetics is the study of inheritance. Most, if not virtually all, human characteristics are regulated at least partially by genes. We will first look at what genes are, then describe some patterns of inheritance.

CHROMOSOMES AND GENES

Each of the cells of an individual (except mature RBCs and egg and sperm) contains 46 chromosomes, the diploid number. These chromosomes are in 23 pairs called **homologous pairs**. One member of each pair has come from the egg and is called maternal, the other member has come from the sperm and is called paternal. The autosomes are the chromosome pairs designated 1 to 22. The sex chromosomes form the remaining pair. In women these are designated XX and in men XY.

Chromosomes are made of DNA and protein; the DNA is the hereditary material. You may wish to refer to Chapter 3 to review DNA structure. The sequence of bases in the DNA of chromosomes is the genetic code for proteins; structural proteins as well as enzymes. The DNA code for one protein is called a gene. For example, a specific region of the DNA of chromosome 11 is the code for the beta chain of hemoglobin. Because an individual has two of chromosome 11, he or she will have two genes for this protein, a maternal gene inherited from the mother and a paternal gene inherited from the father. This is true for virtually all of the 30,000 genes estimated to be found in our chromosomes. In our genetic makeup, each of us has two genes for each protein.

GENOTYPE AND PHENOTYPE

For each gene of a pair, there may be two or more possibilities for its "expression," that is, its precise nature or how it will affect the individual. These possibilities are called **alleles**. A person, therefore, may be said to have two alleles for each protein or trait; the alleles may be the same or may be different.

If the two alleles are the same, the person is said to be **homozygous** for the trait. If the two alleles are different, the person is said to be **heterozygous** for the trait.

The **genotype** is the actual genetic makeup, that is, the alleles present. The **phenotype** is the appearance, or how the alleles are expressed. When a gene has two or more alleles, one allele may be **dominant** over the other, which is called **recessive**. For a person who is heterozygous for a trait, the dominant allele (or gene) is the one that will appear in the phenotype. The recessive allele (or gene) is hidden but is not lost, and may be passed to children. For a recessive trait to be expressed in the phenotype, the person must be homozygous recessive, that is, have two recessive alleles (genes) for the trait.

An example will be helpful here to put all this together and is illustrated in Fig. 21–7. When doing genetics problems, a **Punnett square** is used to show the possible combinations of genes in the egg and sperm for a particular set of parents and their children. Remember that an egg or sperm has only 23 chromosomes and, therefore, has only one gene for each trait.

In this example, the inheritance of eye color has been simplified. Although eye color is determined by many pairs of genes, with many possible phenotypes, one pair is considered the principal pair, with brown eyes dominant over blue eyes. A dominant gene is

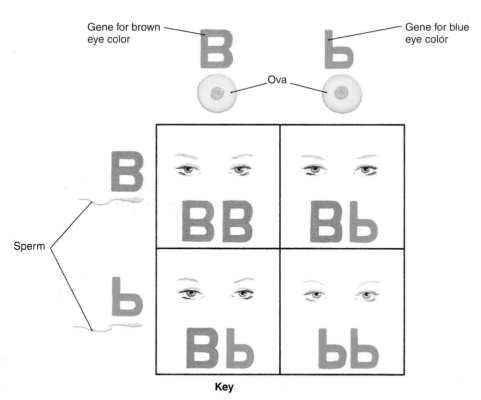

Figure 21–7 Inheritance of eye color. Both mother and father are heterozygous for brown eyes. The Punnett square shows the possible combinations of genes for eye color for each child of these parents. See text for further description.

Key

BB   Genotype: homozygous brown (2 dominant genes)
      Phenotype: brown

Bb   Genotype: heterozygous (1 dominant and 1 recessive gene)
      Phenotype: brown (since brown is dominant)

bb   Genotype: homozygous blue (2 recessive genes)
      Phenotype: blue

usually represented by a capital letter, and the corresponding recessive gene is represented by the same letter, but lowercase. The parents in Fig. 21–7 are both heterozygous for eye color. Their genotype consists of a gene for brown eyes and a gene for blue eyes, but their phenotype is brown eyes.

Each egg produced by the mother has a 50% chance of containing the gene for brown eyes, or an equal 50% chance of containing the gene for blue eyes. Similarly, each sperm produced by the father has a 50% chance of containing the gene for brown eyes and a 50% chance of containing the gene for blue eyes.

Now look at the boxes of the Punnett square; these represent the possibilities for the genetic makeup of each child. For eye color there are three possibilities: a 25% (one of four) chance for homozygous brown eyes, a 50% (two of four) chance for heterozygous brown eyes, and a 25% (one of four) chance for homozygous blue eyes. Notice that BB and Bb have the same phenotype (brown eyes) despite their different genotypes, and that the phenotype of blue eyes is only possible with the genotype bb. Can brown-eyed parents have a blue-eyed child? Yes; if each parent is heterozygous for brown eyes, each child has a 25% chance of inheriting blue eyes. Could these parents have four children with blue eyes? What are the odds of this happening? The answers to these questions will be found in Box 21–7: Solution to Genetics Question.

INHERITANCE: DOMINANT–RECESSIVE

The inheritance of eye color just described is an example of a trait determined by a pair of alleles, one of which may dominate the other. Another example is sickle-cell anemia, which was discussed in Chapter 11. The gene for the beta chain of hemoglobin is on chromosome 11; an allele for normal hemoglobin is dominant, and an allele for sickle-cell hemoglobin is recessive. An individual who is heterozygous is said to have sickle-cell trait; an individual who is homozygous recessive will have sickle-cell anemia. The Punnett square in Fig. 21–8 shows that if both parents are heterozygous, each child has a 25% chance of inheriting the two recessive genes. Table 21–4 lists some other human genetic diseases and their patterns of inheritance.

It is important to remember that in the terminology of genetics, dominant does not mean "common" or "frequent." It simply means that one gene is sufficient for the characteristic to appear in the phenotype. Think back to the ABO blood types. Which type is the most common in a population? Type O is most common, followed by type A, then type B. Type AB is the least common. Here is an instance where the recessive trait, type O, is most frequent in a group of people. Why is type AB the least common, though A and B alleles are dominant over an O allele? Because there are not many B alleles to be found in a population; not many people have a B allele. If you look at Table 21–6 later in this chapter, you will certainly be able to find other dominant traits that are rare.

INHERITANCE: MULTIPLE ALLELES

The best example of this pattern of inheritance is human blood type of the ABO group. For each gene of this blood type, there are three possible alleles: A, B, or O. A person will have only two of these alleles, which may be the same or different. O is the recessive allele; A and B are co-dominant alleles, that is, dominant over O but not over each other.

You already know that in this blood group there are four possible blood types: O, AB, A, and B. Table 21–5 shows the combinations of alleles for each type. Notice that for types O and AB there is only one possible genotype. For types A and B, however, there are

Box 21–7	SOLUTION TO GENETICS QUESTION
Question:	Can parents who are both heterozygous for brown eyes have four children with blue eyes? What are the odds of this happening?
Answer:	Yes. For each child, the odds of having blue eyes are 1 in 4. To calculate the odds of all four children having blue eyes, multiply the odds for each child separately:

1st child   2nd child   3rd child   4th child

$$\frac{1}{4} \times \frac{1}{4} \times \frac{1}{4} \times \frac{1}{4} = \frac{1}{256}$$

The odds are 256 to 1.

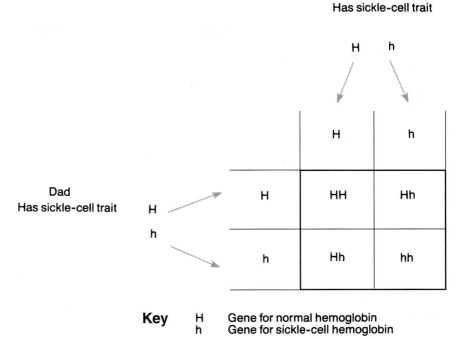

Figure 21–8 Inheritance of sickle-cell anemia (dominant–recessive pattern). See text for description.

Table 21–4	HUMAN GENETIC DISEASES

Disease (Pattern of Inheritance)	Description
Sickle-cell anemia (R)	• The most common genetic disease among people of African ancestry. Sickle-cell hemoglobin forms rigid crystals that distort and disrupt RBCs; oxygen-carrying capacity of the blood is diminished.
Cystic fibrosis (R)	• The most common genetic disease among people of European ancestry. Production of thick mucus clogs the bronchial tree and pancreatic ducts. Most severe effects are chronic respiratory infections and pulmonary failure.
Tay-Sachs disease (R)	• The most common genetic disease among people of Jewish ancestry. Degeneration of neurons and the nervous system results in death by the age of 2 years.
Phenylketonuria or PKU (R)	• Lack of an enzyme to metabolize the amino acid phenylalanine leads to severe mental and physical retardation. These effects may be prevented by the use of a diet (beginning at birth) that limits phenylalanine.
Huntington's disease (D)	• Uncontrollable muscle contractions begin between the ages of 30 and 50 years; followed by loss of memory and personality. There is no treatment that can delay mental deterioration.
Hemophilia (X-linked)	• Lack of Factor 8 impairs chemical clotting; may be controlled with Factor 8 from donated blood.
Duchenne's muscular dystrophy (X-linked)	• Replacement of muscle by adipose or scar tissue, with progressive loss of muscle function; often fatal before age 20 years due to involvement of cardiac muscle.

R = recessive; D = dominant.

Table 21–5	ABO BLOOD TYPES: GENOTYPES
Blood Type	**Possible Genotypes**
O	OO
AB	AB
A	AA or OA
B	BB or OB

two possible genotypes, because both A and B alleles are dominant over an O allele.

Let us now use a problem to illustrate the inheritance of blood type. The Punnett square in Fig. 21–9 shows that Mom has type O blood and Dad has type AB blood. The boxes of the square show the possible blood types for each child. Each child has a 50% chance of having type A blood, and a 50% chance of having type B blood. The genotype, however, will always be heterozygous. Notice that in this example, the blood types of the children will not be the same as those of the parents.

Table 21–6 lists some other human genetic traits, with the dominant and recessive phenotype for each.

INHERITANCE: SEX-LINKED TRAITS

Sex-linked traits may also be called X-linked traits because the genes for them are located only on the X chromosome. The Y does not have corresponding genes for many of the genes on the X chromosome. (The Y chromosome is very small and has only about 20 genes. Some of these genes are active only in the testes and contribute to spermatogenesis. Others are active in many body cells, but their functions are not yet known with certainty.)

The genes for sex-linked traits are recessive, but because there are no corresponding genes on the Y chromosome to mask them, a man needs only one gene to express one of these traits in his phenotype. A woman who has one of these recessive genes on one X chromosome and a dominant gene for normal function on the other X chromosome will not express this trait. She is called a carrier, however, because the gene is part of her genotype and may be passed to children.

Let us use as an example, red-green color blindness. The Punnett square in Fig. 21–10 shows that Mom is carrier of this trait and that Dad has normal color vision. A Punnett square for a sex-linked trait

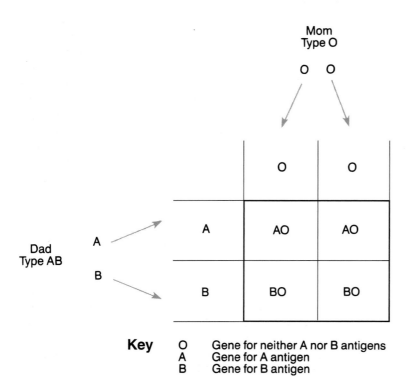

Key	O	Gene for neither A nor B antigens
	A	Gene for A antigen
	B	Gene for B antigen

Figure 21–9 Inheritance of blood type (multiple alleles pattern). See text for description.

Table 21–6 | HUMAN GENETIC TRAITS

Trait	Dominant Phenotype	Recessive Phenotype
ABO blood type	AB, A, B	O
Rh blood type	Rh positive	Rh negative
Hair color	Dark	Light (blond or red)
Change in hair color	Premature gray	Gray later in life
Hair texture	Curly	Straight
Hairline	Widow's peak	Straight
Eye color	Dark	Light
Color vision	Normal	Color blind
Visual acuity	Nearsighted or farsighted	Normal
Skin color	Dark	Light
Freckles	Abundant	Few
Dimples	Present	Absent
Cleft chin	Present	Absent
Ear lobes	Unattached	Attached
Number of fingers/toes	Polydactyly (more than 5 digits)	5 per hand or foot
Mid-digital hair	Present	Absent
Double-jointed thumb	Present	Absent
Bent little finger	Present	Absent
Ability to roll tongue sides up	Able	Unable

uses the X and Y chromosomes with a lower case letter on the X to indicate the presence of the recessive gene. The possibilities for each child are divided equally into daughters and sons. In this example, each daughter has a 50% chance of being a carrier and a 50% chance of not being a carrier. In either case, a daughter will have normal color vision. Each son has a 50% chance of being red-green color blind and a 50% chance of having normal color vision. Men can never be carriers of a trait such as this; they either have it or do not have it.

The inheritance of other characteristics is often not as easily depicted as are the examples shown above. Height, for example, is a multiple gene characteristic, meaning that many pairs of genes contribute. Many pairs of genes result in many possible combinations for genotype and many possible phenotypes. In addition, height is a trait that is influenced by environmental factors such as nutrition. These kinds of circumstances or influences are probably important in many other human characteristics.

Of the estimated 30,000 (or as many as 40,000) human genes, most had been "mapped" as of the end of 2001. This means that they have been precisely located on a particular chromosome. There is still much work to be done, however, and the focus now is on learning what each of these genes is for, that is, the protein the gene codes for, and the function of that protein.

Someday it will be possible to cure genetic diseases by inserting correct copies of malfunctioning genes into the cells of affected individuals. As of 2002, certain disorders of the immune system (which would have been fatal) seem to have been cured in several children by supplying correct copies of their faulty genes. Despite these successes, gene therapy in the United States, because of its complexity and high cost, is still limited to federally-funded experiments performed on individuals or small groups of people. Also unknown at this time, and yet another reason to proceed very slowly, are any possible risks of gene replacement.

Other diseases that may eventually be cured or controlled with gene therapy include cystic fibrosis and hemophilia (for both of which clinical trials are continuing), Parkinson's disease, diabetes, muscular dystrophy, and sickle-cell anemia. Much more research and careful experimentation remain to be done before gene replacement becomes the standard treatment available to everyone with these genetic diseases, but the foundation of this remarkable therapy has been established.

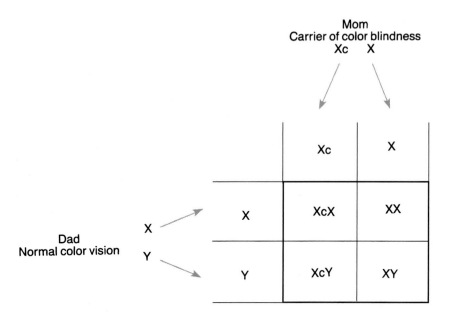

Mom
Carrier of color blindness
Xc   X

Dad
Normal color vision

	Xc	X
X	XcX	XX
Y	XcY	XY

Figure 21–10   Inheritance of red-green color blindness (sex-linked pattern). See text for description.

Key   X   X chromosome with gene for normal color vision
       Y   Y chromosome (has no gene for color vision)
       Xc   X chromosome with gene for red-green color blindness

STUDY OUTLINE

Human Development—growth of a fertilized egg into a human individual

Fertilization—the union of the nuclei of egg and sperm; usually takes place in the fallopian tube

1. Sperm undergo final maturation (capacitation) within the female reproductive tract; the acrosome secretes enzymes to digest the membrane of the ovum.
2. The 23 chromosomes of the sperm join with the 23 chromosomes of the egg to restore the diploid number of 46 in the zygote.
3. A zygote has 22 pairs of autosomes and one pair of sex chromosomes; XX in females, XY in males (see Fig. 21–1).

Implantation (see Fig. 21–2)

1. Within the fallopian tube, the zygote begins mitotic divisions called cleavage to form two-cell, four-cell, eight-cell stages, and so on.
2. A morula is a solid sphere of cells, which divides further to form a hollow sphere called a blastocyst.
3. A blastocyst consists of an outer layer of cells called the trophoblast and an inner cell mass that contains the potential embryo; the cells are stem cells, not yet specialized. The trophoblast secretes enzymes to form a crater in the endometrium into which the blastocyst sinks.

Embryo—weeks 1 through 8 of gestation (see Fig. 21–3)

1. In the embryonic disc, three primary germ layers develop: ectoderm, mesoderm, and endoderm (see Table 21–1).
2. By the eighth week of gestation (end of 2 months), all organ systems are formed (see Table 21–2).

Embryonic Membranes (see Fig. 21–3)

1. The yolk sac forms the first blood cells and the cells that become spermatogonia or oogonia.
2. The amnion surrounds the fetus and contains amniotic fluid; this fluid absorbs shock around the fetus.
3. The chorion develops chorionic villi that will

contain blood vessels that form the fetal portion of the placenta.

Fetus—weeks 9 through 40 of gestation (see Table 21–2)

1. The organ systems grow and mature.
2. The growing fetus brings about structural and functional changes in the mother (see Table 21–3).

Placenta and Umbilical Cord

1. The placenta is formed by the chorion of the embryo and the endometrium of the uterus; the umbilical cord connects the fetus to the placenta.
2. Fetal blood does not mix with maternal blood; fetal capillaries are within maternal blood sinuses (see Fig. 21–5); this is the site of exchanges between maternal and fetal blood.
3. Two umbilical arteries carry blood from the fetus to the placenta; fetal CO_2 and waste products diffuse into maternal blood; oxygen and nutrients enter fetal blood.
4. Umbilical vein returns blood from placenta to fetus.
5. The placenta is delivered after the baby and is called the afterbirth.

Placental Hormones

1. hCG—secreted by the chorion; maintains the corpus luteum so that it secretes estrogen and progesterone during the first few months of gestation. The corpus luteum is too small to secrete sufficient hormones to maintain a full-term pregnancy.
2. Estrogen and progesterone secretion begins within 4 to 6 weeks and continues until birth in amounts great enough to sustain pregnancy.
3. Estrogen and progesterone inhibit FSH and LH secretion during pregnancy and prepare the mammary glands for lactation.
4. Progesterone inhibits contractions of the myometrium until just before birth, when progesterone secretion begins to decrease.
5. Relaxin inhibits contractions of the myometrium and permits stretching of the pubic symphysis.

Parturition and Labor

1. Gestation period ranges from 37 to 42 weeks; the average is 40 weeks.
2. Labor: first stage—dilation of the cervix; uterine contractions force the amniotic sac into the cervix; amniotic sac ruptures and fluid escapes.
3. Labor: second stage—delivery of the infant;

oxytocin causes more powerful contractions of the myometrium. If a vaginal delivery is not possible, a cesarean section may be performed.
4. Labor: third stage—delivery of the placenta; the uterus continues to contract to expel the placenta, then contracts further, decreases in size, and compresses endometrial blood vessels.

The Infant at Birth (see Box 21–6)

1. Umbilical cord is clamped and severed; increased CO_2 stimulates breathing, and lungs are inflated.
2. Foramen ovale closes, and ductus arteriosus constricts; ductus venosus constricts; normal circulatory pathways are established.
3. Jaundice may be present if the infant's immature liver cannot rapidly excrete bilirubin.

Genetics—the study of inheritance chromosomes—46 per human cell; in 23 homologous pairs

1. A homologous pair consists of a maternal and a paternal chromosome of the same type (1 or 2, etc.).
2. There are 22 pairs of autosomes and one pair of sex chromosomes (XX or XY).
3. DNA—the hereditary material of chromosomes.
4. Gene—the genetic code for one protein; an individual has two genes for each protein or trait, one maternal and one paternal.
5. Alleles—the possibilities for how a gene may be expressed.

Genotype—the alleles present in the genetic makeup

1. Homozygous—having two similar alleles (genes).
2. Heterozygous—having two different alleles.

Phenotype—the appearance, or expression of the alleles present

1. Depends on the dominance or recessiveness of alleles or the particular pattern of inheritance involved.

Inheritance—dominant–recessive

1. A dominant gene will appear in the phenotype of a heterozygous individual (who has only one dominant gene). A recessive gene will appear in the phenotype only if the individual is homozygous, that is, has two recessive genes.
2. See Figs. 21–7 and 21–8 for Punnett squares.

Inheritance—multiple alleles

1. More than two possible alleles for each gene: human ABO blood type.
2. An individual will have only two of the alleles (same or different).
3. See Table 21–5 and Fig. 21–9.

Inheritance—sex-linked traits

1. Genes are recessive and found only on the X chromosome; there are no corresponding genes on the Y chromosome.
2. Women with one gene (and one gene for normal functioning) are called carriers of the trait.
3. Men cannot be carriers; they either have the trait or do not have it.
4. See Fig. 21–10.

REVIEW QUESTIONS

1. Where does fertilization usually take place? How many chromosomes are present in a human zygote? Explain what happens during cleavage, and describe the blastocyst stage. (p. 454)

2. Describe the process of implantation, and state where this takes place. (p. 454)

3. How long is the period of embryonic growth? How long is the period of fetal growth? (pp. 454, 457)

4. Name two body structures derived from ectoderm, mesoderm, and endoderm. (p. 458)

5. Name the embryonic membrane with each of these functions: (pp. 455, 457)
   a. Forms the fetal portion of the placenta
   b. Contains fluid to cushion the embryo
   c. Forms the first blood cells for the embryo

6. Explain the function of placenta, umbilical arteries, and umbilical vein. (pp. 458–459)

7. Explain the functions of the placental hormones: hCG, progesterone, and estrogen and progesterone (together). (pp. 459–460)

8. Describe the three stages of labor, and name the important hormone. (p. 460)

9. Describe the major pulmonary and circulatory changes that occur in the infant after birth. (pp. 460–461)

10. What is the genetic material of chromosomes? Explain what a gene is. Explain why a person has two genes for each protein or trait. (p. 464)

11. Define homologous chromosomes, autosomes, and sex chromosomes. (p. 464)

12. Define allele, homozygous, heterozygous, genotype, and phenotype. (p. 465)

13. Genetics Problem: Mom is heterozygous for brown eyes, and Dad has blue eyes. What is the % chance that a child will have blue eyes? Brown eyes? (pp. 465–466)

14. Genetics Problem: Mom is homozygous for type A blood, and Dad is heterozygous for type B blood. What is the % chance that a child will have type AB blood? Type A? Type B? Type O? (p. 468)

15. Genetics Problem: Mom is red-green color blind, and Dad has normal color vision. What is the % chance that a son will be color blind? That a daughter will be color blind? That a daughter will be a carrier? (pp. 469–470)

FOR FURTHER THOUGHT

1. Look at Table 21–1, and for each structure derived from each of the three primary germ layers, try to name a gene or set of genes that will be switched on. The gene or genes may be for a protein or a structure. Then try to name 3 genes that will be active in all of these different types of cells.

2. Women who smoke cigarettes should make special efforts to stop if they wish to have children, in part because nicotine from tobacco causes vasoconstriction. Describe how maternal smoking would affect a fetus.

3. The use of fertility drugs may lead to multiple fertilizations and embryos. With six embryos, or even five, what problems will there be in the maternal uterus?

4. Sometimes during a pregnancy the placenta will become detached. Total detachment is a medical emergency. If detachment is only partial, even a little, there may still be problems for the fetus and the mother. Describe these.

5. Mr. and Mrs. Brown want to have children, but Mr. Brown is hesitant. He had an older brother who died of Duchenne's muscular dystrophy, and he is worried that he may have a gene that can be passed on. "It's recessive," he tells you, "and doesn't always show up; it can skip a generation." What can you tell the Browns?

6. Mr. and Mrs. Gray have 6 children: 3 have type A blood and 3 have type B blood. Can we say with certainty what the two blood types of the parents are? Can we list possible pairs? Can we say with certainty what the parents' blood types are not? (For example, Mr. and Mrs. Gray cannot both be type O.) Make a list of possible pairs, and a list of pairs that are not possible.

7. Your friends, the Kalliomaa family, are of Finnish descent, and they are having a family reunion. Another friend asks you how all of these people in three generations can have blond hair and blue eyes, because these are recessive traits, and dark hair and eyes are dominant. What can you tell your friend to explain this?

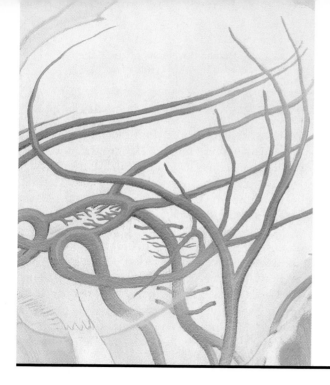

CHAPTER 22

Student Objectives

- Explain how microorganisms are classified and named.
- Describe the distribution of and benefits provided by normal flora.
- Explain what is meant by an infectious disease, and describe the different types of infection.
- Describe the ways in which infectious diseases may be spread.
- Explain how the growth of microorganisms may be controlled and the importance of this to public health.
- Describe the general structure of bacteria, viruses, fungi, and protozoa and the diseases they cause.
- Name the common worm infestations, and name the arthropods that are vectors of disease.

An Introduction to Microbiology and Human Disease

New Terminology

Bacillus (buh-**SILL**-us)

Coccus (**KOK**-us)

Communicable (kuhm-**YOO**-ni-kah-b'l)

Contagious (kun-**TAY**-jus)

Epidemiology (EP-i-DEE-mee-**AH**-luh-jee)

Gram stain (GRAM STAYN)

Infestation (in-fess-**TAY**-shun)

Mycosis (my-**KOH**-sis)

Non-communicable (NON-kuhm-**YOO**-ni-kah-b'l)

Portal of entry (**POR**-tuhl of **EN**-tree)

Portal of exit (**POR**-tuhl of **EG**-zit)

Reservoir (**REZ**-er-vwor)

Spirillum (spih-**RILL**-uhm)

Spirochete (**SPY**-roh-keet)

Vector (**VEK**-ter)

Zoonoses (ZOH-oh-**NOH**-seez)

Related Clinical Terminology

Antitoxin (AN-tee-**TAHK**-sin)

Broad spectrum (BRAWD **SPEK**-trum)

Culture and sensitivity testing (**KUL**-chur and SEN-si-**TIV**-i-tee)

Endotoxin (EN-doh-**TAHK**-sin)

Incubation period (IN-kew-**BAY**-shun)

Narrow spectrum (**NAR**-oh **SPEK**-trum)

Nosocomial infection (no-zoh-**KOH**-mee-uhl)

Opportunistic infection (OP-er-too-**NIS**-tik)

Secondary infection (**SEK**-un-dery)

Subclinical infection (sub-**KLIN**-i-kuhl)

*Terms that appear in **bold type** in the chapter text are defined in the glossary, which begins on page 521.*

Awakening with sniffles and a runny nose… finding a moldy surprise in the refrigerator behind the milk carton… wondering if that milk has gone sour. No matter that we cannot see them, the microbes, including viruses, fungi, and bacteria, are always with us.

Microbiology is the study of microorganisms (also called microbes) and of their place or role in their environment. Sometimes, the environment of microbes is us, people, and that will be our focus. Although there are many perspectives in the field of microbiology, we will concentrate on the microorganisms that affect the functioning of the human body. These microbes include our normal flora and those that are capable of causing human disease. A disease is any disruption of normal body functioning. Many diseases are not caused by microorganisms, but those that are may be called infectious diseases. The microorganisms that cause infectious diseases are called pathogens.

Pathogens may also be called parasites, that is, they live on another living organism called a host and cause harm to the host. Some parasites cause diseases that are fatal to the host, but many others live in a more balanced way with their hosts. These cause illnesses from which the host recovers, and the parasite often survives long enough to be spread to other hosts.

Our introduction to microbiology will begin with a brief description of the classification and naming of microorganisms, followed by a discussion of normal flora. We will then consider infectious diseases, types of infection, and the spread and control of infection. Last, we will describe the types of pathogens in more detail and include the methods we have to treat and control the diseases they cause. For a historical perspective on microbiology, see Box 22–1: The Golden Age of Microbiology, and Box 22–2: Microbiology in the 20th Century.

CLASSIFICATION OF MICROORGANISMS

Bacteria are very simple single-celled organisms and are found virtually everywhere. The natural habitats of bacteria include freshwater, saltwater, soil, and other living organisms. Most bacteria are not harmful to us, and within their normal environments, they have the vital role of decomposing dead organic material and recycling their nutrients. However, a number of bacteria cause human diseases, including strep throat, pneumonia, and meningitis.

Box 22–1   THE GOLDEN AGE OF MICROBIOLOGY

Microorganisms were first seen in the 17th century when simple microscopes were developed. The roles of microorganisms, however, especially in relation to disease, were to remain largely unknown for another two centuries. The years between 1875 and 1900 are sometimes called "The Golden Age of Microbiology" because of the number and significance of the discoveries that were made during this time. The following is only a partial list.

1877 Robert Koch proves that anthrax is caused by a bacterium.
1878 Joseph Lister first grows bacteria in pure culture.
       The oil immersion lens for microscopes is developed.
1879 The bacterium that causes gonorrhea is discovered.
1880 Louis Pasteur develops a vaccine for chicken cholera.
1881 Discovery that staphylococci cause infections.

1882 The cause of tuberculosis is found to be a bacterium.
1883 Diphtheria is found to be caused by a bacterium.
1884 The bacteria that cause tetanus, typhoid fever, and cholera are each isolated. The first description of phagocytosis by white blood cells is published.
1885 Louis Pasteur first uses his vaccine for rabies.
1890 Development of antitoxins to treat tetanus and diphtheria.
1892 Discovery and demonstration of a virus.
1894 The bacterium that causes plague is discovered.
1897 Discovery of the cause of botulism.
       Rat fleas are found to be vectors of plague.
1900 Walter Reed and his associates demonstrate that yellow fever is caused by a virus and that the vector is a mosquito.

Box 22–2   MICROBIOLOGY IN THE 20TH CENTURY

Just a few of the many advances made in microbiology during this century are listed below. Many of them concerned diagnosis, prevention, or treatment of infectious diseases, and some involved using microorganisms and the new genetic technologies.

1928   Discovery of penicillin by Alexander Fleming.

1935   The first of the sulfa drugs is found to be effective against staphylococcal infections.

1938   Penicillin is purified and produced in large quantities.

1941   The fluorescent antibody test is developed.

1943   Streptomycin is discovered and is the first effective drug in the treatment of tuberculosis.

1953   Watson and Crick describe the structure of DNA.

1955   The Salk polio vaccine is first used.

1957   Interferon is discovered.

1959   A vaccine for whooping cough is available.

1962   The Sabin polio vaccine is marketed in the United States.

1963   The measles vaccine becomes available.

1969   A vaccine for rubella is developed.

1976   Legionnaire's disease is discovered and described.

1980   Genetically engineered bacteria produce the hormone insulin.

1981   The first cases of AIDS are described.

1982   The first vaccine for hepatitis B is licensed.

1986   Genetically engineered yeast are used to produce a more effective vaccine for hepatitis B.

Genetically engineered bacteria produce human growth hormone.

Viruses are not cells; they are even smaller and simpler in structure than the bacteria. All viruses are parasites because they can reproduce only within the living cells of a host. Therefore, all viruses cause disease. Common human viral diseases are influenza, the common cold, and chickenpox.

Protozoa are single-celled animals such as amoebas. Most protozoa are free living in fresh or saltwater, where they consume bacteria, fungi, and one another. Human protozoan parasites include those that cause malaria, amebic dysentery, and giardiasis, another intestinal infection.

Fungi may be unicellular or multicellular. Molds and mushrooms are familiar fungi. They decompose organic matter in the soil and freshwater and help recycle nutrients. Fungal diseases of people include yeast infections, ringworm, and more serious diseases such as a type of meningitis.

Worms are multicellular animals. Most are free living and non-pathogenic; within the soil they consume dead organic matter or smaller living things. Worm infestations of people include trichinosis, hookworm disease, and tapeworms.

Arthropods (the name means "jointed legs") are multicellular animals such as lobsters, shrimp, the insects, ticks, and mites. Some insects (such as mosquitoes and fleas) are **vectors** of disease, that is, they spread pathogens from host to host when they bite to obtain blood. Ticks are also vectors of certain diseases, and some mites may cause infestations of the skin.

BINOMIAL NOMENCLATURE

We refer to bacteria and all other living things using two names (binomial nomenclature), the genus and the species. The genus name is placed first, is always capitalized, and is the larger category. The species name is second, is not capitalized, and is the smaller category. Let us use as examples *Staphylococcus aureus* and *Staphylococcus epidermidis*. These two bacteria are in the same genus, *Staphylococcus,* which tells us that they are related or similar to one another. Yet they are different enough to be given their own species names: *aureus* or *epidermidis*. It may be helpful here to think of our own names. Each of us has a family name, which indicates that we are related to other members of our families, and each of us has a first name indicating that we are individuals in this related group. If we wrote our own names using the method of binomial nomenclature, we would write Smith Mary and Smith John.

In scientific articles and books, for the sake of convenience, the genus name is often abbreviated with its first letter. We might read of *S. aureus* as a cause of a food poisoning outbreak or see *E. coli* (*E.* for *Escherichia*) on a lab report as the cause of a patient's urinary tract infection. Therefore, it is important to learn both genus and species names of important pathogens.

NORMAL FLORA

Each of us has a natural population of microorganisms living on and within us. This is our normal flora. These microbes may be further categorized as residents or transients. **Resident flora** are those species that live on or in nearly everyone almost all the time. These residents live in specific sites, and we provide a very favorable environment for them. Some, such as *Staphylococcus epidermidis,* live on the skin. Others, such as *E. coli,* live in the colon and small intestine. When in their natural sites, resident flora do not cause harm to healthy tissue, and some are even beneficial to us. However, residents may become pathogenic if they are introduced into abnormal sites. If *E. coli,* for example, gains access to the urinary bladder, it causes an infection called cystitis. In this situation, *E. coli* is considered an **opportunist**, which is a normally harmless species that has become a pathogen in special circumstances.

Transient flora are those species that are found periodically on or in the body; they are not as well adapted to us as are the residents. *Streptococcus pneumoniae,* for example, is a transient in the upper respiratory tract, where it usually does not cause harm in healthy people. However, transients may become pathogenic when the host's resistance is lowered. In an elderly person with influenza, *S. pneumoniae* may invade the lower respiratory tract and cause a serious or even fatal pneumonia.

The distribution of our normal flora is summarized in Table 22–1. You can see that an important function of normal flora is to inhibit the growth of pathogens in the oral cavity, intestines, and in women, the vagina. The resident bacteria are believed to do this by simply being there and providing competition that makes it difficult for pathogens to establish themselves. An example may be helpful here. Let us use botulism. Typical foodborne botulism is acquired by ingesting the bacterial toxin that has been produced in food. Infants, however, may acquire botulism by ingesting the spores (dormant forms) of the botulism bacteria on foods such as honey or raw vegetables. The infants's colon flora is not yet abundant, and the botulism spores may be able to germinate into active cells

that produce toxin in the baby's own intestine. For older children or adults, botulism spores are harmless if ingested, because the normal colon flora prevents the growth of these bacteria.

Resident flora may be diminished by the use of antibiotics to treat bacterial infections. An antibiotic does not distinguish between the pathogen and the resident bacteria. In such circumstances, without the usual competition, yeasts or pathogenic bacteria may be able to overgrow and create new infections. This is most likely to occur on mucous membranes such as those of the oral cavity and vagina.

INFECTIOUS DISEASE

An infectious disease is one that is caused by microorganisms or by the products (toxins) of microorganisms. To cause an infection, a microorganism must enter and establish itself in a host and begin reproducing.

Several factors determine whether a person will develop an infection when exposed to a pathogen. These include the virulence of the pathogen and the resistance of the host. **Virulence** is the ability of the pathogen to cause disease. Host **resistance** is the total of the body's defenses against pathogens. Our defenses include intact skin and mucous membranes, the sweeping of cilia to clear the respiratory tract, adequate nutrition, and the immune responses of our lymphocytes and macrophages (see Chapter 14).

To illustrate these concepts, let us compare the measles virus and rhinoviruses (common cold). The measles virus has at least a 90% infectivity rate, meaning that for every 100 non-immune people exposed, at least 90 will develop clinical measles. Thus, the measles virus is considered highly virulent, even for healthy people. However, people who have recovered from measles or who have received the measles vaccine have developed an active immunity that increases their resistance to measles. Even if exposed many times, such people probably will not develop clinical measles.

In contrast, the rhinoviruses that cause the common cold are not considered virulent pathogens, and healthy people may have them in their upper respiratory tracts without developing illness. However, fatigue, malnutrition, and other physiological stresses may lower a person's resistance and increase the like-

Table 22–1	DISTRIBUTION OF NORMAL FLORA IN THE HUMAN BODY

Body Site	Description of Flora
Skin	Exposed to the environment; therefore has a large bacterial population and small numbers of fungi, especially where the skin is often moist. Flora are kept in check by the continual loss of dead cells from the stratum corneum.
Nasal cavities	Bacteria, mold spores, and viruses constantly enter with inhaled air; the ciliated epithelium limits the microbial population by continuously sweeping mucus and trapped pathogens to the pharynx, where they are swallowed.
Trachea, bronchi, and lungs	The cilia of the trachea and large bronchial tubes sweep mucus and microbes upward toward the pharynx, where they are swallowed. Very few pathogens reach the lungs, and most of these are destroyed by alveolar macrophages.
Oral cavity	Large bacterial population and small numbers of yeasts and protozoa. Kept in check by lysozyme, the enzyme in saliva that inhibits bacterial reproduction. The resident flora help prevent the growth of pathogens.
Esophagus	Contains the microorganisms swallowed with saliva or food.
Stomach	The hydrochloric acid in gastric juice kills most bacteria. This may not be effective if large numbers of a pathogen or bacterial toxins are present in contaminated food.
Small intestine	The ileum, adjacent to the colon, has the largest bacterial population. The duodenum, adjacent to the stomach, has the smallest.
Large intestine	Contains an enormous population of bacteria, which inhibits the growth of pathogens and produces vitamins. The vitamins are absorbed as the colon absorbs water. Vitamin K is obtained in amounts usually sufficient to meet a person's daily need. Smaller amounts of folic acid, riboflavin, and other vitamins are also obtained from colon flora.
Urinary bladder	Is virtually free of bacteria, as is the upper urethra. The lower urethra, especially in women, has a flora similar to that of the skin.
Vagina	A large bacterial population creates an acidic pH that inhibits the growth of pathogens.
Tissue fluid	Small numbers of bacteria and viruses penetrate mucous membranes or get through breaks in the skin. Most are destroyed in lymph nodules or lymph nodes or by wandering macrophages in tissue fluid.
Blood	Should be free of microorganisms.

lihood of developing a cold upon exposure to these viruses.

Once infected, a person may have a **clinical (apparent** or **symptomatic)** infection, in which symptoms appear. **Symptoms** are observable or measurable changes that indicate illness. For some diseases, **subclinical (inapparent** or **asymptomatic)** infections are possible, in which the person shows no symptoms. Women with the sexually transmitted disease gonorrhea, for example, may have subclinical infections, that is, no symptoms at all. It is important to remember that such people are still **reservoirs** (sources) of the pathogen for others, who may then develop clinical infections.

COURSE OF AN INFECTIOUS DISEASE

When a pathogen establishes itself in a host, there is a period of time before symptoms appear. This is called the **incubation period**. Most infectious diseases have rather specific incubation periods (Table 22–2). Some diseases, however, have more variable incubation periods (see hepatitis in Table 22–2), which may make it difficult to predict the onset of illness after exposure or to trace outbreaks of a disease.

A short time called the prodromal period may follow the incubation period. During this time, vague, non-specific symptoms may begin. These include

Table 22-2	INCUBATION PERIODS OF SOME INFECTIOUS DISEASES

Disease	Incubation Period
Chickenpox	14–16 days
Cholera	1–3 days
Diphtheria	2–6 days
Gas gangrene	1–5 days
Gonorrhea	3–5 days
Hepatitis A	2 weeks–2 months
Hepatitis B	6 weeks–6 months
Hepatitis C	2 weeks–6 months
Herpes simplex	4 days
Influenza	1–3 days
Leprosy	3 months–20+ years
Measles	10–12 days
Meningitis (bacterial)	1–7 days
Mumps	2–3 weeks
Pertussis	5 days–3 weeks
Pinworm	2–6 weeks
Plague	2–6 days
Polio	7–14 days
Rabies	2 weeks–2 months (up to 1 year)
Salmonella food poisoning	12–72 hours
Staphyloccus food poisoning	1–8 hours
Syphilis	10 days–3 months
Tetanus	3 days–5 weeks
Tuberculosis	2–10 weeks

generalized muscle aches, lethargy, and fatigue, or a feeling that "I'm coming down with something."

During the invasion period, the specific symptoms of the illness appear. These might include a high fever, rash, swollen lymph nodes, cough, diarrhea, or such things as the gradual paralysis of botulism. The acme is the height or worst of the disease, and this is followed by the recovery or death of the host.

Some diseases are **self-limiting**; that is, they typically last a certain length of time and are usually followed by recovery. The common cold, chickenpox, and mumps are illnesses that are considered self-limiting.

TYPES OF INFECTION

The terminology of infection may refer to the location of the pathogens in the body, to the general nature of the disease, or to how or where the pathogen was acquired.

A **localized** infection is one that is confined to one area of the body. Examples are the common cold of the upper respiratory tract, boils of the skin, and salmonella food poisoning that affects the intestines.

In a **systemic** infection, the pathogen is spread throughout the body by way of the lymph or blood. Typhoid fever, for example, begins as an intestinal infection, but the bacteria eventually spread to the liver, gallbladder, kidneys, and other organs. Bubonic plague is an infection that begins in lymph nodes, but again the bacteria are carried throughout the body, and fatal plague is the result of pneumonia.

Bacteremia and **septicemia** are terms that are often used synonymously in clinical practice; they mean that bacteria are present in the blood and are being circulated throughout the body. Septicemia is always serious, for it means that the immune defenses have been completely overwhelmed and are unable to stop the spread of the pathogen.

With respect to timing and duration, some infections may be called acute or chronic. An **acute** infection is one that usually begins abruptly and is severe. In contrast, a **chronic** infection often progresses slowly and may last for a long time.

A **secondary** infection is one that is made possible by a primary infection that has lowered the host's resistance. Influenza in an elderly person, for example, may be followed by bacterial pneumonia. This secondary bacterial infection might not have occurred had not the person first been ill with the flu.

Nosocomial infections are those that are acquired in hospitals or other institutions such as nursing homes. The hospital population includes newborns, the elderly, postoperative patients, people with serious chronic diseases, cancer patients receiving chemotherapy, and others whose resistance to disease is lowered. Some hospital-acquired pathogens, such as *Staphylococcus aureus,* are transmitted from patient to patient by healthy hospital personnel. These staff members are reservoirs for *S. aureus* and carry it on their skin or in their upper respiratory tracts. For this reason, proper handwashing is of critical importance for all hospital staff.

Other nosocomial infections, however, are caused by the patient's own normal flora that has been inadvertently introduced into an abnormal body site. Such infections may be called **endogenous,** which literally means "generated from within." Intestinal bacilli such as *E. coli* are also an important cause of nosocomial infections. Without very careful aseptic technique (and sometimes in spite of it), the patient's own intestinal bacteria may contaminate urinary catheters, decubitus ulcers, surgical incisions, chest tubes, and intravenous lines. Such infections are a significant problem in hospitals, and all those involved in any aspect of patient care should be aware of this.

EPIDEMIOLOGY

Epidemiology is the study of the patterns and spread of disease within a population. As you see, this term is related to **epidemic,** which is an outbreak of disease, that is, more than the usual number of cases in a given time period. An **endemic** disease is one that is present in a population, with an expected or usual number of cases in a given time. Influenza, for example, is endemic in large cities during the winter, and public health personnel expect a certain number of cases. In some winters, however, the number of cases of influenza increases, often markedly, and this is an epidemic.

A **pandemic** is an epidemic that has spread throughout several countries. The bubonic plague pandemic of the 14th century affected nearly all of Europe and killed one-fourth of the population. Just after World War I, in 1918 to 1920, an especially virulent strain of the influenza virus spread around the world and caused 20 million deaths. More recently, an epidemic of cholera began in Peru in January 1991, but soon became a pandemic as cholera spread to neighboring South American countries.

To understand the epidemiology of a disease, we must know several things about the pathogen. These include where it lives in a host, the kinds of hosts it can infect, and whether it can survive outside of hosts.

PORTALS OF ENTRY AND EXIT

The **portal of entry** is the way the pathogen enters a host (Fig. 22–1). Breaks in the skin, even very small ones, are potential portals of entry, as are the natural body openings. Pathogens may be inhaled, consumed with food and water, or acquired during sexual activity. Most pathogens that enter the body by way of these natural routes are destroyed by the white blood cells found in and below the skin and mucous membranes, but some may be able to establish themselves and cause disease.

Insects such as mosquitoes, fleas, and lice, and other arthropods, such as ticks, are vectors of disease. They spread pathogens when they bite to obtain a host's blood. Mosquitoes, for example, are vectors of malaria, yellow fever, and encephalitis. Ticks are vectors of Lyme disease and Rocky Mountain spotted fever.

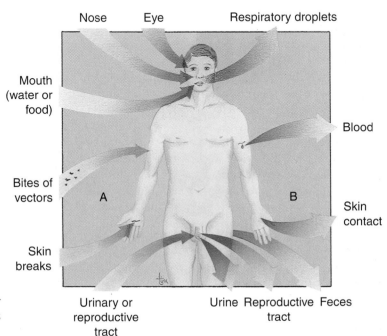

Figure 22–1   **(A)** Portals of entry. **(B)** Portals of exit.

As mentioned previously, it is important to keep in mind that many hospital procedures may provide portals of entry for pathogens. Any invasive procedure, whether it involves the skin or the mucous membranes, may allow pathogens to enter the body. Thus it is essential that all health-care workers follow aseptic technique for such procedures.

The **portal of exit** (see Fig. 22–1) is the way the pathogen leaves the body or is shed from the host. Skin lesions, such as those of chickenpox, contain pathogens that may be transmitted to others by cutaneous contact. Intestinal pathogens such as the hepatitis A virus and the cholera bacteria are excreted in the host's feces, which may contaminate food or water and be ingested by another host (this is called the fecal–oral route of transmission). Respiratory pathogens such as influenza and measles viruses are shed in respiratory droplets from the mouth and nose and may be inhaled by another person. The pathogens of the reproductive tract, such as the bacteria that cause syphilis and gonorrhea, are transmitted to others by sexual contact. Notice that with respect to epidemiology, the pathogen travels from one host's portal of exit to another host's portal of entry.

RESERVOIRS OF INFECTION

Some pathogens cause disease only in people. Measles, whooping cough, syphilis, and bacterial meningitis are strictly human diseases. To acquire such a disease, a person must be exposed to someone who has the illness.

Also of importance is that upon recovery from some diseases, the host may continue to harbor the pathogen and thus be a reservoir of it for others. Such a person is called a **carrier.** Diseases for which the carrier state is possible include typhoid diphtheria, and hepatitis B.

Many other diseases, however, are really animal diseases that people acquire in certain circumstances. These diseases are called **zoonoses** (singular: **zoonosis**) and include plague, Lyme disease, encephalitis, and Rocky Mountain spotted fever, which are spread from animal to person by vectors such as ticks or fleas. Rabies is acquired by contact with infected animal saliva or infected tissue, the virus entering the new host through breaks in the skin. Salmonellosis is a type of food poisoning caused by the intestinal bacilli of animals that contaminate meats such as chicken and turkey. Prevention of such diseases depends upon knowledge of how they are spread.

For example, people who live in areas where Lyme disease is endemic should be aware that the disease is acquired by way of a tick bite. If children and pets are examined for ticks after they have been out of doors, the chance of acquiring Lyme disease is greatly diminished.

Some bacteria are pathogenic only by accident, for their natural habitat is soil or water, where they act as decomposers. The bacteria that cause gas gangrene, tetanus, and botulism are normal soil flora and cause disease when they (or their toxins) contaminate a skin wound, or, in the case of botulism, the toxin is present in food.

SPREAD OF INFECTION

Based on our knowledge thus far, we can classify infectious diseases as noncommunicable or communicable. A **non-communicable** disease is one in which a resident species causes disease under certain conditions or in which a non-resident species causes disease when it enters the body. Such diseases cannot be transmitted directly or indirectly from host to host. Cystitis caused by *E. coli* in a hospital patient, for example, is not communicable to the nurses who care for that patient. Similarly, a nurse caring for a patient with tetanus or botulism need not worry about acquiring these diseases; both are noncommunicable.

A **communicable** disease is one in which the pathogen may be transmitted directly or indirectly from host to host. Direct spread of infection is by way of cutaneous contact (including sexual contact), respiratory droplets, contaminated blood, or placental transmission from mother to fetus. Indirect spread is by way of contaminated food or water, or vectors, or **fomites,** which are inanimate objects that carry the pathogen. Influenza and cold viruses, for example, can survive outside their hosts for a time, so that objects such as eating utensils, door knobs, or childrens toys may be vehicles of transmission for these pathogens.

Some communicable diseases may also be called **contagious,** which means that they are easily spread from person to person by casual cutaneous contact or by respiratory droplets. Chickenpox, measles, and influenza are contagious diseases. In contrast, AIDS is not contagious, because sexual contact, blood contact, or placental transmission is necessary to acquire the virus (HIV). HIV is not spread by cutaneous contact or by respiratory droplets.

METHODS OF CONTROL OF MICROBES

Microorganisms are everywhere in our environment, and although we need not always be aware of their presence, there are times when we must try to diminish or even eliminate them. These situations include the use of chemicals for disinfection, especially in hospitals, and the protection of our food and water supplies.

ANTISEPTICS, DISINFECTANTS, AND STERILIZATION

We are all familiar with the practice of applying iodine, hydrogen peroxide, or alcohol to minor cuts in the skin, and we know the purpose of this: to prevent bacterial infection. The use of such chemicals does indeed destroy many harmful bacteria, although it has no effect on bacterial spores. The chemicals used to prevent infection may be called antiseptics or disinfectants. An **antiseptic** (anti = against; septic = infection) is a chemical that destroys bacteria or inhibits their growth on a living being. The chemicals named above are antiseptics on skin surfaces. A **disinfectant** is a chemical that is used on inanimate objects. Chemicals with antibacterial effects may be further classified as bactericidal or bacteriostatic. **Bactericides** kill bacteria by disrupting important metabolic processes. **Bacteriostatic** chemicals do not destroy bacteria, but rather inhibit their reproduction and slow their growth. Alcohol, for example, is a bactericide that is both an antiseptic and a disinfectant, depending upon the particular surface on which it is used.

Some chemicals are not suitable for use on human skin because they are irritating or damaging, but they may be used on environmental surfaces as disinfectants. Bleach, such as Clorox, and cresols, such as Lysol, may be used in bathrooms, on floors or countertops, and even on dishes and eating utensils (if rinsed thoroughly). These bactericides will also destroy certain viruses, such as those that cause influenza. A dilute (10%) bleach solution will inactivate HIV, the virus that causes AIDS.

In hospitals, environmental surfaces are disinfected, but materials such as surgical instruments, sutures, and dressings must be sterilized. **Sterilization** is a process that destroys all living organisms. Most medical and laboratory products are sterilized by autoclaving. An **autoclave** is a chamber in which steam is generated under pressure. This pressurized steam penetrates the contents of the chamber and kills all microorganisms present, including bacterial spores.

Materials such as disposable plastics that might be damaged by autoclaving are often sterilized by exposure to ionizing radiation. Foods such as meats may also be sterilized by this method. Such food products have a very long shelf life (equivalent to canned food), and this procedure is used for preparing some military field rations.

PUBLIC HEALTH MEASURES

Each of us is rightfully concerned with our own health and the health of our families. People who work in the public health professions, however, consider the health of all of us, that is, the health of a population. Two traditional aspects of public health are ensuring safe food and safe drinking water. Two more recent aspects are tracking and learning about emerging diseases, and preparing defenses against the possible use of biological weapons.

Food

The safety of our food depends on a number of factors. Most cities have certain standards and practices that must be followed by supermarkets and restaurants, and inspections are conducted on a regular basis.

Food companies prepare their products by using specific methods to prevent the growth of microorganisms. Naturally, it is in the best interests of these companies to do so, for they would soon be out of business if their products made people ill. Also of importance is the willingness of companies to recall products that are only suspected of being contaminated. This is all to the benefit of consumers. For example, since 1925 in the United States, only five fatal cases of botulism have been traced to commercially canned food. If we consider that billions of cans of food have been consumed during this time, we can appreciate the high standards the food industry has maintained.

Milk and milk products provide ideal environments for the growth of bacteria because they contain both protein and sugar (lactose) as food sources. For this reason, milk must be **pasteurized**, that is, heated to 145°F (62.9°C) for 30 minutes. Newer methods of pasteurization use higher temperatures for shorter periods of time, but the result is the same:

The pathogens that may be present in milk are killed, although not all bacteria are totally destroyed. Milk products such as cheese and ice cream are also pasteurized, or are made from pasteurized milk.

When a food-related outbreak of disease does take place, public health workers try to trace the outbreak to its source. This stops the immediate spread of disease by preventing access to the contaminated food, and the ensuing publicity on television or in the newspapers may help remind everyone of the need for careful monitoring of food preparation.

Some foods meant to be eaten raw or briefly cooked, such as fruit or rare beef, do carry a small risk. Consumers should realize that food is not sterile, that meat, for example, is contaminated with the animals' intestinal bacteria during slaughtering. Meat should be thoroughly cooked. Fruit and vegetables should be washed or peeled before being eaten raw. (Food-borne diseases, also called food poisoning, are included in the tables of diseases that appear at the end of this chapter.)

Finally, the safety of our food may depend on something we often take for granted: our refrigerators. For example, a Thanksgiving turkey that was carved for dinner at 3 P.M. and left on the kitchen counter until midnight probably should not be used for turkey sandwiches the next day. Although we have to rely on others to ensure that commercially prepared food will be safe, once food reaches our homes, all we really need (besides the refrigerator) is our common sense.

Water

When we turn on a faucet to get a glass of water, we usually do not wonder whether the water is safe to drink. It usually is. Having a reliable supply of clean drinking water depends on two things: diverting human sewage away from water supplies and chlorinating water intended for human consumption.

Large cities have sewer systems for the collection of waste water and its subsequent treatment in sewage plants. Once treated, however, the sludge (solid, particulate matter) from these plants must be disposed of. This is becoming more of a problem simply because there is so much sewage sludge (because there are so many of us). Although the sludge is largely free of pathogens, it ought not be put in landfills, and because ocean dumping is being prohibited in many coastal areas, this is a problem that will be with us for a long time.

Drinking water for cities and towns is usually chlorinated. The added chlorine kills virtually all bacteria that may be present. The importance of chlorination is shown by a 1978 outbreak of enteritis (diarrhea) in a Vermont town of 10,000 people. The chlorination process malfunctioned for 2 days, and 2,000 of the town's inhabitants became ill. (The bacterium was *Campylobacter,* a common intestinal inhabitant of animals.)

You may now be wondering if all those bottled spring waters are safe to drink. The answer, in general, is yes, because the bottling companies do not wish to make people ill and put themselves out of business. Some bottled waters, however, do have higher mold spore counts than does chlorinated tap water. Usually these molds are not harmful when ingested; they are destroyed by the hydrochloric acid in gastric juice.

In much of North America, nearly everyone has easy access to safe drinking water. We might remind ourselves once in a while that our water will not give us typhoid, dysentery, or cholera. These diseases are still very common in other parts of the world, where the nearest river or stream is the laundry, the sewer, and the source of drinking water.

Emerging Diseases and Biological Weapons

The term *emerging diseases* may be a bit misleading, because some of the pathogens are not really new. What has happened is that we have become aware of them. A good example of this is Lyme disease. Lyme disease in the United States was named for the town in Connecticut where a cluster of cases was discovered in the 1970s. When the causative bacteria were later found and the disease fully characterized, health officials realized that the disease had been described in Scandinavia in the early years of the 20th century. Lyme disease was not a new disease after all, merely a newly encountered disease for Americans.

Other emerging diseases are those caused by the Ebola and Marburg viruses, by Hantavirus and West Nile virus, by certain strains of *E. coli,* and by antibiotic-resistant strains of enterococci. The tasks of public health officials are to keep track of all cases of these diseases and to educate medical personnel about them.

Education about a rare disease included page one headlines in American newspapers during October and November 2001. The disease was anthrax, a disease of grazing animals rarely found in people.

Anthrax spores had been mailed to politicians and television anchormen, that is, had been used as a biological weapon. At the time, most physicians had never seen a case of anthrax, and learned about it along with the average citizens. As can be the case when ignorance prevails, panic and hoarding of antibiotics ensued—for a disease that is not contagious. People in other countries with a more agrarian economy were shaking their heads at the American panic, for to them anthrax was simply an occasional and occupational disease of farmers or sheepherders. We in America sometimes ignore the experience of people in the rest of the world, and really should know better.

One good outcome of our anthrax experience and response may be that more money will be alloted for public health programs. The possible use of the smallpox virus as a biological weapon is a great concern, and education, of everyone, is so important. Any improvements to public health policies and procedures that were spurred by the use of anthrax as a weapon will not be at all wasted, but will be applicable to the emerging diseases as well. (See Box 22–3: Microbiology in the 21st Century; you may be able to add to it.)

THE PATHOGENS

In the sections that follow, each group of pathogens will be described with a summary of important characteristics. Examples of specific pathogens will be given to help you become familiar with them.

Tables of important human diseases caused by each group of pathogens are found at the end of this chapter.

BACTERIA (SEE TABLE 22–3)

Bacteria are very simple unicellular organisms. All are microscopic in size, and a magnification of 1000 times is usually necessary to see them clearly. A bacterial cell consists of watery cytoplasm and a single chromosome (made of DNA) surrounded by a cell membrane. Enclosing all of these structures is a cell wall, which is strong and often rigid, giving the bacterium its characteristic shape.

Based on shape, bacteria are classified as one of three groups: coccus, bacillus, or spirillum (Fig. 22–2). A **coccus** (plural: **cocci**) is a sphere; under the microscope, cocci appear round. Certain prefixes may be used to describe the arrangement of spheres. **Staphylo** means clusters; **strepto** refers to chains of cells, and **diplo** means pairs of cells.

A **bacillus** (plural: **bacilli**) is a rod-shaped bacterium; rods may vary in length depending on the genus. A **spirillum** (plural: **spirilla**) is a long cell with one or more curves or coils. Some spirilla, such as those that cause syphilis and Lyme disease, are called **spirochetes**. Many of the bacilli and spirilla are capable of movement because they have **flagella**. These are long, thread-like structures that project from the cell and beat rhythmically.

Bacteria reproduce by the process of **binary fission**, in which the chromosome duplicates itself, and the original cell divides into two identical cells.

Box 22–3 MICROBIOLOGY IN THE 21ST CENTURY

The 21st century has just begun; here is a microbiological perspective.

2001 In sub-Saharan Africa, more than 25 million people have AIDS or are HIV positive.
Anthrax spores are sent through the U.S. mail causing 22 cases of the disease, with 5 fatalities.

2002 In China, the number of AIDS cases increases ever more rapidly.
Multi-drug-resistant strains of *Mycobacterium tuberculosis* proliferate throughout the world.
A strain of *Staphyloccus aureus* is found that is fully resistant to the antibiotic vancomycin.

The presence or absence of oxygen may be important for bacterial reproduction. **Aerobic** bacteria can reproduce only in the presence of oxygen, and **anaerobic** bacteria can reproduce only in the absence of oxygen. **Facultatively anaerobic** bacteria are not inhibited in either situation; they are able to reproduce in either the presence or absence of oxygen. This is obviously an advantage for the bacteria, and many pathogens and potential pathogens are facultative anaerobes.

The Gram Stain

Based on the chemicals in their cell walls, most bacteria can be put into one of two groups, called **gram positive** or **gram negative**. A simple laboratory procedure called the **Gram stain** (Fig. 22–2) shows us the shape of the bacteria and their gram reactions. Gram-positive bacteria appear purple or blue, and gram-negative bacteria appear pink or red. Some bacteria do not stain with the Gram method, but for those that do, each genus is either gram positive or gram negative. This does not change, just as the characteristic shape of the bacteria does not change. The genus *Streptococcus,* for example, is always a gram-positive coccus; the genus *Escherichia* is always a gram-negative bacillus. If a Gram stain is done on a sputum specimen from a patient with pneumonia, and a gram-positive coccus is found, this eliminates all of the gram-negative cocci and bacilli that may also cause pneumonia. The Gram stain, therefore, is often an important first step in the indentification of the pathogen that is causing a particular infection. In Table 22–3 (at the end of this chapter), the gram reaction (where applicable) and shape are included for each pathogen.

Special Characteristics

Although bacteria are simple cells, many have special structural or functional characteristics that help them to survive. Some bacilli and cocci have capsules (see Fig. 22–2); a **capsule** is a gelatinous sheath that encloses the entire cell. Capsules are beneficial to the bacteria because they inhibit phagocytosis by the host's white blood cells. This gives the bacteria time to reproduce and possibly establish themselves in the host. This is *not* beneficial from our point of view (remember that we are the hosts), but bacterial capsules are also **antigenic**, which means that they stimulate antibody production by our lympho-

cytes. This starts the destruction of bacteria by our immune responses. We take advantage of this by using bacterial capsules in some of our vaccines, such as those used to prevent pneumonia and meningitis.

Some bacilli are able to survive unfavorable environments by forming spores. A **spore** is a dormant (inactive) stage that consists of the chromosome and a small amount of cytoplasm surrounded by a thick wall. Spores can survive conditions such as heat (even boiling), freezing, or dehydration, which would kill the vegetative (active) forms of the bacterial cells. Fortunately for us, most pathogens are unable to form spores, but some that do are the causative agents of gas gangrene, botulism, tetanus, and anthrax. These bacteria are decomposers in the soil environment, and their spore-forming ability enables them to survive the extremes of temperature and lack of water that may occur in the soil.

Many bacteria cause disease because they produce **toxins**, which are chemicals that are harmful to host tissues. Often these toxins are the equivalent of our digestive enzymes, which break down the food we eat. Some bacterial toxins such as hemolysins and proteases literally digest host tissues such as red blood cells and proteins. The bacteria then absorb the digested nutrients.

The toxins of other bacteria have very specific effects on certain cells of the host. Botulism and tetanus toxins, for example, are **neurotoxins** that disrupt the functioning of nerve cells, leading to the characteristic symptoms of each disease. The diphtheria toxin causes heart failure, the pertussis (whooping cough) toxin immobilizes the cilia of the respiratory tract, and the cholera enterotoxin causes diarrhea (see also Table 22–3).

The cell walls of gram-negative bacteria are made of chemicals called endotoxins. **Endotoxins** all have the same effects on the host: They cause fever and circulatory shock (low blood pressure and heart failure). **Endotoxin shock** (also called **gram-negative shock)** is a life-threatening condition that may accompany any serious infection with gram-negative bacteria.

Rickettsias and Chlamydias

These two groups of bacteria differ from most other bacteria in that they are obligate intracellular parasites. This means that they can reproduce only within the living cells of a host.

Figure 22–2 **(A–F)** Bacterial shapes and specialized structures (magnification × 2000) **(G)** Gram-positive *Staphylococcus aureus* (× 1000). **(H)** Gram-negative *Neisseria gonorrhoeae* in WBCs (× 1000). **(I)** Gram-negative *Campylobacter jejuni* (× 1000). **(J)** Salmonella enteritidis growing on agar in a Petri dish. The black colonies indicate production of hydrogen sulfide gas. (G–J from Sacher, RA, and McPherson, RA: Widmann's Clinical Interpretation of Laboratory Tests. ed 11, FA Davis, Philadelphia, 2000, color plates 58, 59, 60 and 92, with permission.)

The rickettsias are parasites of mammals (including people) and are often spread by arthropod vectors. In the United States, the most common rickettsial disease is Rocky Mountain spotted fever, which is spread by ticks. In other parts of the world, epidemic typhus, which is spread by body lice, is still an important disease. From a historical perspective, until World War I, more people died of epidemic typhus during times of war than were killed by weapons.

The chlamydias cause several human diseases, including ornithosis (parrot fever) and trachoma, which is the leading cause of blindness throughout the world. In the United States, chlamydial infection of the genitourinary tract has become one of the most prevalent sexually transmitted diseases, with estimates of 4 million new cases each year.

Both rickettsial and chlamydial infections can be treated with antibiotics.

Antibiotics

Antibiotics are chemicals that are used to treat bacterial infections. A **broad-spectrum** antibiotic is one that affects many different kinds of bacteria; a **narrow-spectrum** antibiotic affects just a few kinds of bacteria.

The use of antibiotics is based on a very simple principle: Certain chemicals can disrupt or inhibit the chemical reactions that bacteria must carry out to survive. An antibiotic such as penicillin blocks the formation of bacterial cell walls; without their cell walls, bacteria will die. Other antibiotics inhibit DNA synthesis or protein synthesis. These are vital activities for the bacteria, and without them bacteria cannot reproduce and will die.

It is very important to remember that our own cells carry out chemical reactions that are very similar to some of those found in bacteria. For this reason, our own cells may be damaged by antibiotics. This is why some antibiotics have harmful side effects. The most serious side effects are liver and kidney damage or depression of the red bone marrow. The liver is responsible for detoxifying the medication, which may accumulate and damage liver cells. Similar damage may occur in the kidneys, which are responsible for excreting the medication. The red bone marrow is a very active tissue, with constant mitosis and protein synthesis to produce RBCs, WBCs, and platelets. Any antibiotic that interferes with these processes may decrease production of all of these blood cells. Patients who are receiving any of the potentially toxic antibiotics should be monitored with periodic tests of liver and kidney function or with blood counts to assess the state of the red bone marrow.

Another problem with the use of antibiotics is that bacteria may become resistant to them, and so be unaffected. Bacterial **resistance** means that the bacteria are able to produce an enzyme that destroys the antibiotic, rendering it useless. This is a genetic capability on the part of bacteria, and it is, therefore, passed to new generations of bacteria cells.

Let us use an example with small numbers, and say that of 1000 bacterial cells, 998 are killed by a certain antibiotic. The remaining two bacteria have the gene for an enzyme that breaks the antibiotic molecule, so they survive. What will these two bacteria do? Each will divide by binary fission, becoming two cells, four cells, eight cells, and so on. At the end of 20 divisions

(which under optimum conditions may take less than 24 hours) each bacterium has become more than a million bacteria. And what is true of all of these bacteria? They all have the gene for resistance to that particular antibiotic.

This is exactly what has happened with *Staphylococcus aureus,* most strains of which are resistant to penicillin, and some strains are resistant to many other antibiotics as well. Most of the gram-negative intestinal bacilli are resistant to a great variety of antibiotics. This is why **culture and sensitivity testing** is so important before an antibiotic is chosen to treat these infections.

Education is also important, and health-care personnel must help educate the general public not to demand antibiotics for colds or the flu. These are viral diseases for which antibiotics are useless. What happens is that the antibiotic kills all susceptible bacteria (even beneficial ones) and leaves resistant bacteria to become the most numerous, perhaps to cause serious disease in the future.

To counteract bacterial resistance, new antibiotics are produced that are not inactivated by the destructive bacterial enzymes. Within a few years, however, the usefulness of these new antibiotics will probably diminish as bacteria mutate and develop resistance. This is not a battle that we can ever truly win, because bacteria are living organisms that evolve as their environment changes.

Antibiotics have changed our lives, although we may not always realize that today. A child's strep throat will probably not progress to ear infections and meningitis, and bacterial pneumonia does not have the very high fatality rate that it once did. But, we must keep in mind that antibiotics are not a "cure" for any disease. An infection, especially a serious one, means that the immune system has been overwhelmed by the pathogen. An antibiotic diminishes the number of bacteria to a level with which the immune system can cope. Ultimately, however, the body's own white blood cells must eliminate the very last of the bacteria.

VIRUSES (SEE TABLE 22–4)

Viruses are not cells; their structure is even simpler than that of bacteria, which are the simplest cells. A virus consists of either DNA or RNA surrounded by a protein shell. The protein shell has a shape that is characteristic for each virus (Fig. 22–3). There are no

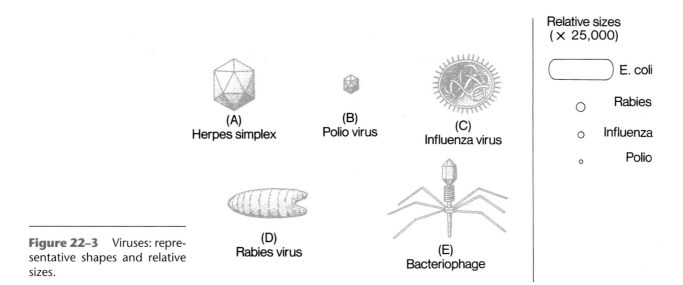

Figure 22–3   Viruses: representative shapes and relative sizes.

enzymes, cytoplasm, cell membranes, or cell walls in viruses, and they can reproduce only when inside the living cells of a host. Therefore, all viruses are obligate intracellular parasites, and they cause disease when they reproduce inside cells. When a virus enters a host cell, it uses the cell's chromosomes, RNA, and enzymes to make new viruses. Several hundred new viruses may be produced from just one virus. The host cell ruptures and dies, releasing the new viruses, which then enter other cells and reproduce.

The severity of a viral disease depends upon the types of cells infected. If the virus affects skin cells, for example, the disease is usually mild and self-limiting, such as chickenpox. Small numbers of skin cells are not crucial to our survival, and these cells can be replaced by mitosis. If, however, the virus affects nerve cells, the disease is more serious and may be fatal. Rabies is such as disease. Neurons are much more vital to us, and they cannot be replaced once they die.

Some viruses, such as those that cause German measles (rubella) and chickenpox, are able to cross the placenta, that is, pass from maternal circulation to fetal circulation. Although the disease may be very mild for the pregnant woman, the virus may severely damage developing fetal organs and cause congenital birth defects such as blindness, heart malformations, and mental retardation. In the most serious cases, fetal infection may result in miscarriage or stillbirth.

Some viruses cause an initial infection, become dormant, then are reactivated, causing another infection months or years later. The herpes viruses that cause cold sores "hide out" in nerves of the face following the initial skin lesion. At some later time when the host's resistance is lowered, the viruses emerge from the nerves and cause another cold sore. The chickenpox virus, which most of us acquire as children, is a herpes virus that may become dormant in nerves for years, and then be reactivated and cause shingles when we are adults.

A few human viruses are known to be tumor viruses, that is, they cause cells to develop abnormally and form tumors. The Epstein-Barr virus, which causes mononucleosis in North America, is associated with Burkitt's lymphoma in Africa and with nasopharyngeal carcinoma in China. There are environmental factors, as yet unknown, that contribute to the development of these cancers in specific parts of the world. Several of the human papilloma viruses have also been associated with cancers of the mouth or larynx, and three of these viruses are found in 90% of cervical carcinomas in women.

Important viral diseases are described in Table 22–4 at the end of this chapter.

Antiviral Medications

The treatment of viral diseases with chemicals poses some formidable challenges. First, viruses are active (reproducing) only within cells, so the medication must be able to enter infected cells to be effective. Second, viruses are such simple structures that the choice of which of their chemical processes to attempt to disrupt is limited. Third, viruses use the host cell's DNA and enzymes for self-replication, and a medication that interferes with DNA or enzymes may kill the host cell even as it kills the virus.

These problems are illustrated by zidovudine (AZT), the first medication that was effective against HIV, the virus that causes AIDS. Zidovudine works by interfering with DNA synthesis, which the virus must carry out to reproduce. The side effects of zidovudine, which are experienced by a significant number of AIDS patients, are caused by the disruption of DNA synthesis in the person's own cells.

Despite these obstacles, a few successful antiviral drugs have been developed. Acyclovir, for example, has proved to be useful in the control (not cure) of herpes viruses. Ribavirin has been quite effective in the treatment of respiratory syncytial virus pneumonia in infants and young children. This is an area of intensive research, and more antiviral medications will undoubtedly be found within the next decade.

FUNGI (SEE TABLE 22–5)

Fungi may be unicellular, such as yeasts, or multicellular, such as the familiar molds and mushrooms. Most fungi are **saprophytes**, that is, they live on dead organic matter and decompose it to recycle the chemicals as nutrients. The pathogenic fungi cause infections that are called **mycoses** (singular: **mycosis**), which may be superficial or systemic.

Yeasts (Fig. 22–4) have been used by people for thousands of years in baking and brewing. In small numbers, yeasts such as *Candida albicans* are part of the resident flora of the skin, mouth, intestines, and vagina. In larger numbers, however, yeasts may cause superficial infections of mucous membranes or the skin, or very serious systemic infections of internal organs. An all-too-common trigger for oral or vaginal yeast infections is the use of an antibiotic to treat a bacterial infection. The antibiotic diminishes the normal bacterial flora, thereby removing competition for the yeasts, which are then able to overgrow. Yeasts may also cause skin infections in diabetics, or in obese people who have skin folds that are always moist. In

A Yeast (x750)   **B** Rhizopus (x40)   **C** Aspergillus (x40)

D Ringworm (x750)   **E** Cryptococcus (x500)   **Figure 22–4** Fungi.

recent years, *Candida* has become an important cause of nosocomial infections. The resistance of hospital patients is often lowered because of their diseases or treatments, and they are more susceptible to systemic yeast infections in the form of pneumonia or endocarditis.

Another superficial mycosis is ringworm (tinea), which may be caused by several species of fungi (see Table 22–5 at the end of this chapter). The name *ringworm* is misleading, because there are no worms involved. It is believed to have come from the appearance of the lesions: circular, scaly patches with reddened edges; the center clears as the lesion grows. Athlete's foot, which is probably a bacterial-fungal infection, is perhaps the most common form of ringworm.

The systemic mycoses are more serious diseases that occur when spores of some fungi gain access to the interior of the body. Most of these fungi grow in a mold-like pattern. The molds we sometimes see on stale bread or overripe fruit look fluffy or fuzzy. The fluff is called a mycelium and is made of many thread-like cellular structures called hyphae. The color of a mold is due to the spore cases (sporangia) in which the reproductive spores are produced (see Fig. 22–4). Each spore may be carried by the air to another site, where it germinates and forms another mycelium.

Because spores of these fungi are common in the environment, they are often inhaled. The immune responses are usually able to prevent infection and healthy people are usually not susceptible to systemic mycoses. Elderly people and those with chronic pulmonary diseases are much more susceptible, however, and they may develop lung infections. The importance of the immune system is clearly evident if we consider people with AIDS. Without the normal immune responses, AIDS patients are very susceptible to invasive fungal diseases, including meningitis caused by *Cryptococcus*.

Antifungal Medications

One of the most effective drugs used to treat serious, systemic mycoses, amphotericin B, has great potential to cause serious side effects. Patients receiving this medication should have periodic tests of liver and kidney function. Newer medications include ketoconazole and fluconazole, which are less toxic to the recipient and may prove to be as effective as amphotericin B.

Superficial mycoses such as ringworm may be treated with certain oral medications. Taken orally, the drug is incorporated into living epidermal cells. When these cells die and reach the stratum corneum, they are resistant to the digestive action of the ringworm fungi. An effective topical spray has also been developed.

There are several effective medications for mucosal yeast infections, but it is important that the trigger for the infection (such as antibiotic therapy) be resolved as well. If not, the yeast infection may recur when the medication is stopped.

PROTOZOA (SEE TABLE 22–6)

Protozoa are unicellular animals, single cells that are adapted to life in freshwater (including soil) and saltwater. Some are human pathogens and are able to form cysts, which are resistant, dormant cells that are able to survive passage from host to host.

Intestinal protozoan parasites of people include *Entamoeba histolytica,* which causes amebic dysentery, and *Giardia lamblia,* which causes diarrhea called giardiasis (Fig. 22–5 and Table 22–6). People acquire these by ingesting food or water contaminated with the cysts of these species. Giardiasis can become a problem in day-care centers if the staff is not careful concerning handwashing and food preparation.

Plasmodium, the genus that causes malaria, affects hundreds of millions of people throughout the world and is probably the most important protozoan parasite. The *Plasmodium* species are becoming increasingly resistant to the standard antimalarial drugs, which are used to prevent disease as well as cure it. Although work is progressing on malaria vaccines, one will probably not be available for several years.

One protozoan of which you have probably heard is *Pneumocystis carinii* (though some researchers believe it is better classified as a fungus), which causes pneumonia in people with AIDS. This species is usually not pathogenic, because the healthy immune system can easily control it. For AIDS patients, however, this form of pneumonia is often the cause of death.

Medications are available that can treat most protozoan infections. Intestinal protozoa, for example, may be treated with metronidazole or furazolidone. The drug pentamidine is used to treat pneumocystis pneumonia, although the underlying cause, AIDS, is not yet curable.

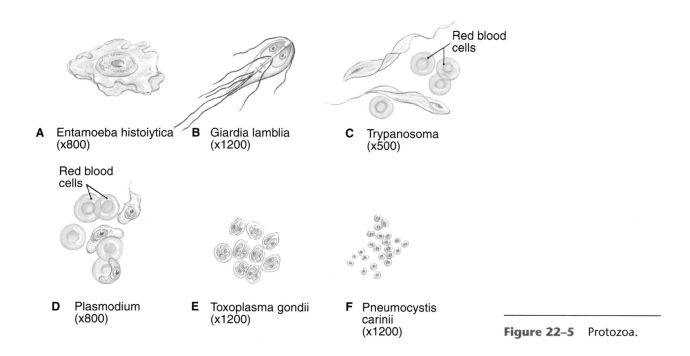

A Entamoeba histoiytica (x800)   **B** Giardia lamblia (x1200)   **C** Trypanosoma (x500)

D Plasmodium (x800)   **E** Toxoplasma gondii (x1200)   **F** Pneumocystis carinii (x1200)

Figure 22–5   Protozoa.

WORMS (HELMINTHS) (SEE TABLE 22–7)

Most worms are simple multicellular animals. The parasitic worms are even simpler than the familiar earthworm, because they live within hosts and use the host's blood or nutrients as food. Many of the parasitic worms have complex life cycles that involve two or more different host species.

The flukes are flatworms that are rare in most of North America but very common in parts of Africa and Asia. People acquire these species by eating aquatic plants or raw fish in which the larval worms have encysted. Within the person, each species lives in a specific site: the intestine, bile ducts, or even certain veins. Although rarely fatal, these chronic worm infestations are often debilitating, and the host person is a source of the eggs of the fluke, which may then infect others.

Tapeworms are also flatworms (Fig. 22–6). Some are 10 to 15 feet long, and the fish tapeworm can be as long as 60 feet. They are as flat as a ribbon, however, and one could easily be held in the palm of the hand. The tapeworm holds on to the lining of a host's small intestine with the suckers and hooks on its scolex (front end). The segments, called proglottids, are produced continuously in most species and

absorb nutrients from the host's digested food. The only function of the proglottids is reproduction: Eggs in one segment are fertilized by sperm from another segment. Mature proglottids containing fertilized eggs break off and are excreted in the host's feces. An intermediate host such as a cow or pig eats food contaminated with human feces, and the eggs hatch within this animal and grow into larval worms that encyst in the animal's muscle tissue. People become infected by eating poorly cooked beef or pork that contains cysts.

Parasitic roundworms of people include hookworm, pinworm, *Ascaris,* and *Trichinella* (see Table 22–7 at the end of this chapter). Medications are available that can eliminate worm infestations. In endemic areas, however, reinfestation is quite common.

ARTHROPODS (SEE TABLE 22–8)

Arthropods such as the scabies mite and head lice are **ectoparasites** that live on the surface of the body. The infestations they cause are very itchy and uncomfortable but not debilitating or life threatening (Fig. 22–7). Of greater importance are the arthropods that are vectors of disease. These are listed in Table 22–8. Mosquitoes, fleas, lice, and flies are all insects. Ticks are not insects but are more closely related to spiders.

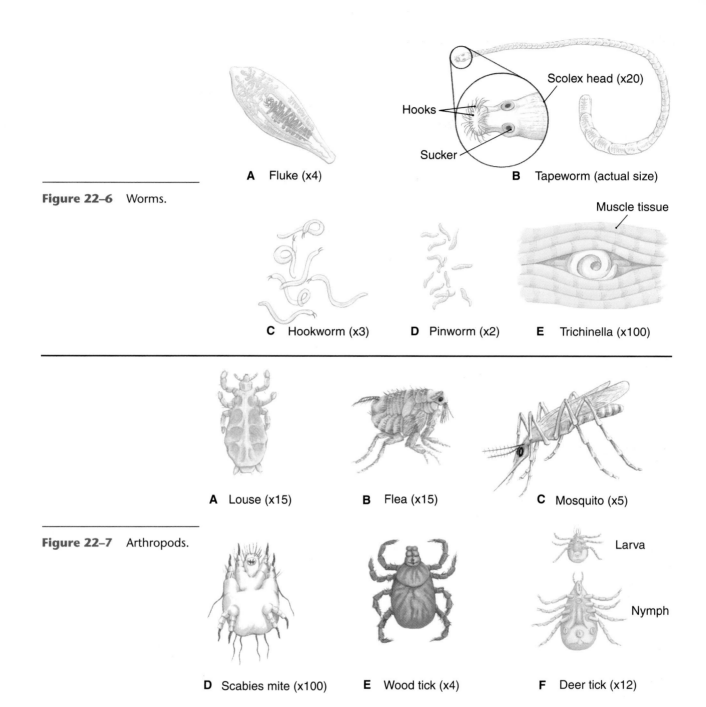

Figure 22–6 Worms.

A Fluke (x4)

B Tapeworm (actual size)

Scolex head (x20)

Hooks

Sucker

Muscle tissue

C Hookworm (x3) **D** Pinworm (x2) **E** Trichinella (x100)

A Louse (x15) **B** Flea (x15) **C** Mosquito (x5)

Figure 22–7 Arthropods.

Larva

Nymph

D Scabies mite (x100) **E** Wood tick (x4) **F** Deer tick (x12)

SUMMARY

The preceding discussion is an introduction to microorganisms and human disease, but it is only part of the story. The rest of this story is the remarkable ability of the human body to resist infection. Although we are surrounded and invaded by potential pathogens, most of us remain healthy most of the time.

The immune responses that destroy pathogens and enable us to remain healthy are described in Chapter 14. Also in that chapter are discussions of vaccines. The development of vaccines represents the practical application of our knowledge of pathogens and of immunity, and it enables us to prevent many diseases. The availability of specific vaccines is noted in the tables of bacterial and viral diseases that follow.

Table 22–3 | DISEASES CAUSED BY BACTERIA

Bacterial Species	Discussion/Disease(s) Caused
Staphylococcus aureus gram (+) coccus	Skin infections such as boils, pneumonia, toxic shock syndrome, osteomyelitis, septicemia. Most strains resistant to penicillin and many strains to related antibiotics as well. An important cause of nosocomial infections, carried on the hands or in the nasal cavities of health-care personnel. Food poisoning characterized by rapid onset (1–8 hours) and vomiting. No vaccine.
Staphylococcus epidermidis gram (+) coccus	Normal skin flora; potential pathogen for those with artificial internal prostheses such as heart valves and joints.
Streptococcus pyogenes gram (+) coccus (Group A streptococci)	Strep throat, otitis media, scarlet fever, endocarditis, puerperal sepsis; possible immunologic complications are rheumatic fever (transient arthritis and permanent damage to heart valves) and glomerulonephritis (transient kidney damage, usually with complete recovery). Rare strains cause necrotizing fasciitis, a potentially fatal hemolytic gangrene. No vaccine.
Streptococcus Group B gram (+) coccus	An important cause of neonatal infection, the bacteria are acquired from the mother during childbirth; risk factors are premature birth and intrapartum fever. May result in pneumonia, meningitis, or septicemia. May be prevented by testing pregnant women for Group B strep colonization and, if present, administering ampicillin. No vaccine.
Streptococcus pneumoniae gram (+) coccus	Pneumonia: accumulation of fluids and white blood cells in the alveoli. The vaccine contains capsules of the most common strains; recommended for the elderly, and for infants to prevent invasive disease. Possible cause of meningitis in adults with predisposing factors such as sickle-cell anemia, alcoholism, asplenism, or head trauma.
Enterococcus faecalis (formerly *Streptococcus faecalis*) and other species gram (+) coccus	Normal colon flora. Has become an important cause of nosocomial infections of the urinary tract. No vaccine. Other species (*E. faecium*) may be acquired from animals. Some strains are resistant to many antibiotics.
Neisseria gonorrhoeae gram (−) coccus	Gonorrhea: inflammation of the mucous membranes of the reproductive and urinary tracts. May cause scarring of reproductive ducts and subsequent sterility; in women may cause pelvic inflammatory disease. Infants of infected women may acquire the bacteria during birth; this is ophthalmia neonatorum and is prevented by antibiotic eyedrops. No vaccine.
Neisseria meningitidis gram (−) coccus	Meningitis: inflammation and edema of the meninges; pressure on the brain may cause death or permanent brain damage. Most common in older children and young adults. Most cases are sporadic, not part of epidemics. The vaccine is given to military recruits. Post-exposure prophylaxis (prevention) involves antibiotics.
Moraxella catarrhalis gram (−) coccobacillus	Otitis media and upper respiratory infection in children; pneumonia in adults, especially the immunocompromised or elderly. No vaccine.
Bacillus anthracis gram (+) bacillus (spore-forming)	Anthrax: spores in soil may be acquired by cattle or sheep. People acquire disease from these animals or from animal products such as wool or leather. The three forms are pulmonary, cutaneous, and gastrointestinal, reflecting the portal of entry. The toxin causes death of tissue, and the pulmonary form may be fatal. Rare in the US, because grazing animals are vaccinated. The vaccine for people was reserved for the military, but has been offered to people thought to be exposed to spores. Anthrax is a potential biological weapon.
Clostridium perfringens gram (+) bacillus (spore-forming)	Gas gangrene: normal soil flora may contaminate wounds; spores require anaerobic environment (dead tissue); toxins destroy more tissue, permitting the bacteria to spread; gas produced collects as bubbles in dead tissue. Food poisoning: from contaminated meat, self-limiting diarrhea.
Clostridium tetani gram (+) bacillus (spore-forming)	Tetanus: normal soil flora may contaminate wounds; spores require anaerobic conditions. The toxin prevents muscle relaxation, resulting in muscle spasms. May be fatal if respiratory muscles are affected. The vaccine contains the toxoid (inactivated toxin) and has made this a rare disease in the U.S. Boosters are strongly recommended for older adults.

Table 22–3 | DISEASES CAUSED BY BACTERIA (Continued)

Bacterial Species	Discussion/Disease(s) Caused
Clostridium botulinum gram (+) bacillus (spore-forming)	Botulism: normal soil flora; spores present in anaerobic food containers germinate and produce the toxin, which causes paralysis. Respiratory paralysis may be fatal without assisted ventilation. May cause infant botulism in children less than 2 years of age who have ingested spores. No vaccine. Treatment is antitoxin (antibodies).
Clostridium difficile gram (+) bacillus (spore-forming)	Diarrhea: the most common identifiable cause of antibiotic-associated diarrhea (pseudomembranous enterocolitis). No vaccine.
Corynebacterium diphtheriae gram (+) bacillus	Diphtheria: toxin causes heart failure and paralysis; a pseudomembrane that grows in the pharynx may cover the larynx and cause suffocation. Vaccination of infants (DTP) has made this a very rare disease in the U.S. Older adults should receive boosters (combined with tetanus: DT).
Listeria monocytogenes gram (+) bacillus	Listeriosis: septicemia and meningitis in the elderly, infants, and unborn; may cause miscarriage or stillbirth. The bacteria are found in soil and in animals such as cattle. In the U.S., food poisoning outbreaks traced to contaminated milk or milk products. Sporadic cases traced to undercooked hot dogs or chicken or to cold cuts from delicatessen counters. No vaccine.
Salmonella typhi gram (−) bacillus	Typhoid fever: intestinal infection with erosion and septicemia; subsequent infection of liver, gallbladder, or kidneys. Upon recovery, the carrier state (bacteria in gallbladder) may occur. Rare in the U.S. because of chlorination of drinking water. The vaccine is used in endemic areas of the world such as Asia.
Salmonella enteritidis and other species gram (−) bacillus	Salmonellosis: food poisoning following consumption of contaminated animal products such as poultry or eggs. Diarrhea is usually self-limiting, but it may be fatal for the elderly. In the U.S. estimates are 4 million cases per year. No vaccine.
Shigella species gram (−) bacillus	Bacillary dysentery: mild to severe diarrhea; may be fatal because of dehydration and circulatory shock. Usually transmitted by food prepared by people with mild cases. No vaccine. An important cause of illness in day-care centers.
Escherichia coli, Serratia marcescens, Proteus vulgaris, and other genera of gram (−) bacilli	Normal colon flora; cause opportunistic infections when introduced into any other part of the body. This group is one of the most common causes of nosocomial infections (urinary tract, pneumonia, skin infections).
Escherichia coli 0157:H7	Hemorrhagic colitis and hemolytic uremic syndrome, potentially fatal. The bacteria may survive in undercooked meat, especially ground beef. A vaccine is in the research stage.
Pseudomonas aeruginosa gram (−) bacillus	Normal soil and water flora; also transient in human intestines. A serious potential pathogen for patients with severe burns, cystic fibrosis (causes pneumonia), or cancer. May even survive in disinfectant solutions. No vaccine.
Yersinia pestis gram (−) bacillus	Bubonic plague: swollen lymph nodes, septicemia, and hemorrhagic pneumonia; often fatal. Animal reservoirs are prairie dogs, ground squirrels, and other rodents. Rats and people are infected by fleas (the vector). In the U.S., the few cases each year occur in the Southwest. The vaccine is no longer available.
Francisella tularensis gram (−) bacillus	Tularemia (rabbit fever): septicemia and pneumonia; not often fatal but very debilitating. Reservoirs are wild animals and birds. People are infected by vectors (ticks, lice, and biting flies), by ingestion of contaminated animal meat, or by inhalation. No vaccine. Tularemia is a potential biological weapon.
Brucella species gram (−) bacillus	Brucellosis (undulant fever): extreme weakness and fatigue, anorexia, a fever that rises and falls. Reservoirs are cattle, sheep, goats, and pigs; people acquire infection by contact with contaminated animal products. In the U.S., this is an occupational disease: meat processing workers, vets, farmers. Vaccines are available for animals.

Table 22–3   DISEASES CAUSED BY BACTERIA (Continued)

Bacterial Species	Discussion/Disease(s) Caused
Haemophilis influenzae gram (−) bacillus	Meningitis in children, especially those less than 2 years of age. Older people may have mild upper respiratory infections or a potentially fatal epiglottitis. The vaccine (Hib) contains the capsules of the bacteria and is recommended for infants beginning at age 2 months. This was the most common cause of meningitis in the U.S., approximately 20,000 cases per year. The vaccine has reduced the annual number of cases to about 1,000.
Haemophilis aegyptius gram (−) bacillus	Conjunctivitis: painful inflammation of the conjunctiva; spread by direct contact or fomites; may occur in epidemics among groups of children. No vaccine.
Bordetella pertussis gram (−) bacillus	Whooping cough (pertussis): paroxysms of violent coughing that may last for several weeks. Adults may have less severe coughing and go undiagnosed. Pneumonia is a complication that may be fatal, especially for children less than 1 year of age. People are the only host, and the vaccine has eliminated epidemics in the U.S. Concern about the safety of the original vaccine has prompted the development of newer vaccines, which may further reduce the annual number of cases.
Vibrio cholerae gram (−) bacillus (comma shaped)	Cholera: profuse watery diarrhea; infection ranges from mild to fatal. Spread of infection is usually by way of water contaminated with human feces. Rare in the U.S.; epidemic in Asia, Africa, and South America. The vaccine is no longer available.
Vibrio parahaemolyticus gram (−) bacillus (comma shaped)	Enteritis: diarrhea and nausea. Acquired by ingestion of raw or lightly cooked seafood; usually self-limiting.
Vibrio vulnificus gram (−) bacillus (comma shaped)	Gangrene and septicemia: acquired from ocean water that contaminates a wound or by the ingestion of raw shellfish. Illness is often severe and protracted, and it may be fatal, especially for people who are immunosuppressed or who have liver disease. No vaccine.
Campylobacter jejuni gram (−) helical bacillus	Enteritis: diarrhea that is often self-limiting but may be severe in the elderly or very young. Reservoirs are animals such as poultry; people acquire infection from contaminated meat. In the U.S., estimates are 2 million cases per year. No vaccine.
Helicobacter pylori gram (−) helical bacillus	Gastric ulcers: most are caused by *H. pylori,* which has also been implicated in cancer of the stomach.
Legionella pneumophilia gram (−) bacillus	Legionellosis, which occurs in two forms: Legionnaire's disease is a pneumonia that may be fatal; Pontiac fever is a mild upper respiratory infection that is usually self-limiting. The bacteria are found in natural water, including soil, and may contaminate air conditioning systems or water supplies. Person-to-person transmission does not seem to occur. Has become an important cause of nosocomial pneumonia. No vaccine.
Mycobacterium tuberculosis acid-fast bacillus	Tuberculosis (TB): formation of tubercles containing bacteria and white blood cells, usually in the lung. Lung tissue is destroyed (caseation necrosis) and is removed by macrophages, leaving large cavities. The bacteria are spread by respiratory droplets from people with active cases. Many people acquire a primary infection that becomes dormant and is without symptoms, yet may be triggered later into an active secondary infection. The BCG vaccine is not used in the U.S., but is in other parts of the world. In the U.S., TB cases are frequent among homeless people, those with AIDS, and in closed populations such as prisons. Strains of the bacteria resistant to the standard TB medications are becoming much more common and pose a difficult treatment problem.
Mycobacterium species acid-fast bacillus	Atypical mycobacterial infections: clinically similar to TB; usually in the lungs. These bacteria are pathogenic for people with AIDS or other forms of immunosuppression, and for those with chronic pulmonary diseases.
Mycobacterium leprae acid-fast bacillus	Leprosy (Hansen's disease): chronic disease characterized by disfiguring skin lesions and nerve damage that may cause paralysis or loss of sensation. The bacteria are acquired by cutaneous contact or respiratory droplets. The incubation period may be several years; children develop clinical disease more rapidly than do adults. A vaccine is in the testing stage.

Table 22–3	DISEASES CAUSED BY BACTERIA (Continued)
Bacterial Species	**Discussion/Disease(s) Caused**
Treponema pallidum spirochete	Syphilis: a sexually transmitted disease that progresses in three stages. Primary syphilis: a painless, hard chancre at the site of entry on skin or mucous membrane. Secondary syphilis: a rash on the skin and mucous membranes (indicates systemic infection). Tertiary syphilis (5 to 40 years later): necrotic lesions (gummas) in the brain, heart valves, aorta, spinal cord, skin, or other organs. Congenital syphilis (the bacteria can cross the placenta) may cause bone and teeth defects, and mental retardation. No vaccine.
Leptospira interrogans spirochete	Leptospirosis: a disease of wild or domestic animals that excrete the bacteria in urine. People acquire the bacteria by contact with contaminated water. Disease is usually mild, resembling intestinal virus infection. Weil's disease is the serious form, with hemorrhages in the liver and kidneys, and jaundice always present, indicating severe liver damage. A vaccine is available for dogs.
Borrelia burgdorferi spirochete	Lyme disease: begins as a flu-like illness, often with a bull's-eye rash at the site of the tick bite. May be followed by cardiac arrhythmias, self-limiting meningitis, or arthritis. Animal reservoirs are deer and field mice; the vector is the deer tick (genus *Ixodes*). The vaccine was taken off the market because of poor sales.
Borrelia vincenti spirochete	Trench mouth (Vincent's gingivitis): an ulcerative infection of the gums and pharynx caused by overgrowth of *Borrelia* and other normal oral flora. Triggered by poor oral hygiene or oral infection, which must be corrected to make antibiotic therapy effective.
Rickettsia prowazekii rickettsia	Epidemic typhus: high fever and delirium, hemorrhagic rash; 40% fatality rate. Vector is the human body louse. Very rare in the U.S. but still endemic in other parts of the world.
Rickettsia typhi rickettsia	Endemic typhus: similar to epidemic typhus but milder; 2% fatality rate. Reservoirs are rats and wild rodents; vectors are fleas. The few cases in the U.S. each year usually occur in the Southeast.
Rickettsia rickettsii rickettsia	Rocky Mountain spotted fever (RMSF): high fever, hemorrhagic rash, and pneumonia; 20% fatality rate. Reservoirs are wild rodents and dogs; vectors are ticks. Despite its name, RMSF in the U.S. is most prevalent in the Southeast coastal states (NC, SC) and in Oklahoma.
Chlamydia trachomatis (serogroups D–K) chlamydia	Genitourinary infection (nongonococcal urethritis): in men, urethritis or epididymitis; in women, cervicitis, although many women are asymptomatic. Complications in women include pelvic inflammatory disease, ectopic pregnancy, and miscarriage. Newborns of infected women may develop conjunctivitis or pneumonia. This is one of the most prevalent sexually transmitted diseases in the U.S. No vaccine.
Chlamydia trachomatis (serogroups A–C) chlamydia	Trachoma: conjunctivitis involving growth of papillae; vascular invasion of the cornea leading to scarring and blindness. Spread by direct contact and fomites. The leading cause of blindness throughout the world, especially in dry, dusty environments.
Chlamydia pneumoniae chlamydia	Pneumonia, usually community-acquired and mild enough to be called "walking pneumonia," with fever, cough, and hoarseness. No vaccine. *C. pneumoniae* as a factor in coronary artery disease has not yet been demonstrated conclusively.
Chlamydia psittaci chlamydia	Psittacosis, also called ornithosis or parrot fever. Reservoirs are wild and domestic birds, which shed the pathogen in feces. Acquired by people by inhalation of fecal dust. Disease ranges from mild upper respiratory infection to a more serious pneumonia. No vaccine.

Table 22–4	DISEASES CAUSED BY VIRUSES
Virus	**Discussion/Disease(s) Caused**
Herpes simplex	Type 1: fever blisters (cold sores) on the lip or in oral cavity; the virus is dormant in nerves of the face between attacks. Spread in saliva; may cause eye infections (self-inoculation). Type 2: genital herpes; painful lesions in the genital area; a sexually transmitted disease. Many people have few or no symptoms but may still spread the virus to sexual partners. No vaccine. Either type may be oral or genital, and may cause systemic infection and herpes encephalitis in newborns, whose immune systems cannot contain the virus.
Herpes varicella-zoster	Chickenpox: the disease of the first exposure; vesicular rash; pneumonia is a possible complication, especially in adults. The virus then becomes dormant in nerves. Shingles: painful, raised lesions on the skin above the affected nerves following reactivation of the dormant virus. Usually occurs in adults. The vaccine is recommended for children.
Human herpes virus 8	Kaposi's sarcoma: a malignancy of blood vessels often seen in people with AIDS; the virus is sexually transmitted. No vaccine.
Human papilloma viruses	More than 100 types, some of which cause genital warts. Several stimulate abnormal growth of cells and are implicated in cervical cancer in women. A vaccine for HPV-16 (the cause of approximately 50% of all cervical cancer) is in the testing stages.
Cytomegalovirus (CMV)	Most people have asymptomatic infection; the virus does no harm but remains in the body. Fetal infection may result in mental retardation, blindness, or deafness. CMV is the most frequent viral infection following organ transplants, and may cause a serious pneumonia. A cause of blindness in people with AIDS. No vaccine.
Epstein-Barr virus (EBV)	Mononucleosis: swollen lymph nodes, fatigue, fever, possible spleen or liver enlargement. Spread by saliva. Has been statistically implicated as a contributing factor to the onset of multiple sclerosis. EBV is linked to Burkitt's lymphoma in Africa and to nasopharyngeal carcinoma in China. No vaccine.
Adenoviruses	Many different types: some cause acute respiratory disease (ARD) similar to the common cold; others cause pharyngoconjunctival fever and may occur in epidemics related to swimming pools. The ARD vaccine is used only in the military.
Rhinoviruses	Common cold: sore throat, runny nose, low fever; usually self-limiting. No vaccine, though several are in the research stage (there are over 100 types of rhinoviruses).
Influenza viruses	Influenza: muscle aches, fever, fatigue, spread in respiratory droplets. Three types: A, B, and C. Type A is responsible for most epidemics. These are mutating viruses, and new vaccines are needed as the virus changes. The most serious complication is secondary bacterial pneumonia.
Respiratory syncytial virus	Pneumonia: especially at risk are infants and young children, esp. those who must be hospitalized. Decades of work have yet to produce an effective vaccine.
Hantaviruses	Hantavirus pulmonary syndrome: fever, cough, pulmonary edema, hypotension. Mortality rate is 40%–50%. Acquired by contact with rodent feces or urine, or inhalation of virus in rodent-infested areas. No vaccine.
Measles virus	Measles (rubeola): fever, sore throat, Koplik's spots (white) on lining of mouth, rash. Complications are ear infections, pneumonia, and measles encephalitis, which may be fatal. The vaccine is given to infants in combination with mumps and rubella (MMR).
Rubella virus	German measles: mild upper respiratory symptoms; a rash may or may not be present. The virus may cross the placenta and cause congenital rubella syndrome (CRS): blindness, deafness, heart defects, mental retardation, or miscarriage. CRS is most likely to occur if the fetus is infected during the first trimester. The vaccine is given to infants (MMR).
Mumps virus	Mumps: fever, swelling of the parotid salivary glands and perhaps the others (asymptomatic infections do occur); the virus is spread in saliva. Complications are rare in children but include pancreatitis, nerve deafness, and mumps encephalitis. Adult men may develop orchitis, inflammation of the testes. Adult women may develop oophoritis, inflammation of the ovaries. The vaccine is given to infants.

Table 22–4	DISEASES CAUSED BY VIRUSES (Continued)

Virus	Discussion/Disease(s) Caused
Polio viruses	Polio: most infections are asymptomatic or mild; major infection may result in paralysis. Two vaccines: IPV (Salk) contains a killed virus and cannot cause polio; booster injections are needed. OPV (Sabin) contains an attenuated virus, is given orally and carries a very small risk of causing polio. In the U.S., polio cases are vaccine related; polio is still endemic in other parts of the world. The WHO has set 2005 as the revised goal for the eradication of polio.
Rabies virus	Rabies: headache, nausea, fever, spasms of the swallowing muscles; seizures; fatal because of respiratory or heart failure; virtually 100% fatal. Reservoirs are wild animals; the virus is present in their saliva. Post-exposure prevention requires Human Rabies Immune Globulin (antibodies) and the rabies vaccine.
Encephalitis viruses	Encephalitis: most infections are mild; CNS involvement is indicated by confusion, lethargy, or coma. Several types of these viruses occur in the U.S. Reservoirs are wild birds and small mammals; vectors are mosquitoes. Vaccines are available for horses and for people whose occupations put them at risk.
West Nile virus	West Nile encephalitis: first found in North America in New York City in 1999 (well known in Africa and the Middle East). Natural reservoirs are birds; several species of mosquitoes are vectors. Symptoms include headache and confusion, but most infections are mild or asymptomatic; fatalities are not common. No vaccine.
Rotaviruses	Enteritis: worldwide the leading cause of diarrhea and potentially fatal dehydration in infants and children. Several vaccines are in the testing stage.
Norwalk viruses	Gastroenteritis: vomiting; called by many "stomach flu." Acquired from food such as shellfish, or from food handled by people with mild cases. No vaccine.
Ebola viruses	Hemorrhagic fever: high fever, systemic hemorrhages, necrosis of the liver; mortality rate 25% to 90%. The viruses also affect monkeys, which may be reservoirs of infection. No vaccine.
Marburg virus	Hemorrhagic fever similar to that caused by Ebola virus. No vaccine.
Yellow fever virus	Yellow fever: hemorrhages in the liver, spleen, kidneys, and other organs. The vector is a mosquito. The vaccine is recommended for travelers to endemic areas: Central and South America and Africa.
Hepatitis viruses: types A, B, and C	Hepatitis: anorexia, nausea, fatigue, jaundice (may not be present in mild cases). HAV is spread by the fecal–oral route; contaminated shellfish or food prepared by people with mild cases. No carriers after recovery. HBV is spread by sexual activity or contact with blood or other body fluids. Carrier state is possible; may lead to liver cancer or cirrhosis. HCV transmission is similar to that of HBV. Carrier state is possible. There are vaccines for hepatitis A and B. Other hepatitis viruses are designated D, E, F, and G.
Human immunodeficiency virus (HIV)	AIDS: destruction of helper T cells and suppression of the immune system; opportunistic infections; invariably fatal, often after many years. HIV is spread by sexual activity, contact with blood, or placental transmission. No vaccine.
Variola major	Smallpox: declared eradicated in the wild by the WHO in 1980. Is a potential biological weapon. A contagious disease characterized by a hemorrhagic rash and internal hemorrhages. Fatality rate is 30% to 50%. In the U.S., childhood vaccination was stopped in 1982.

Table 22–5 | DISEASES CAUSED BY FUNGI

Fungus Genus	Discussion/Disease(s) Caused
Microsporum, Trichophyton, Epidermophyton	Ringworm (tinea): scaly red patches on the skin or scalp; loss of hair. Tinea pedis is athlete's foot. May also infect damaged nails. Spores of these fungi are acquired from people or animals.
Candida (albicans and other species)	Yeast infections: mucosal infections are called thrush; may be oral or vaginal; yeasts have come from resident flora. Systemic infections include pneumonia and endocarditis. Important nosocomial pathogens.
Cryptococcus	Cryptococcosis: pulmonary infection that may progress to meningitis, especially in AIDS patients. Spores are carried in the air from soil or pigeon droppings.
Histoplasma	Histoplasmosis: pulmonary infection that is often self-limiting. Progressive disease involves ulcerations of the liver, spleen, and lymph nodes; usually fatal. Spores are carried by the air from soil.
Coccidioides	Coccidioidomycosis: pulmonary infection that is often self-limiting. Progressive disease involves the meninges, bones, skin, and other organs; high mortality rate. Spores are carried by the air.
Rhizopus	Common bread mold that is harmless to most people, but may cause invasive disease in those with compromised immune systems or poorly controlled diabetes. The spores may be inhaled or ingested and establish themselves in tissues, leading to systemic infection characterized by clotting and necrosis. Also causes digestive disease in cattle and pigs.
Aspergillus	A common mold found on fruits, harmless to healthy people. In those who are immunocompromised it may cause sinusitis, otitis, pneumonia, or more invasive disease.

Table 22–6 | DISEASES CAUSED BY PROTOZOA

Protozoan	Discussion/Disease(s) Caused
Entamoeba histolytica	Amebic dysentery; ulcerative lesions in the colon, bloody diarrhea; abscesses may form in the liver, lungs, or brain. Spread by the fecal–oral route in water or food.
Naegleria species	Amebic meningoencephalitis: inflammation of the meninges and brain; uncommon in the U.S. but almost always fatal. Amebas in fresh water are acquired when swimmers sniff water into the nasal cavities; the amebas move along the olfactory nerves into the brain.
Balantidium coli	Balantidiasis: abdominal discomfort and diarrhea; often mild. Reservoirs are pigs and other domestic animals; spread by the fecal–oral route.
Giardia lamblia	Giardiasis: fatty diarrhea; may be mild. Reservoirs are wild and domestic animals and people. Spread by the fecal–oral route in water or food prepared by people with mild cases. An important cause of diarrhea in day-care centers.
Trichomonas vaginalis	Trichomoniasis: a sexually transmitted disease. Women: causes cervicitis and vaginitis; men are often asymptomatic.
Trypanosoma species	African sleeping sickness: lethargy progressing to coma and death. Reservoirs are wild and domestic animals; vector is the tse tse fly. No vaccine.
Plasmodium species	Malaria: the protozoa reproduce in red blood cells, causing hemolysis and anemia. The vector is the *Anopheles* mosquito. No vaccine yet.
Toxoplasma gondii	Toxoplasmosis: asymptomatic infection in healthy people. Congenital infection: miscarriage or mental retardation, blindness. Reservoirs are cats and grazing animals. Pregnant women may acquire cysts from cat feces or from ingestion of rare beef or lamb.
Cryptosporidium species	Diarrhea: ranges from mild to severe; spread by the fecal–oral route. An important cause of diarrhea in day-care centers and in AIDS patients. Is very resistant to chlorine, may contaminate municipal water supplies or swimming pools and cause extensive epidemics.
Pneumocystis carinii	Pneumonia: only in very debilitated or immunosuppressed persons, such as people with AIDS. Has been classified with the fungi by some researchers, but its antibiotic susceptibity is that of a protozoan. Many people become infected during childhood, but a normal immune system prevents any damage. Such a latent infection may become symptomatic and very serious when cell-mediated immunity is impaired.

Table 22–7 | INFESTATIONS CAUSED BY WORMS

Worm (Genus)	Discussion/Disease(s) Caused
Chinese liver fluke (*Clonorchis*)	Abdominal discomfort; cirrhosis after many years. Adult worms (½ inch) live in bile ducts. Acquired by people from ingestion of raw fish that contains worm cysts.
Tapeworms (*Taenia, Diphyllobothrium*)	Bloating and abdominal discomfort; constipation or diarrhea. People acquire the worms by eating poorly cooked beef, pork, or fish (the alternate hosts) that contain worm cysts.
Pinworm (*Enterobius*)	Adult worms (⅛ inch) live in colon; females lay eggs on perianal skin while host is asleep, causing irritation and itching of skin. Eggs are spread to family members on hands and bed linens. In the U.S., this is probably the most common worm infestation.
Hookworm (*Necator*)	Adult worms (½ inch) live in the small intestine; their food is blood. Heavy infestations cause anemia and fatigue. Eggs are excreted in feces; larval worms burrow through the skin of a bare foot and migrate to the intestine.
Ascaris	Adults are 10–12 inches long, and live in the small intestine. Large numbers of worms may cause intestinal obstruction. Eggs are excreted in feces and are spread to others on hands or vegetation contaminated by human feces.
Trichinella spiralis	Trichinosis: severe muscle pain as migrating worms form cysts that become calcified. Acquired by eating poorly cooked pork (or wild animals) that contains cysts.

Table 22–8　ARTHROPOD VECTORS

Anthropod	Disease (Type of Pathogen)*
Mosquito	Malaria (protozoan) Encephalitis (virus) Yellow fever (virus)
Flea	Plague (bacterium) Endemic typhus (rickettsia)
Body louse	Epidemic typhus (rickettsia) Tularemia (bacterium) Relapsing fever (bacterium)
Tick	Lyme disease (bacterium) Rocky Mountain spotted fever 　(rickettsia) Tularemia (bacterium)
Tse tse fly	African sleeping sickness (protozoan)
Deer fly, horse fly	Tularemia (bacterium)

*These diseases are described in previous tables.

STUDY OUTLINE

Classification of Microorganisms
1. Bacteria—unicellular; some are pathogens.
2. Viruses—not cells; all are parasites.
3. Protozoa—unicellular animals; some are pathogens.
4. Fungi—unicellular (yeasts) or multicellular (molds); most are decomposers.
5. Worms—multicellular animals; a few are parasites.
6. Arthropods—insects, ticks, or mites that are vectors of disease or cause infestations.
   • Binomial nomenclature—the genus and species names.

Normal Flora—see Table 22–1
1. Resident flora—the microorganisms that live on or in nearly everyone, in specific body sites; cause no harm when in their usual sites.
2. Transient flora—the microorganisms that periodically inhabit the body and usually cause no harm unless the host's resistance is lowered.

Infectious Disease
1. Caused by microorganisms or their toxins.
2. Clinical infections are characterized by symptoms; in a subclinical infection, the person shows no symptoms.

3. Course of an infectious disease: Incubation period—the time between the entry of the pathogen and the onset of symptoms. The acme is the worst stage of the disease, followed by recovery or death. A self-limiting disease typically lasts a certain period of time and is followed by recovery.
4. Types of Infection
   • Localized—the pathogen is in one area of the body.
   • Systemic—the pathogen is spread throughout the body by the blood or lymph.
   • Septicemia (bacteremia)—bacteria in the blood.
   • Acute—usually severe or of abrupt onset.
   • Chronic—progresses slowly or is prolonged.
   • Secondary—made possible by a primary infection that lowered host resistance.
   • Nosocomial—a hospital-acquired infection.
   • Endogenous—caused by the person's own normal flora in an abnormal site.

Epidemiology—see Fig. 22–1
1. The study of the patterns and spread of disease.
2. Portal of entry—the way a pathogen enters a host.
3. Portal of exit—the way a pathogen leaves a host.

4. Reservoirs—persons with the disease, carriers after recovery, or animal hosts (for zoonoses).
5. Non-communicable disease—cannot be directly or indirectly transmitted from host to host.
6. Communicable disease—may be transmitted directly from host to host by respiratory droplets, cutaneous or sexual contact, placental transmission, or blood contact. May be transmitted indirectly by food or water, vectors, or fomites.
7. Contagious disease—easily spread from person to person by casual cutaneous contact or respiratory droplets.

Methods of Control of Microbes
1. Antiseptics—chemicals that destroy or inhibit bacteria on a living being.
2. Disinfectants—chemicals that destroy or inhibit bacteria on inanimate objects.
3. Sterilization—a process that destroys all living organisms.
4. Public health measures include laws and regulations to ensure safe food and water.

Bacteria—see Fig. 22–2
1. Shapes: coccus, bacillus, and spirillum.
2. Flagella provide motility for some bacilli and spirilla.
3. Aerobes require oxygen; anaerobes are inhibited by oxygen; facultative anaerobes grow in the presence or absence of oxygen.
4. The gram reaction (positive or negative) is based on the chemistry of the cell wall. The Gram stain is a laboratory procedure used in the identification of bacteria.
5. Capsules inhibit phagocytosis by white blood cells. Spores are dormant forms that are resistant to environmental extremes.
6. Toxins are chemicals produced by bacteria that are poisonous to host cells.
7. Rickettsias and chlamydias differ from other bacteria in that they must be inside living cells to reproduce.
8. Antibiotics are chemicals used in the treatment of bacterial diseases. Broad-spectrum: affects many kinds of bacteria. Narrow-spectrum: affects only a few kinds of bacteria.
9. Bacteria may become resistant to certain antibiotics, which are then of no use in treatment. Resistance is a genetic trait, and will be passed to future generations. Culture and sensitivity testing may be necessary before an antibiotic is chosen to treat an infection.
10. Diseases—see Table 22–3.

Viruses—see Fig. 22–3
1. Not cells; a virus consists of either DNA or RNA surrounded by a protein shell.
2. Must be inside living cells to reproduce, which causes death of the host cell.
3. Severity of disease depends on the types of cells infected; some viruses may cross the placenta and infect a fetus.
4. Antiviral medications must interfere with viral reproduction without harming host cells; few such chemicals are available.
5. Diseases—see Table 22–4.

Fungi—see Fig. 22–4
1. Most are saprophytes, decomposers of dead organic matter. May be unicellular yeasts or multicellular molds.
2. Mycoses may be superficial, involving the skin or mucous membranes, or systemic, involving internal organs such as the lungs or meninges.
3. Effective antifungal medications are available, but some are highly toxic.
4. Diseases—see Table 22–5.

Protozoa—see Fig. 22–5
1. Unicellular animals; some are pathogens.
2. Some are spread by vectors, others by fecal contamination of food or water.
3. Effective medications are available for most diseases.
4. Diseases—see Table 22–6.

Worms—see Fig. 22–6
1. Simple multicellular animals; the parasites are flukes, tapeworms, and some roundworms.
2. May have life cycles that involve other animal hosts as well as people.
3. Effective medications are available for most worm infestations.
4. Diseases—see Table 22–7.

Arthropods—see Fig. 22–7
1. Some cause superficial infestations.
2. Others are vectors of disease—see Table 22–8.

REVIEW QUESTIONS

1. Define resident flora, and explain its importance. (p. 478)

2. State the term described by each statement: (pp. 479–481, 485)
   a. An infection in which the person shows no symptoms
   b. Bacteria that are inhibited by oxygen
   c. A disease that lasts a certain length of time and is followed by recovery
   d. A disease that is usually present in a given population
   e. The presence of bacteria in the blood
   f. An infection made possible by a primary infection that lowers host resistance
   g. A disease of animals that may be acquired by people
   h. Bacteria that are spherical in shape

3. Name these parts of bacterial cell: (pp. 485–486)
   a. Inhibits phagocytosis by white blood cells
   b. Provides motility
   c. The basis for the gram reaction or Gram stain
   d. A form resistant to heat and drying
   e. Chemicals produced that are poisonous to host cells

4. Explain what is meant by a nosocomial infection, and describe the two general kinds with respect to sources of the pathogen. (p. 480)

5. Name five potential portals of entry for pathogens. (p. 481)

6. Name five potential portals of exit for pathogens. (p. 482)

7. Explain the difference between a communicable disease and a contagious disease. (p. 482)

8. Explain the difference between pasteurization and sterilization. (pp. 483–484)

9. Describe the structure of a virus, and explain how viruses cause disease. (pp. 488–489)

10. Describe the differences between yeasts and molds. (pp. 490–491)

11. Describe the difference between superficial and systemic mycoses. (pp. 490–491)

12. Name some diseases that are spread by vectors, and name the vector for each. (p. 502)

FOR FURTHER THOUGHT

1. Smallpox has been eradicated (in the wild). Polio is the next target of world health officials, then measles. What characteristics must a disease or its pathogen have that would allow us even to consider trying to eradicate it? Try to think of five.

2. To understand the epidemiology of a disease, we must know several things about the disease or its agent (pathogen). Again, try to think of five.

3. Many working mothers depend on day-care centers to care for their children. What pathogens are likely to flourish in a day-care center if proper precautions are not taken? There are two general kinds. Besides being sure that all children have the proper vaccinations, what do you think is the most important proper precaution (think: lunchtime)?

4. We're still at the day-care center. Name three diseases that all 2-year-olds should have been vaccinated against. There may be a 6-month-old child in the group who has not yet received certain vaccinations, yet this child may be protected by what we call "herd immunity." Describe what is meant by herd immunity.

5. Explain why leptospirosis may be misdiagnosed as hepatitis (compare the descriptions in the tables of pathogens). Explain the consequences for the patient (notice what kind of pathogen causes each). What does this suggest to us about rare diseases, or the study of rare diseases?

6. Ms. D has had second thoughts about her eyebrow ring, so she has taken it out and now wants the

hole to close. She comes to the clinic on campus because the pierced site is not healing, has become inflamed, red, and painful. Ms. D claims that she keeps the site very clean by applying hydrogen peroxide several times a day. What do you tell her to do?

7. West Nile virus encephalitis was new to North America in 1999. Less than a year later, public health officials could say that most infections were asymptomatic or mild, and only a very small percentage were serious or fatal. How do you think they discovered this?

Units of Measure

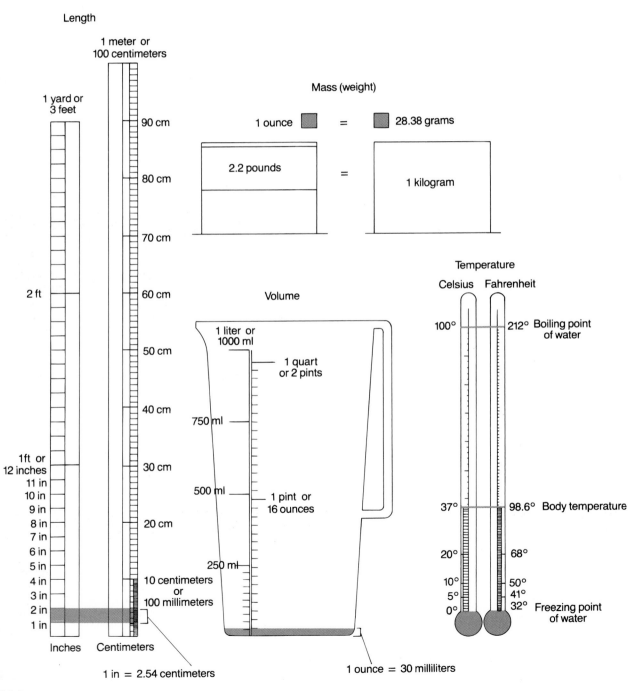

Length

1 meter or
100 centimeters

1 yard or
3 feet

90 cm

80 cm

70 cm

60 cm

2 ft

50 cm

40 cm

750 ml

1ft or
12 inches
11 in
10 in
9 in
8 in
7 in
6 in
5 in
4 in
3 in
2 in
1 in

30 cm

500 ml

20 cm

250 ml

10 centimeters
or
100 millimeters

Inches   Centimeters

1 in = 2.54 centimeters

Mass (weight)

1 ounce [ ] = [ ] 28.38 grams

2.2 pounds = 1 kilogram

Volume

1 liter or
1000 ml

1 quart
or 2 pints

1 pint or
16 ounces

1 ounce = 30 milliliters

Temperature

Celsius   Fahrenheit

100°   212° Boiling point
                  of water

37°   98.6° Body temperature

20°   68°

10°   50°
5°   41°
0°   32° Freezing point
                  of water

Units of Length

	mm	cm	in	ft	yd	M
1 millimeter =	1.0	0.1	0.04	0.003	0.001	0.001
1 centimeter =	10.0	1.0	0.39	0.032	0.011	0.01
1 inch =	25.4	2.54	1.0	0.083	0.028	0.025
1 foot =	304.8	30.48	12.0	1.0	0.33	0.305
1 yard =	914.4	91.44	36.0	3.0	1.0	0.914
1 meter =	1000.0	100.0	39.37	3.28	1.09	1.0

$1 \mu = 1$ mu = 1 micrometer (micron) = 0.001 mm = 0.00004 in.
mm = millimeters; **cm** = centimeters; **in** = inches; **ft** = feet; **yd** = yards; **M** = meters.

Units of Weight

	mg	g	oz	lb	kg
1 milligram =	1.0	0.001	0.00004	0.000002	0.000001
1 gram =	1000.0	1.0	0.035	0.002	0.001
1 ounce =	28,380	28.4	1.0	0.06	0.028
1 pound =	454,000	454.0	16	1.0	0.454
1 kilogram =	1,000,000	1000.0	35.2	2.2	1.0

mg = milligrams; **g** = grams; **oz** = ounces; **lb** = pounds; **kg** = kilograms.

Units of Volume

	ml	in³	oz	qt	l
1 milliliter =	1.0	0.06	0.034	0.001	0.001
1 cubic inch =	16.4	1.0	0.55	0.017	0.016
1 ounce =	29.6	1.8	1.0	0.03	0.029
1 quart =	946.3	57.8	32.0	1.0	0.946
1 liter =	1000.0	61.0	33.8	1.06	1.0

ml = milliliters; **in³** = cubic inches; **oz** = ounces; **qt** = quarts; **l** = liters.

Temperature
Celsius and Fahrenheit

°C	Is Equivalent to	°F
0°C		32°F
5°C		41°F
10°C		50°F
15°C		59°F
20°C		68°F
25°C		77°F
30°C		86°F
35°C		95°F
40°C		104°F
45°C		113°F
50°C		122°F

Abbreviations

The use of abbreviations for medical and scientific terms is timesaving and often standard practice. Some of the most frequently used abbreviations have been listed here. Notice that some have more than one interpretation. It is important to know the abbreviations approved by your institution, use only those, and *never* make up your own abbreviations. If there is any chance of confusion, write out the words.

ABC	airway, breathing, circulation	**CO**	cardiac output; carbon monoxide
ABG	arterial blood gas	**COPD**	chronic obstructive pulmonary disease
ABX	antibiotics	**CP**	cerebral palsy
ACh	acetylcholine	**CPR**	cardiopulmonary resuscitation
ACTH	adrenocorticotropic hormone	**CRF**	chronic renal failure
AD	Alzheimer's disease	**C-section**	cesarean section
ADH	antidiuretic hormone	**CSF**	cerebrospinal fluid
AIDS	acquired immunodeficiency syndrome	**CT (CAT)**	computed (axial) tomography
ALS	amyotrophic lateral sclerosis	**CVA**	cerebrovascular accident
ANS	autonomic nervous system	**CVP**	central venous pressure
ARDS	acute respiratory distress syndrome	**CVS**	chorionic villus sampling
ARF	acute renal failure (acute respiratory failure)	**D & C**	dilation and curettage
ATP	adenosine triphosphate	**DM**	diabetes mellitus (diastolic murmur)
AV	atrioventricular	**DMD**	Duchenne's muscular dystrophy
BAL	blood alcohol level	**DNA**	deoxyribonucleic acid
BBB	blood–brain barrier	**DNR**	do not resuscitate
BMR	basal metabolic rate	**DOA**	date of admission (dead on arrival)
BP	blood pressure	**DRG**	diagnosis-related group
BPH	benign prostatic hypertrophy (hyperplasia)	**Dx**	diagnosis
BPM	beats per minute	**EBV**	Epstein-Barr virus
BS	blood sugar (bowel sounds, breath sounds)	**ECF**	extracellular fluid (extended care facility)
BUN	blood urea nitrogen	**ECG (EKG)**	electrocardiogram
CA	cancer	**EDV**	end-diastolic volume
CAD	coronary artery disease	**EEG**	electroencephalogram
CAPD	continuous ambulatory peritoneal dialysis	**EFM**	electronic fetal monitoring
CBC	complete blood count	**EP**	ectopic pregnancy
CC	creatinine clearance (critical condition, chief complaint)	**ER**	endoplasmic reticulum
		ERT	estrogen replacement therapy
CCCC	closed-chest cardiac compression	**ESR**	erythrocyte sedimentation rate
CF	cystic fibrosis (cardiac failure)	**ESRD**	end-stage renal disease
CHD	coronary heart disease (congenital heart disease)	**ESV**	end-systolic volume
		FAS	fetal alcohol syndrome
		FBG	fasting blood glucose
CHF	congestive heart failure	**FOBT**	fecal occult blood testing
CI	cardiac insufficiency (cerebral infarction)	**FSH**	follicle-stimulating hormone
CNS	central nervous system	**FUO**	fever of unknown origin

Fx	fracture	**PKU**	phenylketonuria
GB	gallbladder	**PMN**	polymorphonuclear leukocyte
GFR	glomerular filtration rate	**PMS**	premenstrual syndrome
GH	growth hormone	**PNS**	peripheral nervous system
GI	gastrointestinal	**PT**	prothrombin time (patient, patient teaching,
HAV	hepatitis A virus		physical therapy)
Hb	hemoglobin	**PTH**	parathyroid hormone
HBV	hepatitis B virus	**PTT**	partial thromboplastin time
HCG	human chorionic gonadotropin	**PVC**	premature ventricular contraction
Hct	hematocrit	**RA**	right atrium
HCV	hepatitis C virus	**RBC**	red blood cell
HDL	high-density lipoprotein	**RBM**	red bone marrow
HLA	human leukocyte antigen	**RDA**	recommended daily allowance
HR	heart rate	**RDS**	respiratory distress syndrome
HRT	hormone replacement therapy	**REM**	rapid eye movement
HSV	herpes simplex virus	**RE(S)**	reticuloendothelial (system)
HTN	hypertension	**Rh**	*Rhesus*
Hx	history	**RIA**	radioimmunoassay
IBD	inflammatory bowel disease	**RLQ**	right lower quadrant
IBS	irritable bowel syndrome	**RNA**	ribonucleic acid
ICF	intracellular fluid	**RV**	right ventricle
ICP	intracranial pressure	**RUQ**	right upper quadrant
ICU	intensive care unit	**Rx**	prescription
ID	intradermal	**SA**	sinoatrial
IDDM	insulin-dependent diabetes mellitus	**SC**	subcutaneous
Ig	immunoglobulin	**SCID**	severe combined immunodeficiency
IM	intramuscular	**SF**	synovial fluid
IV	intravenous	**SIDS**	sudden infant death syndrome
LA	left atrium	**SLE**	systemic lupus erythematosus
LDL	low-density lipoprotein	**SPF**	sun protection factor
LH	luteinizing hormone	**S/S (sx)**	signs and symptoms
LLQ	left lower quadrant	**STD**	sexually transmitted disease
LUQ	left upper quadrant	**SV**	stroke volume
LV	left ventricule	**T₃**	triiodothyronine
mEq/L	milliequivalents per liter	**T₄**	thyroxine
MG	myasthenia gravis	**TIA**	transient ischemic attack
MI	myocardial infarction	**TMJ**	temporomandibular joint
mm³	cubic millimeter	**t-PA**	tissue plasminogen activator
mmHg	millimeters of mercury	**TPN**	total parenteral nutrition
MRI	magnetic resonance imaging	**TSH**	thyroid-stimulating hormone
MS	multiple sclerosis	**TSS**	toxic shock syndrome
MSOF	multisystem organ failure	**Tx**	treatment
MVP	mitral valve prolapse	**UA**	urinalysis
NGU	non-gonococcal urethritis	**URI**	upper respiratory infection
NIDDM	non-insulin-dependent diabetes mellitus	**US**	ultrasound
NPN	non-protein nitrogen	**UTI**	urinary tract infection
OC	oral contraceptive	**UV**	ultraviolet
OTC	over the counter	**VPC**	ventricular premature contraction
PE	pulmonary embolism	**VD**	venereal disease
PET	positron emission tomography	**VS**	vital signs
PG	prostaglandin	**WBC**	white blood cell
PID	pelvic inflammatory disease	**WNL**	within normal limits

Normal Values for Some Commonly Used Blood Tests

Test	Normal Value	Clinical Significance of Variations
Albumin	3.5–5.5 g/100 ml	• Decreases: kidney disease, severe burns
Bilirubin—Total 　　　　Direct 　　　　Indirect	0.3–1.4 mg/100 ml 0.1–0.4 mg/100 ml 0.2–1.0 mg/100 ml	• Increases: liver disease, rapid RBC destruction, biliary obstruction
Calcium	4.3–5.3 mEq/liter	• Increases: hyperparathyroidism • Decreases: hypoparathyroidism, severe diarrhea, malnutrition
Chloride	95–108 mEq/liter	• Decreases: severe diarrhea, severe burns, ketoacidosis
Cholesterol 　HDL cholesterol 　LDL cholesterol	140–199 mg/100 ml 29–77 mg/100 ml <130 mg/100 ml	• Increases: hypothyroidism, diabetes mellitus
Clotting time	5–10 minutes	• Increases: liver disease
Creatinine	0.6–1.5 mg/100 ml	• Increases: kidney disease
Globulins	2.3–3.5 g/100 ml	• Increases: chronic infections
Glucose	70–110 mg/100 ml	• Increases: diabetes mellitus, liver disease, hyperthyroidism, pregnancy
Hematocrit	38%–48%	• Increases: dehydration, polycythemia • Decreases: anemia, hemorrhage
Hemoglobin	12–18 g/100 ml	• Increases: polycythemia, high altitude, chronic pulmonary disease • Decreases: anemia, hemorrhage
P_{CO_2}	35–45 mmHg	• Increases: pulmonary disease • Decreases: acidosis, diarrhea, kidney disease
pH	7.35–7.45	• Increases: hyperventilation, metabolic alkalosis • Decreases: ketoacidosis, severe diarrhea, hypoventilation
P_{O_2}	75–100 mmHg	• Decreases: anemia, pulmonary disease
Phosphorus	1.8–4.1 mEq/liter	• Increases: kidney disease, hypoparathyroidism • Decreases: hyperparathyroidism
Platelet count	150,000–300,000/mm^3	• Decreases: leukemia, aplastic anemia
Potassium	3.5–5.0 mEq/liter	• Increases: severe cellular destruction • Decreases: diarrhea, kidney disease

Test	Normal Value	Clinical Significance of Variations
Prothrombin time	11–15 seconds	• Increases: liver disease, vitamin K deficiency
Red blood cell count	4.5–6.0 million/mm^3	• Increases: polycythemia, dehydration • Decreases: anemia, hemorrhage, leukemia
Reticulocyte count	0.5%–1.5%	• Increases: anemia, following hemorrhage
Sodium	136–142 mEq/liter	• Increases: dehydration • Decreases: kidney disease, diarrhea, severe burns
Urea nitrogen (BUN)	8–25 mg/100 ml	• Increases: kidney disease, high-protein diet
Uric acid	3.0–7.0 mg/100 ml	• Increases: kidney disease, gout, leukemia
White blood cell count	5000–10,000/mm^3	• Increases: acute infection, leukemia • Decreases: aplastic anemia, radiation sickness

Normal Values for Some Commonly Used Urine Tests

Test	Normal Value	Clinical Significance of Variations
Acetone and acetoacetic acid (ketones)	0	• Increases: ketoacidosis, starvation
Albumin	0–trace	• Increases: kidney disease, hypertension
Bilirubin	0	• Increases: biliary obstruction
Calcium	less than 250 mg/24 hrs	• Increases: hyperparathyroidism • Decreases: hypoparathyroidism
Creatinine	1.0–2.0 g/24 hrs	• Increases: infection • Decreases: kidney disease, muscle atrophy
Glucose	0	• Increases: diabetes mellitus
pH	4.5–8.0	• Increases: urinary tract infection, alkalosis, vegetarian diet • Decreases: acidosis, starvation, high-protein diet
Protein	0	• Increases: kidney disease, extensive trauma, hypertension
Specific gravity	1.010–1.025	• Increases: dehydration • Decreases: excessive fluid intake, alcohol intake, severe kidney damage
Urea	25–35 g/24 hrs	• Increases: high-protein diet; excessive tissue breakdown • Decreases: kidney disease
Uric acid	0.4–1.0 g/24 hrs	• Increases: gout, liver disease • Decreases: kidney disease
Urobilinogen	0–4 mg/24 hrs	• Increases: liver disease, hemolytic anemia • Decreases: biliary obstruction

Suggestions for Further Reading

Taber's Cyclopedic Medical Dictionary, 19th ed.
Donald Venes, Editor
F.A. Davis Company, Philadelphia, 2001

Tissues and Organs: A Text-Atlas of Scanning Electron Microscopy
Richard G. Kessel and Randy H. Kardon
W.H. Freeman and Company, San Francisco, 1979

Atlas of Normal Histology, 6th ed.
Mariano S.H. diFiore, edited by Victor P. Eroschenko
Lea & Febiger, Philadelphia, 1989

Principles of Anatomy & Physiology, 9th ed.
Gerard J. Tortora and Sandra R. Grabowski
John Wiley & Sons, New York, 2000

Behold Man: A Photographic Journey Inside the Body
Lennart Nilsson
Little, Brown & Co., Boston, 1973

Life, Death, and in Between: Tales of Clinical Neurology
Harold L. Klawans
Paragon House Publishers, New York, 1992

Toscanini's Fumble and Other Tales of Clinical Neurology
Harold L. Klawans
Bantam Books, New York, 1989

New Guinea Tapeworms and Jewish Grandmothers: Tales of Parasites and People
Robert S. Desowitz
W.W. Norton and Company, New York, 1987

The Malaria Capers: Tales of Parasites and People
Robert S. Desowitz
W.W. Norton and Company, New York, 1993

Genome
Matt Ridley
Harper Collins, New York, 1999

How We Die
Sherwin B. Nuland
Alfred A. Knopf, New York, 1994

Prefixes, Combining Word Roots, and Suffixes Used in Medical Terminology

PREFIXES AND COMBINING WORD ROOTS

a-, an- absent, without (amenorrhea: absence of menstruation)

ab- away from (abduct: move away from the midline)

abdomin/o- abdomen (abdominal aorta: the portion of the aorta in the abdomen)

acou- hearing (acoustic nerve: the cranial nerve for hearing)

ad- toward, near, to (adduct: move toward the midline)

aden/o- gland (adenohypophysis: the glandular part of the pituitary gland)

af- to, toward (afferent: toward a center)

alba- white (albino: an animal lacking coloration)

alg- pain (myalgia: muscle pain)

ana- up, back (anabolism: the constructive phase of metabolism)

angi/o- vessel (angiogram: imaging of blood vessels, as in the heart)

ante- before (antenatal: before birth)

anti- against (antiemetic: an agent that prevents vomiting)

arthr/o- joint (arthritis: inflammation of a joint)

atel- imperfect, incomplete (atelectasis: incomplete expansion of a lung)

auto- self (autoimmune disease: a disease in which immune reactions are directed against part of one's own body)

bi- two, twice (biconcave: concave on each side, as a red blood cell)

bio- life (biochemistry: the chemistry of living organisms)

blasto- growth, budding (blastocyst: a rapidly growing embryonic stage)

brachi/o- arm (brachial artery: the artery that passes through the upper arm)

brachy- short (brachydactyly: abnormally short fingers or toes)

brady- slow (bradycardia: slow heart rate)

bronch- air passage (bronchioles: small air passages in the lungs)

carcin/o- cancer (carcinogen: cancer-causing substance)

cardi/o- heart (cardiopathy: heart disease)

carp/o- wrist (carpals: bones of the wrist)

cata- down (catabolism: the breaking down phase of metabolism)

caud- tail (cauda equina: the spinal nerves that hang below the end of the spinal cord and resemble a horse's tail)

celi/o- abdomen (celiac artery: a large artery that supplies abdominal organs)

cephal/o- head (cephaledema: swelling of the head)

cerebr/o- brain (cerebrum: the largest part of the human brain)

cervic- neck (cervical nerves: the spinal nerves from the neck portion of the spinal cord)

chem/o- chemical (chemotherapy: the use of chemicals to treat disease)

chondr/o- cartilage (chondrocyte: cartilage cell)

circum- around (circumoral: around the mouth)

co-, com-, with, together (congenital: born with)

con-, contra- opposite, against (contraception: the prevention of conception)

cost/o- ribs (intercostal muscles: muscles between the ribs)

crani/o- skull, head (cranial nerves: the nerves that arise from the brain)

cut- skin (cutaneous: pertaining to the skin)

cyan/o- blue (cyanosis: bluish discoloration of the skin due to lack of oxygen)

cyst- bladder, sac (cystic duct: duct of the gallbladder)

cyt/o- cell (hepatocyte: cell of the liver)

dactyl/o- digits, fingers or toes (polydactyly: more than five fingers or toes)

de- down, from (dehydration: loss of water)

derm- skin (dermatologist: a specialist in diseases of the skin)

di- two, twice (disaccharide: a sugar made of two monosaccharides)

diplo- double (diplopia: double vision)

dis- apart, away from (dissect: to cut apart)

duct- lead, conduct (ductus arteriosus: a fetal artery)

dys- difficult, diseased (dyspnea: difficult breathing)

ecto- outside (ectoparasite: a parasite that lives on the body surface)

edem- swelling (edematous: affected with swelling)

endo- within (endocardium: the innermost layer of the heart wall)

enter/o- intestine (enterotoxin: a toxin that affects the intestine and causes diarrhea)

epi- on, over, upon (epidermis: the outer layer of the skin)

erythr/o- red (erythrocyte: red blood cell)

eu- normal, good (eupnea: normal breathing)

ex- out of (excise: to cut out or remove surgically)

exo- without, outside of (exophthalmia: protrusion of the eyeballs)

extra- outside of, in addition to, beyond (extraembryonic membranes: the membranes that surround the embryo-fetus)

fasci- band (fascia: a fibrous connective tissue membrane)

fore- before, in front (forehead: the front of the head)

gastr/o- stomach (gastric juice: the digestive secretions of the stomach lining)

gluco-, glyco- sugar (glycosuria: glucose in the urine)

gyn/o-, gyne/co- woman, female (gynecology: study of the female reproductive organs)

haplo- single, simple (haploid: a single set, as of chromosomes)

hema-, hemato-, hemo- blood (hemoglobin: the protein of red blood cells)

hemi- half (cerebral hemisphere: the right or left half of the cerebrum)

hepat/o- liver (hepatic duct: the duct that takes bile out of the liver)

hetero- different (heterozygous: having two different genes for a trait)

hist/o- tissue (histology: the study of tissues)

homeo- unchanged (homeostasis: the state of body stability)

homo- same (homozygous: having two similar genes for a trait)

hydr/o- water (hydrophobia: fear of water)

hyper- excessive, above (hyperglycemia: high blood glucose level)

hypo- beneath, under, deficient (hypodermic: below the skin)

idio- distinct, peculiar to the individual (idiopathic: of unknown cause, as a disease)

inter- between, among (interventricular septum: the wall between the ventricles of the heart)

intra- within (intracellular: within cells)

is/o equal, the same (isothermal: having the same temperature)

kinesi/o- movement (kinesthetic sense: muscle sense)

labi- lip (herpes labialis: cold sores of the lips)

lacri- tears (lacrimal glands: tear-producing glands)

lact/o- milk (lactation: milk production)

leuc/o, leuk/o- white (leukocyte: white blood cell)

lip/o- fat (liposuction: removal of fat with a suctioning instrument)

macr/o- large (macromolecule: a large molecule such as a protein)

mal- poor, bad (malnutrition: poor nutrition)

medi- middle (mediastinum: a middle cavity, as in the chest)

mega- large (megacolon: abnormally dilated colon)

meta- next to, beyond (metatarsal: bone of the foot next to the ankle)

micr/o- small (microcephaly: small head)

mon/o- one (monozygotic twins: identical twins, from one egg)

morph/o- shape, form (amorphous: without definite shape)

multi- many (multicellular: made of many cells)

my/o- muscle (myocardium: heart muscle)

narco- sleep (narcotic: a drug that produces sleep)

nat/a- birth (neonate: a newborn infant)

neo- new (neoplasty: surgical restoration of parts)

nephr/o- kidney (nephrectomy: removal of a kidney)

neur/o- nerve (neuron: nerve cell)

non- not (non-communicable: unable to spread)

ocul/o- eye (oculomotor nerve: a cranial nerve for eye movement)

olig/o- few, scanty (oliguria: diminished amount of urine)

oo- egg (oogenesis: production of an egg cell)

ophthalmo- eye (ophthalmoscope: instrument to examine the eye)

orth/o- straight, normal, correct (orthostatic: related to standing upright)

oste/o- bone (osteocyte: bone cell)

ot/o- ear (otitis media: inflammation of the middle ear)

ovi-, ovo- egg (oviduct: duct for passage of an egg cell, fallopian tube)

path/o- disease (pathology: the study of disease)

ped/ia- child (pediatric: concerning the care of children)

per- through (permeate: to pass through)

peri- around (pericardium: membranes that surround the heart

phag/o- eat (phagocyte: a cell that engulfs other cells)

phleb/o- vein (phlebitis: inflammation of a vein)

pleuro-, pleura- rib (pleurisy: inflammation of the pleural membranes of the chest cavity)

pneumo- lung (pneumonia: lung infection)

pod- foot (pseudopod: false foot, as in ameboid movement)

poly- many (polysaccharide: a carbohydrate made of many monosaccharides)

post- after (postpartum: after delivery of a baby)

pre- before (precancerous: a growth that probably will become malignant)

pro- before, in front of (progeria: premature old age, before its time)

pseudo- false (pseudomembrane: false membrane)

py/o- pus (pyogenic: pus producing)

pyel/o- renal pelvis (pyelogram: an x-ray of the renal pelvis and ureter)

quadr/i- four (quadriceps femoris: a thigh muscle with four parts)

retro- behind, backward (retroperitoneal: located behind the peritoneum)

rhin/o- nose (rhinoviruses that cause the common cold)

salping/o- fallopian tube (salpingitis: inflammation of a fallopian tube)

sarc/o- flesh, muscle (sarcolemma: membrane of a muscle cell)

sclero- hard (sclerosis: deterioration of tissue with loss of function)

semi- half (semilunar valve: a valve shaped like a half-moon)

steno- narrow (aortic stenosis: narrowing of the aorta)

sub- below, beneath (subcutaneous: below the skin)

supra- above (suprarenal gland: gland above the kidney, the adrenal gland)

sym- together (symphysis: a joint where two bones meet)

syn- together (synapse: the space between two nerve cells)

tachy- fast (tachycardia: rapid heart rate)

thorac/o- chest (thoracic cavity: chest cavity)

thromb/o- clot (thrombosis: formation of a blood clot)

tox- poison (toxicology: the study of poisons)

trans- across (transmural: across the wall of an organ)

tri- three (trigone: a three-sided area on the floor of the urinary bladder)

ultra- excessive, extreme (ultrasonic: sound waves beyond the normal hearing range)

un/i- one (unicellular: made of one cell)

uria-, uro- urine (urinary calculi: stones in the urine)

vas/o- vessel (vasodilation: dilation of a blood vessel)

viscera-, viscero- organ (visceral pleura: the pleural membrane that covers the lungs)

SUFFIXES

-ac pertaining to (cardiac: pertaining to the heart)

-al pertaining to (intestinal: pertaining to the intestine)

-an, -ian characteristic of, pertaining to, belonging to (ovarian cyst: a cyst of the ovary)

-ar relating to (muscular: relating to muscles)

-ary relating to, connected with (salivary: relating to saliva)

-ase enzyme (sucrase: an enzyme that digests sucrose)

-atresia abnormal closure (biliary atresia: closure or absence of bile ducts)

-blast grow, produce (osteoblast: a bone-producing cell)

-cele swelling, tumor (meningocele: a hernia of the meninges)

-centesis puncture of a cavity (thoracocentesis: puncture of the chest cavity to   remove fluid)

-cide kill (bactericide: a chemical that kills bacteria)

-clast destroy, break down (osteoclast: a bone-reabsorbing cell)

-desis binding, stabilizing, fusion (arthrodesis: the surgical immobilization of a joint)

-dipsia thirst (polydipsia: excessive thirst)

-dynia pain (gastrodynia: stomach pain)

-ectasia, -ectasis expansion (atelectasis: without expansion)

-ectomy excision, cutting out (thyroidectomy: removal of the thyroid)

-emia pertaining to blood (hypokalemia: low blood potassium level)

-form structure (spongiform: resembling a sponge)

-gen producing (carcinogen: a substance that produces cancer)

-genesis production of, origin of (spermatogenesis: production of sperm)

-globin protein (myoglobin: a muscle protein)

-gram record, writing (electroencephalogram: a record of the electrical activity of the brain)

-graph an instrument for making records (ultrasonography: the use of ultrasound to produce an image)

-ia condition (pneumonia: condition of inflammation of the lungs)

-iasis diseased condition (cholelithiasis: gall stones)

-ic pertaining to (atomic: pertaining to atoms)

-ile having qualities of (febrile: feverish)

-ism condition, process (alcoholism: condition of being dependent on alcohol)

-ist practitioner, specialist (neurologist: a specialist in diseases of the nervous system)
-itis inflammation (hepatitis: inflammation of the liver)

-lepsy seizure (narcolepsy: a sudden onset of sleep)
-lith stone, crystal (otoliths: stones in the inner ear)
-logy study of (virology: the study of viruses)
-lysis break down (hemolysis: rupture of red blood cells)

-megaly enlargement (splenomegaly: enlargement of the spleen)
-meter a measuring instrument (spirometer: an instrument to measure pulmonary volumes)

-ness state of, quality (illness: state of being ill)

-oid the appearance of (ovoid: resembling an oval or egg)
-ole small, little (arteriole: small artery)
-oma tumor (carcinoma: malignant tumor)
-opia eye (hyperopia: farsightedness)
-ory pertaining to (regulatory: pertaining to regulation)
-ose having qualities of (comatose: having qualities of a coma)
-osis state, condition, action, process (keratosis: abnormal growth of the skin)
-ostomy creation of an opening (colostomy: creation of an opening between the intestine and the abdominal wall)
-otomy cut into (tracheotomy: cut into the trachea)
-ous pertaining to (nervous: pertaining to nerves)

-pathy disease (retinopathy: disease of the retina)
-penia lack of, deficiency (leukopenia: lack of white blood cells)
-philia love of, tendency (hemophilia: a clotting disorder, "love of blood")
-phobia an abnormal fear (acrophobia: fear of heights)
-plasia growth (hyperplasia: excessive growth)
-plasty formation, repair (rhinoplasty: plastic surgery on the nose)

-plegia paralysis (hemiplegia: paralysis of the right or left half of the body)
-poiesis production (erythropoiesis: production of red blood cells)
-ptosis dropping, falling (hysteroptosis: falling of the uterus)

-rrhage burst forth (hemorrhage: loss of blood from blood vessels)
-rrhea discharge, flow (diarrhea: frequent discharge of feces)

-scope instrument to examine (microscope: instrument to examine small objects)
-spasm involuntary contraction (blepharospasm: twitch of the eyelid)
-stasis to be still, control, stop (hemostasis: to stop loss of blood)
-sthenia strength (myasthenia: loss of muscle strength)
-stomy surgical opening (colostomy: a surgical opening in the colon)

-taxia muscle coordination (ataxia: loss of coordination)
-tension pressure (hypertension: high blood pressure)
-tic pertaining to (paralytic: pertaining to paralysis)
-tomy incision, cut into (phlebotomy: incision into a vein)
-tripsy crush (lithotripsy: crushing of stone such as gallstones)
-trophic related to nutrition or growth (autotrophic: capable of making its own food, such as a green plant)
-tropic turning toward (chemotropic: turning toward a chemical)

-ula, -ule small, little (venule: small vein)
-uria urine (hematuria: blood in the urine)

-y condition, process (healthy: condition of health)

Eponymous Terms

An eponym is a person for whom something is named, and an eponymous term is a term that uses that name or eponym. For example, fallopian tube is named for Gabriele Fallopio, an Italian anatomist of the 16th century.

In recent years it has been suggested that eponymous terms be avoided because they are not descriptive and that they be replaced with more informative terms. Such changes, however, occur slowly, because the older terms are so familiar to those of us who teach. Some of us may even use them as opportunities to impart a little history, also known as "telling stories."

In this edition, the most familiar eponymous terms have been retained, with the newer term in parentheses after the first usage. The list below is provided to show the extent of reclassification of eponymous terms as related to basic anatomy and physiology.

Eponymous Term	New Term
Achilles reflex	plantar reflex
Achilles tendon	calcaneal tendon
Adam's apple	thyroid cartilage
ampulla of Vater	hepatopancreatic ampulla
aqueduct of Sylvius	cerebral aqueduct
Auerbach's plexus	myenteric plexus
Bartholin's glands	greater vestibular glands
Bowman's capsule	glomerular capsule
Broca's area	Broca's speech area
Brunner's glands	duodenal submucosal glands
bundle of His	atrioventricular bundle
canal of Schlemm	scleral venous sinus
circle of Willis	cerebral arterial circle
Cowper's glands	bulbourethral glands
crypts of Lieberkuhn	intestinal glands
duct of Santorini	accessory pancreatic duct
duct of Wirsung	pancreatic duct
eustachian tube	auditory tube
fallopian tube	uterine tube
fissure of Rolando	central sulcus
fissure of Sylvius	lateral cerebral sulcus
graafian follicle	vesicular ovarian follicle
Graves' disease	hyperthyroidism
haversian canal	central canal
haversian system	osteon
Heimlich maneuver	abdominal thrust maneuver
islet of Langerhans	pancreatic islet
Krebs cycle	citric acid cycle
Kupffer cells	stellate reticuloendothelial cells

Langerhans cell	non-pigmented granular dendrocyte
Leydig cells	interstitial cells
loop of Henle	loop of the nephron
Meissner's corpuscles	tactile corpuscles
Meissner's plexus	submucosal plexus
nodes of Ranvier	neurofibril nodes
organ of Corti	spiral organ
Pacinian corpuscle	lamellated corpuscle
Peyer's patches	aggregated lymph nodules
Purkinje fibers	cardiac conducting myofibers
Schwann cell	neurolemmocyte
Sertoli cells	sustentacular cells
sphincter of Boyden	sphincter of the common bile duct
sphincter of Oddi	sphincter of the hepatopancreatic ampulla
Stensen's ducts	parotid ducts
Volkmann's canal	perforating canal, nutrient canal
Wernicke's area	posterior speech area
Wharton's duct	submandibular duct
Wormian bone	sutural bone

Glossary

PRONUNCIATION GUIDE

This pronunciation guide is intended to help you pronounce the words that appear in the Glossary. Although it is not a true phonetic key, it does help to suggest the necessary sounds by spelling the sounds of the syllables of frequently encountered words and then using these familiar combinations to "spell out" a pronunciation of the new word being defined in the Glossary.

VOWELS

Long vowel sounds: ay, ee, eye or igh, oh or ow, yoo

The sound spelled as . . .	Is pronounced as it appears in . . .
ay	a as in face
a	a as in atom
aw	au as in cause o as in frost
ah	o as in proper
ee	e as in beat
e	e as in ten
i	i as in it
u	u as in up

CONSONANTS

Consonants are pronounced just as they look, with g pronounced as it appears in gone.

ACCENTS WITHIN WORDS

One accent: boldface capital letters
Two accents: primary accent is in boldface capital
letters; secondary accent is in capital letters

—A—

Abdomen (**AB**-doh-men) Portion of the body between the diaphragm and the pelvis (Chapter 1).

Abdominal cavity(ab-**DAHM**-in-uhl **KAV**-i-tee) Part of the ventral cavity, inferior to the diaphragm and above the pelvic cavity (Chapter 1).

Abducens nerves (ab-**DEW**-senz) Cranial nerve pair VI. Motor to an extrinsic muscle of the eye (Chapter 8).

Abduction (ab-**DUK**-shun) Movement of a bodypart away from the midline of the body (Chapter 7).

ABO group (A-B-O GROOP) The red blood cell types determined by the presence or absence of A and B antigens on the red blood cell membrane; the four types are A, B, AB, and O (Chapter 11).

Absorption (ab-**ZORB**-shun) The taking in of materials by cells or tissues (Chapter 3).

Accessory nerves (ak-**SES**-suh-ree) Cranial nerve pair XI. Motor to the larynx and shoulder muscles (Chapter 8).

Accessory organs (ak-**SES**-suh-ree) The digestive organs that contribute to the process of digestion, although digestion does not take place within them; consist of the teeth, tongue, salivary glands, liver, gallbladder, and pancreas (Chapter 16).

Acetabulum (ASS-uh-**TAB**-yoo-lum) The deep socket in the hip bone that articulates with the head of the femur (from the Latin "little vinegar cup") (Chapter 6).

Acetylcholine (as-**SEE**-tull-KOH-leen) A chemical neurotransmitter released at neuromuscular junctions, as well as by neurons in the central and peripheral nervous systems (Chapter 7).

Acid (**ASS**-id) A hydrogen ion (H⁺) donor; when in solution has a pH less than 7 (Chapter 2).

Acidosis (Ass-i-**DOH**-sis) The condition in which the pH of the blood falls below 7.35 (Chapter 2).

Acne (**AK**-nee) Inflammation of the sebaceous glands and hair follicles (Chapter 5).

Acoustic nerves (uh-**KOO**-stik) Cranial nerve pair VIII. Sensory for hearing and equilibrium (Chapter 8).

Acquired immunity (uh-**KWHY**-erd im-**YOO**-ni-tee) The immunity obtained upon exposure to a pathogen or a vaccine or upon reception of antibodies for a particular pathogen (Chapter 14).

Acromegaly (AK-roh-**MEG**-ah-lee) Hypersecretion of growth hormone in an adult, resulting in excessive growth of the bones of the face, hands, and feet (Chapter 10).

Acrosome (**AK**-roh-sohm) The tip of the head of a sperm cell; contains enzymes to digest the membrane of the ovum (Chapter 20).

Actin (**AK**-tin) A contractile protein in the sarcomeres of muscle fibers (Chapter 7).

Action potential (**AK**-shun poh-**TEN**-shul) The changes in electrical charges on either side of a cell membrane in response to a stimulus; depolarization followed by repolarization (Chapter 7).

Active immunity (**AK**-tiv im-**YOO**-ni-tee) The immunity provided by the production of antibodies after exposure to a foreign antigen; may be natural (recovery from disease) or artificial (reception of a vaccine) (Chapter 14).

Active site theory (**AK**-tiv SITE **THEER**-ree) The process by which an enzyme catalyzes a specific reaction; depends on the shapes of the enzyme and the substrate molecules (Chapter 2).

Active transport (**AK**-tiv **TRANS**-port) The process in which there is movement of molecules against a concentration gradient; that is, from an area of lesser concentration to an area of greater concentration. Requires energy (Chapter 3).

Acute (ah-**KEWT**) 1. Characterized by rapid onset. 2. Sharp or severe, with respect to symptoms; not chronic. (Chapter 22).

Adaptation (A-dap-**TAY**-shun) The characteristic of sensations in which awareness of the sensation diminishes despite a continuing stimulus (Chapter 9).

Addison's disease (**ADD**-i-sonz) Hyposecretion of the hormones of the adrenal cortex, characterized by low blood pressure, dehydration, muscle weakness, and mental lethargy (Chapter 10).

Adduction (ad-**DUK**-shun) The movement of a body part toward the midline of the body (Chapter 7).

Adenohypophysis (uh-DEN-oh-high-**POFF**-e-sis) The anterior pituitary gland (Chapter 10).

Adipocyte (**ADD**-i-poh-site) A cell of adipose tissue, specialized to store fat (Chapter 4).

Adipose tissue (**ADD**-i-pohz **TISH**-yoo) A connective tissue composed primarily of adipocytes; function is fat storage as a source of potential energy (Chapter 4).

Adrenal cortex (uh-**DREE**-nuhl **KOR**-teks) The outer layer of the adrenal glands, which secretes cortisol and aldosterone (Chapter 10).

Adrenal glands (uh-**DREE**-nuhl) The endocrine glands located on the top of the kidneys; each consists of an adrenal cortex, which secretes cortisol and aldosterone, and an adrenal medulla, which secretes epinephrine and norepinephrine (Syn.—suprarenal glands) (Chapter 10).

Adrenal medulla (uh-**DREE**-nuhl muh-**DEW**-lah) The inner layer of the adrenal glands; secretes epinephrine and norepinephrine (Chapter 10).

Adrenocorticotropic hormone (ACTH) (uh-DREE-no-KOR-ti-koh-**TROH**-pik) A hormone produced by the anterior pituitary gland that stimulates the adrenal cortex to secrete cortisol (Chapter 10).

Aerobic (air-**ROH**-bik) Requiring oxygen (Chapter 3).

Afferent (**AFF**-uh-rent) To carry toward a center or main part (Chapter 8).

Afferent arteriole (**AFF**-er-ent ar-**TIR**-ee-ohl) The arteriole that takes blood from the renal artery into a glomerulus; within its wall are juxtaglomerular cells that secrete renin (Chapter 18).

Afterbirth (**AFF**-ter-berth) The placenta delivered shortly after delivery of the infant (Chapter 21).

After-image (**AFF**-ter-IM-ije) The characteristic of sensations in which a sensation remains in the consciousness even after the stimulus has stopped (Chapter 9).

Agglutination (uh-GLOO-ti-**NAY**-shun) Clumping of blood cells or microorganisms; the result of an antigen–antibody reaction (Chapter 11).

AIDS (AYDS) Acquired immunodeficiency syndrome; caused by a virus (HIV) that infects helper T cells and depresses immune responses (Chapter 14).

Albumin (al-**BYOO**-min) A protein synthesized by the liver, which circulates in blood plasma; contributes to the colloid osmotic pressure of the blood (Chapter 11).

Aldosterone (al-**DAH**-ster-ohn) A hormone (mineralocorticoid) secreted by the adrenal cortex that increases the reabsorption of sodium and the excretion of potassium by the kidneys (Chapter 10).

Alimentary tube (AL-i-**MEN**-tah-ree TOOB) The series of digestive organs that extends from the mouth to the anus; consists of the oral cavity, pharynx, esophagus, stomach, small intestine, and large intestine (Chapter 16).

Allele (uh-**LEEL**) One of two or more different genes for a particular characteristic (Chapter 21).

Allergen (**AL**-er-jen) A substance capable of stimulating an allergic response (Chapter 14).

Allergy (**AL**-er-jee) A hypersensitivity to a foreign antigen that usually does not stimulate an immune response in people; the immune response serves no useful purpose (Chapter 14).

Alopecia (AL-oh-**PEE**-she-ah) Loss of hair, especially that of the scalp (Chapter 5).

Alpha cells (**AL**-fah SELLS) The cells of the islets of Langerhans of the pancreas that secrete the hormone glucagon (Chapter 10).

Alveolar type I cell (al-**VEE**-oh-lar TIGHP WON SELL) The simple squamous epithelial cell that forms the walls of the alveoli of the lungs (Chapter 15).

Alveolar type II cell (al-**VEE**-oh-lar TIGHP TOO SELL) The septal cell in the lungs that produces pulmonary surfactant (Chapter 15).

Alveoli (al-**VEE**-oh-lye) The air sacs of the lungs, made of simple squamous epithelium, in which gas exchange takes place (Chapter 15).

Alzheimer's disease (**ALZ**-high-mers) A progressive brain disease, of unknown cause, resulting in loss of memory, intellectual ability, speech, and motor control (Chapter 8).

Amenorrhea (ay-MEN-uh-**REE**-ah) Absence of menstruation (Chapter 20).

Amine/Amino group (ah-**MEEN**/ah-**MEE**-noh) The NH_2 portion of a molecule such as an amino acid (Chapter 12).

Amino acid (ah-**MEE**-noh **ASS**-id) An organic compound that contains an amino, or amine, group (NH_2) and a carboxyl group (COOH). Twenty different amino acids are the subunit molecules of which proteins are made (Chapter 2).

Amniocentesis (AM-nee-oh-sen-**TEE**-sis) A diagnostic procedure in which amniotic fluid is obtained for culture of fetal cells; used to detect genetic diseases or other abnormalities in the fetus (Chapter 21).

Amnion (**AM**-nee-on) An embryonic membrane that holds the fetus suspended in amniotic fluid; fuses with the chorion by the end of the third month of gestation (Chapter 21).

Amniotic fluid (AM-nee-**AH**-tik **FLOO**-id) The fluid contained within the amnion; cushions the fetus and absorbs shock (Chapter 21).

Amphiarthrosis (AM-fee-ar-**THROH**-sis) A slightly movable joint, such as a symphysis (Chapter 6).

Amylase (**AM**-i-lays) A digestive enzyme that breaks down starch to maltose; secreted by the salivary glands and the pancreas (Chapter 16).

Anabolic steroid (AN-ah-**BAH**-lik **STEER**-oyd) A chemical similar in structure and action to the male hormone testosterone; increases protein synthesis, especially in muscles (Chapter 7).

Anabolism (an-**AB**-uh-lizm) Synthesis reactions, in which smaller molecules are bonded together to form larger molecules; require energy (ATP) and are catalyzed by enzymes (Chapter 17).

Anaerobic (AN-air-**ROH**-bik) 1. In the absence of oxygen. 2. Not requiring oxygen (Chapter 7).

Anaphase (**AN**-ah-fayz) The third stage of mitosis, in which the separate sets of chromosomes move toward opposite poles of the cell (Chapter 3).

Anaphylactic shock (AN-uh-fi-**LAK**-tik SHAHK) A type of circulatory shock that is the result of a massive allergic reaction (from the Greek "unguarded") (Chapter 13).

Anastomosis (a-NAS-ti-**MOH**-sis) A connection or joining, especially of blood vessels (Chapter 13).

Anatomic position (AN-uh-**TOM**-ik pa-**ZI**-shun) The position of the body used in anatomic descriptions: The body is erect and facing forward, the arms are at the sides with the palms facing forward (Chapter 1).

Anatomy (uh-**NAT**-uh-mee) The study of the structure of the body and the relationships among the parts (Chapter 1).

Anemia (uh-**NEE**-mee-yah) A deficiency of red blood cells or hemoglobin (Chapter 11).

Aneurysm (**AN**-yur-izm) A localized sac or bubble that forms in a weak spot in the wall of a blood vessel, usually an artery (Chapter 13).

Angiotensin II (AN-jee-oh-**TEN**-sin 2) The final product of the renin-angiotensin mechanism; stimulates vasoconstriction and increased secretion of aldosterone, both of which help raise blood pressure (Chapter 13).

Anion (**AN**-eye-on) An ion with a negative charge (Chapter 2).

Antagonistic muscles (an-**TAG**-on-ISS-tik **MUSS**-uhls) Muscles that have opposite functions with respect to the movement of a joint (Chapter 7).

Anterior (an-**TEER**-ee-your) Toward the front (Syn.—ventral) (Chapter 1).

Antibiotic (AN-ti-bye-**AH**-tik) A chemical medication that stops or inhibits the growth of bacteria or fungi (Chapter 22).

Antibody (**AN**-ti-BAH-dee) A protein molecule produced by plasma cells that is specific for and will bond to a particular foreign antigen (Syn.—gamma globulin, immune globulin) (Chapter 14).

Antibody titer (**AN**-ti-BAH-dee **TIGH**-ter) A diagnostic test that determines the level or amount of a particular antibody in blood or serum (Chapter 14).

Anticodon (**AN**-ti-KOH-don) A triplet of bases on tRNA that matches a codon on mRNA (Chapter 3).

Antidiuretic hormone (ADH) (AN-ti-DYE-yoo-**RET**-ik) A hormone produced by the hypothalamus and stored in the posterior pituitary gland; increases the reabsorption of water by the kidney tubules (Chapter 8).

Antigen (**AN**-ti-jen) A chemical marker that identifies cells of a particular species or individual. May be "self" or "foreign." Foreign antigens stimulate immune responses (Chapter 2).

Antigenic (An-ti-**JEN**-ik) Capable of stimulating antibody production (Chapter 14).

Anti-inflammatory effect (**AN**-ti-in-**FLAM**-uh-tor-ee) To lessen the process of inflammation; cortisol is the hormone that has this effect (Chapter 10).

Antipyretic (**AN**-tigh-pye-**RET**-ik) A medication, such as aspirin, that lowers a fever (Chapter 17).

Antiseptic (**AN**-ti-**SEP**-tik) A chemical that destroys bacteria or inhibits their growth on a living being (Chapter 22).

Antithrombin (**AN**-ti-**THROM**-bin) A protein synthesized by the liver that inactivates excess thrombin to prevent abnormal clotting (Chapter 11).

Antitoxin (**AN**-tee-**TAHK**-sin) Antibodies specific for a bacterial toxin; used in treatment of diseases such as botulism or tetanus (Chapter 7).

Anus (**AY**-nus) The terminal opening of the alimentary tube for the elimination of feces; surrounded by the internal and external anal sphincters (Chapter 16).

Aorta (ay-**OR**-tah) The largest artery of the body; emerges from the left ventricle; has four parts: ascending aorta, aortic arch, thoracic aorta, and abdominal aorta (Chapter 13).

Aortic body (ay-**OR**-tik **BAH**-dee) The site of chemoreceptors in the wall of the aortic arch; detect changes in blood pH and the blood levels of oxygen and carbon dioxide (Chapter 9).

Aortic semilunar valve (ay-**OR**-tik SEM-ee-**LOO**-nar VALV) The valve at the junction of the left ventricle and the aorta; prevents backflow of blood from the aorta to the ventricle when the ventricle relaxes (Chapter 12).

Aortic sinus (ay-**OR**-tik **SIGH**-nus) The site of pressoreceptors in the wall of the aortic arch; detect changes in blood pressure (Chapter 9).

Apgar score (**APP**-gar SKOR) A system of evaluating an infant's condition 1 minute after birth; includes heart rate, respiration, muscle tone, response to stimuli, and color (Chapter 21).

Aphasia (ah-**FAY**-zee-ah) Impairment or absence of the ability to communicate in speech, reading, or writing. May involve word deafness or word blindness (Chapter 8).

Aplastic anemia (ay-**PLAS**-tik un-**NEE**-mee-yah) Failure of the red bone marrow resulting in decreased numbers of red blood cells, white blood cells, and platelets; may be a side effect of some medications (Chapter 11).

Apneustic center (ap-**NEW**-stik **SEN**-ter) The respiratory center in the pons that prolongs inhalation (Chapter 15).

Apocrine gland (**AP**-oh-krin) The type of sweat gland (exocrine) found primarily in the axilla and genital area; actually a modified scent gland (Chapter 5).

Apparent (uh-**PAR**-ent) 1. Readily seen or visible. 2. An infection in which the patient exhibits the symptoms of the disease (Chapter 22).

Appendicitis (uh-PEN-di-**SIGH**-tis) Inflammation of the appendix (Chapter 16).

Appendicular skeleton (AP-en-**DIK**-yoo-lar) The portion of the skeleton that consists of the shoulder and pelvic girdles and the bones of the arms and legs (Chapter 6).

Appendix (uh-**PEN**-diks) A small tubular organ that extends from the cecum; has no known function for people and is considered a vestigial organ (Chapter 16).

Aqueous (**AY**-kwee-us) Pertaining to water; used especially to refer to solutions (Chapter 2).

Aqueous humor (**AY**-kwee-us **HYOO**-mer) The tissue fluid of the eye within the anterior cavity of the eyeball; nourishes the lens and cornea (Chapter 9).

Arachnoid membrane (uh-**RAK**-noid) The middle layer of the meninges, made of web-like connective tissue (from the Greek "spider-like") (Chapter 8).

Arachnoid villi (uh-**RAK**-noid **VILL**-eye) Projections of the cranial arachnoid membrane into the cranial venous sinuses, through which cerebrospinal fluid is reabsorbed back into the blood (Chapter 8).

Areolar connective tissue (uh-**REE**-oh-lar) A tissue that consists of tissue fluid, fibroblasts, collagen and elastin fibers, and wandering WBCs; found in all mucous membranes and in subcutaneous tissue (Syn.—loose connective tissue) (Chapter 4).

Arrhythmia (uh-**RITH**-me-yah) An abnormal or irregular rhythm of the heart (Chapter 12).

Arteriole (ar-**TEER**-ee-ohl) A small artery (Chapter 5).

Arteriosclerosis (ar-TIR-ee-oh-skle-**ROH**-sis) Deterioration of arteries with loss of elasticity that is often a consequence of aging or hypertension; a contributing factor to aneurysm or stroke (Chapter 13).

Artery (**AR**-tuh-ree) A blood vessel that takes blood from the heart toward capillaries (Chapter 13).

Arthropod (**AR**-throw-pod) Invertebrate animals characterized by an exoskeleton and jointed appendages; includes insects, spiders, ticks, mites, and crustaceans (Chapter 22).

Articular cartilage (ar-**TIK**-yoo-lar **KAR**-ti-lidj) The cartilage on the joint surfaces of a bone; provides a smooth surface (Chapter 6).

Articulation (ar-TIK-yoo-**LAY**-shun) A joint (Chapter 6).

Asthma (**AZ**-mah) A respiratory disorder characterized by constriction of the bronchioles, excessive mucus production, and dyspnea; often caused by allergies (Chapter 15).

Astigmatism (uh-**STIG**-mah-**TIZM**) An error of refraction caused by an irregular curvature of the lens or cornea (Chapter 9).

Astrocyte (**ASS**-troh-site) A type of neuroglia that forms the blood–brain barrier to prevent potentially harmful substances from affecting brain neurons (Chapter 8).

Asymptomatic (AY-simp-toh-**MAT**-ik) Without symptoms (Chapter 22).

Atelectasis (AT-e-**LEK**-tah-sis) Collapsed or airless lung, without gas exchange (Chapter 15).

Atherosclerosis (ATH-er-oh-skle-**ROH**-sis) The abnormal accumulation of lipids and other materials in the walls of arteries; narrows the lumen of the vessel and may stimulate abnormal clot formation (Chapter 2).

Atlas (**AT**-las) An irregular bone, the first cervical vertebra; supports the skull (Chapter 6).

Atmospheric pressure (AT-mus-**FEER**-ik) The pressure exerted by the atmosphere on objects on the earth's surface; 760 mmHg at sea level (Chapter 15).

Atom (**A**-tom) The unit of matter that is the smallest part of an element (Chapter 2).

Atomic number (a-**TOM**-ik) Number of protons in the nucleus of an atom (Chapter 2).

Atomic weight (a-**TOM**-ik WAYT) The weight of an atom determined by adding the number of protons and neutrons (Chapter 2).

ATP (Adenosine triphosphate) A specialized nucleotide that traps and releases biologically useful energy (Chapter 2).

Atrial natriuretic hormone (ANH) (**AY**-tree-uhl NAY-tree-yu-**RET**-ik) A peptide hormone secreted by the atria of the heart when blood pressure or blood volume increases; increases loss of sodium ions and water by the kidneys (Chapter 12).

Atrioventricular (AV) node (AY-tree-oh-ven-**TRIK**-yoo-lar NOHD) The second part of the cardiac conduction pathway, located in the lower interatrial septum (Chapter 12).

Atrium (**AY**-tree-um) (Pl.—atria) One of the two upper chambers of the heart that receive venous blood from the lungs or the body (Chapter 12).

Atrophy (**AT**-ruh-fee) Decrease in size of a body part due to lack of use; a wasting (Chapter 7).

Attenuated (uh-**TEN**-yoo-AY-ted) Weakened, or less harmful; used to describe the microorganisms contained in vaccines, which have been treated to reduce their pathogenicity (Chapter 14).

Auditory bones (**AW**-di-tor-ee) The malleus, incus, and stapes in the middle ear (Chapter 6).

Auerbach's plexus (**OW**-er-baks **PLEK**-sus) The autonomic nerve plexus in the external muscle layer of the organs of the alimentary tube; regulates the contractions of the external muscle layer (Syn.—myenteric plexus) (Chapter 16).

Auricle (**AW**-ri-kuhl) The portion of the outer ear external to the skull; made of cartilage covered with skin (Syn.—pinna) (Chapter 9).

Autoclave (**AW**-toh-clayve) A machine that uses steam under pressure for sterilization (Chapter 22).

Autoimmune disease (**AW**-toh-im-**YOON** di-**ZEEZ**) A condition in which the immune system produces antibodies to the person's own tissue (Chapter 6).

Autonomic nervous system (AW-toh-**NOM**-ik **NER**-vuhs) The portion of the peripheral nervous system that consists of visceral motor neurons to smooth muscle, cardiac muscle, and glands (Chapter 8).

Autosomes (**AW**-toh-sohms) Chromosomes other than the sex chromosomes; for people there are 22 pairs of autosomes in each somatic cell (Chapter 21).

Axial skeleton (**AK**-see-uhl) The portion of the skeleton that consists of the skull, vertebral column, and rib cage (Chapter 6).

Axis (**AK**-sis) An irregular bone, the second cervical vertebra; forms a pivot joint with the atlas (Chapter 6).

Axon (**AK**-sahn) The cellular process of a neuron that carries impulses away from the cell body (Chapter 4).

Axon terminal (**AK**-sahn **TER**-mi-nuhl) The end of the axon of a motor neuron, part of the neuromuscular junction (Chapter 7).

—B—

B cell (B SELL) A subgroup of lymphocytes, including memory B cells and plasma cells, both of which are involved in immune responses (Chapter 11).

Bacillus (buh-**SILL**-us) (Pl.—bacilli) A rod-shaped bacterium (Chapter 22).

Bacteremia (bak-tah-**REE**-mee-ah) The presence of bacteria in the blood, which is normally sterile (Chapter 22).

Bacteria (bak-**TIR**-ee-yuh) (Sing.— bacterium) The simple unicellular microorganisms of the class Schizomycetes; may be free living, saprophytic, or parasitic (Chapter 22).

Bactericide (bak-**TEER**-i-sigh'd) A chemical that kills bacteria (Chapter 22).

Bacteriostatic (bak-TEE-ree-oh-**STAT**-ik) Capable of inhibiting the reproduction of bacteria (Chapter 22).

Bacteruria (BAK-tur-**YOO**-ree-ah) The presence of large numbers of bacteria in urine (Chapter 18).

Ball-and-socket joint (BAWL and **SOK**-et) A diarthrosis that permits movement in all planes (Chapter 6).

Bartholin's glands (**BAR**-toh-linz) The small glands in the wall of the vagina; secrete mucus into the vagina and vestibule (Syn.—vestibular glands) (Chapter 20).

Basal ganglia (**BAY**-zuhl **GANG**-lee-ah) Masses of gray matter within the white matter of the cerebral hemispheres; concerned with subconscious aspects of skeletal muscle activity, such as accessory movements (Chapter 8).

Basal metabolic rate (**BAY**-zuhl met-ah-**BAHL**-ik RAYT)

The energy required to maintain the functioning of the body in a resting condition (Chapter 17).

Base (BAYS) A hydrogen ion (H⁺) acceptor, or hydroxyl ion (OH⁻) donor; when in solution has a pH greater than 7 (Chapter 2).

Basilar layer (bah-**SILL**-ar **LAY**-er) The permanent vascular layer of the endometrium that is not lost in menstruation; regenerates the functional layer during each menstrual cycle (Chapter 20).

Basophil (**BAY**-so-fill) A type of white blood cell (granular); contains heparin and histamine (Chapter 11).

Benign (bee-**NINE**) Not malignant (Chapter 3).

Beta cells (**BAY**-tah SELLS) The cells of the islets of Langerhans of the pancreas that secrete the hormone insulin (Chapter 10).

Beta-oxidation (BAY-tah-AHK-si-**DAY**-shun) The process by which the long carbon chain of a fatty acid molecule is broken down into two-carbon acetyl groups to be used in cell respiration; takes place in the liver (Chapter 16).

Bile (BYL) The secretion of the liver that is stored in the gallbladder and passes to the duodenum; contains bile salts to emulsify fats; is the fluid in which bilirubin and excess cholesterol are excreted (Chapter 16).

Bile salts (BYL SAWLTS) The active component of bile that emulsifies fats in the digestive process (Chapter 16).

Bilirubin (**BILL**-ee-roo-bin) The bile pigment produced from the heme portion of the hemoglobin of old red blood cells; excreted by the liver in bile (Chapter 11).

Binary fission (**BYE**-na-ree **FISH**-en) The asexual reproductive process in which one cell divides into two identical new cells (Chapter 22).

Binocular vision (bye-**NOK**-yoo-lur **VI**-zhun) Normal vision involving the use of both eyes; the ability of the brain to create one image from the slightly different images received from each eye (Chapter 9).

Biopsy (**BYE**-op-see) Removal of a small piece of living tissue for microscopic examination; a diagnostic procedure (Chapter 5).

Birth canal (BERTH ka-**NAL**) The vagina during delivery of an infant (Chapter 21).

Blastocyst (**BLAS**-toh-sist) The early stage of embryonic development that follows the morula; consists of the outer trophoblast and the internal inner cell mass and blastocele (cavity) (Chapter 21).

Blister (**BLISS**-ter) A collection of fluid below or within the epidermis (Chapter 5).

Blood (BLUHD) The fluid that circulates in the heart and blood vessels; consists of blood cells and plasma (Chapter 4).

Blood–brain barrier (BLUHD BRAYN) The barrier between the circulating blood and brain tissue, formed by astrocytes and brain capillaries; prevents harmful substances in the blood from damaging brain neurons (Chapter 8).

Blood pressure (BLUHD **PRE**-shure) The force exerted by the blood against the walls of the blood vessels; measured in mmHg (Chapter 13).

Body-mass index (**BAH**-dee mass **IN**-deks) A measure of leanness using height and weight (Chapter 17).

Bond (BAHND) An attraction or force that holds atoms together in the formation of molecules (Chapter 2).

Bone (BOWNE) 1. A connective tissue made of osteocytes in a calcified matrix. 2. An organ that is an individual part of the skeleton (Chapter 4).

Botulism (**BOTT**-yoo-lizm) A disease, characterized by muscle paralysis, caused by the bacterium *Clostridium botulinum* (Chapter 7).

Bowman's capsule (**BOW**-manz **KAP**-suhl) The expanded end of the renal tubule that encloses a glomerulus; receives filtrate from the glomerulus (Chapter 18).

Bradycardia (BRAY-dee-**KAR**-dee-yah) An abnormally slow heart rate; less than 60 beats per minute (Chapter 12).

Brain (BRAYN) The part of the central nervous system within the skull; regulates the activity of the rest of the nervous system (Chapter 8).

Brain stem (BRAYN STEM) The portion of the brain that consists of the medulla, pons, and midbrain (Chapter 8).

Broad-spectrum (BRAWD **SPEK**-trum) An antibiotic that is effective against a wide variety of bacteria (Chapter 22).

Bronchial tree (**BRONG**-kee-uhl TREE) The entire system of air passageways formed by the branching of the bronchial tubes within the lungs; the smallest bronchioles terminate in clusters of alveoli (Chapter 15).

Bronchioles (**BRONG**-kee-ohls) The smallest of the air passageways within the lungs (Chapter 15).

Brush border (BRUSH **BORE**-der) The collective name for the microvilli of the absorptive cells of the mucosa of the small intestine (Chapter 16).

Buffer system (**BUFF**-er **SIS**-tem) A pair of chemicals that prevents significant changes in the pH of a body fluid (Chapter 2).

Bulbourethral glands (BUHL-boh-yoo-**REE**-thruhl) The glands on either side of the prostate gland that open into the urethra; secrete an alkaline fluid that becomes part of semen (Syn.—Cowper's glands) (Chapter 20).

Bundle of His (**BUN**-duhl of HISS) The third part of the cardiac conduction pathway, located in the upper interventricular septum (Chapter 12).

Burn (BERN) Damage caused by heat, flames, chemicals, or electricity, especially to the skin; classified as first degree (minor), second degree (blisters), or third degree (extensive damage) (Chapter 5).

Bursa (**BURR**-sah) A sac of synovial fluid that decreases friction between a tendon and a bone (Chapter 6).

Bursitis (burr-**SIGH**-tiss) Inflammation of a bursa (Chapter 6).

—C—

Calcaneus (kal-**KAY**-nee-us) A short bone, the largest of the tarsals; the heel bone (Chapter 6).

Calciferol (kal-**SIF**-er-awl) A form of vitamin D (Chapter 18).

Calcitonin (KAL-si-**TOH**-nin) A hormone secreted by the thyroid gland that decreases the reabsorption of calcium from bones (Chapter 10).

Callus (**KAL**-us) Thickening of an area of epidermis (Chapter 5).

Calorie (**KAL**-oh-ree) 1. Small calorie: the amount of heat energy needed to change the temperature of 1 gram of water 1 degree centigrade. 2. Large calorie or Calorie: a kilocalorie, used to indicate the energy content of foods (Chapter 17).

Calyx (**KAY**-liks) (Pl.—calyces) A funnel-shaped extension of the renal pelvis that encloses the papilla of a renal pyramid and collects urine (Chapter 18).

Canal of Schlemm (ka-**NAL** of SHLEM) Small veins at the junction of the cornea and iris of the eye; the site of reabsorption of aqueous humor into the blood (Chapter 9).

Canaliculi (KAN-a-**LIK**-yoo-lye) Small channels, such as those in bone matrix, that permit contact between adjacent osteocytes (Chapter 6).

Cancer (**KAN**-ser) A malignant tumor or growth of cells (Chapter 3).

Capacitation (KAH-pas-i-**TAY**-shun) The maturation of sperm within the female reproductive tract; sperm become capable of fertilization (Chapter 21).

Capillary (**KAP**-i-lar-ee) A blood vessel that takes blood from an arteriole to a venule; walls are one cell in thickness to permit exchanges of materials (Chapter 4).

Capsule (**KAP**-suhl) A gelatinous layer located outside the cell wall of some bacteria; provides resistance to phagocytosis (Chapter 22).

Carbohydrate (KAR-boh-**HIGH**-drayt) An organic compound that contains carbon, hydrogen, and oxygen; includes sugars, starches, and cellulose (Chapter 2).

Carbonic anhydrase (kar-**BAHN**-ik an-**HIGH**-drays) The enzyme present in red blood cells and other cells that catalyzes the reaction of carbon dioxide and water to form carbonic acid (Chapter 15).

Carboxyl group (kar-**BAHK**-sul) The COOH portion of a molecule such as an amino acid (Chapter 19).

Carcinogen (kar-**SIN**-oh-jen) A substance that increases the risk of developing cancer (Chapter 3).

Carcinoma (KAR-sin-**OH**-mah) A malignant tumor of epithelial tissue (Chapter 5).

Cardiac cycle (**KAR**-dee-yak **SIGH**-kuhl) The sequence of events in one heartbeat, in which simultaneous contraction of the atria is followed by simultaneous contraction of the ventricles (Chapter 12).

Cardiac muscle (**KAR**-dee-yak **MUSS**-uhl) The muscle tissue that forms the walls of the chambers of the heart (Chapter 4).

Cardiac output (**KAR**-dee-yak **OUT**-put) The amount of blood pumped by a ventricle in 1 minute; the resting average is 5 to 6 liters/min (Chapter 12).

Carotid body (kah-**RAH**-tid **BAH**-dee) The site of chemoreceptors in the wall of the internal carotid artery; detect changes in blood pH and the levels of oxygen and carbon dioxide in the blood (Chapter 9).

Carotid sinus (kah-**RAH**-tid **SIGH**-nus) The site of pressoreceptors in the wall of the internal carotid artery; detect changes in blood pressure (Chapter 9).

Carpals (**KAR**-puhls) The eight short bones of each wrist (Chapter 6).

Carrier (**KAR**-ree-yur) 1. A person who recovers from a disease but continues to be a source of the pathogen and may infect others (Chapter 22). 2. In genetics, a woman with one gene for a sex-linked trait (Chapter 21).

Carrier enzyme (**KA**-ree-er **EN**-zime) An enzyme that is part of a cell membrane and carries out the process of facilitated diffusion of a specific substance (Syn.—transporter) (Chapter 3).

Cartilage (**KAR**-ti-lidj) A connective tissue made of chondrocytes in a protein matrix; is firm yet flexible (Chapter 4).

Catabolism (kuh-**TAB**-uh-lizm) Breakdown or degradation reactions, in which larger molecules are broken down to smaller molecules; often release energy (ATP) and catalyzed by enzymes (Chapter 17).

Catalyst (**KAT**-ah-list) A chemical that affects the speed of a chemical reaction, while remaining itself unchanged; enzymes are catalysts (Chapter 2).

Cataract (**KAT**-uh-rackt) An eye disorder in which the lens becomes opaque and impairs vision (from the Latin "waterfall") (Chapter 9).

Catecholamines (KAT-e-**KOHL**-ah-meens) Epinephrine and norepinephrine, the hormones secreted by the adrenal medulla (Chapter 10).

Cation (**KAT**-eye-on) An ion with a positive charge (Chapter 2).

Cauda equina (**KAW**-dah ee-**KWHY**-nah) The lumbar and sacral spinal nerves that hang below the end of the spinal cord and before they exit from the vertebral canal (Chapter 8).

Cecum (**SEE**-kum) The first part of the large intestine, the dead-end portion adjacent to the ileum (from the Latin "blindness") (Chapter 16).

Cell (SELL) The smallest living unit of structure and function of the body (Chapter 1).

Cell body (SELL **BAH**-dee) The part of a neuron that contains the nucleus (Chapter 4).

Cell-mediated immunity (SELL **MEE**-dee-ay-ted im-**YOO**-ni-tee) The mechanism of immunity that does not involve antibody production, but rather the destruction of foreign antigens by the activities of T cells and macrophages (Chapter 14).

Cell (plasma) membrane (SELL **MEM**-brayn) The membrane made of phospholipids, protein, and cholesterol that forms the outer boundary of a cell and regulates passage of materials into and out of the cell (Chapter 2).

Cell respiration (SELL RES-pi-**RAY**-shun) A cellular process in which the energy of nutrients is released in the form of ATP and heat. Oxygen is required, and carbon dioxide and water are produced (Chapter 2).

Cellulose (**SELL**-yoo-lowse) A polysaccharide produced by plants for their cell walls; it is not digestible by humans but is important as roughage or fiber in the diet (Chapter 2).

Central (**SEN**-truhl) The main part; or in the middle of (Chapter 1).

Central canal (**SEN**-truhl ka-**NAL**) The hollow center of the spinal cord that contains cerebrospinal fluid (Chapter 8).

Central nervous system (**SEN**-tral **NER**-vuhs) The part of the nervous system that consists of the brain and spinal cord (Chapter 8).

Centrioles (**SEN**-tree-ohls) The cell organelles that organize the spindle fibers during cell division (Chapter 3).

Cerebellum (SER-e-**BELL**-uhm) The part of the brain posterior to the medulla and pons; responsible for many of the subconscious aspects of skeletal muscle functioning, such as coordination and muscle tone (Chapter 7).

Cerebral aqueduct (se-**REE**-bruhl **A**-kwi-dukt) A tunnel through the midbrain that permits cerebrospinal fluid to flow from the third to the fourth ventricle (Chapter 8).

Cerebral cortex (se-**REE**-bruhl **KOR**-teks) The gray matter on the surface of the cerebral hemispheres. Includes motor areas, sensory areas, auditory areas, visual areas, taste areas, olfactory areas, speech areas, and association areas (Chapter 8).

Cerebrospinal fluid (se-**REE**-broh-**SPY**-nuhl) The tissue fluid of the central nervous system; formed by choroid plexuses in the ventricles of the brain, circulates in and around the brain and spinal cord, and is reabsorbed into cranial venous sinuses (Chapter 8).

Cerebrovascular accident (SER-e-broh-**VAS**-kyoo-lur) A hemorrhagic or ischemic lesion in the brain, often the result of aneurysm, arteriosclerosis, atherosclerosis, or hypertension (Syn.—stroke) (Chapter 8).

Cerebrum (se-**REE**-bruhm) The largest part of the brain, consisting of the right and left cerebral hemispheres; its many functions include movement, sensation, learning, and memory (Chapter 8).

Cerumen (suh-**ROO**-men) The waxy secretion of ceruminous glands (Chapter 5).

Ceruminous gland (suh-**ROO**-mi-nus) An exocrine gland in the dermis of the ear canal that secretes cerumen (ear wax) (Chapter 5).

Cervical (**SIR**-vi-kuhl) Pertaining to the neck (Chapter 1).

Cervical vertebrae (**SIR**-vi-kuhl **VER**-te-bray) The seven vertebrae in the neck (Chapter 6).

Cervix (**SIR**-viks) The most inferior part of the uterus that projects into the vagina (Chapter 20).

Cesarean section (se-**SAR**-ee-an **SEK**-shun) Removal of the fetus by way of an incision through the abdominal wall and uterus (Chapter 21).

Chemical clotting (**KEM**-i-kuhl **KLAH**-ting) A series of chemical reactions, stimulated by a rough surface or a break in a blood vessel, that result in the formation of a fibrin clot (Chapter 11).

Chemical digestion (**KEM**-i-kuhl dye-**JES**-chun) The breakdown of food accomplished by digestive enzymes; complex organic molecules are broken down to simpler organic molecules (Chapter 16).

Chemoreceptors (KEE-moh-re-**SEP**-ters) 1. A sensory receptor that detects a chemical change. 2. Olfactory receptors, taste receptors, and the carotid and aortic chemoreceptors that detect changes in blood gases and blood pH (Chapter 9).

Chemotherapy (KEE-moh-**THER**-uh-pee) The use of chemicals (medications) to treat disease (Chapter 3).

Chief cells (CHEEF SELLS) The cells of the gastric pits of the stomach that secrete pepsinogen, the inactive form of the digestive enzyme pepsin (Chapter 16).

Chlamydia (kluh-**MID**-ee-ah) A group of simple bacteria; *Chlamydia trachomatis* is a sexually transmitted pathogen that may cause conjunctivitis or pneumonia in infants born to infected women (Chapter 20).

Cholecystokinin (KOH-lee-SIS-toh-**KYE**-nin) A hormone secreted by the duodenum when food enters; stimulates contraction of the gallbladder and secretion of enzyme pancreatic juice (Chapter 16).

Cholesterol (koh-**LESS**-ter-ohl) A steroid that is synthesized by the liver and is part of cell membranes (Chapter 2).

Cholinesterase (KOH-lin-**ESS**-ter-ays) The chemical inactivator of acetylcholine (Chapter 7).

Chondrocyte (**KON**-droh-sight) A cartilage cell (Chapter 4).

Chordae tendineae (**KOR**-day ten-**DIN**-ee-ay) Strands of connective tissue that connect the flaps of an AV valve to the papillary muscles (Chapter 12).

Chorion (**KOR**-ee-on) An embryonic membrane that is formed from the trophoblast of the blastocyst and will develop chorionic villi and become the fetal portion of the placenta (Chapter 21).

Chorionic villi (**KOR**-ee-ON-ik **VILL**-eye) Projections of the chorion that will develop the fetal blood vessels that will become part of the placenta (Chapter 21).

Chorionic villus sampling (KOR-ee-**ON**-ik **VILL**-us) A diagnostic procedure in which a biopsy of the chorionic villi is made; used to detect genetic diseases or other abnormalities in the fetus (Chapter 21).

Choroid layer (**KOR**-oyd) The middle layer of the eyeball, contains a dark pigment derived from melanin that absorbs light and prevents glare within the eye (Chapter 9).

Choroid plexus (**KOR**-oyd **PLEK**-sus) A capillary network in a ventricle of the brain; forms cerebrospinal fluid (Chapter 8).

Chromatin (**KROH**-mah-tin) The thread-like structure of the genetic material when a cell is not dividing; is not visible as individual chromosomes (Chapter 3).

Chromosomes (**KROH**-muh-sohms) Structures made of DNA and protein within the nucleus of a cell. A human cell has 46 chromosomes (Chapter 3).

Chronic (**KRAH**-nik) Characterized by long duration or slow progression (Chapter 22).

Chylomicron (KYE-loh-**MYE**-kron) A small fat globule formed by the small intestine from absorbed fatty acids and glycerol (Chapter 16).

Cilia (**SILLY**-ah) Thread-like structures that project through a cell membrane and sweep materials across the cell surface (Chapter 3).

Ciliary body (**SILLY**-air-ee **BAH**-dee) A circular muscle that surrounds the edge of the lens of the eye and changes the shape of the lens (Chapter 9).

Ciliated epithelium (**SILLY**-ay-ted) The tissue that has cilia on the free surface of the cells (Chapter 4).

Circle of Willis (**SIR**-kuhl of **WILL**-iss) An arterial anastomosis that encircles the pituitary gland and supplies the brain with blood; formed by the two internal carotid arteries and the basilar (two vertebral) artery (Chapter 13).

Circulatory shock (**SIR**-kew-lah-TOR-ee SHAHK) The condition in which decreased cardiac output deprives all tissues of oxygen and permits the accumulation of waste products (Chapter 5).

Cisterna chyli (sis-**TER**-nah **KYE**-lee) A large lymph vessel formed by the union of lymph vessels from the lower body; continues superiorly as the thoracic duct (Chapter 14).

Clavicle (**KLAV**-i-kuhl) The flat bone that articulates with the scapula and sternum (from the Latin "little key") (Syn.—collarbone) (Chapter 6).

Cleavage (**KLEE**-vije) The series of mitotic cell divisions that take place in a fertilized egg; forms the early multicellular embryonic stages (Chapter 21).

Cleft palate (KLEFT **PAL**-uht) A congenital disorder in which the bones of the hard palate do not fuse, leaving an opening between the oral and nasal cavities (Chapter 6).

Clinical infection (**KLIN**-i-kuhl) An infection in which the patient exhibits the symptoms of the disease (Chapter 22).

Clitoris (**KLIT**-uh-ris) An organ that is part of the vulva; a small mass of erectile tissue at the anterior junction of the labia minora; enlarges in response to sexual stimulation (Chapter 20).

Clot retraction (KLAHT ree-**TRAK**-shun) The shrinking of a blood clot shortly after it forms due to the folding of the fibrin strands; pulls the edges of the ruptured vessel closer together (Chapter 11).

Coccus (**KOK**-us) (Pl.—cocci) A spherical bacterium (Chapter 22).

Coccyx (**KOK**-siks) The last four to five very small vertebrae; attachment site for some muscles of the pelvic floor (Chapter 6).

Cochlea (**KOK**-lee-ah) The snail-shell-shaped portion of the inner ear that contains the receptors for hearing in the organ of Corti (Chapter 9).

Codon (**KOH**-don) The sequence of three bases in DNA or mRNA that is the code for one amino acid; also called a triplet code (Chapter 3).

Coenzyme (ko-**EN**-zime) A non-protein molecule that combines with an enzyme and is essential for the functioning of the enzyme; some vitamins and minerals are coenzymes (Chapter 17).

Collagen (**KAH**-lah-jen) A protein that is found in the form of strong fibers in many types of connective tissue (Chapter 4).

Collecting tubule (kah-**LEK**-ting) The part of a renal tubule that extends from a distal convoluted tubule to a papillary duct (Chapter 18).

Colloid osmotic pressure (**KAH**-loyd ahs-**MAH**-tik) The force exerted by the presence of protein in a solution; water will move by osmosis to the area of greater protein concentration (Chapter 13).

Colon (**KOH**-lun) The large intestine (Chapter 16).

Color blindness (**KUHL**-or **BLIND**-ness) The inability to distinguish certain colors, a hereditary trait (Chapter 9).

Columnar (kuh-**LUM**-nar) Shaped like a column; height greater than width; used especially in reference to epithelial tissue (Chapter 4).

Common bile duct (**KOM**-mon BYL DUKT) The duct formed by the union of the hepatic duct from the liver and the cystic duct from the gallbladder, and joined by the main pancreatic duct; carries bile and pancreatic juice to the duodenum (Chapter 16).

Communicable disease (kuhm-**YOO**-ni-kah-b'l) A disease that may be transmitted from person to person by direct or indirect contact (Chapter 22).

Compact bone (**KOM**-pakt BOWNE) Bone tissue made of haversian systems; forms the diaphyses of long bones and covers the spongy bone of other bones (Chapter 6).

Complement (**KOM**-ple-ment) A group of plasma proteins that are activated by and bond to an antigen–antibody complex; complement fixation results in the lysis of cellular antigens (Chapter 14).

Complement fixation test (**KOM**-ple-ment fik-**SAY**-shun)

A diagnostic test that determines the presence of a particular antibody in blood or serum (Chapter 14).

Computed tomography (CT) scan (kom-**PEW**-ted toh-**MAH**-grah-fee SKAN) A diagnostic imaging technique that uses x-rays integrated by computer (Chapter 1).

Concentration gradient (KON-sen-**TRAY**-shun **GRAY**-de-ent) The relative amounts of a substance on either side of a membrane; diffusion occurs with, or along, a concentration gradient, that is, from high concentration to low concentration (Chapter 3).

Conchae (**KONG**-chay) Three pairs of curved, shelf-like bones that extend into the nasal cavities; they increase the surface area of the nasal mucosa (Chapter 6).

Conduction (kon-**DUK**-shun) 1. The heat loss process in which heat energy from the skin is transferred to cooler objects touching the skin. 2. The transfer of any energy form from one substance to another; includes nerve and muscle impulses, and the transmission of vibrations in the ear (Chapter 17).

Condyle (**KON**-dyel) A rounded projection on a bone (Chapter 6).

Condyloid joint (**KON**-di-loyd) A diarthrosis that permits movement in one plane and some lateral movement (Chapter 6).

Cones (KOHNES) The sensory receptors in the retina of the eye that detect colors (the different wavelengths of the visible spectrum of light) (Chapter 9).

Congenital (kon-**JEN**-i-tuhl) Present at birth (Chapter 21).

Conjunctiva (KON-junk-**TIGH**-vah) The mucous membrane that lines the eyelids and covers the white of the eye (Chapter 9).

Conjunctivitis (kon-JUNK-ti-**VIGH**-tis) Inflammation of the conjunctiva, most often due to an allergy or bacterial infection (Chapter 9).

Connective tissue (kah-**NEK**-tiv **TISH**-yoo) Any of the tissues that connects, supports, transports, or stores materials. Consists of cells and matrix (Chapter 4).

Contagious disease (kun-**TAY**-jus) A disease that is easily transmitted from person to person by casual contact (Chapter 22).

Contrast (**KON**-trast) The characteristic of sensations in which a previous sensation affects the perception of a current sensation (Chapter 9).

Contusion (kon-**TOO**-zhun) A bruise; the skin is not broken but may be painful, swollen, and discolored (Chapter 5).

Convection (kon-**VEK**-shun) The heat loss process in which heat energy is moved away from the skin surface by means of air currents (Chapter 17).

Convolution (kon-voh-**LOO**-shun) A fold, coil, roll, or twist; the surface folds of the cerebral cortex (Syn.—gyrus) (Chapter 8).

Cornea (**KOR**-nee-ah) The transparent anterior portion of the sclera of the eye; the first structure that refracts light rays that enter the eye (Chapter 9).

Coronal (frontal) section (koh-**ROH**-nuhl **SEK**-shun) A plane or cut from side to side, separating front and back parts (Chapter 1).

Coronary vessels (**KOR**-ah-na-ree **VESS**-uhls) The blood vessels that supply the myocardium with blood; emerge from the ascending aorta and empty into the right atrium (Chapter 12).

Corpus callosum (**KOR**-pus kuh-**LOH**-sum) The band of white matter that connects the cerebral hemispheres (Chapter 8).

Corpus luteum (**KOR**-pus **LOO**-tee-um) The temporary endocrine gland formed from an ovarian follicle that has released an ovum; secretes progesterone and estrogen (Chapter 10).

Cortex (**KOR**-teks) The outer layer of an organ, such as the cerebrum, kidney, or adrenal gland (Chapter 8).

Cortisol (**KOR**-ti-sawl) A hormone secreted by the adrenal cortex that promotes the efficient use of nutrients in stressful situations and has an anti-inflammatory effect (Chapter 10).

Cough reflex (KAWF) A reflex integrated by the medulla that expels irritating substances from the pharynx, larynx, or trachea by means of an explosive exhalation (Chapter 15).

Covalent bond (ko-**VAY**-lent) A chemical bond formed by the sharing of electrons between atoms (Chapter 2).

Cranial cavity (**KRAY**-nee-uhl **KAV**-i-tee) The cavity formed by the cranial bones; contains the brain; part of the dorsal cavity (Chapter 1).

Cranial nerves (**KRAY**-nee-uhl NERVS) The 12 pairs of nerves that emerge from the brain (Chapter 8).

Cranial venous sinuses (**KRAY**-nee-uhl **VEE**-nus **SIGH**-nuh-sez) Large veins between the two layers of the cranial dura mater; the site of reabsorption of the cerebrospinal fluid (Chapter 8).

Cranium (**KRAY**-nee-um) The cranial bones or bones of the skull that enclose and protect the brain (Chapter 6).

Creatine phosphate (**KREE**-ah-tin **FOSS**-fate) An energy source in muscle fibers; the energy released is used to synthesize ATP (Chapter 7).

Creatinine (kree-**A**-ti-neen) A waste product produced when creatine phosphate is used for energy; excreted by the kidneys in urine (Chapter 7).

Cretinism (**KREE**-tin-izm) Hyposecretion of thyroxine in an infant; if uncorrected, the result is severe mental and physical retardation (Chapter 10).

Cross-section (KRAWS **SEK**-shun) A plane or cut perpendicular to the long axis of an organ (Chapter 1).

Crypts of Lieberkühn (KRIPTS of **LEE**-ber-koon) The digestive glands of the small intestine; secrete digestive enzymes (Chapter 16).

Cuboidal (kew-**BOY**-duhl) Shaped like a cube; used especially in reference to epithelial tissue (Chapter 4).

Culture and sensitivity testing (**KUL**-chur and SEN-si-**TIV**-i-tee) A laboratory procedure to determine the best antibiotic with which to treat a bacterial infection (Chapter 22).

Cushing's syndrome (**KOOSH**-ingz **SIN**-drohm) Hypersecretion of the glucocorticoids of the adrenal cortex, characterized by fragility of skin, poor wound healing, truncal fat deposition, and thin extremities (Chapter 10).

Cutaneous senses (kew-**TAY**-nee-us) The senses of the skin; the receptors are in the dermis (Chapter 9).

Cyanosis (SIGH-uh-**NOH**-sis) A blue, gray, or purple discoloration of the skin caused by hypoxia and abnormal amounts of reduced hemoglobin in the blood (Chapter 15).

Cyclic AMP (**SIK**-lik) A chemical that is the second messenger in the two-messenger theory of hormone action; formed from ATP and stimulates characteristic cellular responses to the hormone (Chapter 10).

Cystic duct (**SIS**-tik DUKT) The duct that takes bile into and out of the gallbladder; unites with the hepatic duct of the liver to form the common bile duct (Chapter 16).

Cystitis (sis-**TIGH**-tis) Inflammation of the urinary bladder; most often the result of bacterial infection (Chapter 18).

Cytochrome transport system (**SIGH**-toh-krohm) The stage of cell respiration in which ATP is formed during reactions of cytochromes with the electrons of the hydrogen atoms that were once part of a food molecule, and metabolic water is formed; aerobic; takes place in the mitochondria of cells (Chapter 17).

Cytokines (**SIGH**-toh-kines) Chemicals released by activated T cells that attract macrophages (Chapter 14).

Cytokinesis (SIGH-toh-ki-**NEE**-sis) The division of the cytoplasm of a cell following mitosis (Chapter 3).

Cytoplasm (**SIGH**-toh-plazm) The cellular material between the nucleus and the cell membrane (Chapter 3).

—D—

Deafness (**DEFF**-ness) Impairment of normal hearing; may be caused by damage to the vibration conduction pathway (conduction), the acoustic nerve or cochlear receptors (nerve), or the auditory area in the temporal lobe (central) (Chapter 9).

Deamination (DEE-am-i-**NAY**-shun) The removal of an amino (NH_2) group from an amino acid; takes place in the liver when excess amino acids are used for energy production; the amino groups are converted to urea (Chapter 16).

Decubitus ulcer (dee-**KEW**-bi-tuss **UL**-ser) The breakdown and death of skin tissue due to prolonged pressure that interrupts blood flow to the area (Syn.—pressure ulcer) (Chapter 5).

Defecation reflex (DEF-e-**KAY**-shun) The spinal cord reflex that eliminates feces from the colon (Chapter 16).

Dehydration (DEE-high-**DRAY**-shun) Excessive loss of water from the body (Chapter 5).

Deltoid (**DELL**-toyd) 1. The shoulder region. 2. The large muscle that covers the shoulder joint (Chapter 1).

Dendrite (**DEN**-dright) The cellular process of a neuron that carries impulses toward the cell body (Chapter 4).

Dentin (**DEN**-tin) The bone-like substance that forms the inner crown and the roots of a tooth (Chapter 16).

Depolarization (DE-poh-lahr-i-**ZAY**-shun) The reversal of electrical charges on either side of a cell membrane in response to a stimulus; negative charge outside and a positive charge inside; brought about by a rapid inflow of sodium ions (Chapter 7).

Dermatology (DER-muh-**TAH**-luh-jee) The study of the skin and skin diseases (Chapter 5).

Dermis (**DER**-miss) The inner layer of the skin, made of fibrous connective tissue (Chapter 5).

Detached retina (dee-**TACHD RET**-in-nah) The separation of the retina from the choroid layer of the eyeball (Chapter 9).

Detrusor muscle (de-**TROO**-ser) The smooth muscle layer of the wall of the urinary bladder; contracts as part of the urination reflex to eliminate urine (Chapter 18).

Diabetes mellitus (DYE-ah-**BEE**-tis mel-**LYE**-tus) Hyposecretion of insulin by the pancreas or the inability of insulin to exert its effects; characterized by hyperglycemia, increased urinary output with glycosuria, and thirst (Chapter 10).

Diagnosis (DYE-ag-**NOH**-sis) The procedures used to identify the cause and nature of a person's illness (Chapter 1).

Diaphragm (**DYE**-uh-fram) The dome-shaped skeletal muscle that separates the thoracic and abdominal cavities; moves downward when it contracts to enlarge the thoracic cavity to bring about inhalation (Chapter 1).

Diaphysis (dye-**AFF**-i-sis) The shaft of a long bone; contains a marrow canal filled with yellow bone marrow (Chapter 6).

Diarthrosis (DYE-ar-**THROH**-sis) A freely movable joint such as hinge, pivot, and ball-and-socket joints; all are considered synovial joints because synovial membrane is present (Chapter 6).

Diastole (dye-**AS**-tuh-lee) In the cardiac cycle, the relaxation of the myocardium (Chapter 12).

Differential WBC count (**DIFF**-er-EN-shul KOWNT) A laboratory test that determines the percentage of each of the five types of white blood cells present in the blood (Chapter 11).

Diffusion (di-**FEW**-zhun) The process in which there is movement of molecules from an area of greater concentration to an area of lesser concentration; occurs because of the free energy (natural movement) of molecules (Chapter 3).

Digestive system (dye-**JES**-tiv **SIS**-tem) The organ system that changes food into simpler organic and inorganic molecules that can be absorbed by the blood and lymph and used by cells; consists of the alimentary tube and accessory organs (Chapter 16).

Diploid number (**DIH**-ployd) The characteristic or usual number of chromosomes found in the somatic (body) cells of a species (human = 46) (Chapter 3).

Disaccharide (dye-**SAK**-ah-ride) A carbohydrate molecule that consists of two monosaccharides bonded together; includes sucrose, maltose, and lactose (Chapter 2).

Disease (di-**ZEEZ**) A disorder or disruption of normal body functioning (Chapter 1).

Disinfectant (DIS-in-**FEK**-tent) A chemical that destroys microorganisms or limits their growth on inanimate objects (Chapter 22).

Dissociation (dih-SEW-see-**AY**-shun) The separation of an inorganic salt, acid, or base into its ions when dissolved in water (Syn.—ionization) (Chapter 2).

Distal (**DIS**-tuhl) Furthest from the origin or point of attachment (Chapter 1).

Distal convoluted tubule (**DIS**-tuhl KON-voh-**LOO**-ted) The part of a renal tubule that extends from a loop of Henle to a collecting tubule (Chapter 18).

Disulfide bond (digh-**SUL**-fyed BAHND) A covalent bond between the sulfur atoms of two amino acids in a protein; helps maintain the three-dimensional shape of the protein (Syn.—disulfide bridge) (Chapter 2).

Diverticulitis (DYE-ver-tik-yoo-**LYE**-tis) Inflammation of diverticula in the intestinal tract (Chapter 16).

DNA (**Deoxyribonucleic acid**) A nucleic acid in the shape of a double helix. Makes up the chromosomes of cells and is the genetic code for hereditary characteristics (Chapter 2).

DNA replication (REP-li-**KAY**-shun) The process by which a DNA molecule makes a duplicate of itself. Takes place before mitosis or meiosis, to produce two sets of chromosomes within a cell (Chapter 3).

Dominant (**DAH**-ma-nent) In genetics, a characteristic that will be expressed even if only one gene for it is present in the homologous pair of chromosomes (Chapter 21).

Dormant (**DOOR**-ment) Temporarily inactive; a state of little metabolic activity (Chapter 22).

Dorsal (**DOR**-suhl) Toward the back (Syn.—posterior) (Chapter 1).

Dorsal cavity (DOR-suhl **KAV**-i-tee) Cavity that consists of the cranial and spinal cavities (Chapter 1).

Dorsal root (**DOR**-suhl ROOT) The sensory root of a spinal nerve (Chapter 8).

Dorsal root ganglion (**DOR**-suhl ROOT **GANG**-lee-on) An enlarged area of the dorsal root of a spinal nerve that contains the cell bodies of sensory neurons (Chapter 8).

Down syndrome (DOWN **SIN**-drohm) A trisomy in which three chromosomes of number 21 are present; characterized by moderate to severe mental retardation and certain physical malformations (Chapter 20).

Duct (DUKT) A tube or channel, especially one that carries the secretion of a gland (Chapter 4).

Ductus arteriosus (**DUK**-tus ar-TIR-ee-**OH**-sis) A short

fetal blood vessel that takes most blood in the pulmonary artery to the aorta, bypassing the fetal lungs (Chapter 13).

Ductus deferens (**DUK**-tus **DEF**-eer-enz) The tubular organ that carries sperm from the epididymis to the ejaculatory duct (Syn.—vas deferens) (Chapter 20).

Ductus venosus (**DUK**-tus ve-**NOH**-sus) A short fetal blood vessel that takes blood from the umbilical vein to the inferior vena cava (Chapter 13).

Duodenum (dew-**AH**-den-um) The first 10 inches of the small intestine; the common bile duct enters (Chapter 16).

Dura mater (**DEW**-rah **MAH**-ter) The outermost layer of the meninges, made of fibrous connective tissue (Chapter 8).

Dwarfism (**DWORF**-izm) The condition of being abnormally small, especially small of stature due to hereditary or endocrine disorder; pituitary dwarfism is caused by a deficiency of growth hormone (Chapter 10).

Dyspnea (**DISP**-nee-ah) Difficult breathing (Chapter 15).

Dysuria (dis-**YOO**-ree-ah) Painful or difficult urination (Chapter 18).

—E—

Ear (EER) The organ that contains the sensory receptors for hearing and equilibrium; consists of the outer ear, middle ear, and inner ear (Chapter 9).

Eccrine gland (**EK**-rin) The type of sweat gland (exocrine) that produces watery sweat; important in maintenance of normal body temperature (Chapter 5).

Ectoderm (**EK**-toh-derm) The outer primary germ layer of cells of an embryo; gives rise to the epidermis and nervous system (Chapter 21).

Ectoparasite (EK-toh-**PAR**-uh-sight) A parasite that lives on the surface of the body (Chapter 22).

Ectopic focus (ek-**TOP**-ik **FOH**-kus) The initiation of a heartbeat by part of the myocardium other than the sinoatrial node (Chapter 12).

Ectopic pregnancy (ek-**TOP**-ik **PREG**-nun-see) Implantation of a fertilized ovum outside the uterus; usually occurs in the fallopian tube but may be in the ovary or abdominal cavity; often results in death of the embryo because a functional placenta cannot be formed in these abnormal sites (Chapter 20).

Eczema (**EK**-zuh-mah) An inflammatory condition of the skin that may include the formation of vesicles or pustules (Chapter 5).

Edema (uh-**DEE**-muh) An abnormal accumulation of tissue fluid; may be localized or systemic (Chapter 19).

Effector (e-**FEK**-tur) An organ such as a muscle or gland that produces a characteristic response after receiving a stimulus (Chapter 8).

Efferent (**EFF**-uh-rent) To carry away from a center or main part (Chapter 8).

Efferent arteriole (**EFF**-er-ent ar-**TIR**-ee-ohl) The arteriole that takes blood from a glomerulus to the peritubular capillaries that surround the renal tubule (Chapter 18).

Ejaculation (ee-JAK-yoo-**LAY**-shun) The ejection of semen from the male urethra (Chapter 20).

Ejaculatory duct (ee-**JAK**-yoo-la-TOR-ee DUKT) The duct formed by the union of the ductus deferens and the duct of the seminal vesicle; carries sperm to the urethra (Chapter 20).

Ejection fraction (ee-**JEK**-shun **FRAK**-shun) The percent of blood in a ventricle that is pumped during systole; a measure of the strength of the heart (Chapter 12).

Elastin (eh-**LAS**-tin) A protein that is found in the form of elastic fibers in several types of connective tissue (Chapter 4).

Electrocardiogram (ECG or EKG) (ee-LEK-troh-**KAR**-dee-oh-GRAM) A recording of the electrical changes that accompany the cardiac cycle (Chapter 12).

Electrolytes (ee-**LEK**-troh-lites) Substances that, in solution, dissociate into their component ions; include acids, bases, and salts (Chapter 19).

Electron (e-**LEK**-trahn) A subatomic particle that has a negative electrical charge; found orbiting the nucleus of an atom (Chapter 2).

Element (**EL**-uh-ment) A substance that consists of only one type of atom; 92 elements occur in nature (Chapter 2).

Embolism (**EM**-boh-lizm) Obstruction of a blood vessel by a blood clot or foreign substance that has traveled to and lodged in that vessel (Chapter 11).

Embryo (**EM**-bree-oh) The developing human individual from the time of implantation until the eighth week of gestation (Chapter 21).

Embryonic disc (EM-bree-**ON**-ik DISK) The portion of the inner cell mass of the early embryo that will develop into the individual (Chapter 21).

Emphysema (EM-fi-**SEE**-mah) The deterioration of alveoli and loss of elasticity of the lungs; normal exhalation and gas exchange are impaired (Chapter 15).

Emulsify (e-**MULL**-si-fye) To physically break up fats into smaller fat globules; the function of bile salts in bile (Chapter 16).

Enamel (en-**AM**-uhl) The hard substance that covers the crowns of teeth and forms the chewing surface (Chapter 16).

Encapsulated nerve ending (en-**KAP**-sul-LAY-ted NERV **END**-ing) A sensory nerve ending enclosed in a specialized cellular structure; the cutaneous receptors for touch and pressure (Chapter 5).

Endemic (en-**DEM**-ik) A disease that occurs continuously or expectedly in a given population (Chapter 22).

Endocardium (EN-doh-**KAR**-dee-um) The simple squamous epithelial tissue that lines the chambers of the heart and covers the valves (Chapter 12).

Endocrine gland (**EN**-doh-krin) A ductless gland that secretes its product (hormone) directly into the blood (Chapter 4).

Endocrine system (**EN**-doh-krin **SIS**-tem) The organ system that consists of the endocrine glands that secrete hormones into the blood (Chapter 10).

Endoderm (**EN**-doh-derm) The inner primary germ layer of cells of an embryo; gives rise to respiratory organs and the lining of the digestive tract (Chapter 21).

Endogenous (en-**DOJ**-en-us) Coming from or produced within the body (Chapter 17).

Endogenous infection (en-**DOJ**-en-us) An infection caused by a person's own normal flora that have been introduced into an abnormal body site (Chapter 22).

Endolymph (**EN**-doh-limf) The fluid in the membranous labyrinth of the inner ear (Chapter 9).

Endometrium (EN-doh-**MEE**-tree-um) The vascular lining of the uterus that forms the maternal portion of the placenta (Chapter 20).

Endoplasmic reticulum (ER) (EN-doh-**PLAZ**-mik re-**TIK**-yoo-lum) A cell organelle found in the cytoplasm; a network of membranous channels that transport materials within the cell and synthesize lipids (Chapter 3).

Endothelium (EN-doh-**THEE**-lee-um) The simple squamous epithelial lining of arteries and veins, continuing as the walls of capillaries (Chapter 13).

Endotoxin (EN-doh-**TAHK**-sin) The toxic portion of the cell walls of gram-negative bacteria; causes fever and shock (Chapter 22).

Endotoxin shock (EN-doh-**TAHK**-sin SHAHK) A state of circulatory shock caused by infection with gram-negative bacteria (Chapter 22).

Energy levels (**EN**-er-jee **LEV**-els) The position of electrons within an atom (Syn.—orbitals or shells) (Chapter 2).

Enteric nervous system (en-**TER**-ik) The nerve fibers and plexuses of the alimentary tube; regulate secretions and contractions, able to function independently of the CNS (Chapter 16).

Enteroendocrine cell (EN-ter-oh-**EN**-doh-krin SELL) A cell of the alimentary tube that secretes hormones (Chapter 16).

Enzyme (**EN**-zime) A protein that affects the speed of a chemical reaction. Also called an organic catalyst (Chapter 2).

Eosinophil (EE-oh-**SIN**-oh-fill) A type of white blood cell (granular); active in allergic reactions and parasitic infections (Chapter 11).

Epicardium (EP-ee-**KAR**-dee-um) The serous membrane on the surface of the myocardium (Syn.—visceral pericardium) (Chapter 12).

Epidemic (EP-i-**DEM**-ik) A disease that affects many people in a given population in a given time with more than the usual or expected number of cases (Chapter 22).

Epidemiology (EP-i-DEE-mee-**AH**-luh-jee) The study of the spread of disease and the factors that determine disease frequency and distribution (Chapter 22).

Epidermis (EP-i-**DER**-miss) The outer layer of the skin, made of stratified squamous epithelium (Chapter 5).

Epididymis (EP-i-**DID**-i-mis) (Pl.—epididymides) The tubular organ coiled on the posterior side of a testis; sperm mature here and are carried to the ductus deferens (Chapter 20).

Epiglottis (EP-i-**GLAH**-tis) The uppermost cartilage of the larynx; covers the larynx during swallowing (Chapter 15).

Epinephrine (EP-i-**NEFF**-rin) A hormone secreted by the adrenal medulla that stimulates many responses to enable the body to react to a stressful situation (Syn.—adrenalin) (Chapter 10).

Epiphyseal disc (e-**PIFF**-i-se-al DISK) A plate of cartilage at the junction of an epiphysis with the diaphysis of a long bone; the site of growth of a long bone (Chapter 6).

Epiphysis (e-**PIFF**-i-sis) The end of a long bone (Chapter 6).

Epithelial tissue (EP-i-**THEE**-lee-uhl **TISH**-yoo) The tissue found on external and internal body surfaces and which forms glands (Chapter 4).

Equilibrium (E-kwe-**LIB**-ree-um) 1. A state of balance. 2. The ability to remain upright and be aware of the position of the body (Chapter 9).

Erythema (ER-i-**THEE**-mah) Redness of the skin (Chapter 5).

Erythroblastosis fetalis (e-RITH-roh-blass-**TOH**-sis fee-**TAL**-is) Hemolytic anemia of the newborn, characterized by anemia and jaundice; the result of an Rh incompatibility of fetal blood and maternal blood; also called Rh disease of the newborn (Chapter 11).

Erythrocyte (e-**RITH**-roh-sight) Red blood cell (Chapter 11).

Erythropoietin (e-RITH-roh-**POY**-e-tin) A hormone secreted by the kidneys in a state of hypoxia; stimulates the red bone marrow to increase the rate of red blood cell production (Chapter 11).

Esophagus (e-**SOF**-uh-guss) The organ of the alimentary tube that is a passageway for food from the pharynx to the stomach (Chapter 16).

Essential amino acids (e-**SEN**-shul ah-**ME**-noh **ASS**-ids) The amino acids that cannot be synthesized by the liver and must be obtained from proteins in the diet (Chapter 16).

Essential fatty acids (e-**SEN**-shul **FA**-tee **ASS**-ids) The fatty acids that cannot be synthesized by the body and must be obtained from fats in the diet (Chapter 17).

Estrogen (**ES**-troh-jen) The sex hormone secreted by a developing ovarian follicle; contributes to the growth of the female reproductive organs and the secondary sex characteristics (Chapter 10).

Ethmoid bone (**ETH**-moyd) An irregular cranial bone that forms the upper part of the nasal cavities and a small part of the lower anterior braincase (Chapter 6).

Eustachian tube (yoo-**STAY**-shee-un TOOB) The air passage between the middle ear cavity and the nasopharynx (Syn.—auditory tube) (Chapter 9).

Exocrine gland (**EK**-so-krin) A gland that secretes its product into a duct to be taken to a cavity or surface (Chapter 4).

Expiration (EK-spi-**RAY**-shun) Exhalation; the output of air from the lungs (Chapter 15).

Expiratory reserve (ek-**SPYR**-ah-tor-ee ree-**ZERV**) The volume of air beyond tidal volume that can be exhaled with the most forceful exhalation; average: 1000–1500 ml (Chapter 15).

Extension (eks-**TEN**-shun) To increase the angle of a joint (Chapter 7).

External (eks-**TER**-nuhl) On the outside; toward the surface (Chapter 1).

External anal sphincter (eks-**TER**-nuhl **AY**-nuhl **SFINK**-ter) The circular skeletal muscle that surrounds the internal anal sphincter and provides voluntary control of defecation (Chapter 16).

External auditory meatus (eks-**TER**-nuhl **AW**-di-TOR-ee me-**AY**-tuss) The ear canal; the portion of the outer ear that is a tunnel in the temporal bone between the auricle and the eardrum (Chapter 9).

External respiration (eks-**TER**-nuhl RES-pi-**RAY**-shun) The exchange of gases between the air in the alveoli and the blood in the pulmonary capillaries (Chapter 15).

External urethral sphincter (yoo-**REE**-thruhl **SFINK**-ter) The skeletal muscle of the pelvic floor encircling the urethra; provides voluntary control of urination (Chapter 18).

Extracellular fluid (EKS-trah-**SELL**-yoo-ler **FLOO**-id) The water found outside cells; includes plasma, tissue fluid, lymph, and other fluids (Chapter 2).

Extrinsic factor (eks-**TRIN**-sik **FAK**-ter) Vitamin B_{12}, obtained from food and necessary for DNA synthesis, especially by stem cells in the red bone marrow (Chapter 11).

Extrinsic muscles (eks-**TRIN**-sik) The six muscles that move the eyeball (Chapter 9).

—F—

Facial bones (**FAY**-shul) The 14 irregular bones of the face (Chapter 6).

Facial nerves (**FAY**-shul) Cranial nerve pair VII; sensory for taste, motor to facial muscles and the salivary glands (Chapter 8).

Facilitated diffusion (fuh-**SILL**-ah-tay-ted di-**FEW**-zhun) The process in which a substance is transported through a membrane in combination with a carrier or transporter molecule (Chapter 3).

Facultative anaerobe (**FAK**-uhl-tay-tive **AN**-air-robe) A bacterium that is able to reproduce either in the presence or absence of oxygen (Chapter 22).

Fallopian tube (fuh-**LOH**-pee-an TOOB) The tubular organ that propels an ovum from the ovary to the uterus by means of ciliated epithelium and peristalsis of its smooth muscle layer (Syn.—uterine tube) (Chapter 20).

Fascia (**FASH**-ee-ah) A fibrous connective tissue membrane that covers individual skeletal muscles and certain organs (Chapter 4).

Fatty acid (**FA**-tee **ASS**-id) A lipid molecule that consists of an even-numbered carbon chain of 12–24 carbons with hydrogens; may be saturated or unsaturated; an end product of the digestion of fats (Chapter 2).

Femur (**FEE**-mur) The long bone of the thigh (Chapter 6).

Fertilization (FER-ti-li-**ZAY**-shun) The union of the nuclei of an ovum and a sperm cell; restores the diploid number (Chapter 3).

Fetal alcohol syndrome (**FEE**-tuhl **AL**-koh-hol) Birth defects or developmental abnormalities in infants born to women who chronically consumed alcohol during the gestation period (Chapter 21).

Fever (**FEE**-ver) An abnormally high body temperature, caused by pyrogens; may accompany an infectious disease or severe physical injury (Chapter 17).

Fever blister (**FEE**-ver **BLISS**-ter) An eruption of the skin caused by the Herpes simplex virus (Syn.—cold sore) (Chapter 5).

Fiber (**FIGH**-ber) Cellulose in the diet that provides exercise for the colon and helps prevent constipation (Chapter 2).

Fibrillation (fi-bri-**LAY**-shun) Very rapid and uncoordinated heartbeats; ventricular fibrillation is a life-threatening emergency due to ineffective pumping and decreased cardiac output (Chapter 12).

Fibrin (**FYE**-brin) A thread-like protein formed by the action of thrombin on fibrinogen; the substance of which a blood clot is made (Chapter 11).

Fibrinogen (fye-**BRIN**-o-jen) A protein clotting factor produced by the liver; converted to fibrin by thrombin (Chapter 11).

Fibrinolysis (FYE-brin-**AHL**-e-sis) 1. The dissolving of a fibrin clot by natural enzymes, after the clot has served its purpose. 2. The clinical use of clot-dissolving enzymes to dissolve abnormal clots (Chapter 11).

Fibroblast (**FYE**-broh-blast) A connective tissue cell that produces collagen and elastin fibers (Chapter 4).

Fibrous connective tissue (**FYE**-brus) The tissue that consists primarily of collagen fibers. Its most important physical characteristic is its strength (Chapter 4).

Fibula (**FIB**-yoo-lah) A long bone of the lower leg; on the lateral side, thinner than the tibia (Chapter 6).

Filtration (fill-**TRAY**-shun) The process in which water and dissolved materials move through a membrane from an area of higher pressure to an area of lower pressure (Chapter 3).

Fimbriae (**FIM**-bree-ay) Finger-like projections at the end of the fallopian tube that enclose the ovary (Chapter 20).

Fissure (**FISH**-er) A groove or furrow between parts of an organ such as the brain (Syn.—sulcus) (Chapter 8).

Flagellum (flah-**JELL**-um) (Pl.—flagella) A long, thread-like projection through a cell membrane; provides motility for the cell (Chapter 3).

Flexion (**FLEK**-shun) To decrease the angle of a joint (Chapter 7).

Flexor reflex (**FLEKS**-er **REE**-fleks) A spinal cord reflex in which a painful stimulus causes withdrawal of a body part (Chapter 8).

Fluorescent antibody test (floor-**ESS**-ent **AN**-ti-BAH-dee) A diagnostic test that uses fluorescently tagged antibodies to determine the presence of a particular pathogen in the blood or other tissue specimen (Chapter 14).

Flutter (**FLUH**-ter) A very rapid yet fairly regular heartbeat (Chapter 12).

Follicle-stimulating hormone (FSH) (**FAH**-li-kuhl) A gonadotropic hormone produced by the anterior pituitary gland that initiates the production of ova in the ovaries or sperm in the testes (Chapter 10).

Fomites (**FOH**-mights; **FOH**-mi-teez) Inanimate objects capable of transmitting infectious microorganisms from one host to another (Chapter 22).

Fontanel (FON-tah-**NELL**) An area of fibrous connective tissue membrane between the cranial bones of an infant's skull, where bone formation is not complete (Chapter 6).

Foramen (for-**RAY**-men) A hole or opening, as in a bone (from the Latin "to bore") (Chapter 6).

Foramen ovale (for-**RAY**-men oh-**VAHL**-ee) An opening in the interatrial septum of the fetal heart that permits blood to flow from the right atrium to the left atrium, bypassing the fetal lungs (Chapter 13).

Fossa (**FAH**-sah) A shallow depression in a bone (from the Latin "ditch") (Chapter 6).

Fovea (**FOH**-vee-ah) A depression in the retina of the eye directly behind the lens; contains only cones and is the area of best color vision (Chapter 9).

Fracture (**FRAK**-chur) A break in a bone (Chapter 6).

Free nerve ending (FREE NERV **END**-ing) The end of a sensory neuron; the receptor for the sense of pain, heat, or cold in the skin and pain in the viscera (Chapter 5).

Free radical (FREE **RA**-di-kuhl) A molecule with an unpaired electron that is very reactive; formed during normal metabolism and contributes to the natural deterioration (aging) of cells (Chapter 17).

Frontal bone (**FRUN**-tuhl) The flat cranial bone that forms the forehead (Chapter 6).

Frontal lobes (**FRUN**-tuhl LOWBS) The most anterior parts of the cerebrum; contain the motor areas for voluntary movement and the motor speech area (Chapter 8).

Frontal section (**FRUN**-tuhl **SEK**-shun) A plane separating the body into front and back portions (Syn.—coronal section) (Chapter 1).

Frostbite (**FRAWST**-bite) The freezing of part of the body, resulting in tissue damage or death (gangrene) (Chapter 17).

Fructose (**FRUHK**-tohs) A monosaccharide, a six-carbon sugar that is part of the sucrose in food; converted to glucose by the liver (Chapter 2).

Functional layer (**FUNK**-shun-ul **LAY**-er) The vascular layer of the endometrium that is lost in menstruation, then regenerated by the basilar layer (Chapter 20).

Fungus (**FUNG**-gus) Any of the organisms of the kingdom Fungi; they lack chlorophyll; may be unicellular or multicellular; saprophytic or parasitic; include yeasts, molds, and mushrooms (Chapter 22).

—G—

Galactose (guh-**LAK**-tohs) A monosaccharide, a six-carbon sugar that is part of the lactose in food; converted to glucose by the liver (Chapter 2).

Gallbladder (**GAWL**-bla-der) An accessory organ of digestion; a sac located on the undersurface of the liver; stores and concentrates bile (Chapter 16).

Gallstones (**GAWL**-stohns) Crystals formed in the gallbladder or bile ducts; the most common type is made of cholesterol (Chapter 16).

Gametes (**GAM**-eets) The male or female reproductive cells, sperm cells or ova, each with the haploid number of chromosomes (Chapter 3).

Gamma globulins (**GA**-mah **GLAH**-byoo-lins) Antibodies (Chapter 14).

Ganglion (**GANG**-lee-on) A group of neuron cell bodies located outside the CNS (Chapter 8).

Ganglion neurons (**GANG**-lee-on **NYOOR**-onz) The neurons that form the optic nerve; carry impulses from the retina to the brain (Chapter 9).

Gastric juice (**GAS**-trik JOOSS) The secretion of the gastric pits of the stomach; contains hydrochloric acid, pepsin, gastrin, and mucus (Chapter 16).

Gastric pits (**GAS**-trik PITS) The glands of the mucosa of the stomach; secrete gastric juice (Chapter 16).

Gastric ulcer (**GAS**-trik **UL**-ser) An erosion of the gastric mucosa and submucosa (Chapter 16).

Gastrin (**GAS**-trin) A hormone secreted by the G cells of the gastric mucosa when food enters the stomach; stimulates the secretion of gastric juice (Chapter 16).

Gene (JEEN) A segment of DNA that is the genetic code for a particular protein and is located in a definite position on a particular chromosome (Chapter 3).

Genetic code (je-**NET**-ik KOHD) The DNA code for proteins that is shared by all living things; the sequence of bases of the DNA in the chromosomes of cells (Chapter 2).

Genetic disease (je-**NET**-ik di-**ZEEZ**) A hereditary disorder that is the result of an incorrect sequence of bases in the DNA (gene) of a particular chromosome. May be passed to offspring (Chapter 3).

Genetic immunity (je-**NET**-ik im-**YOO**-ni-tee) The immunity provided by the genetic makeup of a species; reflects the inability of certain pathogens to cause disease in certain host species (Chapter 14).

Genome (**JEE**-nohm) The total genetic information

contained in the chromosomes of a cell of a species (Chapter 3).

Genotype (**JEE**-noh-type) The genetic makeup of an individual; the genes that are present (Chapter 21).

Gestation (jes-**TAY**-shun) The length of time from conception to birth; the human gestation period averages 280 days (Chapter 21).

Giantism (**JIGH**-an-tizm) Excessive growth of the body or its parts; may be the result of hypersecretion of growth hormone in childhood (Chapter 10).

Gingiva (jin-**JIGH**-vah) The gums; the tissue that covers the upper and lower jaws around the necks of the teeth (Chapter 16).

Gland (GLAND) A cell or group of epithelial cells that are specialized to secrete a substance (Chapter 4).

Glaucoma (glaw-**KOH**-mah) An eye disease often characterized by increased intraocular pressure due to excessive accumulation of aqueous humor; may result in optic nerve damage and blindness (Chapter 9).

Gliding joint (**GLY**-ding) A diarthrosis that permits a sliding movement (Chapter 6).

Globulins (**GLAH**-byoo-lins) Proteins that circulate in blood plasma; alpha and beta globulins are synthesized by the liver; gamma globulins (antibodies) are synthesized by lymphocytes (Chapter 11).

Glomerular filtration (gloh-**MER**-yoo-ler fill-**TRAY**-shun) The first step in the formation of urine; blood pressure in the glomerulus forces plasma, dissolved materials, and small proteins into Bowman's capsule; this fluid is then called renal filtrate (Chapter 18).

Glomerular filtration rate (gloh-**MER**-yoo-ler fill-**TRAY**-shun RAYT) The total volume of renal filtrate that the kidneys form in 1 minute; average is 100–125 ml/minute (Chapter 18).

Glomerulus (gloh-**MER**-yoo-lus) A capillary network that is enclosed by Bowman's capsule; filtration takes place from the glomerulus to Bowman's capsule (from the Latin "little ball") (Chapter 18).

Glossopharyngeal nerves (GLAH-so-fuh-**RIN**-jee-uhl) Cranial nerve pair IX. Sensory for taste and cardiovascular reflexes. Motor to salivary glands (Chapter 8).

Glottis (**GLAH**-tis) The opening between the vocal cords; an air passageway (Chapter 15).

Glucagon (**GLOO**-kuh-gahn) A hormone secreted by the pancreas that increases the blood glucose level (Chapter 10).

Glucocorticoids (**GLOO**-koh-**KOR**-ti-koids) The hormones secreted by the adrenal cortex that affect the metabolism of nutrients; cortisol is the major hormone in this group (Chapter 10).

Gluconeogenesis (**GLOO**-koh-nee-oh-**JEN**-i-sis) The conversion of excess amino acids to simple carbohydrates or to glucose to be used for energy production (Chapter 10).

Glucose (**GLOO**-kos) A hexose monosaccharide that is the primary energy source for body cells (Chapter 2).

Glycerol (**GLISS**-er-ol) A three-carbon molecule that is one of the end products of the digestion of fats (Chapter 2).

Glycogen (**GLY**-ko-jen) A polysaccharide that is the storage form for excess glucose in the liver and muscles (Chapter 2).

Glycogenesis (GLY-koh-**JEN**-i-sis) The conversion of glucose to glycogen to be stored as potential energy (Chapter 10).

Glycogenolysis (GLY-koh-jen-**AHL**-i-sis) The conversion of stored glycogen to glucose to be used for energy production (Chapter 10).

Glycolysis (gly-**KAHL**-ah-sis) The first stage of the cell respiration of glucose, in which glucose is broken down to two molecules of pyruvic acid and ATP is formed; anaerobic; takes place in the cytoplasm of cells (Chapter 17).

Glycosuria (GLY-kos-**YOO**-ree-ah) The presence of glucose in urine; often an indication of diabetes mellitus (Chapter 18).

Goblet cell (**GAHB**-let) Unicellular glands that secrete mucus; found in the respiratory and GI mucosa (Chapter 4).

Goiter (**GOY**-ter) An enlargement of the thyroid gland, often due to a lack of dietary iodine (Chapter 10).

Golgi apparatus (**GOHL**-jee) A cell organelle found in the cytoplasm; synthesizes carbohydrates and packages materials for secretion from the cell (Chapter 3).

Gonadotropic hormone (GAH-nah-doh-**TROH**-pik) A hormone that has its effects on the ovaries or testes (gonads); FSH and LH (Chapter 10).

Gonorrhea (GAH-nuh-**REE**-ah) A sexually transmitted disease caused by the bacterium *Neisseria gonorrhoeae;* may also cause conjunctivitis in newborns of infected women (Chapter 20).

Graafian follicle (**GRAF**-ee-uhn **FAH**-li-kuhl) A mature ovarian follicle that releases an ovum (Chapter 20).

Gram negative (GRAM **NEG**-uh-tiv) Bacteria that appear red or pink after Gram staining (Chapter 22).

Gram positive (GRAM **PAHS**-uh-tiv) Bacteria that appear purple or blue after Gram staining (Chapter 22).

Gram stain (GRAM STAYN) A staining procedure for bacteria to make them visible microscopically and to determine their gram reaction, which is important in the identification of bacteria (Chapter 22).

Graves' disease (GRAYVES) Hypersecretion of thyroxine, believed to be an autoimmune disease; symptoms reflect the elevated metabolic rate (Chapter 10).

Gray matter (GRAY) Nerve tissue within the central nervous system that consists of the cell bodies of neurons (Chapter 8).

Growth hormone (GH) (GROHTH **HOR**-mohn) A hormone secreted by the anterior pituitary gland that increases the rate of cell division and protein synthesis (Chapter 10).

Gyrus (**JIGH**-rus) A fold or ridge, as in the cerebral cortex (Syn.—convolution) (Chapter 8).

—H—

Hair (HAIR) An accessory skin structure produced in a hair follicle (Chapter 5).

Hair cells (HAIR SELLS) Cells with specialized cilia found in the inner ear; the receptors for hearing (cochlea), static equilibrium (utricle and saccule), and motion equilibrium (semicircular canals) (Chapter 9).

Hair follicle (HAIR **FAH**-li-kuhl) The structure within the skin in which a hair grows (Chapter 5).

Hair root (HAIR ROOT) The site of mitosis at the base of a hair follicle; new cells become the hair shaft (Chapter 5).

Haploid number (**HA**-ployd) Half the usual number of chromosomes found in the cells of a species. Characteristic of the gametes of the species (human = 23) (Chapter 3).

Hard palate (HARD **PAL**-uht) The anterior portion of the palate formed by the maxillae and the palatine bones (Chapter 6).

Haustra (**HOWS**-trah) The pouches of the colon (Chapter 16).

Haversian system (ha-**VER**-zhun) The structural unit of compact bone, consisting of a central haversian canal surrounded by concentric rings of osteocytes within matrix (Chapter 4).

Heart murmur (HART **MUR**-mur) An abnormal heart sound heard during the cardiac cycle; often caused by a malfunctioning heart valve (Chapter 12).

Heat exhaustion (HEET eks-**ZAWS**-chun) A state of weakness and dehydration caused by excessive loss of body water and sodium chloride in sweat; the result of exposure to heat or of strenuous exercise (Chapter 17).

Heat stroke (HEET STROHK) An acute reaction to heat exposure in which there is failure of the temperature-regulating mechanisms; sweating ceases, and body temperature rises sharply (Chapter 17).

Heimlich maneuver (**HIGHM**-lik ma-**NEW**-ver) A procedure used to remove foreign material lodged in the pharynx, larynx, or trachea (Chapter 15).

Helix (**HEE**-liks) A coil or spiral. Double helix is the descriptive term used for the shape of a DNA molecule: two strands of nucleotides coiled around each other and resembling a twisted ladder (Chapter 2).

Hematocrit (hee-**MAT**-oh-krit) A laboratory test that determines the percentage of red blood cells in a given volume of blood; part of a complete blood count (Chapter 11).

Hematuria (HEM-uh-**TYOO**-ree-ah) The presence of blood (RBCs) in urine (Chapter 18).

Hemodialysis (HEE-moh-dye-**AL**-i-sis) A technique for providing the function of the kidneys by passing the blood through tubes surrounded by solutions that selectively remove waste products and excess minerals; may be life-saving in cases of renal failure (Chapter 18).

Hemoglobin (**HEE**-muh-**GLOW**-bin) The protein in red blood cells that contains iron and transports oxygen in the blood (Chapter 7).

Hemolysis (he-**MAHL**-e-sis) Lysis or rupture of red blood cells; may be the result of an antigen–antibody reaction or of increased fragility of red blood cells in some types of anemia (Chapter 11).

Hemophilia (HEE-moh-**FILL**-ee-ah) A hereditary blood disorder characterized by the inability of the blood to clot normally; hemophilia A is caused by a lack of clotting factor 8 (Chapter 11).

Hemopoietic tissue (HEE-moh poy-**ET**-ik) A blood-forming tissue; the red bone marrow and lymphatic tissue (Chapter 4).

Hemorrhoids (**HEM**-uh-royds) Varicose veins of the anal canal (Chapter 13).

Hemostasis (HEE-moh-**STAY**-sis) Prevention of blood loss; the mechanisms are chemical clotting, vascular spasm, and platelet plug formation (Chapter 11).

Heparin (**HEP**-ar-in) A chemical that inhibits blood clotting, an anticoagulant; produced by basophils. Also used clinically to prevent abnormal clotting, such as following some types of surgery (Chapter 11).

Hepatic duct (hep-**PAT**-ik DUKT) The duct that takes bile out of the liver; joins the cystic duct of the gallbladder to form the common bile duct (Chapter 16).

Hepatic portal circulation (hep-**PAT**-ik **POOR**-tuhl) The pathway of systemic circulation in which venous blood from the digestive organs and the spleen circulates through the liver before returning to the heart (Chapter 13).

Hepatitis (HEP-uh-**TIGH**-tis) Inflammation of the liver, most often caused by the hepatitis viruses A, B, or C (Chapter 16).

Herniated disc (**HER**-nee-ay-ted DISK) Rupture of an intervertebral disc (Chapter 6).

Herpes simplex (**HER**-peez **SIM**-pleks) A virus that causes lesions in the skin or mucous membranes of the mouth (usually type 1) or genital area (usually type 2); genital herpes may cause death or mental retardation of infants of infected women (Chapter 20).

Heterozygous (HET-er-oh-**ZYE**-gus) Having two different alleles for a trait (Chapter 21).

Hexose sugar (**HEKS**-ohs) A six-carbon sugar, such as glucose, that is an energy source (in the process of cell respiration) (Chapter 2).

Hilus (**HIGH**-lus) An indentation or depression on the surface of an organ such as a lung or kidney (Chapter 15).

Hinge joint (HINJ) A diarthrosis that permits movement in one plane (Chapter 6).

Hip bone (HIP BOWNE) The flat bone that forms half of the pelvic bone; consists of the upper ilium, the lower posterior ischium, and the lower anterior pubis (Chapter 6).

Histamine (**HISS**-tah-meen) An inflammatory chemical released by damaged tissues; stimulates increased capillary permeability and vasodilation (Chapter 5).

Hives (**HIGHVZ**) A very itchy eruption of the skin, usually the result of an allergy (Chapter 5).

Hodgkin's disease (**HODJ**-kinz) A malignancy of the lymphatic tissue; a lymphoma (Chapter 14).

Homeostasis (HOH-mee-oh-**STAY**-sis) The state in which the internal environment of the body remains relatively stable by responding appropriately to changes (Chapter 1).

Homologous pair (hoh-**MAHL**-ah-gus) A pair of chromosomes, one maternal and one paternal, that contain genes for the same characteristics (Chapter 21).

Homozygous (HOH-moh-**ZYE**-gus) Having two similar alleles for a trait (Chapter 21).

Hormone (**HOR**-mohn) The secretion of an endocrine gland that has specific effects on particular target organs (Chapter 4).

Human leukocyte antigens (HLA) (**HYOO**-man **LOO**-koh-sight **AN**-ti-jens) The antigens on white blood cells that are representative of the antigens present on all the cells of the individual; the "self" antigens that are controlled by several genes on chromosome number 6; the basis for tissue typing before an organ transplant is attempted (Chapter 11).

Humerus (**HYOO**-mer-us) The long bone of the upper arm (Chapter 6).

Humoral immunity (**HYOO**-mohr-uhl im-**YOO**-ni-tee) The mechanism of immunity that involves antibody production and the destruction of foreign antigens by the activities of B cells, T cells, and macrophages (Syn.—antibody-mediated immunity) (Chapter 14).

Hyaline membrane disease (**HIGH**-e-lin **MEM**-brayn) A pulmonary disorder of premature infants whose lungs have not yet produced sufficient pulmonary surfactant to permit inflation of the alveoli (Chapter 15).

Hydrochloric acid (HIGH-droh-**KLOR**-ik **ASS**-id) An acid secreted by the parietal cells of the gastric pits of the stomach; activates pepsin and maintains a pH of 1–2 in the stomach (Chapter 16).

Hydrogen bond (**HIGH**-droh-jen BAHND) A weak bond that helps maintain the three-dimensional shape of proteins and nucleic acids (Chapter 2).

Hymen (**HIGH**-men) A thin fold of mucous membrane that partially covers the vaginal orifice (Chapter 20).

Hypercalcemia (HIGH-per-kal-**SEE**-mee-ah) A high blood calcium level (Chapter 10).

Hyperglycemia (HIGH-per-gligh-**SEE**-mee-ah) A high blood glucose level (Chapter 10).

Hyperkalemia (HIGH-per-kuh-**LEE**-mee-ah) A high blood potassium level (Chapter 19).

Hypernatremia (HIGH-per-nuh-**TREE**-mee-ah) A high blood sodium level (Chapter 19).

Hyperopia (HIGH-per-**OH**-pee-ah) Farsightedness; an

error of refraction in which only distant objects are seen clearly (Chapter 9).

Hypertension (HIGH-per-**TEN**-shun) An abnormally high blood pressure, consistently above 130/85 mmHg (Chapter 13).

Hypertonic (HIGH-per-**TAHN**-ik) Having a greater concentration of dissolved materials than the solution used as a comparison (Chapter 3).

Hypertrophy (high-**PER**-troh-fee) Increase in size of a body part, especially of a muscle following long-term exercise or overuse (Chapter 7).

Hypocalcemia (HIGH-poh-kal-**SEE**-mee-ah) A low blood calcium level (Chapter 10).

Hypoglossal nerves (HIGH-poh-**GLAH**-suhl) Cranial nerve pair XII. Motor to the tongue (Chapter 8).

Hypoglycemia (HIGH-poh-gligh-**SEE**-mee-ah) A low blood glucose level (Chapter 10).

Hypokalemia (HIGH-poh-kuh-**LEE**-mee-ah) A low blood potassium level (Chapter 19).

Hyponatremia (HIGH-poh-nuh-**TREE**-mee-ah) A low blood sodium level (Chapter 19).

Hypophyseal portal system (high-POFF-e-**SEE**-al **POR**-tuhl) The pathway of circulation in which releasing factors from the hypothalamus circulate directly to the anterior pituitary gland (Chapter 10).

Hypophysis (high-**POFF**-e-sis) The pituitary gland (Chapter 10).

Hypotension (HIGH-poh-**TEN**-shun) An abnormally low blood pressure, consistently below 90/60 mmHg (Chapter 13).

Hypothalamus (HIGH-poh-**THAL**-uh-muss) The part of the brain superior to the pituitary gland and inferior to the thalamus; its many functions include regulation of body temperature and regulation of the secretions of the pituitary gland (Chapter 8).

Hypothermia (HIGH-poh-**THER**-mee-ah) 1. The condition in which the body temperature is abnormally low due to excessive exposure to cold. 2. A procedure used during some types of surgery to lower body temperature to reduce the patient's need for oxygen (Chapter 17).

Hypotonic (HIGH-po-**TAHN**-ik) Having a lower concentration of dissolved materials than the solution used as a comparison (Chapter 3).

Hypovolemic shock (HIGH-poh-voh-**LEEM**-ik SHAHK) A type of circulatory shock caused by a decrease in blood volume (Chapter 13).

Hypoxia (high-**PAHK**-see-ah) A deficiency or lack of oxygen (Chapter 2).

—I—

Idiopathic (ID-ee-oh-**PATH**-ik) A disease or disorder of unknown cause (Chapter 11).

Ileocecal valve (ILL-ee-oh-**SEE**-kuhl VALV) The tissue of the ileum that extends into the cecum and acts as a sphincter; prevents the backup of fecal material into the small intestine (Chapter 16).

Ileum (**ILL**-ee-um) The third and last portion of the small intestine, about 11 feet long (Chapter 16).

Ilium (**ILL**-ee-um) The upper, flared portion of the hip bone (Chapter 6).

Immunity (im-**YOO**-ni-tee) The state of being protected from an infectious disease, usually by having been exposed to the infectious agent or a vaccine (Chapter 11).

Impetigo (IM-pe-**TYE**-go) A bacterial infection of the skin that occurs most often in children (Chapter 5).

Implantation (IM-plan-**TAY**-shun) Embedding of the embryonic blastocyst in the endometrium of the uterus 6 to 8 days after fertilization (Chapter 21).

Inactivator (in-**AK**-ti-vay-tur) A chemical that inactivates a neurotransmitter to prevent continuous impulses (Chapter 8).

Inapparent infection (**IN**-uh-PAR-ent) An infection without symptoms (Syn.—subclinical, asymptomatic) (Chapter 22).

Incubation period (IN-kew-**BAY**-shun) In the course of an infectious disease, the time between the entry of the pathogen and the onset of symptoms (Chapter 22).

Incus (**ING**-kuss) The second of the three auditory bones in the middle ear; transmits vibrations from the malleus to the stapes (Chapter 9).

Infarct (**IN**-farkt) An area of tissue that has died due to lack of a blood supply (Chapter 12).

Infection (in-**FEK**-shun) A disease process caused by the invasion and multiplication of a microorganism (Chapter 22).

Inferior (in-**FEER**-ee-your) Below or lower (Chapter 1).

Inferior vena cava (**VEE**-nah **KAY**-vah) The vein that returns blood from the lower body to the right atrium (Chapter 12).

Infestation (in-fess-**TAY**-shun) The harboring of parasites, especially worms or arthropods (Chapter 22).

Inflammation (in-fluh-**MAY**-shun) The reactions of tissue to injury (Chapter 5).

Inguinal canal (**IN**-gwi-nuhl ka-**NAL**) The opening in the lower abdominal wall that contains a spermatic cord in men and the round ligament of the uterus in women; a natural weak spot that may be the site of hernia formation (Chapter 20).

Inhibin (in-**HIB**-in) A protein hormone secreted by the sustentacular cells of the testes and by the ovaries; inhibits secretion of follicle-stimulating hormone (Chapter 10).

Inorganic (**IN**-or-GAN-ik) A chemical compound that does not contain carbon–hydrogen covalent bonds; includes water, salts, and oxygen (Chapter 1).

Insertion (in-**SIR**-shun) The more movable attachment point of a muscle to a bone (Chapter 7).

Inspiration (in-spi-**RAY**-shun) Inhalation; the intake of air to the lungs (Chapter 15).

Inspiratory reserve (in-**SPYR**-ah-tor-ee ree-**ZERV**) The volume of air beyond tidal volume that can be inhaled with the deepest inhalation; average: 2000–3000 ml (Chapter 15).

Insulin (**IN**-syoo-lin) A hormone secreted by the pancreas that decreases the blood glucose level by increasing storage of glycogen and use of glucose by cells for energy production (Chapter 10).

Integumentary system (in-TEG-yoo-**MEN**-tah-ree) The organ system that consists of the skin and its accessory structures and the subcutaneous tissue (Chapter 5).

Intensity (in-**TEN**-si-tee) The degree to which a sensation is felt (Chapter 9).

Intercostal muscles (IN-ter-**KAHS**-tuhl **MUSS**-uhls) The skeletal muscles between the ribs; the external intercostals pull the ribs up and out for inhalation; the internal intercostals pull the ribs down and in for a forced exhalation (Syn.—spareribs) (Chapter 15).

Intercostal nerves (IN-ter-**KAHS**-tuhl NERVS) The pairs of peripheral nerves that are motor to the intercostal muscles (Chapter 15).

Interferon (in-ter-**FEER**-on) A chemical produced by T cells or by cells infected with viruses; prevents the reproduction of viruses (Chapter 14).

Internal (in-**TER**-nuhl) On the inside, or away from the surface (Chapter 1).

Internal anal sphincter (in-**TER**-nuhl **AY**-nuhl **SFINK**-ter) The circular smooth muscle that surrounds the anus; relaxes as part of the defecation reflex to permit defecation (Chapter 16).

Internal respiration (in-**TER**-nuhl RES-pi-**RAY**-shun) The exchange of gases between the blood in the systemic capillaries and the surrounding tissue fluid and cells (Chapter 15).

Internal urethral sphincter (yoo-**REE**-thruhl **SFINK**-ter) The smooth muscle sphincter at the junction of the urinary bladder and the urethra; relaxes as part of the urination reflex to permit urination (Chapter 18).

Interneuron (**IN**-ter-NYOOR-on) A nerve cell entirely within the central nervous system (Chapter 8).

Interphase (**IN**-ter-fayz) The period of time between mitotic divisions during which DNA replication takes place (Chapter 3).

Interstitial cells (in-ter-**STISH**-uhl SELLS) The cells in the testes that secrete testosterone when stimulated by LH (Chapter 20).

Intestinal glands (in-**TESS**-tin-uhl) 1. The glands of the small intestine that secrete digestive enzymes. 2. The glands of the large intestine that secrete mucus (Chapter 16).

Intracellular fluid (IN-trah-**SELL**-yoo-ler **FLOO**-id) The water found within cells (Chapter 2).

Intramuscular injection (in-trah-**MUSS**-kew-ler in-**JEK**-shun) An injection of a medication into a muscle (Chapter 7).

Intrapleural pressure (in-trah-**PLOOR**-uhl) The pressure within the potential pleural space; always slightly below atmospheric pressure, about 756 mmHg (Chapter 15).

Intrapulmonic pressure (in-trah-pull-**MAHN**-ik) The air pressure within the bronchial tree and alveoli; fluctuates below and above atmospheric pressure during breathing (Chapter 15).

Intrinsic factor (in-**TRIN**-sik **FAK**-ter) A chemical produced by the parietal cells of the gastric mucosa; necessary for the absorption of vitamin B_{12} (Chapter 11).

***In vitro* fertilization** (IN **VEE**-troh FER-ti-li-**ZAY**-shun) Fertilization outside the body, in which sperm and ova are mixed in laboratory glassware; early embryos may then be introduced into the uterus for implantation (Chapter 20).

Involuntary muscle (in-**VAHL**-un-tary **MUSS**-uhl) Another name for smooth muscle tissue (Chapter 4).

Ion (**EYE**-on) An atom or group of atoms with an electrical charge (Chapter 2).

Ionic bond (eye-**ON**-ik) A chemical bond formed by the loss and gain of electrons between atoms (Chapter 2).

Iris (**EYE**-ris) The colored part of the eye, between the cornea and lens; made of two sets of smooth muscle fibers that regulate the size of the pupil, the opening in the center of the iris (from the Latin "rainbow") (Chapter 9).

Ischemic (iss-**KEY**-mik) Lack of blood to a body part, often due to an obstruction in circulation (Chapter 12).

Ischium (**ISH**-ee-um) The lower posterior part of the hip bone (Chapter 6).

Islets of Langerhans (**EYE**-lets of **LAHNG**-er-hanz) The endocrine portions of the pancreas that secrete insulin and glucagon (Syn.—pancreatic islets) (Chapter 10).

Isometric exercise (EYE-so-**MEH**-trik) Contraction of muscles without movement of a body part (Chapter 7).

Isotonic (EYE-so-**TAHN**-ik) Having the same concentration of dissolved materials as the solution used as a comparison (Chapter 3).

Isotonic exercise (EYE-so-**TAHN**-ik) Contraction of muscles with movement of a body part (Chapter 7).

—J—

Jaundice (**JAWN**-diss) A condition characterized by a yellow color in the whites of the eyes and in light skin; caused by an elevated blood level of bilirubin. May be hepatic, pre-hepatic, or post-hepatic in origin (Chapter 11).

Jejunum (je-**JOO**-num) The second portion of the small intestine, about 8 feet long (Chapter 16).

Joint capsule (JOYNT **KAP**-suhl) The fibrous connective tissue sheath that encloses a joint (Chapter 6).

Juxtaglomerular cells (JUKS-tah-gloh-**MER**-yoo-ler SELLS) Cells in the wall of the afferent arteriole that secrete renin when blood pressure decreases (Chapter 18).

—K—

Keratin (**KER**-uh-tin) A protein produced by epidermal cells; found in the epidermis, hair, and nails (from the Greek "horn") (Chapter 5).

Keratinocyte (KER-un-**TIN**-oh-sight) A cell of the epidermis, produces keratin before dying (Chapter 5).

Ketoacidosis (KEY-toh-ass-i-**DOH**-sis) A metabolic acidosis that results from the accumulation of ketones in the blood when fats and proteins are used for energy production (Chapter 10).

Ketones (**KEY**-tohns) Organic acid molecules that are formed from fats or amino acids when these nutrients are used for energy production; include acetone and acetoacetic acid (Chapter 10).

Ketonuria (KEY-ton-**YOO**-ree-ah) The presence of ketones in urine (Chapter 18).

Kidneys (**KID**-nees) The two organs on either side of the vertebral column in the upper abdomen that produce urine to eliminate waste products and to regulate the volume, pH, and fluid–electrolyte balance of the blood (Chapter 6).

Kilocalorie (KILL-oh-**KAL**-oh-ree) A Calorie, which is one thousand calories; used to indicate the energy content of foods or the energy expended in activity (See: Calorie) (Chapter 17).

Kinesthetic sense (KIN-ess-**THET**-ik) Muscle sense (Chapter 9).

Krebs cycle (KREBS **SIGH**-kuhl) The stage of cell respiration comprising a series of reactions in which pyruvic acid or acetyl CoA is broken down to carbon dioxide and ATP is formed; aerobic; takes place in the mitochondria of cells (Syn.—citric acid cycle) (Chapter 17).

Kupffer cells (**KUP**-fer SELLS) The macrophages of the liver; phagocytize pathogens and old red blood cells (Chapter 16).

Kyphosis (kye-**FOH**-sis) An exaggerated thoracic curvature of the vertebral column (Chapter 6).

—L—

Labia majora (**LAY**-bee-uh muh-**JOR**-ah) The outer folds of skin of the vulva; enclose the labia minora and the vestibule (Chapter 20).

Labia minora (**LAY**-bee-uh min-**OR**-ah) The inner folds of the vulva; enclose the vestibule (Chapter 20).

Labor (**LAY**-ber) The process by which a fetus is expelled from the uterus through the vagina to the exterior of the body (Chapter 21).

Labyrinth (**LAB**-i-rinth) 1. A maze; an interconnected series of passageways. 2. In the inner ear, the bony labyrinth is a series of tunnels in the temporal bone lined with membrane called the membranous labyrinth (Chapter 9).

Lacrimal glands (**LAK**-ri-muhl) The glands that secrete tears, located at the upper, outer corner of each eyeball (Chapter 9).

Lactase (**LAK**-tays) A digestive enzyme that breaks down lactose to glucose and galactose; secreted by the small intestine (Chapter 16).

Lacteals (lak-**TEELS**) The lymph capillaries in the villi of the small intestine, which absorb the fat-soluble end products of digestion (Chapter 14).

Lactic acid (**LAK**-tik **ASS**-id) The chemical end product of anaerobic cell respiration; contributes to fatigue in muscle cells (Chapter 7).

Lactose (**LAK**-tohs) A disaccharide made of one glucose and one galactose molecule (Syn.—milk sugar) (Chapter 2).

Lactose intolerance (**LAK**-tohs in-**TAHL**-er-ense) The inability to digest lactose due to a deficiency of the enzyme lactase; may be congenital or acquired (Chapter 16).

Langerhans cell (**LAHNG**-er-hanz SELL) A phagocytic cell of the epidermis (Chapter 5).

Large intestine (LARJ in-**TESS**-tin) The organ of the alimentary tube that extends from the small intestine to the anus; absorbs water, minerals, and vitamins and eliminates undigested materials (Syn.—colon) (Chapter 16).

Laryngopharynx (la-RIN-goh-**FA**-rinks) The lower portion of the pharynx that opens into the larynx and the esophagus; a passageway for both air and food (Chapter 15).

Larynx (**LA**-rinks) The organ that is an airway between the pharynx and the trachea; contains the vocal cords for speech (Syn.—voice box) (Chapter 15).

Lateral (**LAT**-er-uhl) Away from the midline, or at the side (Chapter 1).

Lens (LENZ) The oval structure of the eye posterior to the pupil, made of transparent protein; the only adjustable portion of the refraction pathway for the focusing of light rays (Chapter 9).

Lesion (**LEE**-zhun) An area of pathologically altered tissue; an injury or wound (Chapter 5).

Leukemia (loo-**KEE**-mee-ah) Malignancy of blood-forming tissues, in which large numbers of immature and non-functional white blood cells are produced (Chapter 11).

Leukocyte (**LOO**-koh-sight) White blood cell; the five kinds are neutrophils, eosinophils, basophils, lymphocytes, and monocytes (Chapter 11).

Leukocytosis (LOO-koh-sigh-**TOH**-sis) An elevated white blood cell count, often an indication of infection (Chapter 11).

Leukopenia (LOO-koh-**PEE**-nee-ah) An abnormally low white blood cell count; may be the result of aplastic anemia, or a side effect of some medications (Chapter 11).

Ligament (**LIG**-uh-ment) A fibrous connective tissue structure that connects bone to bone (Chapter 6).

Lipase (**LYE**-pays) A digestive enzyme that breaks down emulsified fats to fatty acids and glycerol; secreted by the pancreas (Chapter 16).

Lipid (**LIP**-id) An organic chemical insoluble in water; includes true fats, phospholipids, and steroids (Chapter 2).

Lipoprotein (li-poh-**PRO**-teen) A large molecule that is a combination of proteins, triglycerides, and cholesterol; formed by the liver to circulate lipids in the blood (Chapter 16).

Lithotripsy (LITH-oh-**TRIP**-see) Crushing of gallstones or renal calculi by an instrument that uses ultrasonic waves applied to the exterior of the body (Chapter 16).

Liver (**LIV**-er) The organ in the upper right and center of the abdominal cavity; secretes bile for the emulsification of fats in digestion; has many other functions related to the metabolism of nutrients and the composition of blood (Chapter 16).

Liver lobule (**LIV**-er **LAH**-byool) The structural unit of the liver; a columnar hexagon of liver cells and sinusoids surrounding a central vein; includes the smallest bile ducts (Chapters 16).

Localized infection (**LOH**-kuhl-IZ'D) An infection confined to one body organ or site (Chapter 22).

Longitudinal section (LAWNJ-i-**TOO**-din-uhl **SEK**-shun) A plane or cut along the long axis of an organ or the body (Chapter 1).

Loop of Henle (LOOP of **HEN**-lee) The part of a renal tubule that extends from the proximal convoluted tubule to the distal convoluted tubule (Chapter 18).

Lordosis (lor-**DOH**-sis) An exaggerated lumbar curvature of the vertebral column (Chapter 6).

Lower esophageal sphincter (e-SOF-uh-**JEE**-uhl **SFINK**-ter) The circular smooth muscle at the lower end of the esophagus; prevents backup of stomach contents (Syn.—cardiac sphincter) (Chapter 16).

Lower respiratory tract (**LOH**-er **RES**-pi-rah-TOR-ee TRAKT) The respiratory organs located within the chest cavity (Chapter 15).

Lumbar puncture (**LUM**-bar **PUNK**-chur) A diagnostic procedure that involves removal of cerebrospinal fluid from the lumbar meningeal sac to assess the pressure and constituents of cerebrospinal fluid (Chapter 8).

Lumbar vertebrae (**LUM**-bar **VER**-te-bray) The five large vertebrae in the small of the back (Chapter 6).

Lungs (LUHNGS) The paired organs in the thoracic cavity in which gas exchange takes place between the air in the alveoli and the blood in the pulmonary capillaries (Chapter 15).

Luteinizing hormone (LH or ICSH) (LOO-tee-in-**EYE**-zing) A gonadotropic hormone produced by the anterior pituitary gland that, in men, stimulates secretion of testosterone by the testes or, in women, stimulates ovulation and secretion of progesterone by the corpus luteum in the ovary (Chapter 10).

Lymph (LIMF) The water found within lymphatic vessels (Chapter 2).

Lymph node (LIMF NOHD) A small mass of lymphatic tissue located along the pathway of a lymph vessel; produces lymphocytes and monocytes and destroys pathogens in the lymph (Chapter 14).

Lymph nodule (LIMF **NAHD**-yool) A small mass of lymphatic tissue located in a mucous membrane; produces lymphocytes and monocytes and destroys pathogens that penetrate mucous membranes (Chapter 14).

Lymphatic tissue (lim-**FAT**-ik **TISH**-yoo) A hemopoietic tissue that produces lymphocytes and monocytes; found in the spleen and lymph nodes and nodules (Chapter 11).

Lymphocyte (**LIM**-foh-sight) A type of white blood cell (agranular); T cells and B cells are involved in specific immune responses; natural killer cells are nonspecific (Chapter 11).

Lysosome (**LYE**-soh-zome) A cell organelle found in the cytoplasm; contains enzymes that digest damaged cell parts or material ingested by the cell (Chapter 3).

Lysozyme (**LYE**-soh-zyme) An enzyme in tears and saliva that inhibits the growth of bacteria in these fluids (Chapter 9).

—M—

Macrophage (**MAK**-roh-fahj) A phagocytic cell derived from monocytes; capable of phagocytosis of pathogens, dead or damaged cells, and old red blood cells; also involved in recognition of foreign antigens (Chapter 11).

Macula lutea (**MAK**-yoo-lah **LOO**-tee-ah) A spot in the center of the retina; contains the fovea (Chapter 9).

Magnetic resonance imaging (MRI) (mag-**NET**-ik **REZ**-ah-nanse **IM**-ah-jing) A diagnostic imaging technique that uses a magnetic field and a computer to integrate the images of internal organs (Chapter 1).

Malignant (muh-**LIG**-nunt) Tending to spread and become worse; used especially with reference to cancer (Chapter 3).

Malleus (**MAL**-ee-us) The first of the three auditory bones in the middle ear; transmits vibrations from the eardrum to the incus (Chapter 9).

Maltase (**MAWL**-tays) A digestive enzyme that breaks down maltose to glucose; secreted by the small intestine (Chapter 16).

Maltose (**MAWL**-tohs) A disaccharide made of two glucose molecules (Chapter 2).

Mammary glands (**MAM**-uh-ree) The glands of the female breasts that secrete milk; secretion and release of milk are under hormonal control (Chapter 20).

Mammography (mah-**MOG**-rah-fee) A diagnostic procedure that uses radiography to detect breast cancer (Chapter 20).

Mandible (**MAN**-di-buhl) The lower jaw bone (Chapter 6).

Manubrium (muh-**NOO**-bree-um) The upper part of the sternum (Chapter 6).

Marrow canal (**MA**-roh ka-**NAL**) The cavity within the diaphysis of a long bone; contains yellow bone marrow (Chapter 4).

Mastoid sinus (**MASS**-toyd) An air cavity within the mastoid process of the temporal bone (Chapter 6).

Matrix (**MAY**-triks) The non-living intercellular material that is part of connective tissues (Chapter 4).

Matter (**MAT**-ter) Anything that occupies space; may be solid, liquid, or gas; may be living or non-living (Chapter 2).

Maxilla (mak-**SILL**-ah) The upper jaw bone (Chapter 6).

Mechanical digestion (muh-**KAN**-i-kuhl dye-**JES**-chun) The physical breakdown of food into smaller pieces, which increases the surface area for the action of digestive enzymes (Chapter 16).

Medial (**MEE**-dee-uhl) Toward the midline, or in the middle (Chapter 1).

Mediastinum (ME-dee-ah-**STYE**-num) The area or space between the lungs; contains the heart and great vessels (Chapter 12).

Medulla (muh-**DEW**-lah) (muh-**DULL**-ah) 1. The part of the brain superior to the spinal cord; regulates vital functions such as heart rate, respiration, and blood pressure. 2. The inner part of an organ, such as the renal medulla or the adrenal medulla (Chapter 8).

Megakaryocyte (MEH-ga-**KA**-ree-oh-sight) A cell in the red bone marrow that breaks up into small fragments called platelets, which then circulate in peripheral blood (Chapter 11).

Meiosis (my-**OH**-sis) The process of cell division in which one cell with the diploid number of chromosomes divides twice to form four cells, each with the haploid number of chromosomes (Chapter 3).

Meissner's plexus (**MIZE**-ners **PLEK**-sus) The autonomic nerve plexus in the submucosa of the organs of the alimentary tube; regulates secretions of the glands in the mucosa of these organs (Syn.—submucosal plexus) (Chapter 16).

Melanin (**MEL**-uh-nin) A protein pigment produced by melanocytes. Absorbs ultraviolet light; gives color to the skin, hair, iris, and choroid layer of the eye (Chapter 5).

Melanocyte (muh-**LAN**-o-sight) A cell in the lower epidermis that synthesizes the pigment melanin (Chapter 5).

Melanoma (MEL-ah-**NOH**-mah) Malignant pigmented mole or nevus (Chapter 5).

Melatonin (mel-ah-**TOH**-nin) A hormone produced by the pineal gland; influences sleep cycles (Chapter 10).

Membrane (**MEM**-brayn) A sheet of tissue; may be made of epithelial tissue or connective tissue (Chapter 4).

Meninges (me-**NIN**-jeez) The connective tissue membranes that line the dorsal cavity and cover the brain and spinal cord (Chapter 1).

Meningitis (MEN-in-**JIGH**-tis) Inflammation of the meninges, most often the result of bacterial infection (Chapter 8).

Menopause (**MEN**-ah-paws) The period during life in which menstrual activity ceases; usually occurs between the ages of 45 and 55 years (Chapter 20).

Menstrual cycle (**MEN**-stroo-uhl **SIGH**-kuhl) The periodic series of changes that occur in the female reproductive tract; the average cycle is 28 days (Chapter 20).

Menstruation (MEN-stroo-**AY**-shun) The periodic discharge of a bloody fluid from the uterus that occurs at regular intervals from puberty to menopause (Chapter 20).

Mesentery (**MEZ**-en-TER-ee) The visceral peritoneum (serous) that covers the abdominal organs; a large fold attaches the small intestine to the posterior abdominal wall (Chapter 1).

Mesoderm (**MEZ**-oh-derm) The middle primary germ layer of cells of an embryo; gives rise to muscles, bones, and connective tissues (Chapter 21).

Metabolic acidosis (MET-uh-**BAH**-lik ass-i-**DOH**-sis) A condition in which the blood pH is lower than normal, caused by any disorder that increases the number of acidic molecules in the body or increases the loss of alkaline molecules (Chapter 15).

Metabolic alkalosis (MET-uh-**BAH**-lik al-kah-**LOH**-sis) A condition in which the blood pH is higher than normal, caused by any disorder that decreases the number of acidic molecules in the body or increases the number of alkaline molecules (Chapter 15).

Metabolism (muh-**TAB**-uh-lizm) All the reactions that take place within the body; includes anabolism and catabolism (Chapter 17).

Metacarpals (MET-uh-**KAR**-puhls) The five long bones in the palm of the hand (Chapter 6).

Metaphase (**MET**-ah-fayz) The second stage of mitosis, in which the pairs of chromatids line up on the equator of the cell (Chapter 3).

Metastasis (muh-**TASS**-tuh-sis) The spread of disease from one part of the body to another (Chapter 3).

Metatarsals (MET-uh-**TAR**-suhls) The five long bones in the arch of the foot (Chapter 6).

Microglia (my-kroh-**GLEE**-ah) A type of neuroglia capable of movement and phagocytosis of pathogens (Chapter 8).

Micron (**MY**-kron) A unit of linear measure equal to 0.001 millimeter (Syn.—micrometer) (Chapter 3).

Microvilli (MY-kro-**VILL**-eye) Folds of the cell membrane on the free surface of an epithelial cell; increase the surface area for absorption (Chapter 3).

Micturition (MIK-tyoo-**RISH**-un) Urination; the voiding or elimination of urine from the urinary bladder (Chapter 18).

Midbrain (**MID**-brayn) The part of the brain between the pons and hypothalamus; regulates visual, auditory, and righting reflexes (Chapter 8).

Mineral (**MIN**-er-al) An inorganic element or compound; many are needed by the body for normal metabolism and growth (Chapter 17).

Mineralocorticoids (MIN-er-al-oh-**KOR**-ti-koidz) The hormones secreted by the adrenal cortex that affect fluid–electrolyte balance; aldosterone is the major hormone in this group (Chapter 10).

Minute respiratory volume (**MIN**-uht RES-pi-rah-**TOR**-ee **VAHL**-yoom) The volume of air inhaled and exhaled in 1 minute; calculated by multiplying tidal volume by number of respirations per minute (Chapter 15).

Mitochondria (MY-toh-**KAHN**-dree-ah) The cell organelles in which aerobic cell respiration takes place and energy (ATP) is produced; found in the cytoplasm of a cell (Chapter 3).

Mitosis (my-**TOH**-sis) The process of cell division in which one cell with the diploid number of chromosomes divides once to form two identical cells, each with the diploid number of chromosomes (Chapter 3).

Mitral valve (**MY**-truhl VALV) The left AV valve (bicuspid valve), which prevents backflow of blood from the left ventricle to the left atrium when the ventricle contracts (Chapter 12).

Mixed nerve (MIKSD NERV) A nerve that contains both sensory and motor neurons (Chapter 8).

Molecule (**MAHL**-e-kuhl) A chemical combination of two or more atoms (Chapter 2).

Monocyte (**MAH**-no-sight) A type of white blood cell (agranular); differentiates into a macrophage, which is capable of phagocytosis of pathogens and dead or damaged cells (Chapter 11).

Monosaccharide (MAH-noh-**SAK**-ah-ride) A carbohydrate molecule that is a single sugar; includes the hexose and pentose sugars (Chapter 2).

Morula (**MOR**-yoo-lah) An early stage of embryonic development, a solid mass of cells (Chapter 21).

Motility (moh-**TILL**-e-tee) The ability to move (Chapter 3).

Motion sickness (**MOH**-shun) Queasiness that accompanies repetitive or unexpected motion (Chapter 9).

Motor area (**MOH**-ter) Part of the cerebral cortex of the frontal lobe; generates the impulses necessary for voluntary movement (Chapter 7).

Motor neuron (**MOH**-ter **NYOOR**-on) A nerve cell that carries impulses from the central nervous system to an effector (Syn.—efferent neuron) (Chapter 8).

Mucosa (mew-**KOH**-suh) A mucous membrane, the epithelial lining of a body cavity that opens to the environment (Chapter 4).

Mucous membrane (**MEW**-kuss **MEM**-brayn) The epithelial tissue lining of a body tract that opens to the environment (Chapter 4).

Mucus (**MEW**-kuss) The thick fluid secreted by mucous membranes or mucous glands (Chapter 4).

Multicellular (MULL-tee-**SELL**-yoo-lar) Consisting of more than one cell; made of many cells (Chapter 4).

Multiple sclerosis (**MULL**-ti-puhl skle-**ROH**-sis) A progressive nervous system disorder, possibly an autoimmune disease, characterized by the degeneration of the myelin sheaths of CNS neurons (Chapter 8).

Muscle fatigue (**MUSS**-uhl fah-**TEEG**) The state in which muscle fibers cannot contract efficiently, due to a lack of oxygen and the accumulation of lactic acid (Chapter 7).

Muscle fiber (**MUSS**-uhl **FYE**-ber) A muscle cell (Chapter 7).

Muscle sense (**MUSS**-uhl SENSE) The conscious or unconscious awareness of where the muscles are, and their degree of contraction, without having to look at them (Chapter 7).

Muscle tissue (**MUSS**-uhl **TISH**-yoo) The tissue specialized for contraction and movement of parts of the body (Chapter 4).

Muscle tone (**MUSS**-uhl TONE) The state of slight contraction present in healthy muscles (Chapter 7).

Muscular dystrophy (**MUSS**-kyoo-ler **DIS**-truh-fee) A genetic disease characterized by the replacement of muscle tissue by fibrous connective tissue or adipose tissue, with progressive loss of muscle functioning; the most common form is Duchenne's muscular dystrophy (Chapter 7).

Muscular system (**MUSS**-kew-ler) The organ system that consists of the skeletal muscles and tendons; its functions are to move the skeleton and produce body heat (Chapter 7).

Mutation (mew-**TAY**-shun) A change in DNA; a genetic change that may be passed to offspring (Chapter 3).

Myalgia (my-**AL**-jee-ah) Pain or tenderness in a muscle (Chapter 7).

Myasthenia gravis (MY-ass-**THEE**-nee-yuh **GRAH**-viss) An autoimmune disease characterized by extreme muscle weakness and fatigue following minimal exertion (Chapter 7).

Mycosis (my-**KOH**-sis) (Pl.—mycoses) An infection caused by a pathogenic fungus (Chapter 22).

Myelin (**MY**-uh-lin) A phospholipid produced by Schwann cells and oligodendrocytes that forms the myelin sheath of axons and dendrites (Chapter 2).

Myelin sheath (**MY**-uh-lin SHEETH) The white, segmented, phospholipid sheath of most axons and dendrites; provides electrical insulation and increases the speed of impulse transmission (Chapter 4).

Myocardial infarction (MI) (MY-oh-**KAR**-dee-yuhl in-**FARK**-shun) Death of part of the heart muscle due to lack of oxygen; often the result of an obstruction in a coronary artery (Syn.—heart attack) (Chapter 12).

Myocardium (MY-oh-**KAR**-dee-um) The cardiac muscle tissue that forms the walls of the chambers of the heart (Chapter 4).

Myofibril (MY-oh-**FYE**-bril) A linear arrangement of sarcomeres within a muscle fiber (Chapter 7).

Myoglobin (**MY**-oh-GLOW-bin) The protein in muscle fibers that contains iron and stores oxygen in muscle fibers (Chapter 7).

Myometrium (MY-oh-**MEE**-tree-uhm) The smooth muscle layer of the uterus; contracts for labor and delivery of an infant (Chapter 20).

Myopathy (my-**AH**-puh-thee) A disease or abnormal condition of skeletal muscles (Chapter 7).

Myopia (my-**OH**-pee-ah) Nearsightedness; an error of refraction in which only near objects are seen clearly (Chapter 9).

Myosin (**MY**-oh-sin) A contractile protein in the sarcomeres of muscle fibers (Chapter 7).

Myxedema (MIK-suh-**DEE**-mah) Hyposecretion of thyroxine in an adult; decreased metabolic rate results in physical and mental lethargy (Chapter 10).

—N—

Nail follicle (NAYL **FAH**-li-kuhl) The structure within the skin of a finger or toe in which a nail grows; mitosis takes place in the nail root (Chapter 5).

Narrow-spectrum (**NAR**-oh **SPEK**-trum) An antibiotic that is effective against only a few kinds of bacteria (Chapter 22).

Nasal cavities (**NAY**-zuhl **KAV**-i-tees) The two air cavities within the skull through which air passes from the nostrils to the nasopharynx; separated by the nasal septum (Chapter 15).

Nasal mucosa (**NAY**-zuhl mew-**KOH**-sah) The lining of the nasal cavities; made of ciliated epithelium that warms and moistens the incoming air and sweeps mucus, dust, and pathogens toward the nasopharynx (Chapter 15).

Nasal septum (**NAY**-zuhl **SEP**-tum) The vertical plate made of bone and cartilage that separates the two nasal cavities (Chapter 15).

Nasolacrimal duct (**NAY**-zo-**LAK**-ri-muhl) A duct that carries tears from the lacrimal sac to the nasal cavity (Chapter 9).

Nasopharynx (**NAY**-zo-**FA**-rinks) The upper portion of the pharynx above the level of the soft palate; an air passageway (Chapter 15).

Natural killer cell (**NATCH**-er-al **KILL**-er SELL) A type of lymphocyte that is not specific; kills pathogens and tumor cells by direct contact (Chapter 14).

Negative feedback mechanism (**NEG**-ah-tiv **FEED**-bak) A control system in which a stimulus initiates a response that reverses or reduces the stimulus, thereby stopping the response until the stimulus occurs again and there is a need for the response (Chapter 1).

Nephritis (ne-**FRY**-tis) Inflammation of the kidney; may be caused by bacterial infection or toxic chemicals (Chapter 18).

Nephron (**NEFF**-ron) The structural and functional unit of the kidney that forms urine; consists of a renal corpuscle and a renal tubule (Chapter 18).

Nerve (NERV) A group of neurons, together with blood vessels and connective tissue (Chapter 8).

Nerve tissue (NERV **TISH**-yoo) The tissue specialized to generate and transmit electrochemical impulses that have many functions in the maintenance of homeostasis (Chapter 4).

Nerve tract (NERV TRAKT) A group of neurons that share a common function within the central nervous system; a tract may be ascending (sensory) or descending (motor) (Chapter 8).

Nervous system (**NERV**-us **SIS**-tem) The organ system that regulates body functions by means of electrochemical impulses; consists of the brain, spinal cord, cranial nerves, and spinal nerves (Chapter 8).

Neuralgia (new-**RAL**-jee-ah) Sharp, severe pain along the course of a nerve (Chapter 8).

Neuritis (new-**RYE**-tis) Inflammation of a nerve (Chapter 8).

Neuroglia (new-**ROG**-lee-ah) The non-neuronal cells of the central nervous system (Chapter 4).

Neurohypophysis (NEW-roo-high-**POFF**-e-sis) The posterior pituitary gland (Chapter 10).

Neurolemma (NEW-roh-**LEM**-ah) The sheath around peripheral axons and dendrites, formed by the cytoplasm and nuclei of Schwann cells; is essential for the regeneration of damaged peripheral neurons (Chapter 8).

Neuromuscular junction (NYOOR-oh-**MUSS**-kew-lar **JUNK**-shun) The termination of a motor neuron on the sarcolemma of a muscle fiber; the synapse is the microscopic space between the two structures (Chapter 7).

Neuron (**NYOOR**-on) A nerve cell; consists of a cell body, an axon, and dendrites (Chapter 4).

Neuropathy (new-**RAH**-puh-thee) Any disease or disorder of the nerves (Chapter 8).

Neurotoxin (NEW-roh-**TOK**-sin) A chemical that disrupts an aspect of the functioning of the nervous system (Chapter 7).

Neurotransmitter (NYOOR-oh-**TRANS**-mih-ter) A chemical released by the axon of a neuron, which crosses a synapse and affects the electrical activity of the postsynaptic membrane (neuron or muscle cell or gland) (Chapter 4).

Neutron (**NEW**-trahn) A subatomic particle that has no electrical charge; found in the nucleus of an atom (Chapter 2).

Neutrophil (**NEW**-troh-fill) A type of white blood cell (granular); capable of phagocytosis of pathogens (Chapter 11).

Nevus (**NEE**-vus) A pigmented area of the skin; a mole (Chapter 5).

Night blindness (NITE **BLIND**-ness) The inability to see well in dim light or at night; may result from a vitamin A deficiency (Chapter 9).

Nine areas (NYNE) The subdivision of the abdomen into

nine equal areas to facilitate the description of locations (Chapter 1).

Non-communicable disease (NON-kuhm-**YOO**-ni-kah-b'l) A disease that cannot be directly or indirectly transmitted from host to host (Chapter 22).

Non-essential amino acids (NON-e-**SEN**-shul ah-**ME**-noh **ASS**-ids) The amino acids that can be synthesized by the liver (Chapter 16).

Norepinephrine (NOR-ep-i-**NEFF**-rin) A hormone secreted by the adrenal medulla that causes vasoconstriction throughout the body, which raises blood pressure in stressful situations (Chapter 10).

Normal flora (**NOR**-muhl **FLOOR**-uh) 1. The population of microorganisms that is usually present in certain parts of the body. 2. In the colon, the bacteria that produce vitamins and inhibit the growth of pathogens (Chapter 16).

Normoblast (**NOR**-mow-blast) A red blood cell with a nucleus, an immature stage in red blood cell formation; usually found in the red bone marrow and not in peripheral circulation (Chapter 11).

Nosocomial infection (no-zoh-**KOH**-mee-uhl) An infection acquired in a hospital or other health-care institution (Chapter 22).

Nuclear membrane (**NEW**-klee-er **MEM**-brayn) The double-layer membrane that encloses the nucleus of a cell (Chapter 3).

Nucleic acid (new-**KLEE**-ik **ASS**-id) An organic chemical that is made of nucleotide subunits. Examples are DNA and RNA (Chapter 2).

Nucleolus (new-**KLEE**-oh-lus) A small structure made of DNA, RNA, and protein. Found in the nucleus of a cell; produces ribosomal RNA (Chapter 3).

Nucleotide (**NEW**-klee-oh-tide) An organic compound that consists of a pentose sugar, a phosphate group, and one of five nitrogenous bases (adenine, guanine, cytosine, thymine, or uracil); the subunits of DNA and RNA (Chapter 2).

Nucleus (**NEW**-klee-us) 1. The membrane bound part of a cell that contains the hereditary material in chromosomes. 2. The central part of an atom containing protons and neutrons (Chapters 2, 3).

—O—

Occipital bone (ok-**SIP**-i-tuhl) The flat bone that forms the back of the skull (Chapter 6).

Occipital lobes (ok-**SIP**-i-tuhl LOWBS) The most posterior part of the cerebrum; contain the visual areas (Chapter 8).

Oculomotor nerves (OK-yoo-loh-**MOH**-tur) Cranial nerve pair III. Motor to the extrinsic muscles of the eye, the ciliary body, and the iris (Chapter 8).

Olfactory nerves (ohl-**FAK**-tuh-ree) Cranial nerve pair I. Sensory for smell (Chapter 8).

Olfactory receptors (ohl-**FAK**-tuh-ree ree-**SEP**-ters) The sensory receptors in the upper nasal cavities that detect vaporized chemicals, providing a sense of smell (Chapter 9).

Oligodendrocyte (ah-li-goh-**DEN**-droh-sight) A type of neuroglia that produces the myelin sheath around neurons of the central nervous system (Chapter 8).

Oligosaccharide (ah-lig-oh-**SAK**-ah-ride) A carbohydrate molecule that consists of from 3–20 monosaccharides bonded together; form "self" antigens on cell membranes (Chapter 2).

Oliguria (AH-li-**GYOO**-ree-ah) Decreased urine formation and output (Chapter 18).

Oogenesis (Oh-oh-**JEN**-e-sis) The process of meiosis in the ovary to produce an ovum (Chapter 3).

Opportunistic infection (OP-er-too-**NIS**-tik) An infection caused by a microorganism that is usually a saprophyte but may become a parasite under certain conditions, such as lowered host resistance (Chapter 22).

Opsonization (OP-sah-ni-**ZAY**-shun) The action of antibodies or complement that upon binding to a foreign antigen attracts macrophages and facilitates phagocytosis (from the Greek "to purchase food") (Chapter 14).

Optic chiasma (**OP**-tik kye-**AS**-muh) The site of the crossing of the medial fibers of each optic nerve, anterior to the pituitary gland; important for binocular vision (Chapter 9).

Optic disc (**OP**-tik DISK) The portion of the retina where the optic nerve passes through; no rods or cones are present (Syn.—blind spot) (Chapter 9).

Optic nerves (**OP**-tik) Cranial nerve pair II. Sensory for vision (Chapter 8).

Oral cavity (**OR**-uhl **KAV**-i-tee) The cavity in the skull bounded by the hard palate, cheeks, and tongue (Chapter 16).

Orbit (**OR**-bit) The cavity in the skull that contains the eyeball (Syn.—eye socket) (Chapter 9).

Organ (**OR**-gan) A structure with specific functions; made of two or more tissues (Chapter 1).

Organ of Corti (**KOR**-tee) (spiral organ) The structure in the cochlea of the inner ear that contains the receptors for hearing (Chapter 9).

Organ system (**OR**-gan **SIS**-tem) A group of related organs that work together to perform specific functions (Chapter 1).

Organelle (OR-gan-**ELL**) An intracellular structure that has a specific function (Chapter 3).

Organic (or-**GAN**-ik) A chemical compound that contains carbon–hydrogen covalent bonds; includes carbohydrates, lipids, proteins, and nucleic acids (Chapter 1).

Origin (**AHR**-i-jin) 1. The more stationary attachment point of a muscle to a bone. 2. The beginning (Chapter 7).

Oropharynx (OR-oh-**FA**-rinks) The middle portion of the pharynx behind the oral cavity; a passageway for both air and food (Chapter 15).

Osmolarity (ahs-moh-**LAR**-i-tee) The concentration of osmotically active particles in a solution (Chapter 19).

Osmoreceptors (AHS-moh-re-**SEP**-ters) Specialized cells in the hypothalamus that detect changes in the water content of the body (Chapter 10).

Osmosis (ahs-**MOH**-sis) The diffusion of water through a selectively permeable membrane (Chapter 3).

Osmotic pressure (ahs-**MAH**-tik) Pressure that develops when two solutions of different concentration are separated by a selectively permeable membrane. A hypertonic solution that would cause cells to shrivel has a higher osmotic pressure. A hypotonic solution that would cause cells to swell has a lower osmotic pressure (Chapter 3).

Ossification (AHS-i-fi-**KAY**-shun) The process of bone formation; bone matrix is produced by osteoblasts during the growth or repair of bones (Chapter 6).

Osteoarthritis (AHS-tee-oh-ar-**THRY**-tiss) The inflammation of a joint, especially a weight-bearing joint, that is most often a consequence of aging (Chapter 6).

Osteoblast (**AHS**-tee-oh-BLAST) A bone-producing cell; produces bone matrix for the growth or repair of bones (Chapter 6).

Osteoclast (**AHS**-tee-oh-KLAST) A bone-destroying cell; reabsorbs bone matrix as part of the growth or repair of bones (Chapter 6).

Osteocyte (**AHS**-tee-oh-sight) A bone cell (Chapter 4).

Osteomyelitis (AHS-tee-oh-my-uh-**LYE**-tiss) Inflammation of a bone caused by a pathogenic microorganism (Chapter 6).

Osteoporosis (AHS-tee-oh-por-**OH**-sis) A condition in which bone matrix is lost and not replaced, resulting in weakened bones that are then more likely to fracture (Chapter 6).

Otitis media (oh-**TIGH**-tis **MEE**-dee-ah) Inflammation of the middle ear (Chapter 9).

Otoliths (**OH**-toh-liths) Microscopic crystals of calcium carbonate in the utricle and saccule of the inner ear; are pulled by gravity (Chapter 9).

Oval window (**OH**-vul **WIN**-doh) The membrane-covered opening through which the stapes transmits vibrations to the fluid in the inner ear (Chapter 9).

Ovary (**OH**-vuh-ree) The female gonad that produces ova; also an endocrine gland that produces the hormones estrogen and progesterone (Chapter 10).

Ovum (**OH**-vuhm) (Pl.—ova) An egg cell, produced by an ovary (Chapter 20).

Oxygen debt (**OKS**-ah-jen DET) The state in which there is not enough oxygen to complete the process of cell respiration; lactic acid is formed, which contributes to muscle fatigue (Syn.—recovery oxygen uptake) (Chapter 7).

Oxytocin (OK-si-**TOH**-sin) A hormone produced by the hypothalamus and stored in the posterior pituitary gland; stimulates contraction of the myometrium during labor and release of milk by the mammary glands (Chapter 8).

—P—

Palate (**PAL**-uht) The roof of the mouth, which separates the oral cavity from the nasal cavities (Chapter 16).

Palpitation (pal-pi-**TAY**-shun) An irregular heartbeat of which the person is aware (Chapter 12).

Pancreas (**PAN**-kree-us) 1. An endocrine gland located between the curve of the duodenum and the spleen; secretes insulin and glucagon. 2. An exocrine gland that secretes digestive enzymes for the digestion of starch, fats, and proteins (Chapter 10).

Pancreatic duct (PAN-kree-**AT**-ik DUKT) The duct that takes pancreatic juices to the common bile duct (Chapter 16).

Pandemic (pan-**DEM**-ik) An epidemic that affects several countries at the same time (Chapter 22).

Papillae (pah-**PILL**-ay) 1. Elevated, pointed projections. 2. On the tongue, the projections that contain taste buds (Chapter 16).

Papillary layer (**PAP**-i-lar-ee **LAY**-er) The uppermost layer of the dermis; contains capillaries to nourish the epidermis (Chapter 5).

Papillary muscles (**PAP**-i-lar-ee **MUSS**-uhls) Columns of myocardium that project from the floor of a ventricle and anchor the flaps of the AV valve by way of the chordae tendineae (Chapter 12).

Paralysis (pah-**RAL**-i-sis) Complete or partial loss of function, especially of a muscle (Chapter 7).

Paralytic ileus (**PAR**-uh-LIT-ik **ILL**-ee-us) Paralysis of the intestines that may occur following abdominal surgery (Chapter 16).

Paranasal sinus (PAR-uh-**NAY**-zuhl **SIGH**-nus) An air cavity in the frontal, maxilla, sphenoid, or ethmoid bones; opens into the nasal cavities (Chapter 6).

Paraplegia (PAR-ah-**PLEE**-gee-ah) Paralysis of the legs (Chapter 8).

Parasite (**PAR**-uh-sight) An organism that lives on or in another living organism, called a host, to which it causes harm (from the Greek for "to eat at another's table") (Chapter 22).

Parasympathetic (PAR-ah-SIM-puh-**THET**-ik) The division of the autonomic nervous system that dominates during non-stressful situations (Chapter 8).

Parathyroid glands (PAR-ah-**THIGH**-royd) The four endocrine glands located on the posterior side of the thyroid gland; secrete parathyroid hormone (Chapter 10).

Parathyroid hormone (PTH) (PAR-ah-**THIGH**-royd) A hormone secreted by the parathyroid glands; increases the reabsorption of calcium from bones and the absorption of calcium by the small intestine and kidneys (Chapter 10).

Parietal (puh-**RYE**-uh-tuhl) 1. Pertaining to the walls of a body cavity (Chapter 1). 2. The flat bone that forms the crown of the cranial cavity (from the Latin "wall") (Chapter 6).

Parietal cells (puh-**RYE**-uh-tuhl SELLS) The cells of the gastric pits of the stomach that secrete hydrochloric acid and the intrinsic factor (Chapter 16).

Parietal lobes (puh-**RYE**-uh-tuhl LOWBS) The parts of the cerebrum posterior to the frontal lobes; contain the sensory areas for cutaneous sensation and conscious muscle sense (Chapter 8).

Parkinson's disease (**PAR**-kin-sonz) A progressive disorder of the basal ganglia, characterized by tremor, muscle weakness and rigidity, and a peculiar gait (Chapter 8).

Parotid glands (pah-**RAH**-tid) The pair of salivary glands located just below and in front of the ears (Chapter 16).

Partial pressure (**PAR**-shul **PRES**-shur) 1. The pressure exerted by a gas in a mixture of gases. 2. The value used to measure oxygen and carbon dioxide concentrations in the blood or other body fluid (Chapter 15).

Parturition (PAR-tyoo-**RISH**-uhn) The act of giving birth (Chapter 21).

Passive immunity (**PASS**-iv im-**YOO**-ni-tee) The immunity provided by the reception of antibodies from another source; may be natural (placental, breast milk) or artificial (injection of gamma globulins) (Chapter 14).

Pasteurization (PAS-tyoor-i-**ZAY**-shun) The process of heating a fluid to moderate temperatures in order to destroy pathogenic bacteria (Chapter 22).

Patella (puh-**TELL**-ah) The kneecap, a short bone (from the Latin "flat dish") (Chapter 6).

Patellar reflex (puh-**TELL**-ar **REE**-fleks) A stretch reflex integrated in the spinal cord, in which a tap on the patellar tendon causes extension of the lower leg (Syn.—knee-jerk reflex) (Chapter 8).

Pathogen (**PATH**-oh-jen) A microorganism capable of producing disease; includes bacteria, viruses, fungi, protozoa, and worms (Chapters 14, 22).

Pathophysiology (PATH-oh-FIZZ-ee-**AH**-luh-jee) The study of diseases as they are related to functioning (Chapter 1).

Pelvic cavity (**PELL**-vik **KAV**-i-tee) Inferior portion of the ventral cavity, below the abdominal cavity (Chapter 1).

Penis (**PEE**-nis) The male organ of copulation when the urethra serves as a passage for semen; an organ of elimination when the urethra serves as a passage for urine (Chapter 20).

Pentose sugar (**PEN**-tohs) A five-carbon sugar (monosaccharide) that is a structural part of the nucleic acids DNA, RNA, and ATP (Chapter 2).

Pepsin (**PEP**-sin) The enzyme found in gastric juice that begins protein digestion; secreted by chief cells (Chapter 16).

Peptidases (**PEP**-ti-day-ses) Digestive enzymes that break down polypeptides to amino acids; secreted by the small intestine (Chapter 16).

Peptide bond (**PEP**-tyde) A chemical bond that links two amino acids in a protein molecule (Chapter 2).

Pericardium (PER-ee-**KAR**-dee-um) The three membranes that enclose the heart, consisting of an outer fibrous layer and two serous layers (Chapter 12).

Perichondrium (PER-ee-**KON**-dree-um) The fibrous connective tissue membrane that covers cartilage (Chapter 4).

Perilymph (**PER**-i-limf) The fluid in the bony labyrinth of the inner ear (Chapter 9).

Periodontal membrane (PER-ee-oh-**DON**-tal) The membrane that lines the tooth sockets in the upper and lower jaws; produces a bone-like cement to anchor the teeth (Chapter 16).

Periosteum (PER-ee-**AHS**-tee-um) The fibrous connective tissue membrane that covers bone; contains osteoblasts for bone growth or repair (Chapter 4).

Peripheral (puh-**RIFF**-uh-ruhl) Extending from a main part; closer to the surface (Chapter 1).

Peripheral nervous system (puh-**RIFF**-uh-ruhl **NERV**-vuhs) The part of the nervous system that consists of the cranial nerves and spinal nerves (Chapter 8).

Peripheral resistance (puh-**RIFF**-uh-ruhl ree-**ZIS**-tense) The resistance of the blood vessels to the flow of blood; changes in the diameter of arteries have effects on blood pressure (Chapter 13).

Peristalsis (per-i-**STALL**-sis) Waves of muscular contraction (one-way) that propel the contents through a hollow organ (Chapter 2).

Peritoneum (PER-i-toh-**NEE**-um) The serous membrane that lines the abdominal cavity (Chapter 1).

Peritonitis (per-i-toh-**NIGH**-tis) Inflammation of the peritoneum (Chapter 16).

Peritubular capillaries (PER-ee-**TOO**-byoo-ler) The capillaries that surround the renal tubule and receive the useful materials reabsorbed from the renal filtrate; carry blood from the efferent arteriole to the renal vein (Chapter 18).

Pernicious anemia (per-**NISH**-us uh-**NEE**-mee-yah) An anemia that is the result of a deficiency of vitamin B_{12} or the intrinsic factor (Chapter 11).

Peyer's patches (**PYE**-erz) The lymph nodules in the mucosa of the small intestine, especially in the ileum (Chapter 14).

pH A symbol of the measure of the concentration of hydrogen ions in a solution. The pH scale extends from 0–14, with a value of 7 being neutral. Values lower than 7 are acidic; values higher than 7 are alkaline (basic) (Chapter 2).

Phagocytosis (FAG-oh-sigh-**TOH**-sis) The process by which a moving cell engulfs a particle; especially, the ingestion of microorganisms by white blood cells (Chapter 3).

Phalanges (fuh-**LAN**-jees) The long bones of the fingers and toes. There are 14 in each hand or foot (from the Latin "line of soldiers") (Chapter 6).

Phantom pain (**FAN**-tum PAYN) Pain following amputation of a limb that seems to come from the missing limb (Chapter 9).

Pharynx (**FA**-rinks) A muscular tube located behind the nasal and oral cavities; a passageway for air and food (Chapter 15).

Phenotype (**FEE**-noh-type) The appearance of the individual as related to genotype; the expression of the genes that are present (Chapter 21).

Phlebitis (fle-**BY**-tis) Inflammation of a vein (Chapter 13).

Phospholipid (**FOSS**-foh-LIP-id) An organic compound in the lipid group that is made of one glycerol, two fatty acids, and a phosphate molecule; forms the bilayer of cell membranes (Chapter 2).

Phrenic nerves (**FREN**-ik NERVZ) The pair of peripheral nerves that are motor to the diaphragm (Chapter 15).

Physiology (FIZZ-ee-**AH**-luh-jee) The study of the functioning of the body and its parts (Chapter 1).

Pia mater (**PEE**-ah **MAH**-ter) The innermost layer of the meninges, made of thin connective tissue on the surface of the brain and spinal cord (Chapter 8).

Pilomotor muscle (**PYE**-loh-MOH-ter) A smooth muscle attached to a hair follicle; contraction pulls the follicle upright, resulting in "goose bumps" (Syn.—arrector pili muscle) (Chapter 5).

Pineal gland (**PIN**-ee-uhl) An endocrine gland on the posterior wall of the third ventricle of the brain; secretes melatonin (Chapter 10).

Pinocytosis (PIN-oh-sigh-**TOH**-sis) The process by which a stationary cell ingests very small particles or a liquid (Chapter 3).

Pituitary gland (pi-**TOO**-i-TER-ee) An endocrine gland located below the hypothalamus, consisting of anterior and posterior lobes (Syn.—hypophysis) (Chapter 10).

Pivot joint (**PI**-vot) A diarthrosis that permits rotation (Chapter 6).

Placenta (pluh-**SEN**-tah) The organ formed in the uterus during pregnancy, made of both fetal and maternal tissue; the site of exchanges of materials between fetal blood and maternal blood (Chapter 13).

Plane (PLAYN) An imaginary flat surface that divides the body in a specific way (Chapter 1).

Plasma (**PLAZ**-mah) The water found within the blood vessels. Plasma is 52%–62% of the total blood (Chapter 2).

Plasma cell (**PLAZ**-mah SELL) A cell derived from an activated B cell that produces antibodies to a specific antigen (Chapter 14).

Plasma proteins (**PLAZ**-mah **PRO**-teenz) The proteins that circulate in the liquid portion of the blood; include albumin, globulins, and clotting factors (Chapter 11).

Platelets (**PLAYT**-lets) Blood cells that are fragments of larger cells (megakaryocytes) of the red bone marrow; involved in blood clotting and other mechanisms of hemostasis (Syn.—thrombocytes) (Chapter 4).

Pleural membranes (**PLOOR**-uhl **MEM**-braynz) The serous membranes of the thoracic cavity (Chapter 1).

Plica circulares (**PLEE**-ka SIR-kew-**LAR**-es) The circular folds of the mucosa and submucosa of the small intestine; increase the surface area for absorption (Chapter 16).

Pneumonia (new-**MOH**-nee-ah) Inflammation of the lungs caused by bacteria, viruses, or chemicals (Chapter 15).

Pneumotaxic center (NEW-moh-**TAK**-sik **SEN**-ter) The respiratory center in the pons that helps bring about exhalation (Chapter 15).

Pneumothorax (NEW-moh-**THAW**-raks) The accumulation of air in the potential pleural space, which increases intrapleural pressure and causes collapse of a lung (Chapter 15).

Podocytes (**POH**-doh-sights) The cells that form the inner layer of Bowman's capsule of the renal corpuscle; adjacent foot processes form pores that make the layer very permeable (Chapter 18).

Polarization (POH-lahr-i-**ZAY**-shun) The distribution of ions on either side of a membrane; in a resting neuron or muscle cell, sodium ions are more abundant outside the cell, and potassium and negative ions are more abundant inside the cell, giving the membrane a positive charge outside and a relative negative charge inside (Chapter 7).

Polypeptide (PAH-lee-**PEP**-tyde) A short chain of amino acids, not yet a specific protein (Chapter 2).

Polysaccharide (PAH-lee-**SAK**-ah-ryde) A carbohydrate molecule that consists of many monosaccharides (usually glucose) bonded together; includes glycogen, starch, and cellulose (Chapter 2).

Polyuria (PAH-li-**YOO**-ree-ah) Increased urine formation and output (Chapter 18).

Pons (PONZ) The part of the brain anterior and superior to the medulla; contributes to the regulation of respiration (from the Latin "bridge") (Chapter 8).

Pore (POR) An opening on a surface to permit the passage of materials (Chapter 3).

Portal of entry (**POR**-tuhl of **EN**-tree) The way a pathogen enters the body, such as natural body openings or breaks in the skin (Chapter 22).

Portal of exit (**POR**-tuhl of **EG**-zit) The way a pathogen leaves a host, such as in respiratory droplets, feces, or reproductive secretions (Chapter 22).

Positive feedback (**PAHS**-ah-tiv **FEED**-bak) A control system that requires an external event to stop or reverse the stimulus (Chapter 1).

Positron emission tomography (PET) (**PAHS**-i-tron eh-**MISH**-shun toh-**MAH**-grah-fee) An imaging technique that depicts rate of metabolism or blood flow in organs or tissues (Chapter 1).

Posterior (poh-**STEER**-ee-your) Toward the back (Syn.—dorsal) (Chapter 1).

Postganglionic neuron (POST-gang-lee-**ON**-ik) In the

autonomic nervous system, a neuron that extends from a ganglion to a visceral effector (Chapter 8).

Precapillary sphincter (pree-**KAP**-i-lar-ee **SFINK**-ter) A smooth muscle cell at the beginning of a capillary network that regulates the flow of blood through the network (Chapter 13).

Preganglionic neuron (PRE-gang-lee-**ON**-ik) In the autonomic nervous system, a neuron that extends from the CNS to a ganglion and synapses with a postganglionic neuron (Chapter 8).

Presbyopia (PREZ-bee-**OH**-pee-ah) Farsightedness that is a consequence of aging and the loss of elasticity of the lens (Chapter 9).

Pressoreceptors (**PRESS**-oh-ree-SEP-ters) The sensory receptors in the carotid sinuses and aortic sinus that detect changes in blood pressure (Chapter 9).

Primary bronchi (**PRY**-ma-ree **BRONG**-kye) The two branches of the lower end of the trachea; air passageways to the right and left lungs (Chapter 15).

Prime mover (PRYME **MOO**-ver) The muscle responsible for the main action when a joint is moved (Chapter 7).

Prions (**PREE**-ons) Proteinaceous infectious particles that are the cause of lethal disease of the nervous system in people and animals (Chapter 2).

Progesterone (proh-**JESS**-tuh-rohn) The sex hormone secreted by the corpus luteum of the ovary and by the placenta; contributes to the growth of the endometrium and the maintenance of pregnancy (Chapter 10).

Projection (proh-**JEK**-shun) The characteristic of sensations in which the sensation is felt in the area where the receptors were stimulated (Chapter 9).

Prolactin (proh-**LAK**-tin) A hormone produced by the anterior pituitary gland that stimulates milk production by the mammary glands (Chapter 10).

Pronation (pro-**NAY**-shun) Turning the palm downward, or lying face down (Chapter 7).

Prophase (**PROH**-fayz) The first stage of mitosis, in which the pairs on chromatids become visible (Chapter 3).

Proprioceptor (**PROH**-pree-oh-SEP-ter) A sensory receptor in a muscle that detects stretching of the muscle (Syn.—stretch receptor) (Chapter 7).

Prostaglandins (PRAHS-tah-**GLAND**-ins) Locally acting hormone-like substances produced by virtually all cells from the phospholipids of their cell membranes; the many types have many varied functions (Chapter 10).

Prostate gland (**PRAHS**-tayt) A muscular gland that surrounds the first inch of the male urethra; secretes an alkaline fluid that becomes part of semen; its smooth muscle contributes to ejaculation (Chapter 20).

Prostatic hypertrophy (prahs-**TAT**-ik high-**PER**-truh-fee) Enlargement of the prostate gland; may be benign or malignant (Chapter 20).

Protein (**PRO**-teen) An organic compound made of amino acids linked by peptide bonds (Chapter 2).

Proteinuria (PRO-teen-**YOO**-ree-ah) The presence of protein in urine (Chapter 18).

Prothrombin (proh-**THROM**-bin) A clotting factor synthesized by the liver and released into the blood; converted to thrombin in the process of chemical clotting (Chapter 11).

Proton (**PRO**-tahn) A subatomic particle that has a positive electrical charge; found in the nucleus of an atom (Chapter 2).

Protozoa (PROH-tuh-**ZOH**-ah) (Sing.— protozoan) The simplest animal-like microorganisms in the kingdom Protista; usually unicellular, some are colonial; may be free living or parasitic (Chapter 22).

Proximal (**PROK**-si-muhl) Closest to the origin or point of attachment (Chapter 1).

Proximal convoluted tubule (**PROK**-si-muhl KON-voh-**LOO**-ted) The part of a renal tubule that extends from Bowman's capsule to the loop of Henle (Chapter 18).

Pruritus (proo-**RYE**-tus) Severe itching (Chapter 5).

Puberty (**PEW**-ber-tee) The period during life in which members of both sexes become sexually mature and capable of reproduction; usually occurs between the ages of 10 and 14 years (Chapter 20).

Pubic symphysis (**PEW**-bik **SIM**-fi-sis) The joint between the right and left pubic bones, in which a disc of cartilage separates the two bones (Chapter 6).

Pubis (**PEW**-biss) The lower anterior part of the hip bone (Syn.—pubic bone) (Chapter 6).

Pulmonary artery (**PULL**-muh-NER-ee **AR**-tuh-ree) The artery that takes blood from the right ventricle to the lungs (Chapter 12).

Pulmonary edema (**PULL**-muh-NER-ee uh-**DEE**-muh) Accumulation of tissue fluid in the alveoli of the lungs (Chapter 15).

Pulmonary semilunar valve (**PULL**-muh-NER-ee SEM-ee-**LOO**-nar VALV) The valve at the junction of the right ventricle and the pulmonary artery; prevents backflow of blood from the artery to the ventricle when the ventricle relaxes (Chapter 12).

Pulmonary surfactant (**PULL**-muh-NER-ee sir-**FAK**-tent) A lipoprotein secreted by the alveoli in the lungs; reduces the surface tension within alveoli to permit inflation (Chapter 15).

Pulmonary veins (**PULL**-muh-NER-ee VAYNS) The four veins that return blood from the lungs to the left atrium (Chapter 12).

Pulp cavity (PUHLP) The innermost portion of a tooth that contains blood vessels and nerve endings (Chapter 16).

Pulse (PULS) The force of the heartbeat detected at an arterial site such as the radial artery (Chapter 12).

Pulse deficit (PULS **DEF**-i-sit) The condition in which the radial pulse count is lower than the rate of the heartbeat heard with a stethoscope; may occur in some types of heart disease in which the heartbeat is weak (Chapter 13).

Pulse pressure (PULS **PRES**-shur) The difference between systolic and diastolic blood pressure; averages about 40 mmHg (Chapter 13).

Punnett square (**PUHN**-net SKWAIR) A diagram used to determine the possible combinations of genes in the offspring of a particular set of parents (Chapter 21).

Pupil (**PYOO**-pil) The opening in the center of the iris; light rays pass through the aqueous humor in the pupil (Chapter 9).

Purkinje fibers (purr-**KIN**-jee) Specialized cardiac muscle fibers that are part of the cardiac conduction pathway (Chapter 12).

Pyloric sphincter (pye-**LOR**-ik **SFINK**-ter) The circular smooth muscle at the junction of the stomach and the duodenum; prevents backup of intestinal contents into the stomach (from the Greek "gatekeeper") (Chapter 16).

Pyloric stenosis (pye-**LOR**-ik ste-**NOH**-sis) Narrowing of the opening between the stomach and duodenum caused by hypertrophy of the pyloric sphincter; a congenital disorder (Chapter 16).

Pyrogen (**PYE**-roh-jen) Any microorganism or substance that causes a fever; includes bacteria, viruses, or chemicals released during inflammation (called endogenous pyrogens); activates the heat production and conservation mechanisms regulated by the hypothalamus (Chapter 17).

—Q—

QRS wave The portion of an ECG that depicts depolarization of the ventricles (Chapter 12).

Quadrants (**KWAH**-drants) A division into four parts, used especially to divide the abdomen into four areas to facilitate description of locations (Chapter 1).

Quadriplegia (KWA-dri-**PLEE**-jee-ah) Paralysis of all four limbs (Chapter 17).

—R—

Radiation (RAY-dee-**AY**-shun) 1. The heat loss process in which heat energy from the skin is emitted to the cooler surroundings. 2. The emissions of certain radioactive elements; may be used for diagnostic or therapeutic purposes (Chapter 17).

Radius (**RAY**-dee-us) The long bone of the forearm on the thumb side (from the Latin "a spoke") (Chapter 6).

Range-of-motion exercises (RANJE of **MOH**-shun) Movements of joints through their full range of motion; used to preserve mobility or to regain mobility following an injury (Chapter 7).

Receptor (ree-**SEP**-tur) A specialized cell or nerve ending that responds to a particular change such as light, sound, heat, touch, or pressure (Chapter 5).

Receptor site (ree-**SEP**-ter SIGHT) An arrangement of molecules, often part of the cell membrane, that will accept only molecules with a complementary shape (Chapter 3).

Recessive (ree-**SESS**-iv) In genetics, a characteristic that will be expressed only if two genes for it are present in the homologous pair of chromosomes (Chapter 21).

Recovery oxygen uptake (ree-**KOV**-e-ree **OKS**-ah-jen **UP**-tayk) Oxygen debt (Chapter 7).

Red blood cells (RED BLUHD SELLS) The most numerous cells in the blood; carry oxygen bonded to the hemoglobin within them (Syn.—erythrocytes) (Chapter 4).

Red bone marrow (RED BOWN **MAR**-row) A hemopoietic tissue found in flat and irregular bones; produces all the types of blood cells (Chapter 6).

Reduced hemoglobin (re-**DOOSD HEE**-muh-GLOW-bin) Hemoglobin that has released its oxygen in the systemic capillaries (Chapter 11).

Referred pain (ree-**FURD** PAYNE) Visceral pain that is projected and felt as cutaneous pain (Chapter 9).

Reflex (**REE**-fleks) An involuntary response to a stimulus (Chapter 8).

Reflex arc (**REE**-fleks ARK) The pathway nerve impulses follow when a reflex is stimulated (Chapter 8).

Refraction (ree-**FRAK**-shun) The bending of light rays as they pass through the eyeball; normal refraction focuses an image on the retina (Chapter 9).

Relaxin (ree-**LAKS**-in) A hormone produced by the corpus luteum and placenta; inhibits contractions of the myometrium (Chapter 20).

Releasing hormones (ree-**LEE**-sing **HOR**-mohns) Hormones released by the hypothalamus that stimulate secretion of hormones by the anterior pituitary gland (SYN-releasing factors) (Chapter 10).

Remission (ree-**MISH**-uhn) Lessening of severity of symptoms (Chapter 8).

Renal artery (**REE**-nuhl **AR**-te-ree) The branch of the abdominal aorta that takes blood into a kidney (Chapter 18).

Renal calculi (**REE**-nuhl **KAL**-kew-lye) Kidney stones; made of precipitated minerals in the form of crystals (Chapter 18).

Renal corpuscle (**REE**-nuhl **KOR**-pus'l) The part of a nephron that consists of a glomerulus enclosed by a Bowman's capsule; the site of glomerular filtration (Chapter 18).

Renal cortex (**REE**-nuhl **KOR**-teks) The outermost tissue layer of the kidney; consists of renal corpuscles and convoluted tubules (Chapter 18).

Renal failure (**REE**-nuhl **FAYL**-yer) The inability of the kidneys to function properly and form urine; causes include severe hemorrhage, toxins, and obstruction of the urinary tract (Chapter 18).

Renal fascia (**REE**-nuhl **FASH**-ee-ah) The fibrous connective tissue membrane that covers the kidneys and the surrounding adipose tissue and helps keep the kidneys in place (Chapter 18).

Renal filtrate (**REE**-nuhl **FILL**-trayt) The fluid formed from blood plasma by the process of filtration in the renal corpuscles; flows from Bowman's capsules through the renal tubules where most is reabsorbed; the filtrate that enters the renal pelvis is called urine (Chapter 18).

Renal medulla (**REE**-nuhl muh-**DEW**-lah) The inner tissue layer of the kidney; consists of loops of Henle and collecting tubules; the triangular segments of the renal medulla are called renal pyramids (Chapter 18).

Renal pelvis (**REE**-nuhl **PELL**-vis) The most medial area of the kidney; a cavity formed by the expanded end of the ureter at the hilus of the kidney (Chapter 18).

Renal pyramids (**REE**-nuhl **PEER**-ah-mids) The triangular segments of the renal medulla; the papillae of the pyramids empty urine into the calyces of the renal pelvis (Chapter 18).

Renal tubule (**REE**-nuhl **TOO**-byool) The part of a nephron that consists of a proximal convoluted tubule, loop of Henle, distal convoluted tubule, and collecting tubule; the site of tubular reabsorption and tubular secretion (Chapter 18).

Renal vein (**REE**-nuhl VAYN) The vein that returns blood from a kidney to the inferior vena cava (Chapter 18).

Renin-angiotensin mechanism (**REE**-nin AN-jee-oh-**TEN**-sin) A series of chemical reactions initiated by a decrease in blood pressure that stimulates the kidneys to secrete the enzyme renin; culminates in the formation of angiotensin II (Chapter 10).

Repolarization (RE-pol-lahr-i-**ZAY**-shun) The restoration of electrical charges on either side of a cell membrane following depolarization; positive charge outside and a negative charge inside brought about by a rapid outflow of potassium ions (Chapter 7).

Reproductive system (REE-proh-**DUK**-tive **SIS**-tem) The male or female organ system that produces gametes, ensures fertilization, and in women, provides a site for the developing embryo-fetus (Chapter 20).

Reservoir (**REZ**-er-vwor) 1. A person or animal who harbors a pathogen and is a source of the pathogen for others (Chapter 22). 2. A storage site (Chapter 7).

Resident flora (**REZ**-i-dent **FLOOR**-uh) Part of normal flora; those microorganisms on or in nearly everyone in specific body sites nearly all the time (Chapter 22).

Residual air (ree-**ZID**-yoo-al) The volume of air that remains in the lungs after the most forceful exhalation; important to provide for continuous gas exchange; average: 1000–1500 ml (Chapter 15).

Resistance (re-**ZIS**-tenss) The total of all of the body's defenses against pathogens; includes non-specific barriers such as unbroken skin and specific mechanisms such as antibody production (Chapter 22).

Respiratory acidosis (RES-pi-rah-**TOR**-ee ass-i-**DOH**-sis) A condition in which the blood pH is lower than normal, caused by disorders that decrease the rate or efficiency of respiration and permit the accumulation of carbon dioxide (Chapter 15).

Respiratory alkalosis (RES-pi-rah-**TOR**-ee al-kah-**LOH**-sis) A condition in which the blood pH is higher than normal, caused by disorders that increase the rate of respiration and decrease the level of carbon dioxide in the blood (Chapter 15).

Respiratory pump (**RES**-pi-rah-**TOR**-ee) A mechanism that increases venous return; pressure changes during breathing compress the veins that pass through the thoracic cavity (Chapter 13).

Respiratory system (**RES**-pi-rah-TOR-ee **SIS**-tem) The organ system that moves air into and out of the lungs so that oxygen and carbon dioxide may be exchanged between the air and the blood (Chapter 15).

Resting potential (**RES**-ting poh-**TEN**-shul) The difference in electrical charges on either side of a cell membrane not transmitting an impulse; positive charge outside and a negative charge inside (Chapter 7).

Reticulocyte (re-**TIK**-yoo-loh-sight) A red blood cell that contains remnants of the endoplasmic reticulum, an immature stage in red blood cell formation; makes up about 1% of the red blood cells in peripheral circulation (Chapter 11).

Reticuloendothelial system (re-TIK-yoo-loh-en-doh-**THEE**-lee-al) Former name for the tissue macrophage system, the organs or tissues that contain macrophages (RE cells) that phagocytize old red blood cells; the liver, spleen, and red bone marrow (Chapter 11).

Retina (**RET**-i-nah) The innermost layer of the eyeball that contains the photoreceptors, the rods and cones (Chapter 9).

Retroperitoneal (RE-troh-PER-i-toh-**NEE**-uhl) Located behind the peritoneum (Chapter 18).

Reuptake (ree-**UP**-tayk) The reabsorption of a substance that was just secreted; used with respect to some neurotransmitters (Chapter 8).

Rh factor (R-H **FAK**-ter) The red blood cell types determined by the presence or absence of the Rh (D) antigen on the red blood cell membranes; the two types are Rh positive and Rh negative (Chapter 11).

Rheumatoid arthritis (**ROO**-muh-toyd ar-**THRY**-tiss) Inflammation of a joint; an autoimmune disease. The joint damage may progress to fusion and immobility of the joint (Chapter 6).

Rhodopsin (roh-**DOP**-sin) The chemical in the rods of the retina that breaks down when light waves strike it; this chemical change initiates a nerve impulse (Chapter 9).

RhoGAM (**ROH**-gam) The trade name for the Rh (D) antibody administered to an Rh-negative woman who has delivered an Rh-positive infant; it will destroy any fetal red blood cells that may have entered maternal circulation (Chapter 11).

Ribosome (**RYE**-boh-sohme) A cell organelle found in the cytoplasm; the site of protein synthesis (Chapter 3).

Ribs (RIBZ) The 24 flat bones that, together with the sternum, form the rib cage. The first seven pairs are true ribs, the next three pairs are false ribs, and the last two pairs are floating ribs (Chapter 6).

Rickets (**RIK**-ets) A deficiency of vitamin D in children, resulting in poor and abnormal bone growth (Chapter 6).

RNA (ribonucleic acid) A nucleic acid that is a single strand of nucleotides; essential for protein synthesis within cells; messenger RNA (mRNA) is a copy of the genetic code of DNA; transfer RNA (tRNA) aligns amino acids in the proper sequence on the mRNA (Chapter 2).

Rods (RAHDZ) The sensory receptors in the retina of the eye that detect the presence of light (Chapter 9).

Round window (ROWND **WIN**-doh) The membrane-covered opening of the inner ear that bulges to prevent pressure damage to the organ of Corti (Chapter 9).

Rugae (**ROO**-gay) Folds of the mucosa of organs such as the stomach, urinary bladder, and vagina; permit expansion of these organs (Chapter 16).

—S—

Saccule (**SAK**-yool) A membranous sac in the vestibule of the inner ear that contains receptors for static equilibrium (Chapter 9).

Sacroiliac joint (SAY-kroh-**ILL**-ee-ak) The slightly movable joint between the sacrum and the ilium (Chapter 6).

Sacrum (**SAY**-krum) The five fused sacral vertebrae at the base of the spine (Chapter 6).

Saddle joint (**SA**-duhl) The carpometacarpal joint of the thumb, a diarthrosis (Chapter 6).

Sagittal section (**SAJ**-i-tuhl **SEK**-shun) A plane or cut from front to back, separating right and left parts (from the Latin "arrow") (Chapter 1).

Saliva (sah-**LYE**-vah) The secretion of the salivary glands; mostly water and containing the enzyme amylase (Chapter 16).

Salivary glands (**SAL**-i-va-ree) The three pairs of exocrine glands that secrete saliva into the oral cavity; parotid, submandibular, and sublingual pairs (Chapter 16).

Salt (SAWLT) A chemical compound that consists of a positive ion other than hydrogen and a negative ion other than hydroxyl (Chapter 2).

Saltatory conduction (**SAWL**-tah-taw-ree kon-**DUK**-shun) The rapid transmission of a nerve impulse from one node of Ranvier to the next; characteristic of myelinated neurons (Chapter 8).

Saprophyte (**SAP**-roh-fight) An organism that lives on dead organic matter; a decomposer (Chapter 22).

Sarcolemma (SAR-koh-**LEM**-ah) The cell membrane of a muscle fiber (Chapter 7).

Sarcomere (**SAR**-koh-meer) The unit of contraction in a skeletal muscle fiber; a precise arrangement of myosin and actin filaments between two Z lines (Chapter 7).

Sarcoplasmic reticulum (SAR-koh-**PLAZ**-mik re-**TIK**-yoo-lum) The endoplasmic reticulum of a muscle fiber; is a reservoir for calcium ions (Chapter 7).

Saturated fat (**SAT**-uhr-ay-ted) A true fat that is often solid at room temperature and of animal origin (Chapter 2).

Scapula (**SKAP**-yoo-luh) The flat bone of the shoulder that articulates with the humerus (Syn.—shoulder blade) (Chapter 6).

Schwann cell (SHWAHN SELL) A cell of the peripheral nervous system that forms the myelin sheath and neurolemma of peripheral axons and dendrites (Chapter 4).

Sclera (**SKLER**-ah) The outermost layer of the eyeball, made of fibrous connective tissue; the anterior portion is the transparent cornea (Chapter 9).

Scoliosis (SKOH-lee-**OH**-sis) A lateral curvature of the vertebral column (Chapter 6).

Scrotum (**SKROH**-tum) The sac of skin between the upper thighs in males; contains the testes, epididymides, and part of the ductus deferens (Chapter 20).

Sebaceous gland (suh-**BAY**-shus) An exocrine gland in the dermis that produces sebum (Chapter 5).

Sebum (**SEE**-bum) The lipid (oil) secretion of sebaceous glands (Chapter 5).

Secondary infection (**SEK**-un-DAR-ee) An infection made possible by a primary infection that has lowered the host's resistance (Chapter 22).

Secondary sex characteristics (**SEK**-un-DAR-ee SEKS) The features that develop at puberty in males or females; they are under the influence of the sex hormones but are not directly involved in reproduction. Examples are growth of facial or body hair and growth of muscles (Chapter 20).

Secretin (se-**KREE**-tin) A hormone secreted by the duodenum when food enters; stimulates secretion of bile by the liver and secretion of bicarbonate pancreatic juice (Chapter 16).

Secretion (see-**KREE**-shun) The production and release of a cellular product with a useful purpose (Chapter 4).

Section (**SEK**-shun) The cutting of an organ or the body to make internal structures visible (Chapter 1).

Selectively permeable (se-**LEK**-tiv-lee **PER**-me-uh-buhl) A characteristic of cell membranes; permits the passage of some materials but not of others (Chapter 3).

Self-limiting disease (self-**LIM**-i-ting) A disease that typically lasts a certain period of time and is followed by recovery (Chapter 22).

Semen (**SEE**-men) The thick, alkaline fluid that contains sperm and the secretions of the seminal vesicles, prostate gland, and bulbourethral glands (Chapter 20).

Semicircular canals (SEM-eye-**SIR**-kyoo-lur) Three oval canals in the inner ear that contain the receptors that detect motion (Chapter 9).

Seminal vesicles (**SEM**-i-nuhl **VESS**-i-kulls) The glands located posterior to the prostate gland and inferior to the urinary bladder; secrete an alkaline fluid that enters the ejaculatory ducts and becomes part of semen (Chapter 20).

Seminiferous tubules (sem-i-**NIFF**-er-us) The site of spermatogenesis in the testes (Chapter 20).

Sensation (sen-**SAY**-shun) A feeling or awareness of conditions outside or inside the body, resulting from the stimulation of sensory receptors and interpretation by the brain (Chapter 9).

Sensory neuron (**SEN**-suh-ree **NYOOR**-on) A nerve cell that carries impulses from a receptor to the central nervous system. (Syn.—afferent neuron) (Chapter 8).

Septic shock (**SEP**-tik **SHAHK**) A type of circulatory shock that is a consequence of a bacterial infection (Chapter 13).

Septicemia (SEP-tih-**SEE**-mee-ah) The presence of bacteria in the blood (Chapter 5).

Septum (**SEP**-tum) A wall that separates two cavities, such as the nasal septum between the nasal cavities or the interventricular septum between the two ventricles of the heart (Chapter 12).

Serous fluid (**SEER**-us **FLOO**-id) A fluid that prevents friction between the two layers of a serous membrane (Chapter 4).

Serous membrane (**SEER**-us **MEM**-brayn) An epithelial membrane that lines a closed body cavity and covers the organs in that cavity (Chapter 4).

Sex chromosomes (SEKS **KROH**-muh-sohms) The pair of chromosomes that determines the gender of an individual; designated XX in females and XY in males (Chapter 21).

Sex-linked trait (SEKS LINKED TRAYT) A genetic characteristic in which the gene is located on the X chromosome (Chapter 7).

Simple (**SIM**-puhl) Having only one layer, used especially to describe certain types of epithelial tissue (Chapter 4).

Sinoatrial (SA) node (**SIGH**-noh-AY-tree-al NOHD) The first part of the cardiac conduction pathway, located in the wall of the right atrium; initiates each heartbeat (Chapter 12).

Sinusoid (**SIGH**-nuh-soyd) A large, very permeable capillary; permits proteins or blood cells to enter or leave the blood (Chapter 13).

Skeletal muscle pump (**SKEL**-e-tuhl **MUSS**-uhl) A mechanism that increases venous return; contractions of the skeletal muscles compress the deep veins, especially those of the legs (Chapter 13).

Skeletal system (**SKEL**-e-tuhl) The organ system that consists of the bones, ligaments, and cartilage; supports the body and is a framework for muscle attachment (Chapter 6).

Skin (SKIN) An organ that is part of the integumentary system; consists of the outer epidermis and the inner dermis (Chapter 5).

Sliding filament theory (**SLY**-ding **FILL**-ah-ment) The sequence of events that occurs within sarcomeres when a muscle fiber contracts (Chapter 7).

Small intestine (SMAWL in-**TESS**-tin) The organ of the alimentary tube between the stomach and the large intestine; secretes enzymes that complete the digestive process and absorbs the end products of digestion (Chapter 16).

Smooth muscle (SMOOTH **MUSS**-uhl) The muscle tissue that forms the walls of hollow internal organs. Also called visceral or involuntary muscle (Chapter 4).

Sneeze reflex (SNEEZ) A reflex integrated by the medulla that expels irritating substances from the nasal cavities by means of an explosive exhalation (Chapter 15).

Sodium-potassium pumps (**SEW**-dee-um pa-**TASS**-ee-um) The active transport mechanisms that maintain a high sodium ion concentration outside the cell and a high potassium ion concentration inside the cell (Chapter 7).

Soft palate (SAWFT **PAL**-uht) The posterior portion of the palate that is elevated during swallowing to block the nasopharynx (Chapter 15).

Solute (**SAH**-loot) The substance that is dissolved in a solution (Chapter 3).

Solution (suh-**LOO**-shun) The dispersion of one or more compounds (solutes) in a liquid (solvent) (Chapter 2).

Solvent (**SAHL**-vent) A liquid in which substances (solutes) will dissolve (Chapter 2).

Somatic (soh-**MA**-tik) Pertaining to structures of the body wall, such as skeletal muscles and the skin (Chapter 8).

Somatostatin (SOH-mat-oh-**STAT**-in) 1. Growth hormone inhibiting hormone (GHIH); produced by the hypothalamus. 2. The hormone produced by the delta cells of the pancreas (Chapter 10).

Somatotropin (SOH-mat-oh-**TROH**-pin) Growth hormone (Chapter 10).

Specialized fluids (**SPEH**-shul-eyezd **FLOO**-ids) Specific compartments of extracellular fluid; include cerebrospinal fluid, synovial fluid, aqueous humor in the eye, and others (Chapter 2).

Spermatic cord (sper-**MAT**-ik KORD) The cord that suspends the testis; composed of the ductus deferens, blood vessels, and nerves (Chapter 20).

Spermatogenesis (SPER-ma-toh-**JEN**-e-sis) The process of meiosis in the testes to produce sperm cells (Chapter 3).

Spermatozoa (sper-MAT-oh-**ZOH**-ah) (Sing.—spermatozoon) Sperm cells; produced by the testes (Chapter 20).

Sphenoid bone (**SFEE**-noyd) The flat bone that forms part of the anterior floor of the cranial cavity and encloses the pituitary gland (Chapter 6).

Sphincter (**SFINK**-ter) A circular muscle that regulates the size of an opening (Chapter 7).

Spinal cavity (**SPY**-nuhl **KAV**-i-tee) The cavity within the vertebral column that contains the spinal cord and meninges; part of the dorsal cavity (Syn.—vertebral canal or cavity) (Chapter 1).

Spinal cord (**SPY**-nuhl KORD) The part of the central nervous system within the vertebral canal; transmits impulses to and from the brain (Chapter 8).

Spinal cord reflex (**SPY**-nuhl KORD **REE**-fleks) A reflex integrated in the spinal cord, in which the brain is not directly involved (Chapter 8).

Spinal nerves (**SPY**-nuhl NERVS) The 31 pairs of nerves that emerge from the spinal cord (Chapter 8).

Spinal shock (**SPY**-nuhl SHAHK) The temporary or permanent loss of spinal cord reflexes following injury to the spinal cord (Chapter 8).

Spirillum (spih-**RILL**-uhm) (Pl.—spirilla) A bacterium with a spiral shape (Chapter 22).

Spirochete (**SPY**-roh-keet) Spiral bacteria of the order Spirochaetales (Chapter 22).

Spleen (SPLEEN) An organ located in the upper left abdominal quadrant behind the stomach; consists of lymphatic tissue that produces lymphocytes and monocytes; also contains macrophages that phagocytize old red blood cells (Chapter 14).

Spongy bone (**SPUN**-jee BOWNE) Bone tissue not organized into haversian systems; forms most of short, flat, and irregular bones and forms epiphyses of long bones (Chapter 6).

Spontaneous fracture (spahn-**TAY**-nee-us) A fracture that occurs without apparent trauma; often a consequence of osteoporosis (Chapter 6).

Spore (SPOOR) 1. A bacterial form that is dormant and highly resistant to environmental extremes such as heat. 2. A unicellular fungal reproductive form (Chapter 22).

Squamous (**SKWAY**-mus) Flat or scale-like; used especially in reference to epithelial tissue (Chapter 4).

Stapes (**STAY**-peez) The third of the auditory bones in the middle ear; transmits vibrations from the incus to the oval window of the inner ear (Chapter 9).

Starch (STARCH) A polysaccharide produced by plants; digested to glucose, a source of energy for cell respiration (Chapter 2).

Starling's Law of the Heart (**STAR**-lingz LAW) The force of contraction of cardiac muscle fibers is determined by the length of the fibers; the more cardiac muscle fibers are stretched, the more forcefully they contract (Chapter 12).

Stem cell (STEM SELL) 1. An embryonic cell capable of differentiating into any of the specialized cells of an organism (Chapter 3). 2. The unspecialized cell found in red bone marrow and lymphatic tissue that is the precursor cell for all types of blood cells (Chapter 11). 3. Any unspecialized adult cell with the potential to differentiate (Chapter 3).

Stenosis (ste-**NOH**-sis) An abnormal constriction or narrowing of an opening or duct (Chapter 12).

Sterilization (STIR-ill-i-**ZAY**-shun) The process of completely destroying all of the microorganisms on or in a substance or object (Chapter 22).

Sternum (**STIR**-num) The flat bone that forms part of the anterior rib cage; consists of the manubrium, body, and xiphoid process (Syn.—breastbone) (Chapter 6).

Steroid (**STEER**-oyd) An organic compound in the lipid group; includes cholesterol and certain hormones (Chapter 2).

Stimulus (**STIM**-yoo-lus) A change, especially one that affects a sensory receptor or that brings about a response in a living organism (Chapter 9).

Stomach (**STUM**-uk) The sac-like organ of the alimentary tube between the esophagus and the small intestine; is a reservoir for food and secretes gastric juice to begin protein digestion (Chapter 16).

Stratified (**STRA**-ti-fyed) Having two or more layers (Chapter 4).

Stratum corneum (**STRA**-tum **KOR**-nee-um) The outermost layer of the epidermis, made of many layers of dead, keratinized cells (Chapter 5).

Stratum germinativum (**STRA**-tum JER-min-ah-**TEE**-vum) The innermost layer of the epidermis; the cells undergo mitosis to produce new epidermis (Syn.—stratum basale) (Chapter 5).

Streptokinase (STREP-toh-**KYE**-nase) An enzyme produced by bacteria of the genus *Streptococcus* that is used clinically to dissolve abnormal clots, such as those in coronary arteries (Chapter 11).

Stretch receptor (STRETCH ree-**SEP**-ter) A sensory receptor in a muscle that detects stretching of the muscle (Syn.—proprioceptor) (Chapter 7).

Stretch reflex (STRETCH **REE**-fleks) A spinal cord reflex in which a muscle that is stretched will contract (Chapter 8).

Striated muscle (**STRY**-ay-ted **MUSS**-uhl) The muscle tissue that forms the skeletal muscles that move bones (Syn.—voluntary, skeletal muscle) (Chapter 4).

Stroke volume (STROHK **VAHL**-yoom) The amount of blood pumped by a ventricle in one beat; the resting average is 60–80 ml/beat (Chapter 12).

Subarachnoid space (SUB-uh-**RAK**-noid) The space between the arachnoid membrane and the pia mater; contains cerebrospinal fluid (Chapter 8).

Subclinical infection (sub-**KLIN**-i-kuhl) An infection in which the person shows no symptoms (Syn.—inapparent, asymptomatic) (Chapter 22).

Subcutaneous (SUB-kew-**TAY**-nee-us) Below the skin; the tissues between the dermis and the muscles (Chapter 5).

Sublingual glands (sub-**LING**-gwal) The pair of salivary glands located below the floor of the mouth (Chapter 16).

Submandibular glands (SUB-man-**DIB**-yoo-lar) The pair of salivary glands located at the posterior corners of the mandible (Chapter 16).

Submucosa (SUB-mew-**KOH**-sah) The layer of connective tissue and blood vessels located below the mucosa (lining) of a mucous membrane (Chapter 16).

Substrates (**SUB**-strayts) The substances acted upon, as by enzymes (Chapter 2).

Sucrase (**SOO**-krays) A digestive enzyme that breaks down sucrose to glucose and fructose; secreted by the small intestine (Chapter 16).

Sucrose (**SOO**-krohs) A disaccharide made of one glucose and one fructose molecule (Syn.—cane sugar, table sugar) (Chapter 2).

Sulcus (**SUHL**-kus) A furrow or groove, as between the gyri of the cerebrum (Syn.—fissure) (Chapter 8).

Superficial (soo-per-**FISH**-uhl) Toward the surface (Chapter 1).

Superficial fascia (soo-per-**FISH**-uhl **FASH**-ee-ah) The subcutaneous tissue, between the dermis and the muscles. Consists of areolar connective tissue and adipose tissue (Chapter 4).

Superior (soo-**PEER**-ee-your) Above, or higher (Chapter 1).

Superior vena cava (**VEE**-nah **KAY**-vah) The vein that returns blood from the upper body to the right atrium (Chapter 12).

Supination (SOO-pi-**NAY**-shun) Turning the palm upward, or lying face up (Chapter 7).

Suspensory ligaments (suh-**SPEN**-suh-ree **LIG**-uh-ments) The strands of connective tissue that connect the ciliary body to the lens of the eye (Chapter 9).

Sustentacular cells (SUS-ten-**TAK**-yoo-lar SELLS) The cells of the testes that secrete inhibin (Chapter 20).

Suture (**SOO**-cher) A synarthrosis, an immovable joint between cranial bones or facial bones (from the Latin "seam") (Chapter 6).

Sympathetic (SIM-puh-**THET**-ik) The division of the autonomic nervous system that dominates during stressful situations (Chapter 8).

Sympathomimetic (SIM-pah-tho-mi-**MET**-ik) Having the same effects as sympathetic impulses, as has epinephrine, a hormone of the adrenal medulla (Chapter 10).

Symphysis (**SIM**-fi-sis) An amphiarthrosis in which a disc of cartilage is found between two bones, as in the vertebral column (Chapter 6).

Symptomatic infection (**SIMP**-toh-MAT-ik) An infection in which the patient exhibits the symptoms of the disease (Chapter 22).

Synapse (**SIN**-aps) The space between the axon of one neuron and the cell body or dendrite of the next neuron or between the end of a motor neuron and an effector cell (Chapter 4).

Synaptic knob (si-**NAP**-tik NAHB) The end of an axon of a neuron that releases a neurotransmitter (Chapter 8).

Synarthrosis (SIN-ar-**THROH**-sis) An immovable joint, such as a suture (Chapter 6).

Synergistic muscles (SIN-er-**JIS**-tik **MUSS**-uhls) Muscles that have the same function, or a stabilizing function, with respect to the movement of a joint (Chapter 7).

Synovial fluid (sin-**OH**-vee-uhl **FLOO**-id) A thick slippery fluid that prevents friction within joint cavities (Chapter 6).

Synovial membrane (sin-**OH**-ve-uhl **MEM**-brayn) The connective tissue membrane that lines joint cavities and secretes synovial fluid (Chapter 4).

Synthesis (**SIN**-the-siss) The process of forming complex molecules or compounds from simpler compounds or elements (Chapter 2).

Syphilis (**SIFF**-i-lis) A sexually transmitted disease caused by the bacterium *Treponema pallidum;* may also cause congenital syphilis in newborns of infected women (Chapter 20).

Systemic infection (sis-**TEM**-ik) An infection that has spread throughout the body from an initial site (Chapter 22).

Systole (**SIS**-tuh-lee) In the cardiac cycle, the contraction of the myocardium; ventricular systole pumps blood into the arteries (Chapter 12).

—T—

T cells (T SELLS) A subgroup of lymphocytes; include helper T cells, cytotoxic T cells, and suppressor T cells, all of which are involved in immune responses (Chapter 11).

T tubule (TEE **TOO**-byool) A transverse tubule, a fold of the sarcolemma; carries the action potential to the interior of a muscle fiber (Chapter 7).

Tachycardia (TAK-ee-**KAR**-dee-yah) An abnormally rapid heart rate; more than 100 beats per minute (Chapter 12).

Taenia coli (**TAY**-nee-uh **KOH**-lye) The longitudinal muscle layer of the colon; three bands of smooth muscle fibers that extend from the cecum to the sigmoid colon (Chapter 16).

Talus (**TAL**-us) One of the tarsals; articulates with the tibia (Chapter 6).

Target organ (**TAR**-get **OR**-gan) The organ (or tissue) in which a hormone exerts its specific effects. (Chapter 10).

Tarsals (**TAR**-suhls) The seven short bones in each ankle (Chapter 6).

Taste buds (TAYST BUDS) Structures on the papillae of the tongue that contain the chemoreceptors for the detection of chemicals (food) dissolved in saliva (Chapter 9).

Tears (TEERS) The watery secretion of the lacrimal glands; wash the anterior surface of the eyeball and keep it moist (Chapter 9).

Teeth (TEETH) Bony projections in the upper and lower jaws that function in chewing (Chapter 16).

Telophase (**TELL**-ah-fayz) The fourth stage of mitosis, in which two nuclei are re-formed (Chapter 3).

Temporal bone (**TEM**-puh-ruhl) The flat bone that forms the side of the cranial cavity and contains middle and inner ear structures (Chapter 6).

Temporal lobes (**TEM**-puh-ruhl LOWBS) The lateral parts of the cerebrum; contain the auditory, olfactory, and taste areas (Chapter 8).

Tendon (**TEN**-dun) A fibrous connective tissue structure that connects muscle to bone (Chapter 7).

Teratogen (te-**RAH**-toh-jen) Anything that causes developmental abnormalities in an embryo; may be a chemical or microorganism to which an embryo is exposed by way of the mother (Chapter 21).

Testes (**TES**-teez) (Sing.—testis) The male gonads that produce sperm cells; also endocrine glands that secrete the hormone testosterone (Chapter 10).

Testosterone (tes-**TAHS**-ter-ohn) The sex hormone secreted by the interstitial cells of the testes; responsible for the maturation of sperm, growth of the male reproductive organs, and the secondary sex characteristics (Chapter 10).

Tetanus (**TET**-uh-nus) 1. A sustained contraction of a muscle fiber in response to rapid nerve impulses; the basis for all useful movements. 2. A disease, characterized by severe muscle spasms, caused by the bacterium *Clostridium tetani* (Chapter 7).

Thalamus (**THAL**-uh-muss) The part of the brain superior to the hypothalamus; regulates subconscious aspects of sensation (Chapter 8).

Theory (**THEER**-ree) A statement that is the best explanation of all the available evidence on a particular process or mechanism. A theory is *not* a guess (Chapter 3).

Thoracic cavity (thaw-**RASS**-ik **KAV**-i-tee) Part of the ventral cavity, superior to the diaphragm (Chapter 1).

Thoracic duct (thaw-**RASS**-ik DUKT) The lymph vessel that empties lymph from the lower half and upper left quadrant of the body into the left subclavian vein (Chapter 14).

Thoracic vertebrae (thaw-**RASS**-ik **VER**-te-bray) The 12 vertebrae that articulate with the ribs (Chapter 6).

Threshold level–renal (**THRESH**-hold **LE**-vuhl) The concentration at which a substance in the blood *not* normally excreted by the kidneys begins to appear in the urine; for several substances, such as glucose, in the renal filtrate, there is a limit to how much the renal tubules can reabsorb (Chapter 18).

Thrombocyte (**THROM**-boh-sight) Platelet; a fragment of a megakaryocyte (Chapter 11).

Thrombocytopenia (THROM-boh-SIGH-toh-**PEE**-nee-ah) An abnormally low platelet count (Chapter 11).

Thrombus (**THROM**-bus) A blood clot that obstructs blood flow through a blood vessel (Chapter 11).

Thymus (**THIGH**-mus) An organ made of lymphatic tissue located inferior to the thyroid gland; large in the fetus and child, and shrinks with age; produces T cells and hormones necessary for the maturation of the immune system (Chapter 14).

Thyroid cartilage (**THIGH**-roid **KAR**-ti-ledj) The largest and most anterior cartilage of the larynx; may be felt in the front of the neck (Chapter 15).

Thyroid gland (**THIGH**-roid) An endocrine gland on the anterior side of the trachea below the larynx; secretes thyroxine, triiodothyronine, and calcitonin (Chapter 10).

Thyroid-stimulating hormone (TSH) A hormone secreted by the anterior pituitary gland that causes the thyroid gland to secrete triiodothyronine and thyroxine (Chapter 10).

Thyroxine (T4) (thigh-**ROK**-sin) A hormone secreted by the thyroid gland that increases energy production and protein synthesis (Chapter 10).

Tibia (**TIB**-ee-yuh) The larger long bone of the lower leg (Syn.—shinbone) (Chapter 6).

Tidal volume (**TIGH**-duhl **VAHL**-yoom) The volume of air in one normal inhalation and exhalation; average: 400–600 ml (Chapter 15).

Tissue (**TISH**-yoo) A group of cells with similar structure and function (Chapter 1).

Tissue fluid (**TISH**-yoo **FLOO**-id) The water found in intercellular spaces. Also called interstitial fluid (Chapter 2).

Tissue macrophage system (**TISH**-yoo **MAK**-roh-fayj) The organs or tissues that contain macrophages that phagocytize old red blood cells: the liver, spleen, and red bone marrow (Chapter 11).

Tissue typing (**TISH**-yoo **TIGH**-ping) A laboratory procedure that determines the HLA types of a donated organ, prior to an organ transplant (Chapter 11).

Titin (**TIGH**-tin) The protein in sarcomeres that anchors myosin filaments to the Z lines (Chapter 7).

Tongue (TUHNG) A muscular organ on the floor of the oral cavity; contributes to chewing and swallowing and contains taste buds (Chapter 16).

Tonsillectomy (TAHN-si-**LEK**-toh-mee) The surgical removal of the palatine tonsils and/or adenoid (Chapter 14).

Tonsils (**TAHN**-sills) The lymph nodules in the mucosa of the pharynx, the palatine tonsils, and the adenoid; also the lingual tonsils on the base of the tongue (Chapter 14).

Toxin (**TAHK**-sin) A chemical that is poisonous to cells (Chapter 22).

Toxoid (**TAHK**-soyd) An inactivated bacterial toxin that is no longer harmful yet is still antigenic; used as a vaccine (Chapter 14).

Trace element (TRAYS **EL**-uh-ment) Those elements needed in very small amounts by the body for normal functioning (Chapter 2).

Trachea (**TRAY**-kee-ah) The organ that is the air passageway between the larynx and the primary bronchi (Syn.—windpipe) (Chapter 15).

Transamination (TRANS-am-i-**NAY**-shun) The transfer of an amino (NH_2) group from an amino acid to a carbon chain to form a non-essential amino acid; takes place in the liver (Chapter 16).

Transient flora (**TRAN**-zee-ent **FLOOR**-uh) Part of normal flora; those microorganisms that may inhabit specific sites in the body for short periods of time (Chapter 22).

Transitional (trans-**ZI**-shun-uhl) Changing from one form to another (Chapter 4).

Transitional epithelium (tran-**ZI**-shun-uhl) A type of epithelium in which the surface cells change from rounded to flat as the organ changes shape (Chapter 4).

Transporter (trans-**POOR**-ter) A protein that is part of a cell membrane and necessary for the facilitated diffusion of a substance such as glucose (Chapter 3).

Transverse section (trans-**VERS SEK**-shun) A plane or cut from front to back, separating upper and lower parts (Chapter 1).

Tricuspid valve (try-**KUSS**-pid VALV) The right AV valve, which prevents backflow of blood from the right ventricle to the right atrium when the ventricle contracts (Chapter 12).

Trigeminal nerves (try-**JEM**-in-uhl) Cranial nerve pair V; sensory for the face and teeth; motor to chewing muscles (Chapter 8).

Triglyceride (try-**GLI**-si-ryde) An organic compound, a true fat, that is made of one glycerol and three fatty acids (Chapter 2).

Trigone (**TRY**-gohn) Triangular area on the floor of the urinary bladder bounded by the openings of the two ureters and the urethra (Chapter 18).

Triiodothyronine (T3) (TRY-eye-oh-doh-**THIGH**-roh-neen) A hormone secreted by the thyroid gland that increases energy production and protein synthesis (Chapter 10).

Trisomy (**TRY**-suh-mee) In genetics, having three homologous chromosomes instead of the usual two (Chapter 20).

Trochlear nerves (**TROK**-lee-ur) Cranial nerve pair IV; motor to an extrinsic muscle of the eye (Chapter 8).

Trophoblast (**TROH**-foh-blast) The outermost layer of the embryonic blastocyst; will become the chorion, one of the embryonic membranes (Chapter 21).

Tropomyosin (TROH-poh-**MYE**-oh-sin) A protein that inhibits the contraction of sarcomeres in a muscle fiber (Chapter 7).

Troponin (**TROH**-poh-nin) A protein that inhibits the contraction of the sarcomeres in a muscle fiber (Chapter 7).

True fat (TROO FAT) An organic compound in the lipid group that is made of glycerol and fatty acids (Chapter 2).

Trypsin (**TRIP**-sin) A digestive enzyme that breaks down proteins into polypeptides; secreted by the pancreas (Chapter 16).

Tubal ligation (**TOO**-buhl lye-**GAY**-shun) A surgical procedure to remove or sever the fallopian tubes; usually done as a method of contraception in women (Chapter 20).

Tubular reabsorption (**TOO**-byoo-ler REE-ab-**SORP**-shun) The processes by which useful substances in the renal filtrate are returned to the blood in the peritubular capillaries (Chapter 18).

Tubular secretion (**TOO**-byoo-ler se-**KREE**-shun) The processes by which cells of the renal tubules secrete

substances into the renal filtrate to be excreted in urine (Chapter 18).

Tunica (**TOO**-ni-kah) A layer or coat, as in the wall of an artery (Chapter 13).

Tympanic membrane (tim-**PAN**-ik) The eardrum, the membrane that is stretched across the end of the ear canal; vibrates when sound waves strike it (Chapter 9).

Typing and cross matching (**TIGH**-ping and **KROSS**-match-ing) A laboratory test that determines whether or not donated blood is compatible, with respect to the red blood cell types (Chapter 11).

—U—

Ulna (**UHL**-nuh) The long bone of the forearm on the little finger side (Chapter 6).

Ultrasound (**UHL**-tra-sownd) 1. Inaudible sound. 2. A technique used in diagnosis in which ultrasound waves provide outlines of the shapes of organs or tissues (Chapter 21).

Umbilical arteries (uhm-**BILL**-i-kull **AR**-tuh-rees) The fetal blood vessels contained in the umbilical cord that carry deoxygenated blood from the fetus to the placenta (Chapter 13).

Umbilical cord (um-**BILL**-i-kull KORD) The structure that connects the fetus to the placenta; contains two umbilical arteries and one umbilical vein (Chapter 13).

Umbilical vein (uhm-**BILL**-i-kull VAYN) The fetal blood vessel contained in the umbilical cord that carries oxygenated blood from the placenta to the fetus (Chapter 13).

Unicellular (YOO-nee-**SELL**-yoo-lar) Composed of one cell (Chapter 4).

Unsaturated fat (un-**SAT**-uhr-ay-ted) A true fat that is often liquid at room temperature; often of plant origin (Chapter 2).

Upper respiratory tract (**UH**-per **RES**-pi-rah-TOR-ee TRAKT) The respiratory organs located outside the chest cavity (Chapter 15).

Urea (yoo-**REE**-ah) A nitrogenous waste product formed in the liver from the deamination of amino acids or from ammonia (Chapter 5).

Uremia (yoo-**REE**-me-ah) The condition in which blood levels of nitrogenous waste products are elevated; caused by renal insufficiency or failure (Chapter 18).

Ureter (**YOOR**-uh-ter) The tubular organ that carries urine from the renal pelvis (kidney) to the urinary bladder (Chapter 18).

Urethra (yoo-**REE**-thrah) The tubular organ that carries urine from the urinary bladder to the exterior of the body (Chapter 18).

Urinary bladder (**YOOR**-i-NAR-ee **BLA**-der) The organ that stores urine temporarily and contracts to eliminate urine by way of the urethra (Chapter 18).

Urinary system (**YOOR**-i-**NAR**-ee **SIS**-tem) The organ system that produces and eliminates urine; consists of the kidneys, ureters, urinary bladder, and urethra (Chapter 18).

Urine (**YOOR**-in) The fluid formed by the kidneys from blood plasma (Chapter 18).

Uterus (**YOO**-ter-us) The organ of the female reproductive system in which the placenta is formed to nourish a developing embryo-fetus (Chapter 20).

Utricle (**YOO**-tri-kuhl) A membranous sac in the vestibule of the inner ear that contains receptors for static equilibrium (Chapter 9).

—V—

Vaccine (vak-**SEEN**) A preparation of a foreign antigen that is administered by injection or other means in order to stimulate an antibody response to provide immunity to a particular pathogen (Chapter 14).

Vagina (vuh-**JIGH**-nah) The muscular tube that extends from the cervix of the uterus to the vaginal orifice; serves as the birth canal (Chapter 20).

Vagus nerves (**VAY**-gus) Cranial nerve pair X; sensory for cardiovascular and respiratory reflexes; motor to larynx, bronchioles, stomach, and intestines (Chapter 8).

Valence (**VAY**-lens) The combining power of an atom when compared to a hydrogen atom; expressed as a positive or negative number (Chapter 2).

Valve (VALVE) A structure in a cavity or tube that closes upon, and thus prevents, backflow of the fluid therein (from the Latin "a leaf of a double door") (Chapter 12).

Varicose vein (**VAR**-i-kohs VAYN) An enlarged, abnormally dilated vein; most often occurs in the legs (Chapter 13).

Vasectomy (va-**SEK**-tuh-me) A surgical procedure to remove or sever the ductus deferens; usually done as a method of contraception in men (Chapter 20).

Vasoconstriction (**VAY**-zoh-kon-**STRIK**-shun) A decrease in the diameter of a blood vessel caused by contraction of the smooth muscle in the wall of the vessel (Chapter 5).

Vasodilation (**VAY**-zoh-dye-**LAY**-shun) An increase in the diameter of a blood vessel caused by relaxation of the smooth muscle in the wall of the vessel (Chapter 5).

Vasomotor center (**VAY**-zoh **MOH**-ter) The part of the medulla that regulates the diameter of arteries and veins; contributes to normal blood pressure (Chapter 8).

Vector (**VEK**-ter) An arthropod that transmits pathogens from host to host, usually when it bites to obtain blood (Chapter 22).

Vein (VAYN) A blood vessel that takes blood from capillaries back to the heart (Chapter 13).

Venous return (**VEE**-nus ree-**TURN**) The amount of blood returned by the veins to the heart; is directly related to cardiac output, which depends on adequate venous return (Chapter 12).

Ventilation (**VEN**-ti-**LAY**-shun) The movement of air into and out of the lungs (Chapter 15).

Ventral (**VEN**-truhl) Toward the front (Syn.—anterior) (Chapter 1).

Ventral cavity (**VEN**-truhl **KAV**-i-tee) Cavity that consists of the thoracic, abdominal, and pelvic cavities (Chapter 1).

Ventral root (**VEN**-truhl ROOT) The motor root of a spinal nerve (Chapter 8).

Ventricle (**VEN**-tri-kul) 1. A cavity, such as the four ventricles of the brain that contain cerebrospinal fluid. 2. One of the two lower chambers of the heart that pump blood to the body or to the lungs (Chapter 8).

Venule (**VEN**-yool) A small vein (Chapter 13).

Vertebra (**VER**-te-brah) One of the bones of the spine or backbone (Chapter 6).

Vertebral canal (**VER**-te-brahl ka-**NAL**) The spinal cavity that contains and protects the spinal cord (Chapter 6).

Vertebral column (**VER**-te-brahl **KAH**-luhm) The spine or backbone (Chapter 6).

Vestibule (**VES**-ti-byool) 1. The bony chamber of the inner ear that contains the utricle and saccule (Chapter 9). 2. The female external genital area between the labia minor that contains the openings of the urethra, vagina, and Bartholin's glands (Chapter 20).

Vestigial organ (ves-**TIJ**-ee-uhl) An organ that is reduced in size and function when compared with that of evolutionary ancestors; includes the appendix, ear muscles that move the auricle, and wisdom teeth (Chapter 16).

Villi (**VILL**-eye) 1. Folds of the mucosa of the small intestine that increase the surface area for absorption; each villus contains a capillary network and a lacteal (Chapter 16). 2. Projections of the chorion, an embryonic membrane that forms the fetal portion of the placenta (Chapter 21).

Virulence (**VIR**-yoo-lents) The ability of a microorganism to cause disease; the degree of pathogenicity (Chapter 22).

Virus (**VIGH**-rus) The simplest type of microorganism, consisting of either DNA or RNA within a protein shell; all are obligate intracellular parasites (Chapter 14).

Visceral (**VISS**-er-uhl) Pertaining to organs within a body cavity, especially thoracic and abdominal organs (Chapter 8).

Visceral effectors (**VISS**-er-uhl e-**FEK**-turs) Smooth muscle, cardiac muscle, and glands; receive motor nerve fibers of the autonomic nervous system; responses are involuntary (Chapter 8).

Visceral muscle (**VIS**-ser-uhl **MUSS**-uhl) Another name for smooth muscle tissue (Chapter 4).

Vital capacity (**VY**-tuhl kuh-**PASS**-i-tee) The volume of air involved in the deepest inhalation followed by the most forceful exhalation; average: 3500–5000 ml (Chapter 15).

Vitamin (**VY**-tah-min) An organic molecule needed in small amounts by the body for normal metabolism or growth (Chapter 17).

Vitreous humor (**VIT**-ree-us **HYOO**-mer) The semi-solid, gelatinous substance in the posterior cavity of the eyeball; helps keep the retina in place (Chapter 9).

Vocal cords (**VOH**-kul KORDS) The pair of folds within the larynx that are vibrated by the passage of air, producing sounds that may be turned into speech (Chapter 15).

Voluntary muscle (**VAHL**-un-tary **MUSS**-uhl) Another name for striated or skeletal muscle tissue (Chapter 4).

Vomer (**VOH**-mer) The flat bone that forms the lower, posterior portion of the nasal septum (from the Latin "plowshare") (Chapter 6).

Vomiting (**VAH**-mi-ting) Ejection through the mouth of stomach and intestinal contents (Chapter 16).

Vulva (**VUHL**-vah) The female external genital organs (Chapter 20).

—W–X–Y–Z—

Wart (WART) An elevated, benign skin lesion caused by a virus (Chapter 5).

White blood cells (WIGHT BLUHD SELLS) The cells that destroy pathogens that enter the body and provide immunity to some diseases; the five types are neutrophils, eosinophils, basophils, lymphocytes, and monocytes (Syn.—leukocytes) (Chapter 4).

White matter (WIGHT) Nerve tissue within the central nervous system that consists of myelinated axons and dendrites of interneurons (Chapter 8).

Worm (WURM) An elongated invertebrate; parasitic worms include tapeworms and hookworm (Chapter 22).

Xiphoid process (**ZYE**-foyd) The most inferior part of the sternum (from the Greek "sword-like") (Chapter 6).

Yellow bone marrow (**YELL**-oh BOWN **MAR**-roh) Primarily adipose tissue, found in the marrow cavities of the diaphyses of long bones and in the spongy bone of the epiphyses of adult bones (Chapter 6).

Yolk sac (YOHK SAK) An embryonic membrane that forms the first blood cells for the developing embryo (Chapter 21).

Z line (ZEE LYEN) The lateral boundary of a sarcomere in muscle tissue; anchors myosin and actin filaments (Chapter 7).

Zoonoses (ZOH-oh-**NOH**-seez) (Sing.— zoonosis) Diseases of animals that may be transmitted to people under certain conditions (Chapter 22).

Zygote (**ZYE**-goht) A fertilized egg, formed by the union of the nuclei of egg and sperm; the diploid number of chromosomes (46 for people) is restored (Chapter 20).

Index

C

Q